THE WESTMINSTER SERIES

General Editor: W. A. J. FARNDALE

VOLUME 7

NEW ASPECTS OF THE MENTAL HEALTH SERVICES

THE WESTMINSTER SERIES

General Editor: W. A. J. FARNDALE

NEW ASPECTS
OF THE
MENTAL HEALTH SERVICES

Edited by

HUGH FREEMAN

*Consultant Psychiatrist, Salford Royal Hospital
and City of Salford; Honorary Consultant,
National Association for Mental Health
and Editor of 'Mental Health'*

and

JAMES FARNDALE

*Senior Lecturer in Hospital Administration,
City of Westminster College*

PERGAMON PRESS

OXFORD · LONDON · EDINBURGH · NEW YORK
TORONTO · SYDNEY · PARIS · BRAUNSCHWEIG

Pergamon Press Ltd., Headington Hill Hall, Oxford
4 & 5 Fitzroy Square, London W.1
Pergamon Press (Scotland) Ltd., 2 & 3 Teviot Place, Edinburgh 1
Pergamon Press Inc., 44–01 21st Street, Long Island City, New York 11101
Pergamon of Canada, Ltd., 6 Adelaide Street East, Toronto, Ontario
Pergamon Press (Aust.) Pty. Ltd., 20–22 Margaret Street, Sydney, N.S.W.
Pergamon Press S.A.R.L., 24 rue des Écoles, Paris 5e
Vieweg & Sohn GmbH, Burgplatz 1, Braunschweig

First edition 1967

Library of Congress Catalog Card No. 67–22823

Printed in Great Britain by A. Wheaton & Co. Ltd, Exeter
3128/67

Contents

List of Contributors

APTE, ROBERT Z., M.S.W., Lecturer, School of Social Work, University of California, U.S.A. Formerly Research Student, London School of Economics.

BALDWIN, J. A., M.A., M.B., CH.B., Senior Research Fellow, Department of Mental Health, University of Aberdeen, Scotland.

BENNETT, DOUGLAS, M.D., D.P.M., Physician, Bethlem Royal and Maudsley Hospitals, London, S.E.5.

BRAITHWAITE, E. G., M.A., LL.B., Secretary, South-west Metropolitan Regional Hospital Board, London, W.2.

BUDGE, UNA V., S.R.N., R.M.N., S.T. DIP., Principal Tutor, Tooting Bec Hospital, London.

CHICK, J. D., B.A., Corpus Christi College, Cambridge.

COOPER, BRIAN, M.D., D.P.M., Lecturer, Institute of Psychiatry, Maudsley Hospital, London, S.E.5.

CRAFT, MICHAEL, M.D., M.R.C.P.E., D.P.M., Consultant Psychiatrist, North and Mid-Wales Psychiatric Services, Lecturer in Medical Psychology, University of Wales, Bangor.

CUTHBERT, T. M., M.R.C.S., L.R.C.P., D.P.M., Physician Superintendent, St. Luke's Hospital, Middlesbrough, Yorks.

DENHAM, JOHN, M.D., D.P.M., Medical Director, St. Clement's Hospital, London, E.3.

DAVIDSON, HENRY A., M.D., Superintendent, Essex County Hospital, Cedar Grove, N.J., U.S.A., Clinical Professor of Psychiatry, New Jersey College of Medicine, Editor of *Mental Hygiene*.

DOWNHAM, E. T., M.D., D.P.M., Consultant Psychiatrist, Burnley General Hospital, Burnley, Lancs.

DOWNING, JOSEPH J., M.D., Programme Chief, Mental Health Services Division, San Mateo County Department of Public Health and Welfare, San Mateo, Calif., U.S.A.

EARLY, D. F., L.R.C.P.I., D.P.H., D.P.M., Consultant Psychiatrist, Glenside Hospital, Stapleton, Bristol.

ELDER, ALEX T., PH.D., M.D., M.R.C.P.G., D.P.H., Deputy Chief Medical Officer, Ministry of Health and Social Services, Belfast, Northern Ireland.

FIELD, MARK G., Professor of Sociology, College of Liberal Arts, Boston University, Boston, Mass., U.S.A.

GATHERER, A., M.D., CH.B., D.P.H., D.I.H., Medical Officer of Health, County Borough of Reading.

GILSENAN, B. M. C., M.D., D.P.M., Consultant Psychiatrist, Shenley Hospital, St. Albans, Herts.

GLATT, M. M., M.D., D.P.M., Consultant Psychiatrist, St. Bernard's Hospital, Southall, Middx.

GOLDBERG, E. M., A.A.P.S.W., Senior Lecturer (Research), the National Institute for Social Work Training, London, W.C.1.

GORE, CHARLES, P., M.D., M.R.C.P.I., D.P.M., Consultant Psychiatrist, Scalebor Park, Ilkley, Yorks.

HAMILTON, MARIAN W., M.A., Lecturer, Department of Psychiatry, University of Manchester.

HAMILTON, W. J., M.B., M.A.N.Z.C.P., D.P.M., Psychiatrist, The Royal Brisbane Hospital, Brisbane, Australia.

HANSON, PHILIP G., M.S., P.R.D., Clinical Assistant Professor of Psychology, Baylor University School of Medicine, Houston, Texas, U.S.A.

HOENIG, J., M.D., D.P.M., Reader, Department of Psychiatry, University of Manchester.

HUNTER, T. D., F.H.A., Group Secretary and Treasurer, the Royal Edinburgh Hospital, Edinburgh, Scotland.

JOHNSON, DALE L., PH.D., Associate Professor, Department of Psychology, University of Houston, Texas, U.S.A.

JONES, KATHLEEN, M.A., PH.D., Professor of Social Administration, University of York.

JONES, MAXWELL, C.B.E., M.D., M.R.C.P.E., D.P.M., Physician Superintendent, Dingleton Hospital, Melrose, Roxburghshire, Scotland.

JUEL-NIELSEN, NIELS, M.D., Arhus State Hospital, Risskov, Denmark.

KAHN, J. H., M.D., D.P.M., Consultant in charge of Community Mental Health Services and Medical Director of the Child Guidance Clinic, London Borough of Newham.

*KIDD, H. B., M.B., B.CHIR., D.P.M., Medical Superintendent, the Towers Hospital, Leicester.

KRAMER, BERNARD M., PH.D., Associate Professor of Preventive Medicine, Tufts University School of Medicine, Boston, Mass., U.S.A.

KUSHLICK, ALBERT, M.B., M.R.C.P., Director of Research in Subnormality, Wessex Regional Hospital Board, Winchester, Hants.

MAY, ANTHONY R., M.B., M.R.C.P.E., D.P.M., Principal Medical Officer, Ministry of Health, London, S.E.1.

MCKERRACHER, D. G., M.D., Professor of Psychiatry, University of Saskatchewan, Saskatoon, Canada.

MILLER, LOUIS, M.D., Director of Mental Health Services, Ministry of Health, Jerusalem, Israel.

MITTLER, PETER, M.A., Lecturer in Psychology, Birkbeck College, University of London, W.C.1.

MORGAN, ROGER, M.B., B.S., D.P.M., Director of Rehabilitation, St. Wulstan's Hospital, Malvern, Worcs.

MOUNTNEY, GEORGE, A.A.P.S.W., Senior Mental Welfare Officer, Health Department, Salford 5, Lancs.

NIELSEN, JOHANNES, M.D., Arhus State Hospital, Risskov, Denmark.

ROTHAUS, PAUL, PR.D., Clinical Assistant Professor of Psychology, Baylor University School of Medicine, Houston, Texas, U.S.A.

SCHMIDT, K. E., M.D., M.R.C.S., L.R.C.P., D.P.M., Medical Superintendent, Sarawak Mental Hospital, Kuching, Sarawak, Malaysia.

SHELDON, A. P., M.A., M.B., B. CHIR., S.M. (HYG.), Laboratory of Community Psychiatry, Harvard Medical School, Boston, Mass., U.S.A.

SMITH, COLIN M., M.D., F.R.C.P.C., D.P.M., Associate Professor of Psychiatry, University of Saskatchewan, Saskatoon, Canada.

SHEPHERD, MICHAEL, M.A., D.M., M.R.C.P., D.P.M., Reader, Institute of Psychiatry, London, S.E.5.

STRÖMGREN, ERIK, Professor, Arhus State Hospital, Risskov, Denmark.

SUSSER, MERVYN, M.B., CH.B., M.R.C.P.E., Professor of Epidemiology, School of Public Health, Columbia University, New York, U.S.A.

TAYLOR, WALLIS, B.SC. (ECON), PH.D., Senior Lecturer in Social Statistics, University of Manchester.

WARD, BRIAN, M.B., CH.B., D.P.M., Medical Superintendent, Winwick Hospital, Lancs.

WEEKS, K. F., M.B., B.S., D.P.M., Consultant Psychiatrist, Plymouth Clinical Area.

WING, J. K., M.D., PH.D., D.P.M., Director, Medical Research Council Social Psychiatry Research Unit and Honorary Physician, Maudsley Hospital, London, S.E.5.

WOODWARD, MARY, M.A., PH.D., Lecturer in Psychology, University College of Swansea, South Wales.

WRIGHT, S. L., M.D., M.R.C.P., D.P.H., Medical Officer of Health, London Borough of Croydon.

Contributors from public authorities wish to state that their authorities accept no responsibility for any statement or expression of opinion contained in their articles.

* Dr. Kidd died in August 1965.

Editors' Preface

IT IS now three years since the publication of our previous volume, *Trends in the Mental Health Services*. We expressed the hope then that such a collection of data and opinions would be of real value to those professional workers who were operating or studying psychiatric services. The result was very encouraging to us, both in the opinions of reviewers and in the many comments received personally. This volume is still in regular use in universities, hospitals, local authority departments and other public bodies. It is also supplemented by other volumes in the Westminster Series, dealing with day hospitals, the National Health Service in general and social welfare services.

This time, we hope to have achieved the aims which were expressed in the preface to our 1963 volume—to maintain continuity, to cover new ground and to extend that part which deals with services outside Great Britain. We have also taken the opportunity to introduce a number of other changes. In particular, readers will find that the great majority of papers have been specially written for this volume, though a small number, which we have felt to be of particular interest and importance, have been reprinted from journals. Owing to the greater length of this present book, we have also been able to deal with many subjects in much greater depth and we hope that this also will increase the value of the collection.

As before, the papers have been divided into several sections and the first deals with a series of significant general topics, rather than with specific services. It is opened by a very important and comprehensive paper by Dr. Wing, who was one of our contributors last time. This summarizes all the reliable information about the results of treating schizophrenia under present-day conditions and no one is better qualified to do so than Dr. Wing, since much of the material comes from the research unit which he directs himself. This paper will discourage any facile optimism about the treatment of schizophrenia today, and its final conclusions are of the greatest significance for future planning. There is also a very comprehensive bibliography, which research students will find of tremendous value. Dr. Wing is followed by another author who has done important research work in the field of schizophrenia—Miss E. M. Goldberg. This work was stimulated by a finding of the Medical Research Council Social Psychiatry Research Unit in 1958 that the performance of male schizophrenics discharged from mental hospitals showed a relationship to the type of family setting to which they returned. [1] Miss Goldberg and her colleagues have investigated this important matter in great depth and her conclusions are particularly valuable when considered together with those of Dr. Wing. Under present conditions, schizophrenia can never be regarded merely as a disease requiring particular forms of medical treatment. It is a phenomenon profoundly influenced by social and interpersonal factors, so that the problems of its management extend into many different aspects of social policy. This same theme will be found in the next paper, which is by a hospital administrator, Mr. T. D. Hunter. He looks beyond the current administrative problems of hospitals to the broad social forces which have moulded medical care during the last two centuries. Readers will find in this paper a store of stimulating ideas and a valuable collection of references, though certainly more questions are raised than can yet be answered in practical terms. Mr. Hunter's approach will be seen to differ from that taken later in the book by one of our medical contributors, Dr. Gilsenan.

Returning to the topic of schizophrenia, we again welcome one of our previous contributors, Dr. Bennett, who has done most valuable work in the fields of rehabilitation and community care. Here, he deals with the place of drug therapy, particularly in relation to patients in the community, and its influence relative to that of social forces. This is another important review, which readers will wish to consider together with the first two papers. It is followed by a reprinted paper from Drs. Shepherd and Cooper of the Institute of Psychiatry, London. Their summary of epidemiological methods and knowledge certainly deserves the more permanent place it has found in this volume. Another review is that by Dr. Glatt of the problem of alcoholism in Britain, and of the extent of facilities for treating it. Dr. Glatt is the acknowledged pioneer of hospital alcoholic units in this country and it is a privilege to include him amongst our contributors. The very comprehensive information in this article should be of great value to those involved in setting up services for alcoholics. This paper is followed by one in which Dr. Early summarizes his important work in the field of social and industrial rehabilitation. No one in this country has shown greater energy or ingenuity than Dr. Early in restoring the severely handicapped to a place in normal society, and this makes his conclusions all the more useful to readers. Next in this section, Professor Susser discusses some theoretical aspects of community care of psychiatric illness. This is a most thoughtful paper, aiming to discover some of the fundamental process in this important field. Dr. Cuthbert deals, on the basis of personal experience, with the advisory bodies of the National Health Service, particularly in their relationship to mental health services. His account is by no means uncritical, though less so than that of an earlier contributor to one of the Westminster Series. [2] Finally in this section, Dr. Elder writes authoritatively on the mental health services of Northern

Ireland—a subject insufficiently known about, even elsewhere in the United Kingdom.

The next section of this book deals with services outside Britain, though it begins with a paper by a British author. Dr. Michael Craft described his remarkably successful service for the subnormal of North Wales in our last volume (*Trends in the Mental Health Services*) and this time he compares British ideas and practices in the care of the mentally subnormal with those of the U.S.S.R. and U.S.A. (In this book, the word "subnormal", which is officially used in Britain, can be regarded as interchangable with "retarded", as used in North America.) This paper is followed by certainly the most exotic of our contributions—Dr. Schmidt's remarkable account of his almost single-handed struggle to establish a mental health service for the country of Sarawak. Readers will be as much impressed by Dr. Schmidt's ingenuity in using non-medical personnel as by his description of the astonishing ethnic variety of this area. This is undoubtedly a case where bricks have been made without straw. The next paper comes from a very active psychiatric centre, whose head contributed to our last volume. Drs. Smith and McKerracher describe one of their many enterprising projects at the Department of Psychiatry, University of Saskatchewan. Their aim of integrating general practitioners more fully into psychiatric care is one that is universally accepted, but involves particular problems in this case because of the great distances and relatively sparse population in the province they serve. Their paper is followed by one from Australia. Dr. Hamilton has been a local pioneer in establishing a psychiatric day hospital in Brisbane and he describes very fully and frankly what this has achieved so far and what the difficulties have been. His experience will be valuable to professional workers in many areas who still lack facilities for day care. Dr. Downing, who contributes the subsequent paper, is particularly welcome to our list of authors as the initiator of one of the most significant programmes of psychiatric care in the United States. San Mateo County is relatively fortunate in the extent of its local resources and in its attractiveness as an area for professional staff. Nevertheless, it has certainly shown what can be achieved outside the state mental hospital and its experience will be widely used in the preparation of new mental health centres under the Kennedy legislation. It is with these centres that Dr. Downing is particularly concerned here. He is followed by Dr. Louis Miller who, as Director of Mental Health Services at the Israel Ministry of Health, is particularly well equipped to describe community mental health services in his country. For those accustomed to dealing with stable and fairly homogeneous populations, Dr. Miller's account of the problems resulting from mass immigration, clashing of cultures and the aftermath of persecution will come as a chastening thought. There is certainly much to be learned about the sociological and anthropological aspects of psychiatry from the experience of this microcosm.

Next, Professor Mark Field, who is a distinguished expert on the health services of the U.S.S.R., contributes a reprinted paper which contrasts the basic approaches of the U.S.S.R. and U.S.A. towards the care of psychiatric illness. This includes a good deal of important data as well as significant comment on matters of principle. The next author, Dr. Henry Davidson, is acknowledged to be one of the most stimulating writers on the American psychiatric scene and is the author of a number of well-known books. We referred in the preface to our last volume to the disastrous results of trained psychiatric manpower being drawn largely into private individual psycho-therapy, particularly in the U.S.A., and this is a theme which Dr. Davidson takes up most strongly. He has been a powerful champion of the psychotic patient needing public care, particularly in the pages of the *American Journal of Psychiatry*, and the few replies so far to his arguments have been feeble and unconvincing. Dr. Bernard M. Kramer was also one of our previous contributors. Here, he includes a short but fertile essay, picking out the important positive and negative factors which affect the relationship between hospital and community. The following paper is the first we have included from continental Europe and is by three Danish authors. The Samsø Project, with which they are concerned, is a most important epidemiological study, and many students will wish to compare their data with that from other areas.

This section continues with an account by Professor Johnson and his colleagues of an original and successful programme which they have de-veloped and have called the Human Relations Training Laboratory. This will be seen to have affinities to both the living–learning experience of the thera-peutic community and to many of the concepts of behaviour therapy, based on learning theory. It is, however, unique in many respects, and both its theo-retical background and its practical details are important for mental health workers everywhere who face the problem of providing "effective and economical psychiatric treatment" for large numbers. The final contribution on the international scene comes from an unusual source for a book of this kind. Mr. Chick is a Cambridge undergraduate, intending to enter one of the psychiatric professions, who received a bursary to study some aspect of French life. He chose the community mental health service in the Thirteenth *Arrondissement* of Paris. This is well known by name in English-speaking countries, but very little has been written here about its practical details. Mr. Chick obtained much first-hand knowledge of the service, by working within it, and his description of the organization and facilities is a valuable contribution.

Our third section deals more specifically with the psychiatric hospital. It begins with a reprinted paper which embodies a most important piece of research; this should be considered together with the statistical material in our 1963 volume. To test out the assumptions included in the 1962 Hospital Plan, Drs. Gore, Jones, Taylor and Ward carried out a census of all psychiatric in-patients in a complete hospital region. It will be very clear to readers that the resulting data did not in any way bear out the assumptions of the Hospital Plan, and it now seems astonishing that some work of this sort was not done before the Plan was drawn up. Dr. Baldwin is also concerned with statistical studies on demand for and use of psychiatric hospital beds. His methods, however, are most sophisticated and this paper will be found to be both highly informative and full of stimulating questions about readily accepted clichés in this field. This is followed by a paper which will certainly be regarded as one of the most important in the present collection, and one by an acknowledged master of his subject. The name of Maxwell Jones is inevitably linked with the principle of the therapeutic community, and we are privileged to include here a comprehensive account by Dr. Jones of his recent important work at Dingleton Hospital. The next paper is a powerful plea for the continuing role of the independent psychiatric hospital as the centre of a comprehensive mental health service. Its author, the late Dr. Humphrey Kidd, will almost certainly be recalled with affection and respect by many readers of this volume. This was his last written work, and it is full of the dynamism and human sympathy for which he was well known. However, Dr. Kidd's views on the role of the medical superintendent differed from those of our next author. Dr. Gilsenan believes that psychiatric hospitals must evolve from the old authoritarian structure, with a superintendent at the top, to the tripartite structure which is accepted for general hospitals. In this matter, we appear to have no coherent national policy at the moment, though the trend seems to be running strongly in the direction Dr. Gilsenan maps out. We mentioned earlier that Mr. Hunter, in his paper, finds the tripartite structure deficient as a final model, but perhaps it will have to be achieved first, before we move on to higher things.

It is important that both doctors and administrators should take a close interest in the recruitment, training and qualifications of their nursing staff, whose work is so vital and often so little supervised by those nominally responsible. We are glad, therefore, to include an article by Miss Una Budge, who is Principal Tutor in a large psychiatric hospital and has had wide experience in training men and women to become psychiatric nurses. Miss Budge's hospital forms part of the South-west Metropolitan Hospital Region which, owing to its inheritance of many of the hospitals built by the former London County Council, has the greatest number of psychiatric beds of any hospital region in this country. Mr. Braithwaite, who is the Secretary of this Board, deals in his paper with the vast administrative problems that have been faced since the region was constituted in 1947. The next paper records a remarkable piece of independent research, which Dr. Roger Morgan carried out whilst working as a junior member of the medical staff of a psychiatric hospital. It is obviously important, in view of the severe overall shortage of professional staff, to know what is actually done by those we have. But as far as doctors are concerned, this does not seem to have been attempted before and Dr. Morgan, who undertook the investigation without any official help, deserves all the more credit for his initiative. His findings should certainly be important in any discussion of medical staffing in psychiatric hospitals. The final paper in this section comes from Mr. Mittler and Dr. Woodward, who deal with the education of children in hospitals for the subnormal. These authors have done important work in connection with I.Q. levels and the care of subnormality, and the present paper records a valuable investigation of present facilities.

Our final section deals with extramural psychiatric services. Dr. Kahn, who also contributed to our last volume, has the distinction of having created an entirely unique service in this country. Its principles were outlined in *Trends in the Mental Health Services,* but we are now fortunate in being able to include a detailed description of how the mental health service in Newham has evolved. There is much to be learnt here of the way in which non-psychiatric personnel can play a useful role in the promotion of mental health. The next paper is by Drs. May and Wright, who were the main architects of a pioneering service of district psychiatry in the former County Borough of Croydon. The principles they state and the results of their practical experience should be of wide interest. As an appendix, there is a brief paper by Drs. May and Sheldon which describes the work of the day hospital in the Croydon psychiatric service. The accompanying data give statistical details which are not readily available in relation to the work of most day hospitals. The paper by Dr. Hoenig and Miss Hamilton represents part of a major investigation into the operation of general hospital psychiatric units in the Manchester Region, where they have been most intensively developed so far. One of the fundamental problems in connection with all services of this sort is whether they involve the transfer of too great a burden to the community, in comparison with more traditional care by psychiatric hospitals. In this paper, a method is worked out whereby this problem can be assessed numerically and the results are given for the services which were investigated. This is a paper of considerable importance in connection with future research and we have little doubt that it will attract wide attention. It is particularly useful to have as the next contribution a personal account by Dr. Downham of one of the services which was studied. This is the administrative and clinical background to the research material, and it is impressive to read how an effective programme of comprehensive psychiatry was created from the most unpromising beginnings. Dr. Denham, who contributes the next paper, is another pioneer. He has been associated with the development of a remarkable organization in the East End of London—the Psychiatric Rehabilitation Association. Though this is in some respects a self-help group, it has been guided and encouraged by Dr. Denham and his professional associates. Since there are still so many gaps in our provision for psychiatric patients in the community, much could surely be achieved by fostering organizations similar to the P.R.A. in other areas.

One of the main vehicles towards the development of community care in this country has been the psychiatric hostel—at least as far as plans are concerned. Yet virtually nothing was known, in terms of real data, of the operation of these facilities at the time local health authorities were given the duty of providing them. Their enthusiasm to act as pioneers in this field has varied very greatly and it is not surprising that such hostels as already exist do not follow a single pattern. Mr. Apte, an American social worker, has been carrying out the first systematic research in this field and we are fortunate in being able to publish some of his data for the first time. The importance of this particular project has been emphasized by Professor Richard Titmus.[3] Another most significant research programme is being carried out in the Wessex Hospital Region by Dr. Kushlick. We are privileged to include here a major paper by Dr. Kushlick on the epidemiological problems of mental subnormality and on the implications for future care of the subnormal. His data and his proposals should arouse very wide interest. In contrast, Dr. Gatherer provides a detailed descriptive account of an experiment in mental health education. The Northamptonshire Project of 1963 was a remarkably successful community-wide enterprise, not least in managing to avoid any "anti-effect", such as can only too easily be aroused. There has certainly been nothing comparable to it in this country and probably not elsewhere. Public education is an essential aspect of a comprehensive mental health service, and therefore Dr. Gatherer's experience should be of great value to all professional workers in mental health. Dr. Weeks and his colleagues have been fortunate in being able to operate their mental health service from a new purpose-built headquarters (circumstances which are rare enough in this country). They have also been wise enough to establish a prospective research programme to study the effects of their new arrangements for psychiatric treatment in the Plymouth area over a number of years. Those who hope to be able to provide new buildings for other services will find their experience most useful. This is followed by a further paper, bringing up to date the studies which one of us (W. A. J. F.) has been carrying out for a number of years into the structure and operations of day hospitals in the country. Finally, the personal experience of one of us (H. L. F.) in developing a community care service for an English city is described in a paper written jointly with the Senior Mental Welfare Officer for the area, Mr. George Mountney.

Whilst this volume has had the same general aims as its predecessor, we hope that its particular function will have been in two main directions: firstly, in providing major reviews of a number of basic issues in the field of mental health services; secondly, in the detailed descriptions of pioneering models whose experience can be drawn on by those developing services elsewhere. Much of this information appears for the first time in an accessible and comprehensive form. May we once again thank our contributors for their ready co-operation and express our appreciation to the editors of those journals who kindly allowed us to reproduce their papers.

H. L. FREEMAN
W. A. J. FARNDALE

Acknowledgements. The editors wish to thank the following publications for kindly agreeing to the reproduction of papers originally published by them— *Community Mental Health Journal, Comprehensive Psychiatry, Journal of Neurology, Neurosurgery and Psychiatry, The Lancet, Medical Care, Review of Soviet Medical Sciences*. The index was prepared by Colin F. Sutton, B.Sc.

References

1. BROWN, G. W., CARSTAIRS, G. M. and TOPPING, G. G. (1958), *Lancet*, ii, 685.
2. MARCUS, A. (1964), in *Trends in the National Health Service* (ed. Farndale, W. A. J.), Oxford, Pergamon Press.
3. TITMUS, R. M. (1965), Supplement No. 49 to *Canada's Mental Health*, Ottawa, Department of National Health and Welfare.

SECTION A
GENERAL ASPECTS OF THE SERVICES

1. The Modern Management of Schizophrenia

J. K. WING

The Statistics of Schizophrenia

During the 3 months 1 January to 31 March 1965, 1569 people from Camberwell (a socially mixed but predominantly residential district in south-east London) came into contact with psychiatric services. Expressed as a crude proportion of Camberwell residents (175,304 in 1961), this means that 0.9% of the population were in contact with a psychiatrist. The numbers are shown in more detail in Table 1.*

TABLE 1.

Three-month Administrative Prevalence of Schizophrenia and Other Psychiatric Conditions: Camberwell, London

	In spell of contact on 31.12.64				Began new episode: 1.1.65–31.3.65			
	Schizophrenia		Other diagnoses		Schizophrenia		Other diagnoses	
Out-patient or day-patient	87	(50)	449	(256)	39	(22)	367	(209)
In-patient								
Short-stay	24	(14)	67	(38)	27	(15)	54	(31)
Medium-stay	22	(12)	67	(38)	—		—	
Long-stay	233	(133)	133	(76)	—		—	
Total	366	(209)	716	(408)	66	(37)	421	(240)

(Figures in brackets are crude rates per 100,000.)

*A Cumulative Psychiatric Diseases Register has been set up to cover the services likely to be contacted by patients from Camberwell. Probably fewer than 5% of patients are missed. An episode is regarded as ended when a patient has not contacted a psychiatrist for 3 months: a subsequent contact begins a new episode. Patients in a spell of contact on 31 December 1964 were therefore in-patients, day-patients, or out-patients who had been in contact before that day and attended at least once after it, within a period of 3 months. Patients who began a new spell of *out-patient* contact between 1 January and 31 March 1965 might also have been admitted to hospital at some time during the 3 months: the figures in Table 1 show the situation at the first contact only, and are therefore unduplicated. Patients with mental subnormality are excluded throughout.

3

Over one-quarter of these patients were suffering from some form of schizophrenia: $0\cdot25\%$ of the total population. This figure is similar to the 1-year prevalence of active cases found in the Eastern Health District of Baltimore in 1936 ($0\cdot29\%$: Lemkau, Tietze and Cooper, 1943), and to the 1-day prevalence, including recovered cases, found on the Danish island of Bornholm in 1935 ($0\cdot27\%$: Strömgren, 1938). Although these rates are not strictly comparable, numbers of a similar order have been found everywhere in the world where intensive studies have been made. Table 1 shows that only 13% of Camberwell patients attending out-patient clinics and day hospitals had been given the diagnosis, but that 29% of short- and medium-stay beds, and no fewer than 64% of long-stay beds, were occupied by patients with schizophrenia. These figures illustrate two of the outstanding features of the disease—its severity and its chronicity.

Patients with "no fixed abode" (in practice, individuals referred from Camberwell Reception Centre, and people without an address sent to the Observation Ward by Camberwell police) are not included in Table 1. They are, of course, particularly common in large conurbations. One hundred and sixty-one of them were in hospital on 31 December 1965 (54% with schizophrenia and 74% long-stay), and another 38 were referred to a psychiatrist during the subsequent 3 months. The latter figure represents only a small fraction of the reception centre population who are in need of psychiatric attention (10,000 individuals pass through the centre in a year).

Jones and Miles (1964), in a study of Anglesey, found 216 schizophrenic patients ($0\cdot42\%$) during the prevalence year, 1960. Forty-five of these were known only to their general practitioners (that is, they had never seen a psychiatrist). The residual prevalence ($0\cdot33\%$) is very similar to the estimated 1-year rate for Camberwell ($0\cdot31\%$). The Anglesey figure suggests that a general practitioner's list of 2500 people will contain 4 or 5 schizophrenic patients who are or have been under psychiatric care, 4 who are in hospital and 2 who have never seen a psychiatrist.

These static figures are not very much different from what they would have been before the Second World War, and none of them gives a hint of the revolution which is supposed to have overtaken English psychiatry since then. During the 1930's, about one-third of schizophrenic patients admitted to English mental hospitals were likely to stay for at least 2 years, and probably for the remainder of their lives. Before that, the proportion was about two-thirds (Brown, 1960). Of patients first admitted in 1954 or 1955, however, only 12–13% remained for as long as 2 years and even they still had a good chance of eventual discharge (Brooke, 1963). The process of accumulation which has filled our mental hospitals with long-stay schizophrenics has been slowed almost to a standstill. When it is realized that one-half of the mental hospital population is suffering from schizophrenia, and that two-thirds of the long-stay patients have this disease (these proportions can be worked out from Table 1), it becomes readily understandable that the number of occupied beds must be going down. Tooth and Brooke (1961) demonstrated this in a famous paper. Their figures showed that bed occupancy in mental hospitals in England and Wales reached a peak in 1954, and has since declined steadily. Brown, Parkes and Wing (1961) studied cohorts of schizophrenic and other patients admitted to three mental hospitals serving adjacent areas in Greater London in 1951 and 1956, with a 3-year follow-up period. The total length of stay (including re-admissions) decreased from 17 to 11·4 months out of 36. In 1951, 446 schizophrenic patients were admitted (41% of them first admissions); in 1956 the admission cohort was 715 (only 33% first admissions). Of the 307 patients in the earlier cohort who were discharged within 2 years, 50% were re-admitted during the follow-up period. The equivalent proportion of the 1956 cohort was 64% of 625. Brill and Patton (1962) showed a very similar pattern in the New York state mental hospital statistics.

These statistical trends seemed to draw attention to 1955 as the important point at which changes began to take place. Many therapeutic innovations seemed to be coming together to produce a new spirit of hope among mental hospital staff. This was the period when reserpine and chlorpromazine were introduced, when the idea of the therapeutic community began to seem relevant to long-stay wards as well as to special institutions, when the "open door" began to symbolize a new attitude to the care of chronic psychotic patients, and when practical methods of rehabilitation and resettlement began to have an impact on discharge rates. Most mental hospitals have a back ward which was "opened up" at about this time (L. Wing, 1956; Ytrehus, 1959), and senior nurses still look back with pride at an achievement which they regard as the best thing they have done.

Oram and Knowles (1964) studied the accumulation of long-stay patients in Fulbourn Hospital, Cambridge, where the records enabled them to go back to 1900 in looking for trends. They found that the absolute numbers of patients becoming long-stay (i.e. staying as long as 2 years) increased steadily throughout the century, with the consequent development of severe over-crowding, but that expressed as a proportion of the catchment area population, the rate of recruitment to long-stay status actually *declined* steadily. That is to say, the pressures of overcrowding became such that the numbers of long-stay patients *had* to be kept down, otherwise, as the general population increased in size, the hospital could not have functioned at all. Administrative considerations of this kind have played at least as important a part as therapeutic ones in apparently medical decisions such as whether to admit or discharge a patient.

Brown (1959a) showed that patients who were visited in Banstead or Long Grove hospitals during the first 4 weeks after admission in 1951 were much more likely to be discharged within 2 years than patients who were not visited. This distinction was lost in the 1956 cohort of admissions because, by that time, the decision about discharge no longer depended on whether the patient had interested relatives. A follow-up study of patients discharged from London mental hospitals in 1959 (Wing *et al.*, 1964) showed that, at the time of discharge, most schizophrenic patients were confident about the future, did not regard themselves as ill, thought their families would welcome them (but were not very bothered if they had no relatives) and, above all, *wanted to leave*. The decision had passed out of the hands of their medical advisers and was taken principally by the patients themselves.

This analysis of some of the statistics relating to schizophrenia shows the complexity of the factors underlying what appear to be straightforward trends. The lesson to be learned (it cannot be too often repeated at this moment in psychiatric history) is that administrative indices give no necessary indication of clinical condition. The fact that the mental hospital bed occupancy is decreasing does *not* necessarily mean that patients (particularly schizophrenic patients) are less ill than they used to be, any more than the reverse trends of the 1880's and 1890's (Bockhoven, 1956; Jones, 1960) meant that schizophrenia was increasing in malignancy then. To establish the truth about the efficacy of new methods of management, there is no substitute for the laborious process of directly measuring morbidity.

Several follow-up studies made at various times during the past half-century enable us to follow at least the social progress of the condition. The proportion of patients who were alive, out of hospital, socially competent and free from severe symptoms of the illness in the Heidelberg series described by Mayer-Gross (1932), 16 years after admission in 1912 or 1913, was 35%. In the Maudsley series studied by Guttman, Mayer-Gross and Slater (1939), the equivalent proportion was 43%, 3 years after admission in 1934 and 1935. Harris *et al.* (1956) studied early cases admitted to the Maudsley between 1945 and 1948, and found 50% socially recovered 5 years later. Kelly and Sargant (1965), following up schizophrenic patients admitted to a general hospital unit between 1956 and 1961, found that two-thirds were socially independent 2 years after discharge. Thus there is evidence of an improvement in the social prognosis of early schizophrenia which appears to indicate a clinical improvement as well.

A discussion of modern methods of management, therefore, seems to fall into two convenient parts, one dealing with long-stay schizophrenic patients, most of whom accumulated before the present era of early discharge and community care, the other concerned with patients who are admitted nowadays, and who can expect to leave hospital within a few months.

The Problem of "Institutionalism"

The social organization of mental hospitals during the first half of this century was largely concerned with the safe custody of the inmates, at a low cost to public funds. This had not always been the case. The "moral treatment" practised in many asylums 100 years earlier was based on principles (such as non-restraint and early discharge), which would be generally accepted today (Bockhoven, 1956; Conolly, 1856; Deutsch, 1949; Jones, 1954; Rees, 1957). This period did not last long. The hallmarks of the era that followed were large and overcrowded hospitals, with a high proportion of chronic wards, in which long-stay patients led a restricted and inactive life. Belknap (1956) and Dunham and Weinberg (1960) have described two American state mental hospitals which seem to sum up all that was worst in the custodial era. The main functions were to prevent a mentally ill individual from harming himself or others and to ensure that he could not escape. Routines of supervision and control were developed which would leave nothing to chance—hence the railed airing-courts, the locked doors, the windows that would only open 2 inches and the warning whistles carried by attendants. Given the twin facts of a large patient population and a small inadequately trained staff, it was inevitable that procedures which were adopted for the control of a few potentially dangerous patients should be generalized to the amenable majority. As Goffman pointed out, much time and trouble can be saved "if everyone's soiled clothing can be indiscriminately placed in one bundle, and laundered clothing can be redistributed, not according to ownership, but according to rough size". These are the perennial problems of large custodial institutions, and they are not confined to mental hospitals (Goffman, 1961; Sykes, 1958).

What *is* unique is the contribution of the mental hospital population itself to the culture of the institution (Sommer, 1959). Schizophrenic patients, for example, by reason of their numbers and prolonged residence, acquire, transmit and partially determine the peculiar social atmosphere of the mental hospital community. "Institutionalism", in fact, is a very complicated concept which cannot be reduced to any single line of cause and effect. There are at least three components of disability in patients said to be "institutionalized".

The first, and most overlooked, is a factor of selection. Individuals who have not built up strong ties in an outside community through marriage or work or family or other social interests, or who are vulnerable because of poverty or age or social position, or who have never been much concerned with problems of personal liberty and decision taking, or who actively prefer an environment where social interaction can be minimal, may have both an increased likelihood of admission and a decreased chance of discharge. Such factors need not keep anyone in hospital nowadays, as Brown (1959a) showed in his study of visiting, but they have certainly been important in the past. The premorbid personality of schizophrenic patients is quite often distinguished by factors of this kind (Brooke, 1959; Goldberg and Morrison, 1963; Wardle, 1962).

The second component in "institutionalism" is the disease process itself. The bowed head and shoulders, the shuffling gait, the apathetic faces, the social withdrawal and disinterest, the loss of spontaneity, initiative and individuality described so graphically by Barton (1959) may be seen in patients who have never been in an institution in their lives. Studies of intellectual performance seem to show that the damage is often relatively sudden in onset, rather than gradual in development as would be the case if it were the result of imposed social isolation (Kendig and Richmond, 1940; Foulds and Dixon, 1962). There is little evidence either of gradual clinical deterioration (Wing, 1962). This is not to say, of course, that the social surroundings do not affect clinical state; indeed, there is evidence to the contrary. Wing and Freudenberg (1961) found that severely handicapped schizophrenic patients responded immediately, during controlled periods of social stimulation, by an increase in output on an industrial task in a sheltered workshop, and that this activity was accompanied by a decrease in abnormalities of behaviour such as immobility, mannerisms and restlessness. Ward behaviour was unaffected, however, and workshop behaviour returned to its previous level as soon as the social stimulation was withdrawn.

Evidence on a larger scale, but of a less experimental kind, was provided by a comparative study of three mental hospitals, in which 100 randomly selected chronic schizophrenic women under the age of 60 years were interviewed to obtain standard descriptions of mental state. Ward behaviour scales were completed by senior nurses, and a sociologist collected systematic information about the specific social environment of each patient (Wing and Brown, 1961). Relatively hard indices, such as the proportion of patients in the samples who owned various items of clothing, showed up large differences between the three social *milieux*. At hospital A, 80% owned an overcoat or raincoat; at hospital B, 95%; at hospital C, 30%. The differences were more marked when less obvious items were considered; for example, the proportions owning articles of make-up such as lipstick or face powder were 71%, 55% and 34% respectively. Potentially dangerous items illustrated even larger discrepancies—55%, 18% and 8% respectively owned either a pair of scissors or a nail-file. Other social measurements, such as nurses' attitudes to various aspects of patients' performance, or the amount of locker space available, or the restrictiveness of the ward routines to which patients were exposed, or a time-budget of daily activities (in particular, the amount of waking time during which patients were completely unoccupied—an average of 5 hours 39 minutes at hospital C) all gave similar results. Hospitals A and C were at opposite poles, while B was intermediate (conditions for the patients who had been resident up to 10 years were similar to those at A, while conditions for patients with more than 20 years' residence were similar to those at C). Thus, there was an opportunity to test the hypothesis that social conditions were related to clinical state. In fact, the association was found to be very close, all the clinical measurements being distributed in much the same way as the social variables. The mean scores representing socially withdrawn and correlated behaviours, for example, were 2·9, 4·6 and 5·4 at the three hospitals, and the proportions of patients who were mute or almost mute at interview were 6%, 14% and 24%.

These data cannot be used to prove the case because of the possibility of differential admission or discharge practices (though there was no evidence for these, or for differences in drug treatment which would explain the results), but a strong case could be made that the social conditions under which a patient lived affected his mental state. Nevertheless, even at the hospital with the best social conditions, where rehabilitation procedures had been most thoroughly applied, at least 60% of the sample were severely handicapped. Barton (1959) puts forward the response to rehabilitation as the only means of distinguishing between "institutional neurosis" and chronic schizophrenia. As we shall see in the next section, the contribution of the disease process to residual disabilities in long-stay schizophrenic patients, according to this criterion, is substantial.

The third component in "institutionalism" is that contributed by the social pressures of the institution, acting gradually over many years, even on patients whose premorbid personality was lively and sociable and in whom the disease has not run a severe course. The demonstration of such a factor presents problems because of the difficulty of following patients over long periods of time and watching changes which occur gradually. However, a partial test can be made by comparing patients who have been in hospital for various periods from 2 to 40 years. The selective factor, mentioned earlier, is likely to operate principally during the first 2 years after admission, while the effect of age can be controlled, in part, by looking for differences within age-groups and also by excluding patients over the age of 60. Under these conditions, it is difficult to demonstrate much change in clinical condition with length of stay, but changes in attitudes, in plans for the future, in knowledge of the outside world and in contact with visitors are very marked (Wing, 1962). Within the 30–39 age group of schizophrenic patients at two mental hospitals, for example, 77% of those who had been resident for 2–4 years had some wish to leave, compared with 38% of those resident for 5–9 years, and 17% of those resident for 10 years or more. A similar trend was found when age, date of first admission, or clinical condition were taken into account. The attitudes of short-stay patients at the point of discharge, referred to earlier, were in striking contrast—nearly everyone wanted to leave.

Thus at the heart of this component of the syndrome of institutionalism, lies a gradually increasing dependence on the hospital way of life and inability to lead any other. Habits which are a necessity in everyday life in an industrial society—travelling to work, clocking in on time, following workshop routines and getting on with workmates, conforming to the standards of the social group in dress and manners—are not regularly practised in many mental hospitals. In their place, new habits develop, which are maladaptive so far as outside society is concerned. As time goes on, relatives die or move away or simply cease to visit, and the patient's whole world may come to be bounded by the walls of the institution, or even by those of a single ward (Sommer and Osmond, 1961).

This kind of deterioration seems to have occurred in most mental hospitals, irrespective of the present social environment. In the comparative study of three mental hospitals, mentioned earlier, there was a decline in wish to leave with increase in length of stay, in all three samples. Hospital A contained more patients who wanted to be discharged than hospital B, which in turn contained more than hospital C—the differences were just significant. This does seem to prove, at least, that improving the social conditions does not necessarily mean that patients will be more likely to want to stay. All three hospitals shared the same heritage of custodial staff attitudes and practices, though they had progressed at different rates towards the common goal. Most patients, in each hospital, were "institutionalized".

This analysis of institutionalism may serve as a realistic introduction to the problems of rehabilitation and the therapeutic community which are discussed in the next section.

Rehabilitation of the Long-stay Patient

For many of the long-stay patients now in mental hospitals, the original aim of their doctors has been fulfilled; they are amenable, institutionalized, content to remain in hospital for the rest of their lives. The fact that the goal has now become resettlement in the community, in a job which will make them self-supporting, is a change imposed from outside—the patients themselves did not initiate it, nor did their relatives. The easy adjustment to the routines and limitations of the institution, which used to be a sign of success, is now a handicap to be overcome by using methods of rehabilitation.

It is clear from what has been said in the previous section that, from the point of view of resettlement, most long-stay patients are handicapped in three basic ways:

(a) They have disabilities which were present even before the onset of florid symptoms, such as handicapping personality traits or lack of manual or intellectual skills.

(b) They have disabilities which are basically part of their illness, such as incoherent thought processes, delusional motivation or catatonic slowness and apathy.

(c) They have "secondary" handicaps, which have accumulated because they have been ill and because of their own and other people's reactions to the illness.

These disabilities fuse together into the characteristic picture of "institutionalism", but if a rational plan of rehabilitation is to be set up, an attempt must be made to separate the various components and decide which ones, if any, can be reduced. A realistic goal can then be adopted and the patient's progress constantly assessed against it.

Although the first job of the rehabilitation team is to describe, classify and measure handicaps, very little use has been made of the considerable literature on psychological deficit. Investigators have been mainly concerned with two fundamental types of dysfunction in schizophrenia—represented by the clinical symptoms of affective blunting and disordered associations. The former has been described in terms of intellectual slowness (e.g. by Babcock, 1933, and by numerous investigators since), but it was always apparent that patients often *could* undertake complex tasks if they would co-operate (e.g. Hunt, 1936). A series of studies was then reported showing that patients could be motivated to perform better (e.g. Peters and Jenkins, 1954), and describing the basic problem as an inability to maintain a "set" (e.g. Rodnick and Shakow, 1940). Recent theories have returned to the possibility, suggested by Babcock, that "attention" itself is fundamentally disturbed in schizophrenia (Venables, 1960). The other classical symptom—disturbance of associations—has also received a great deal of investigation (e.g. Cameron and Magaret, 1951) though its relation to affective blunting has hardly been considered since Jung's early discussion (1906). Studies of industrial output have shown that a characteristic of the learning curve in schizophrenic patients is a slow and linear improvement with practice, which contrasts markedly with the more usual negatively accelerated form seen in normal people and imbeciles (O'Connor, 1957; Wing and Freudenberg, 1961). This result proffers the useful advice that if schizophrenics' progress is slow, at least it is steady and prolonged.

The techniques of investigation of these psychobiological studies have yet to be seriously applied to the assessment of disability for practical purposes, but on a cruder level, the handicaps are very evident. When schizophrenic and non-schizophrenic workers at an Industrial Rehabilitation Unit were compared, for example, the former were described by occupational supervisors to be slow, lacking in initiative and to have an impaired capacity for independent judgement. They could not make complicated decisions and they lacked manual skill. Even the least handicapped patients from a good mental hospital were socially withdrawn at the industrial rehabilitation unit though they were not unfriendly when approached (Wing, Bennett and Denham, 1964). Secondary handicaps were even more obvious—difficulty in using public transport, inability to manage money, bewilderment when faced by everyday procedures which most people in an industrial society take in their stride.

The concept of handicap is essential to the rational application of re-habilitation procedures. The aim is to prevent, reduce or manage handicaps in such a way that the patient's assets can be maximized and his manner of life be as near as possible to what it would have been if he had not become ill (or even, if possible, better than that). The value of thinking in terms of handicap is that, if residual disability seems to be irreducible, all that happens is a shift of gear from techniques designed to reduce handicap to techniques designed to compensate for them.

The experiment by Wing and Freudenberg (1961) shows that it is possible to demonstrate clinical changes as a result of social activation. Work is an alternative to immobility, manneristic behaviour or ineffectual restlessness. However, although the response to extra social stimulation was clear-cut and without latency, the relapse to the former rate of working (and therefore to the former level of behavioural abnormality) was equally striking and immediate. There was also a marked reaction to "random" environmental changes, such as the substitution of an unknown for a known supervisor (the sort of thing that is constantly happening in a hospital environment). It is a sound principle of rehabilitation to give exercise to functions which have become disused following illness or injury, in the hope that partial or com-plete recovery may eventually occur. A large part of institutionalism in chronic schizophrenics may be due to the fact that affectively blunted patients may not actively use their faculties and, in a crowded and understaffed ward, it is difficult to give the proper medical and nursing attention which would keep residual mental and physical functions at the optimum level. Such active remedial care may have to be kept up for very long periods of time, and a practical exercise for advocates of the therapeutic community would be to devise social situations in which nursing and occupational supervisors will not tire of this basic duty.

Further evidence that social activation (the injection of motivation) is the fundamental groundwork on which other rehabilitation procedures can build comes from the comparative study of samples of chronic schizophrenic patients in three mental hospitals. The surveys were repeated in 1962 and 1964 and a preliminary analysis of the data shows that in hospital C, where there was most room for change, both social and clinical improvement has taken place. However, the only social change which is directly associated with clinical improvement is a reduction in the amount of time spent doing nothing. Other changes, such as a decrease in ward restrictiveness, or an increase in the number of personal possessions or a favourable change in attitude on the part of nursing staff, occur just as much in patients who were clinically no different, as in patients who were better. This illustrates the value of distinguishing different types of handicap, because changes which enrich the social environment are directed mainly at secondary rather than primary disabilities, and a failure to produce clinical improvement does *not* mean that they have been unsuccessful.

Group techniques have been recommended as particularly suitable for the re-education of chronic schizophrenic patients. The idea of the therapeutic community, which did not arise within the mental hospital but in a totally different setting and in response to quite different problems (Main, 1946; Jones, 1952), has also been taken over (Freeman, Cameron and McGhie, 1958; Clark, Hooper and Oram, 1962; Martin, 1962; Jones, 1962). Apart from the article by Hooper (1962), there has been very little effort at systematic and detailed quantification, either of the social procedures involves, or of the results. Certainly nothing like a controlled experiment has been undertaken. Some of the earlier social treatments, such as "total push", which *were* rigorously investigated, did not come out very well (Bennett and Robertson, 1955; Galioni, Adams and Tallman, 1953; Maas, Varon and Rosenthal, 1951), and it may be that schizophrenic patients are particularly resistant to group pressures. A certain caution is obviously called for in assessing some of the claims recently put forward. The difficulty is due, in large part, to the flexibility of the concepts used—"increased communication", for example, which can take a different meaning according to the personality and energy of the group leader (Etzioni, 1960). There is no doubt that, in order to create the right conditions for medical, nursing and occupational staff to undertake the rehabilitation of long-stay schizophrenic patients, the social organization of the hospital and its various departments has to be radically changed, and the attitudes of staff at all levels re-educated (Bennett, Folkard and Nicholson, 1961). In this sense, "administrative therapy" (Clark, 1964) is an important and valuable concept. It should not detract, however, from a realization that much of the pioneering work in this field was carried out by Physician Superintendents who had the power and the influence to carry through their ideas. It is unlikely that the functions of an energetic reformer can be built into the social structure of an institution (Superintendents could also be autocratic mediocrities), but a partial substitute can be derived from a knowledge of the ways in which social processes affect the manifestations of illness, and how they can be used to prevent the accumulation of secondary handicaps and to promote resettlement.

Perhaps the most thoroughly studied techniques have been those of industrial rehabilitation. In a pilot experiment (Wing and Giddens, 1959; Wing, 1960), it was found that the practical results of offering courses at an industrial rehabilitation unit to moderately-handicapped chronic schizophrenic patients with some wish to leave hospital were fairly good. In particular, attitudes to work became much more realistic. When the project was extended to include patients up to 60 years of age, and patients who had not actually expressed a wish to leave hospital, the results were naturally less striking, but they enabled the limits of this form of treatment to be drawn (Wing, Bennett and Denham, 1964). Out of 45 patients, 24 were employed outside hospital 1 year after completing the course. Three were giving rise to some anxiety, but the remaining 21 (10 of them in sheltered employment) were working satisfactorily. The rest were unemployed. Eight patients were living outside hospital and behaving normally. Six others had caused difficulty in their lodgings, hostel or home, but not seriously enough to warrant their return to hospital. A further 3 patients were living in Rowton Houses and their adjustment was precarious. The remaining 28 patients were still in hospital. All the patients remained handicapped in some way, though in some cases the disability was slight. At least 6 patients became more severely ill at the I.R.U. and another 10 showed a milder form of adverse reaction—a finding also noted by Stone and Eldred (1959)—but taken over the whole period of the investigation, no patient was worse for having been to the I.R.U. and at least half benefited considerably. Those who went to Remploy factories were not more handicapped, or more difficult to deal with, than physically disabled men who started work at the same time. If anything, the comparison was in favour of the schizophrenics.

The patients came from two hospitals, which differed from each other in the amount of preparation which was given before the course started. Adequate preparation seemed to decrease the likelihood of adverse reactions and increase the proportion of patients who benefited. If the results could be applied to the equivalent mental hospital population of long-stay moderately handicapped men under 60, about 6000 people would be represented, of whom over 1500 might be expected to be satisfactorily resettled in open employment and another 1500 to be settled in Remploy or other sheltered factories.

Clearly, an I.R.U. course is only one step in the process of rehabilitation (and it may, in many cases, be unnecessary). It will be useless without skilled preliminary work and active and prolonged after-care. But the I.R.U. does provide three features which are difficult to reproduce in a mental hospital— a realistic industrial setting, a majority of non-institutionalized workers, and specific training in work habits. In this setting, a realistic trial can be made of a patient's capacity to travel, clock in, mix without causing social embarrassment, manage a financial budget, and work to a required standard. If the patient can make this demonstration (to himself as much as to the staff), he may change his views of the possibility of resettlement and begin to acquire realistic attitudes, particularly about work. In neither the pilot study, nor the main project, did attitudes to discharge change realistically, but this may very well be another example of the general principle that each handicap must be tackled separately. The patients were living in hospital throughout the I.R.U. course, and no hostel was available which would have provided an equivalent social pressure directed specifically at attitude to discharge.

Rehabilitation and sheltered workshops are now being set up extensively in mental hospitals, as well as outside them (Carstairs, O'Connor and Rawnsley, 1956; Wadsworth, Scott and Tonge, 1958; Early, 1960; Morgan, Cushing and Manton, 1965). There is a clear danger that some enthusiastic proponents will run through the "cream" of the long-stay population, achieving a good discharge rate and success at follow-up and making exaggerated claims on this basis, with the inevitable reaction from critics of reform, who will be able to point out that later endeavours do not fulfil these high expectations, and thus herald an eventual disillusionment with all such methods. This process has occurred before. There is, in fact, in all mental hospitals where social innovations have not yet made much headway, a group of patients who could probably be discharged without much preparation or after-care (Garratt, Lowe and McKeown, 1957; Rawnsley, Loudon and Miles, 1962). When these have been discharged there are still some relatively easy problems to tackle before getting down to the really difficult (and highly skilled) work of rehabilitation. Catterson, Bennett and Freudenberg (1963) calculated that only 13% of their sample of long-stay schizophrenic patients under the age of 60 were anywhere near a point at which discharge could be considered. They pointed out that

> the working and living arrangements of many of the remaining patients could be duplicated outside the hospital boundaries if a series of hostels and workshops were set up. The only disadvantage would lie in the lack of extensive hospital grounds which, at present, constitute a buffer area between the hospital and community, where patients can move freely without their idiosyncracies of behaviour being immediately noticeable to the public. Such arrangements do not mean that the patient has been "resettled" and they are, in principle, no different from what is already being provided in a good hospital, since the patient is not self-supporting.

Early (1965) has specified more precisely the component parts of a rehabilitation service for chronically handicapped patients, in which it is explicitly recognized that patients may not reach equivalent points in industrial and domestic resettlement at the same time. The essence of the scheme is that a series of agencies should be provided which will allow the patient to make progress without having to adjust to large changes in level of required performance. Thus the "ladder" of domestic resettlement leads from the high-supervision ward, via "workers' villa", predischarge ward or night hospital, to various types of community hostel, supervised lodgings or family care, and finally to full domestic independence. A similarly wide range of occupational facilities is also available and a patient can be at completely different levels on the two "ladders".

The organization of these agencies presents problems which will be discussed in a later section, but it should be emphasized that only one new principle is involved. All these services are already present, in embryo at least, in good psychiatric hospitals. The new suggestion is that they should be geographically dispersed throughout the community and closely coordinated with other social and occupational agencies, such as those of the Ministry of Labour or the services for the physically handicapped. No working model of this kind is yet available for study, though the Bristol services perhaps come closest to it.

As the long-stay population "runs down", the focus of interest shifts to other problems and there is a danger that the importance of rehabilitation (which has come to be thought of as applicable principally in a hospital setting) will be forgotten. The best remedy for this is to consider the problems of the short-stay schizophrenic patient.

Early Discharge and the Prevention of Chronic Disability

The most obvious justification for a policy of early discharge from mental hospitals is that it prevents the accumulation of the chronic handicaps which together make up the picture of "institutionalism". In so far as the syndrome *is* the result of prolonged exposure to an understimulating and perhaps positively harmful social environment, it is a tautology that it will be pre-vented, but this only illustrates the semantic hazards of coining new phrases. We have seen that there are at least two other kinds of handicap, one which existed before the patient was admitted in the first place, and the other which is not particularly affected by length of stay. As for secondary handicaps, they are dependent on the other two kinds, and probably always develop to some extent when a patient is chronically ill. They have been described in physically handicapped individuals who have not been institutionalized (Hewitt, 1949; Fowler, 1955; Feintuch, 1955; Wing, 1965) and cannot be wished away simply by discharging a patient. The form they take will, however, depend on what happens after discharge.

The administrative division of the Health Service between three separate hierarchies—hospital, local authority and general practitioner—has be-devilled all attempts to provide a comprehensive and continuous care system. The problem has been tackled in various ways. In Nottingham, the Physician Superintendent of Mapperley Hospital (whose interest in community care began before the Second World War while the hospital was administered by the local authority) is Advisory Medical Officer of Mental Health. He is concerned not only with the medical problem of patients in the hospital and its numerous clinics (which extend into every field of psychiatry) but with the mental health of the city of Nottingham. The core of the integration between local government and hospital services is the system of shared duties between mental welfare officers and social workers. Both types of worker take responsibility for patients in the hospital *and* in the community and act as a combined team. The policy is now beginning to be extended to psychiatric nurses. A network of supporting services, such as day hospitals, hostels and old people's homes, has been set up (Macmillan, 1958 and 1961).

A similar system is being developed in Croydon (May, 1965), in Plymouth (Weeks, 1965) and elsewhere.

A wealth of other models of community care now exists in the United Kingdom but, so far, there has been little attempt at evaluation. The survey by Sainsbury and Grad (1962) is an exception, but the number of schizophrenic patients is not large enough to make possible an evaluation of this particular problem. The same is true of the preliminary report by Hoenig and Hamilton (1965).

A study of schizophrenic patients discharged from London mental hospitals in 1959 and 1960 disclosed considerable morbidity during the follow-up year. Only 17% had severe symptoms at discharge, but 54% subsequently deteriorated in clinical condition and 49% were re-admitted at least once. There was a sudden social crisis, in which the police, neighbours, or members of the general public were involved, in 41% of cases, usually following a period of severe distress at home (Wing *et al.*, 1964). Most of these patients had an established disease, and the services provided were very sketchy. The family doctor, M.W.O. and out-patient clinic were the only community services generally used, but their main function appeared to be to arrange re-admission when a social crisis became unavoidable. Thirty-eight per cent attended an employment exchange, but half of those who were found work in this way lost it, or left it within a month or two. Unemployment was common. Active domiciliary supervision and adequate day hospital accommodation were not available, and sheltered workshop facilities were offered to only two patients (Parkes, Brown and Monck, 1962; Monck, 1963).

These results illustrate the difficult problems of active supervision and after-care in a large conurbation, but they are not entirely unrepresentative of those found elsewhere. Smith, Pumphrey and Hall (1963), for example, studied the incidents which resulted in requests for the admission of 100 schizophrenic patients and found that 53 patients actually committed or threatened to commit a dangerous act and the behaviour of a further 38 was socially unacceptable. The authors emphasized that the majority of the incidents were extreme and that most of the families had reached the limits of their tolerance.

The London follow-up study already mentioned was primarily concerned to test a hypothesis which had arisen out of earlier work (Brown, 1959b), which has considerable relevance to the question of the management of schizophrenic patients after discharge from hospital. Ratings of the emotional involvement of a key relative (usually the mother or wife) with the patient were made at a joint interview at home, shortly after the patient left hospital, and were then used to predict outcome. Of those who were only mildly ill when they left hospital, 64% deteriorated in clinical state if they returned to homes where the key relative was highly involved, compared with only 14% of the "low involvement" group. The equivalent proportions among those

who were still moderately or severely ill at the time of discharge were 81 %
and 40% (Brown *et al.*, 1962). This result requires confirmation and further
investigation, but it is sufficiently striking to warrant discussion of its implications for "community psychiatry". However, some results from another,
more extensive, follow-up study will be presented first.

Three hundred and thirty-nine schizophrenic patients admitted to three
mental hospitals in 1956 were selected for study. Data were collected from
hospital and out-patient records, mental welfare officers, employment exchanges and the Ministry of Pensions. A visit to the patient's home was made
5 years after the key admission. In this way, a fairly detailed picture was
built up of 5 years in the life of each patient.

The three hospitals were chosen because the first was well known for its
emphasis on rehabilitation, the second for its comprehensive community
services, and the third because it was representative of the large number where
no integration between hospital and community services had been attempted.

One hundred and eleven patients were first admitted in 1956. By that time
the early discharge policy had become firmly established at all three hospitals,
but particularly at the second, where it had been pioneered and where
patients spent a total of only 6 months, including re-admissions, throughout
the whole 5 years. At the other two hospitals the average stay during the
follow-up period was about 1 year. Thus "institutionalism", in the sense of a
condition brought about by a prolonged stay in a mental hospital, was
almost completely prevented and could not be regarded as an important
factor determining outcome in the community. Various indices gave a
similar picture of clinical outcome in each of the three groups: just over
one-quarter of the patients were still severely ill 5 years after first admission,
and another quarter were still handicapped by less severe symptoms.

There were no differences in the proportion of first-admitted patients
employed at the time of follow-up—about two-thirds in each cohort. Total
unemployment during the 5 years also showed up no differences. However,
the group which spent less time in hospital also spent more time in the
community unemployed and gave rise to rather more problems from the
point of view of relatives. About two-thirds of all admissions and readmissions, in each area, were preceded by an episode of severely disturbed
behaviour (i.e. by a social crisis).

The outcome for the 228 patients who had been in hospital before 1956
was not, of course, as good as that for the first-admitted patients, but again
there was very little difference between the three cohorts. About one-half of
the previously admitted patients, in each area, were still very severely ill at
the time of follow-up, and a further quarter were still handicapped though to
a lesser extent. Nearly one-third, however, were working competently and
showed no psychotic symptoms during the final 6 months of the follow-up
period (Brown *et al.*, 1966).

In some ways, the results are encouraging, since the prognosis (particularly in early schizophrenia) is better than it has ever been before. But it is clear that a substantial proportion of patients remains handicapped, and that the community services were not able to prevent the morbidity or the burden on many of the families. It is the management of these patients which constitutes the major challenge to the developing community services. The remainder of this chapter is devoted to a discussion of some of the most difficult problems which must be solved, if the term "community care" is to have any meaning.

The Modern Management of Schizophrenia

(A) DRUG ADMINISTRATION

It has been shown in several studies that about 40% of schizophrenic patients fail to take their medication as advised (Renton et al., 1963; Parkes, Brown and Monck, 1962; Brown et al., 1966). This is about the same proportion as in diabetes or tuberculosis. Some patients have the feeling that it is wrong to be "dependent" on drugs, others do not consider themselves ill, others again complain of the side-effects of the phenothiazines (particularly lassitude and obesity).

There is little doubt that patients who do not take drugs regularly as advised are more likely to relapse than those who stick closely to instructions. Whether this is because patients stop taking the drugs as they become ill, or because stopping the drug makes them ill, is not clear from the studies quoted. However, evidence from adequately controlled trials does show that several of the phenothiazines are more effective than a placebo, at least in the short run (N.I.M.H., 1964; Goldberg, Klerman and Cole, 1965; Pasamanick et al., 1964; Scarpitti et al., 1964). It is therefore worth considering how best to supervise drug administration in each individual case, whether through the relatives, or the general practitioner, or a public health or psychiatric nurse. Many general practitioners prefer to reduce the dose advised by the hospital consultant and some change to one of the minor tranquillizers which acts as a placebo only.

(B) EMPLOYMENT

Although the Ministry of Labour services acted quite effectively in the case of the rehabilitation projects for long-stay patients (which were, of course, specially organized and supervised), routine experience with groups of short-stay patients has not been encouraging. In the three-hospital follow-up study, for example, only 15 patients out of 339 were referred to an industrial rehabilitation unit, and only 4 of these could be considered at all successful. Since the basic requirement for rehabilitation procedures, that they should be continuous, was not fulfilled in any of these instances, and there was no preparation before the I.R.U. course nor special supervision afterwards, these cases cannot be considered tests of the I.R.U. system.

Extremely few patients, in any of the published series, have been found sheltered work. Disablement resettlement officers have had to bear much of the brunt of trying to find handicapped patients work, and the results have not been very successful. The efforts of social workers have met with even less success. By far the best results have come from patients returning to the jobs they held before entering hospital, or finding work themselves.

In the comparative study of three groups of long-stay in-patients, it was shown that one of the key variables differentiating the hospitals was the amount of inactivity allowed. Schizophrenic patients do tend to lapse into inertia when left to their own devices, and the proportion of waking time spent doing absolutely nothing was found to be 21%, 26% and 43% at the three hospitals. These figures can be compared with data from the time-budget analysis in the comparative follow-up study. Twenty-one first-admitted patients who were outside hospital, but either severely disturbed or unemployed during the final 6 months of the 5-year follow-up period, spent 30% of their daytime hours doing nothing. The equivalent figure for previously admitted patients was 38% ($N = 53$).

It would be pointless to apportion blame in these matters, but the fact remains that handicapped patients in the community were often not as well looked after as long-stay patients in a hospital which was proud of its rehabilitation programme. "Integration" and "co-ordination" are acceptable words to use when describing community services, but they are rarely apt when applied to the co-operation between hospital, local authority and Ministry of Labour services in carrying out a plan of rehabilitation which must often last several years.

In fact, everything that was said about the rehabilitation of long-stay patients applies with equal force to the care of handicapped patients in the community. Rehabilitation consists in attempting to order the environment in such a way that primary disabilities are minimized, and secondary handicaps are prevented or kept to the lowest level possible. Rehabilitation efforts in hospital must be continuously applied if hard-won progress is not to be lost, and the same seems to be true after the patient has been discharged. Unfortunately, it is precisely at the point of discharge that efforts *do* tend to be relaxed. Even when some contact is kept with the patient after discharge, there is little systematic attempt to measure handicaps, in order to plan the kinds of non-hospital environment which are most likely to minimize morbidity.

(C) THE FAMILY PROBLEMS OF SCHIZOPHRENIC PATIENTS

About one-third of the relatives of first-admitted patients, and two-thirds of the relatives of patients who had been previously admitted, reported one or more problems at the time of follow-up, because of having the patient at home. Frequently mentioned were the health of the informant and the health of children in the household, and the main reported cause was the patient's disturbed behaviour.

Nevertheless, the large majority of relatives accepted the patient's presence at home without complaint. Fewer than 20% of the patients were permanently rejected during the follow-up period. Mothers in particular, although the majority were over 60 (40% were over 70), were very tolerant. Husbands or wives were less accepting and the divorce rate was three to four times that of the general population.

This general toleration and lack of complaint has been used as a justification for the early discharge policy, but in fact, the relatives are not always given a choice. They did not complain in the days when schizophrenic patients remained in hospital for long years, but no one now thinks that this fact justified that system. It remains a medical responsibility to give advice, and if relatives were told that patients would be better off in hospital, many of them would undoubtedly accept that as well. They are often not told this, although community rehabilitation facilities are so tenuous; which reflects the psychiatrist's view of what is available in hospital. Given the choice between poor hospital facilities and poor community services he is tempted to make no long-term recommendation at all, and fortunately the relatives make no complaint.

The way out of the impasse is to provide better community services, but this will prove expensive, above all in the provision of skilled personnel to run them.

The study of Brown et al. (1962) raises the question of whether the social environment provided by the family is always conducive to the patient's recovery. It is a frequent criticism of the "revolving door" policy that the patient recovers rapidly in hospital because some noxious influence has been removed, but that as soon as he begins to get better he is allowed to go straight back into the pathological environment. This is certainly one interpretation of the data, though Brown and his colleagues were very careful not to give strong backing to it, since other interpretations are equally possible. In particular, the possibility that the patient's abnormal behaviour provokes characteristic reactions in otherwise normal relatives has not been sufficiently considered. Brown et al. thought that only about one-third of the relatives they interviewed were markedly abnormal, though this proportion is higher than would be expected. Several controlled studies of disturbed communication in the families of schizophrenic patients have now been published, and both environmental theories (Beavers *et al.*, 1965; Singer and Wynne, 1963) and genetic theories (Phillips *et al.*, 1965) have been put forward to account for the results.

(D) TECHNIQUES OF MANAGEMENT

The outstanding feature of the course of schizophrenia is the "social crisis". When a patient is admitted to hospital, his behaviour usually becomes normal quite quickly, perhaps because of the re-establishment of drug treatment, or because of removal from an environment which provokes abnormality, or because the hospital environment is controlling in a way that the home environment is not. We have seen that schizophrenic behaviour does characteristically respond in this immediate way to controlled changes in social stimulation (Wing and Freudenberg, 1961), and it may be hoped that one day the dynamics of the process will be so well understood that it will be possible to prescribe social conditions which do not allow the crises to develop. There may, of course, be a biological process at work which is independent of social conditions—severe fluctuations in behaviour are quite common among a small group of long-stay patients, for example, even in a good mental hospital. The larger proportion of moderately-handicapped long-stay schizophrenics usually remain stable in behaviour for many years, under the non-stressful conditions of the "workers' wards", but they may then show a reactivation of symptoms in response to a sudden change in the level of social stimulation (Wing, Bennett and Denham, 1964; Stone and Eldred, 1959). Something of the same kind may therefore be happening to cause social crises after the patient leaves hospital. The family is, indeed, a "social *milieu*" equivalent to the hospital ward. However, there is no evidence, as yet, on which to base a rational family therapy.

The most successful technique appears to be a steady impersonal stimulation. Understimulation (as in the oldfashioned back ward) or overstimulation (as in the hothouse atmosphere of a highly charged emotional relationship with an abnormal parent) are equally harmful. A balance is fairly easy to achieve in a hospital workshop, in which the supervisor's approach to the patient is interpreted "neutrally" as it were (W. V. Wadsworth, personal communication). It is much more difficult for the patient's relatives to achieve, because they are necessarily emotionally involved with the patient, and find it difficult to treat him professionally. Yet, if the analogy between the social environment of the family and the hospital ward is taken seriously, this is precisely what they are being asked to do. They are not only husbands, wives or parents, they are nurses as well. The stresses and strains of this dual role have never been adequately investigated.

The basic problem for the "community team" is to interrupt the sequence of behaviours and reactions which lead to a social crisis. At the moment, the crisis is a means of identifying families who need help, but all too frequently the help is given only at the point of crisis, and the large bulk of the submerged iceberg is ignored. Mental welfare officers were not, for example, more likely to be in routine contact with families which contained a severely disturbed patient (in one follow-up series) than with families which had no immediate problems. For a moment, at a time of crisis, the community care official has the opportunity of looking below the surface. Unfortunately, he is rarely in a position to remember what he has seen, or to apply practical measures of prevention, after the crisis is over, so that it does not occur again.

Assuming that adequate resources (particularly of highly skilled and experienced staff, and a comprehensive range of rehabilitation agencies) were available, what would be the best manner of organization? The staff functions would be threefold:

(a) To obtain sufficient information about the behaviour of each patient on an active list, and about the relationships between family members, to give a really complete picture of handicaps and problems.

(b) To construct a plan on the basis of this information for minimizing handicaps and problems and maximizing assets, through the use of advice on techniques of management and, equally important, advice on which rehabilitation agencies, or what kind of practical help, were most appropriate at any given stage. This plan would have to be brought up to date from time to time, in the light of the progress made by the family.

(c) To obtain the trust of patient and relatives so that full information could be obtained and so that the advice given would be acceptable.

The present organization of community services manifestly does not prevent social crises or family problems. The first essential is an active list, so that families at risk are known and the responsibility for minimizing morbidity falls clearly on the community team. The second essential is that the team (composed of doctor, nurse, social worker and occupational adviser) should gain specialist experience. This does not mean that they must confine their attention to schizophrenia, since the problems involved are probably not dissimilar in many other psychiatric conditions. Nor does it mean that the work will be dreary because of the exclusion of "interesting" short-term conditions. This self-fulfilling doctrine has been built up through decades of neglect, and it will not be dispelled until specialist rehabilitation teams have adequate services at their disposal and have been able to build up a theoretical as well as an empirical fund of knowledge. The "firm" system, in which a team is supposed to deal with both short-term and long-term conditions, merely ensures that the acute problems with their rapid turnover, urgent demands and satisfying tendency to rapid improvement, occupy the centre of attention to the exclusion of patients with chronic handicaps.

The latter present the more difficult problems, requiring an equal degree of judgement and skill. It is one of the paradoxes of the present organization of psychiatric services that the more complicated the problem, the less likely is it to receive skilled and intensive attention. The situation is, of course, even worse in the United States (Bellak, 1964).

There is also disagreement about the development of specialist roles for the different members of the team. The position presented here requires the development of different types of skill by doctor, nurse, social worker and occupational expert, in sharp contradistinction to the therapeutic community approach, in which roles depend more on the personality of the participants. The psychiatric nurse, for example, is trained to look after patients who cannot care for themselves, to administer drugs, to anticipate and manage disturbed behaviour and to support the patient in his day-to-day difficulties. This is exactly what relatives are often called upon to do at home, and it seems wasteful to confine the nurse's expertise to brief periods while the patient is in hospital. The role of social worker has a quite different emphasis to that of a nurse. The social worker is the one who has to collect information, to advise the family on the various types of help available and which of these is most appropriate for a particular problem and also, in rather rare cases, to attempt to alter family relationships (Goldberg, 1960). These different types of activity require complementary skills. They are based, at the moment, on experience and apprenticeship rather than on theory, and they are still developing. Naturally, the functions of members of the team will overlap—all will contribute information, all will participate in the attempt to gain the family's trust, all will represent an outward authority, which may help the patient to see his behaviour through the eyes of the community.

Conclusion

McKeown (1961) has pointed out that, with the concentration of mortality at the very beginning and the very end of the natural human life-span, the centre of attention in social medicine and public health will increasingly be focused on the problems of chronic morbidity in children and adults. Social psychiatry is a part of social medicine, and a large proportion of all severe psychiatric conditions is chronic, although while psychiatric staff have time to deal only with recurrent exacerbations and crises, they will not realize to the full the fascination and reward obtainable from studying the process longitudinally, and trying to ameliorate it.

This article has perhaps been describing not so much the *modern* management of schizophrenia as the *future* management of the condition. Very few of the services which seem desirable, both for long-stay and for short-stay patients, are in existence as yet. British psychiatry, however, has progressed further along this road than most, perhaps because of the empirical temper and willingness to experiment of British psychiatrists, and perhaps because the social services in general have been regarded, since the time of the Minority Report to the Poor Law Commission (1909), as the responsibility of the whole nation.

References

BABCOCK, H. (1933), *Dementia Praecox: A Psychological Study*, New York.
BARTON, R. (1959), *Institutional Neurosis*, Bristol, Wright.
BEAVERS, W. R., BLAUMBERG, S., TIMKEN, K. R. and WEINER, M. F. (1965), Communication patterns of mothers of schizophrenics, *Family Process*, **4**, 95–104.
BELKNAP, I. (1956), *Human Problems of a State Mental Hospital*, New York, McGraw-Hill.
BELLAK, L. (1964), *Handbook of Community Psychiatry*, New York, Grune & Stratton.
BENNETT, D. H. and ROBERTSON, J. P. S. (1955), The effects of habit training on chronic schizophrenic patients, *J. Ment. Sci.* **101**, 664.
BENNETT, D. H., FOLKARD, S. and NICHOLSON, AUDREY (1961), Resettlement unit in a mental hospital, *Lancet*, **ii**, 539.
BOCKHOVEN, J. S. (1956), Moral treatment in American psychiatry, *J. Nerv. Ment. Dis.* **124**, 167, 292.
BRILL, H. and PATTON, R. E. (1962), Clinical-statistical analysis of population changes in New York state mental hospitals since introduction of psychotropic drugs, *Amer. J. Psychiat.* **119**, 20.
BROOKE, EILEEN (1959), National statistics in epidemiology of mental illness, *J. Ment. Sci.* **105**, 893.
BROOKE, EILEEN (1963), Factors affecting the demand for psychiatric beds, *Lancet*, **ii**, 1211.
BROWN, G. W. (1959a), Social factors influencing the length of hospital stay of schizophrenic patients, *Brit. Med. J.* **ii**, 1300.
BROWN, G. W. (1959b), Experiences of discharged chronic schizophrenic mental hospital patients in various types of living group, *Milbank Mem. Fund Quart.* **37**, 105.
BROWN, G. W. (1960), Length of hospital stay and schizophrenia, *Acta Psychiat.* **35**, 414.
BROWN, G. W., PARKES, C. and WING, J. K. (1961), Admissions and re-admissions to three London mental hospitals, *J. Ment. Sci.* **107**, 1070.
BROWN, G. W., BONE, MARGARET, DALISON, BRIDGET and WING, J. K. (1966), *Schizophrenia and Social Care: A Comparative Follow-up Study of 339 Schizophrenic Patients*, London, O.U.P. (to be published).
BROWN, G. W., MONCK, E. M., CARSTAIRS, G. M. and WING, J. K. (1962), The influence of family life on the course of schizophrenic illness, *Brit. J. Prev. Soc. Med.* **16**, 55.
CAMERON, N. and MAGARET, A. (1951), *Behaviour Pathology*, New York.
CARSTAIRS, G. M., O'CONNOR, N. and RAWNSLEY, K. (1956), The organization of a hospital workshop for chronic psychotic patients, *Brit. J. Prev. Soc. Med.* **10**, 136.
CATTERSON, A. G., BENNETT, D. H. and FREUDENBERG, R. K. (1963), A survey of long-stay schizophrenic patients, *Brit. J. Psychiat.* **109**, 750.
CLARK, D. H. (1964), *Administrative Therapy*, London, Tavistock.
CLARK, D. H., HOOPER, D. F. and ORAM, E. G. (1962), Creating a therapeutic community in a psychiatric ward, *Human Relations*, **15**, 123.
CONOLLY, J. (1856), *The Treatment of the Insane without Mechanical Restraints*, London.
DEUTSCH, A. (1949), *The Mentally Ill in America*, New York, Columbia Univ. Press.
DUNHAM, H. W. and WEINBERG, S. K. (1960), *The Culture of the State Mental Hospital*, Detroit, Wayne State Univ. Press.
EARLY, D. F. (1960), The Industrial Therapy Organization (Bristol): A development of work in hospital, *Lancet*, **ii**, 754.
EARLY, D. F. (1963), The Industrial Therapy Organization (Bristol): The first two years, *Lancet*, **i**, 435.

EARLY, D. F. (1965), Domestic Resettlement, and Industrial Resettlement. Chapters in *Psychiatric Hospital Care* (ed. Freeman, H. L.), London, Bailliere, Tindall & Cassell.

ETZIONI, A. (1960), Interpersonal and structural factors in the study of mental hospitals, *Psychiat.* **23**, 13.

FEINTUCH, A. (1955), Improving the employability and attitudes of "difficult-to-place" persons, *Psychol. Monogr. Gen. and Appl.* **69**, No. 7.

FOULDS, G. A. and DIXON, PENELOPE (1962), The nature of intellectual deficit in schizophrenia, *Brit. J. Soc. Clin. Psychol.* **1**, 199.

FOWLER, P. B. S. (1955), The pathology of rehabilitation, *Lancet*, **i**, 467.

FREEMAN, T., CAMERON, J. L. and McGHIE, A. (1958), *Chronic Schizophrenia*, London, Tavistock.

GALIONI, E. F., ADAMS, F. H. and TALLMAN, T. F. (1953), Intensive treatment of backward patients. A controlled pilot study, *Amer. J. Psychiat.* **109**, 576.

GARRATT, F. N., LOWE, C. R. and McKEOWN, T. (1957), Investigation of the medical and social needs of patients in mental hospitals, *Brit. J. Prev. Soc. Med.* **11**, 163.

GOFFMAN, E. (1961), *Asylums*, New York, Anchor Books.

GOLDBERG, E. M. (1960), Parents and psychotic sons, *Brit. J. Psychiat. Soc. Work*, **5**, 2.

GOLDBERG, E. M. and MORRISON, S. L. (1963), Schizophrenia and social class, *Brit. J. Psychiat*, **109**, 785.

GOLDBERG, S. C., KLERMAN, G. L. and COLE, J. O. (1965), Changes in schizophrenic psychopathology and ward behaviour as a function of phenothiazine treatment, *Brit. J. Psychiat.* **111**, 120.

GUTTMAN, E., MAYER-GROSS, W. and SLATER, E. (1939), Short-distance prognosis of schizophrenia, *J. Neurol. Psychiat.* **2**, 1.

HARRIS, A., NORRIS, V., LINKER, I. and SHEPHERD, M. (1956), Schizophrenia: a prognostic and social study, *Brit. J. Prev. Soc. Med.* **10**, 107.

HEWITT, M. (1949), The unemployed disabled man, *Lancet*, **ii**, 523.

HOENIG, J. and HAMILTON, MARIAN (1965), Extramural care of psychiatric patients, *Lancet*, **i**, 1322.

HOOPER, D. (1962), Changing the milieu in a psychiatric ward, *Human Relations*, **15**, 111.

HUNT, J. McV. (1936), Psychological experiments with disordered persons, *Psychol. Bull.* **33**, 1.

JONES, D. A. and MILES, H. L. (1964), The Anglesey Mental Health Survey. Chapter in *Problems and Progress in Medical Care* (ed. McLachlan, G., Nuffield Prov. Hosp. Trust), London, O.U.P.

JONES, KATHLEEN (1954), *Lunacy, Law and Conscience, 1744–1845*, London, Routledge.

JONES, KATHLEEN (1960), *Mental Health and Social Policy*, London, Routledge.

JONES, MAXWELL (1952), *Social Psychiatry: A Study of Therapeutic Communities*, London.

JONES, MAXWELL (1962), *Social Psychiatry: In the Community, in Hospitals and in Prisons*, Springfield, Thomas.

JUNG, C. G. (1906), The psychology of dementia praecox (trans. Brill, A. A.), *Nerv. Ment. Dis. Monogr.* 1936.

KELLY, D. and SARGANT, W. (1965), Present treatment of schizophrenia, *Brit. Med. J.* **1**, 147.

KENDIG, I. and RICHMOND, W. V. (1940), *Psychological Studies in Dementia Praecox*, Michigan, Ann Arbor.

LEMKAU, P., TIETZE, C. and COOPER, M. (1943), A survey of the prevalence and incidence of mental disorders in sample populations, *Pub. Health Rep.* **58**, 1909.

MAAS, H. S., VARON, E. and ROSENTHAL, D. (1951), A technique for studying the social behaviour of schizophrenics, *J. Abnorm. Soc. Psychol.* **46**, 119.

MACMILLAN, D. (1958), Hospital–community relationships. In *An Approach to the Prevention of Disability from Chronic Psychoses*, New York, Milbank Mem. Fund.

MACMILLAN, D. (1961), Community mental health services and the mental hospital: The Mapperley Hospital scheme, *World Mental Health*, **13**, 12.

MAIN, T. F. (1946), The hospital as a therapeutic institution, *Bull. Menninger Clin.* **10**, 66.

MARTIN, D. V. (1962), *Adventure in Psychiatry*, Oxford, Cassirer.

MAY, A. R. (1965), Principles underlying community care. In *Psychiatric Hospital Care* (ed. Freeman, H. L.), London, Bailliere, Tindall & Cassell.

MAYER-GROSS, W. (1932), in *Handbuch der Geisteskrankheiten*, **9**, 534 (ed. Bumke, O.), Berlin.
MCKEOWN, T. (1961), The next 40 years in public health, *Millbank Mem. Fund Quarterly*, **39**, 564.
MONCK, E. M. (1963), Employment experiences of 127 discharged schizophrenic men in London, *Brit. J. Prev. Soc. Med.* **17**, 101.
MORGAN, R., CUSHING, D. and MANTON, N. S. (1965), A regional psychiatric rehabilitation hospital, *Brit. J. Psychiat.* **111**, 955.
NATIONAL INSTITUTE OF MENTAL HEALTH—P.S.C. Collaborative Study Group (1964), Phenothiazine treatment in acute schizophrenia, *Arch. Gen. Psychiat.* **10**, 246.
O'CONNOR, N. (1957), Reminiscence and work decrement in catatonic and paranoid schizophrenics, *Brit. J. Med. Psychol.* **30**, 188.
ORAM, E. G. and KNOWLES, M. C. (1964), The Chronically Mentally Ill—Movements in a Rural Area: 1900–1961. Chapter in *Problems and Progress in Medical Care* (ed. McLachlan, G., Nuffield Prov. Hosp. Trust), London, O.U.P.
PARKES, C. M., BROWN, G. W. and MONCK, E. M. (1962), The general practitioner and the schizophrenic patient, *Brit. Med. J.* **i**, 972.
PASAMANICK, B. *et al.* (1964), Home versus hospital care for schizophrenia, *J. Amer. Med. Ass.* **187**, 177.
PETERS, H. N. and JENKINS, R. L. (1954), Improvement of chronic schizophrenic patients with guided problem-solving motivated by hunger, *Psychiat. Quart. Supp.* **28**, 84.
PHILLIPS, J. E., JACOBSON, N. and TURNER, W. J. (1965), Conceptual thinking in schizophrenics and their relatives, *Brit. J. Psychiat.* **111**, 823.
RAWNSLEY, K., LOUDON, J. and MILES, H. L. (1962), The attitudes of relatives of patients in mental hospitals, *Brit. J. Prev. Soc. Med.* **16**, 1.
REES, J. P. (1957), Back to moral treatment, *J. Ment. Sci.* **103**, 303.
RENTON, C. A., FORREST, A. D., AFFLECK, J. W. and CARSTAIRS, G. M. (1963), A follow-up of schizophrenic patients in Edinburgh, *Acta Psychiat.* **39**, 548.
RODNICK, E. H. and SHAKOW, D. (1940), Set in the schizophrenic, as measured by a composite reaction time index, *Amer. J. Psychiat.* **97**, 214.
SAINSBURY, P. and GRAD, JACQUELINE (1962), An Evaluation of Treatment and Services. In *The Burden on the Community: the Epidemiology of Mental Illness. A Symposium*, London.
SCARPITTI, F. R. *et al.* (1964), Problems in a home care study for schizophrenics, *Arch. Gen. Psychiat.* **10**, 143.
SINGER, M. T. and WYNNE, L. C. (1963), Differentiating characteristics of parents of childhood schizophrenics, childhood neurotics and young adult schizophrenics, *Amer. J. Psychiat.* **120**, 234–43.
SMITH, K., PUMPHREY, M. and HALL, J. O. (1963), "The last straw": the decisive incidents resulting in the request for hospitalization in 100 schizophrenic patients, *Amer. J. Psychiat.* **120**, 228.
SOMMER, R. (1959), Patients who grow old in a mental hospital, *Geriatrics*, **14**, 581.
SOMMER, R. and OSMOND, H. (1961), Symptoms of institutional care, *Social Problems*, **8**, 254.
STONE, A. A. and ELDRED, S. H. (1959), Delusion formation during the activation of chronic schizophrenic patients, *Arch. Gen. Psychiat.* **1**, 177.
STRÖMGREN, E. (1938), Beiträge zur psychiatrischen Erblehre, *Acta Psychiat*, Supp. 19.
SYKES, G. M. (1958), *The Society of Captives*, Princeton, Princeton Univ. Press.
TOOTH, G. and BROOKE, EILEEN (1961), Trends in the mental hospital population and their effect on future planning, *Lancet*, **i**, 710.
VENABLES, P. H. (1960), The effect of auditory and visual stimuli on the skin potential response of schizophrenics, *Brain*, **83**, 77.
WADSWORTH, W. V., SCOTT, R. F. and TONGE, W. L. (1958), A hospital workshop, *Lancet*, **ii**, 896.
WARDLE, C. (1962), Social Factors in the Major Functional Psychoses. In *Society: Problems and Methods of Study* (eds. Welford, A.T. *et al.*), London, Routledge.
WATERS, M. A. and NORTHOVER, J. (1965), Rehabilitated long-stay schizophrenics in the community, *Brit. J. Psychiat.* **111**, 258.

WEEKS, K. F. (1965), The Plymouth Nuffield Clinic—a Community Mental Health Centre. In *Psychiatric Hospital Care* (ed. Freeman, H. L.), London, Bailliere, Tindall & Cassell.

WING, J. K. (1960), Pilot experiment on the rehabilitation of long-hospitalized male schizophrenic patients, *Brit. J. Prev. Soc. Med.* **14,** 173.

WING, J. K. (1962), Institutionalism in mental hospitals, *Brit. J. Soc. Clin. Psychol.* **1,** 38.

WING, J. K. (1965), Social and psychological changes in a rehabilitation unit, *Soc. Psychiat.* **1,** 21.

WING, J. K. and BROWN, G. W. (1961), Social treatment of chronic schizophrenia: a comparative survey of three mental hospitals, *J. Ment. Sci.* **107,** 847.

WING, J. K. and FREUDENBERG, R. K. (1961), The response of severely ill chronic schizophrenic patients to social stimulation, *Amer. J. Psychiat.* **118,** 311.

WING, J. K. and GIDDENS, R. G. T. (1959), Industrial rehabilitation of male chronic schizophrenics, *Lancet,* **ii,** 505.

WING, J. K., BENNETT, D. H. and DENHAM, J. (1964), *The Industrial Rehabilitation of Longstay Schizophrenic Patients,* Medical Research Council, Report No. 42, London, H.M.S.O.

WING, J. K., MONCK, ELIZABETH, BROWN, G. W. and CARSTAIRS, G. M. (1964), Morbidity in the community of schizophrenic patients discharged from London mental hospitals in 1959, *Brit. J. Psychiat.* **110,** 10.

WING, LORNA (1956), The use of reserpine in chronic psychotic patients: a controlled trial, *J. Ment. Sci.* **102,** 530.

WING, LORNA and WING, J. K. (1965), The Camberwell Psychiatric Diseases Register. Unpublished document.

YTREHUS, A. (1959), Environmental therapy of chronic schizophrenic patients, *Acta Psychiat. Neurol.* **34,** 126.

2. The Families of Schizophrenic Patients

E. M. GOLDBERG

Introduction

While a study of schizophrenia and social class was in progress (Goldberg and Morrison, 1963) among young male patients, their frequent re-admissions to hospital and the difficulties of caring for them in the community became very obvious. The impression was gained that the patients' living conditions and especially their family environment played an important part in their recurring difficulties. Although serious disturbances in the patient's social relationships were often clearly revealed during his stay in hospital, yet on his discharge he had to face the self-same problems and stressful relationships with very little support from either doctors or social workers. It was decided to investigate these problems further and a systematic follow-up study was carried out.

Some findings from this follow-up study were reported in a previous paper (Goldberg, 1966). Home circumstances were found to be related to the amount of time the patient spent in hospital as well as to the frequency of his re-admissions. The more unfavourable the home was, in terms of family relationships and the presence of mental disturbance in other members of the family, the longer the stay in hospital and the more often were patients re-admitted.

It also emerged that patients who went home to their parents on discharge had a poorer work record than those who went to other kin or into lodgings. Patients who returned to families in which relationships were disturbed, and in which other relatives were mentally ill, had a poorer work record than those who returned to well-functioning families which were free from mental illness.

In this paper, the family environment and its effect on these patients is described in greater detail. Ways in which social workers can be of help in the varying family situations are explored and some tentative suggestions are made about how the medical and social services might be organized to deal more effectively with the needs of these patients and their families.

Other Family Studies

Many family studies of schizophrenic patients and their families have been carried out or are in progress both in the United States and in this country. They are mainly of two kinds. First, there are studies based on prolonged and intensive observation or treatment of comparatively small samples of families. The investigators use psychoanalytical concepts, as well as sociological notions about social roles, means of communication and cultural prescriptions of the society in which the family functions. Bateson *et al.* (1956), Laing and Esterson (1964), Lidz and Fleck (1960), Jackson and Weakland (1961), Wynne *et al.* (1958) belong to this group. Although each uses idiosyncratic language and concepts, the basic findings of these investigators are similar; in brief, they are as follows.

The personalities of both parents are usually considered to be severely disturbed, their marriages are beset by chronic strife, or, if peaceful, are maintained at the expense of the children. The ties between parents and children are of a pathological nature and the "generation barriers" are often violated, one parent either competing with the child for the spouse's attention or establishing a special bond with the child at the expense of the spouse. The close ties between parent and child often lead to an intensification of oedipal rivalries, rather than to their resolution. The schizophrenic patient is said to be confronted by insurmountable problems of sexual and social identification (Fleck *et al.*, 1959).

The pattern of communication in these families is described as one of irrationality and contradiction, the most famous formulation being Bateson's "double-bind" hypothesis (Bateson *et al.*, 1956). This attempts to explain the schizophrenic's reaction in terms of communication theory. The double-bind characterizes a special type of relationship, from which the growing child cannot escape. The child is subjected to contradictory messages that require him to deny important aspects of himself and his experience. Such a communication is the command, "I order you to disobey me". Clearly, this command cannot be obeyed without violating one or another part of the statement. The dilemma is extreme when the child expects punishment to follow either choice, and especially when there is a third negative injunction which prohibits him from escaping from the situation. Such a system of communication, it is suggested, may lead to schizophrenic behaviour in the double-bound individual. His only escape is to strip his own messages of meaning, thus preventing the other person from understanding his response. This may eventually lead to an inability to discriminate the true meaning of one's own or others' communications.

It is also suggested that the irrational family patterns help to isolate these families culturally, if only because so much energy is bound up in the emotional involvements inside the family.

Most of the investigators mentioned regard the social and psychological factors as the primary cause of the disease. They all believe strongly in the possibilities of psychotherapeutic treatment of the family, and research usually includes therapeutic experiments.

Currently, several groups of research workers, both in the U.S.A. and in Great Britain, are trying to test hypotheses about the processes of social interaction prevailing in families containing schizophrenic patients by means of standardized psychological procedures. (For example, see Wynne and Singer, 1963.)

The second group of studies, in particular those of Brown *et al.* (1962) in this country and Freeman and Simmons (1963) in the U.S.A., are based on larger samples of patients than the studies just mentioned and include a wide age-range. The investigators are not primarily concerned with aetiology and experiments in treatment, but aim at an accurate observation of the nature of the interaction between the patient and his environment. Their approach differs from that of the first group. Clearly stated hypotheses were tested, by comparing the outcome after 1 year in the community with predictions based on observations of family attitudes at the point of discharge. Although these researchers do not use psychoanalytical concepts or communication theory, they also find certain pathological relationships and attitudes within the family which are significantly related to the exacerbation of illness in the patient. Brown *et al.* (1962) call this constellation "high emotional involvement between the key relative and the patient". Freeman and Simmons similarly find some association between deterioration of the patient and unfavourable family attitudes. The family situations to be discussed in this paper largely confirm the findings of both groups of investigators.

Background of Present Study

The data presented here are part of a study of 101 men under 30, who were admitted consecutively to a mental hospital on the eastern outskirts of London between January 1958 and December 1960, and whose discharges took place between April 1958 and September 1961. These patients, therefore, were at risk for varying periods, which has obvious disadvantages when trying to estimate outcome. On the other hand, it was possible to follow the progress of a representative series of patients from admission, through varying periods of 1–4 years, the mean length being 2 years and 8 months.*

* It was actually shown in a previous paper (Goldberg, 1966) that the differences in the patients' adjustments were not a function of the varying periods of observation.

THE SAMPLE

The study was confined to males under the age of 30. Foreign-born and Irish patients whose families resided in Eire, epileptics, and severely subnormal patients were excluded. (For further details of sampling and diagnostic criteria, see Goldberg and Morrison, 1963.)

DIAGNOSIS

The psychiatrist at the hospital classified the patients as "definitely schizophrenic" (S), "possibly schizophrenic" (PS), or "definitely not schizophrenic" (NS).

The NS group included various types of anxiety state and behaviour disorder. For the purposes of this paper, I shall only consider the "definitely schizophrenic" patients (52) and the "not schizophrenic" patients (33), leaving out the 16 "possibly schizophrenic" patients.

AGE AND CIVIL STATE

The average age of the S patients* on entry to the sample—the "key admission"—was somewhat higher than those of the NS patients (Table 1).

TABLE 1.

Sample of Consecutive Male Admissions to a District Mental Hospital.
Age Distribution by Diagnosis (January 1958–December 1960)

Age	Schizophrenic Patients	Not Schizophrenic Patients	Total
15–19	4	9	13
20–24	14	16	30
25–29	34	8	42
Total	52	33	85
Mean age (years)	25	22	24

This is largely explained by the fact that less than half the S patients were first admissions, while about two-thirds of the NS patients were first admissions (Table 2).

* The mean age of S patients whose key admission was their first ever was 23.

TABLE 2.

*Number of Admissions to a Mental
Hospital before "Key Admission"*[a]

Previous Admissions	S Patients	NS Patients
0	23	23
1	12	7
2	7	1
3+	10	2
Total	52	33

[a] Key admission = the first admission
observed on entry to the study.

Only one of the S patients and five of the NS patients were married on admission to hospital. All the others were single.

RESIDENCE AND SOCIAL CLASS

About half the patients lived in a working-class county borough, adjoining metropolitan East London and the Docks, and about half lived in a thriving, rapidly developing suburb in an eastern home county. The schizophrenic patients showed the well-known preponderance of unskilled and semi-skilled labourers in the Registrar General's Social Classes IV and V, compared with the average for young men of their age living in the Greater London area. Their fathers had a more balanced class distribution, as had the NS patients and their families. Most of the patients thus came from "ordinary" homes, in respect of the occupational status of the head of the household (Goldberg and Morrison, 1963).

SOCIO-ECONOMIC CIRCUMSTANCES

The majority of patients lived with their parents in reasonable material circumstances. None of the parental families had housing problems. Three NS married men experienced acute housing difficulties. Economic hardship was clearly evident in about one-fifth of the S families. Two widows were too unstable to go out to work and a third was too old. Their sons remained virtually unemployable. One family, in which all members were mentally unstable and unable to earn a regular living, was in serious and chronic financial difficulties. In another family the irregular income of the parents, who were artists, had to provide for two mentally ill sons and a student son.

At least five unemployed S patients proved a drain on their families' slender resources. Two of these patients refused to apply for any kind of assistance. The economic situation was very different in the NS group, since most patients were able to work on discharge. Only two psychopaths with young families got into serious debt.

Method of Follow-up

Soon after admission, the parents of all the patients in the sample were visited at least twice. Both fathers and mothers were seen. A very detailed social history was obtained and family relationships were explored and, as far as possible, observed. In addition to the information gathered in interviews, school reports were obtained.

The follow-up inquiry was directed to parents or other key relatives. This clearly is not the best way of carrying out a follow-up study, which should include the patients themselves as well as their relatives. However, since the original contact had been mainly with the parents, it was advisable to continue the investigation in the same manner. Follow-up visits were paid, irrespective of whether the patients were in or out of hospital. It was left to the discretion of the parents to tell the patient of the visit. Many parents of patients who were well and working felt that it was best not to mention the visit and these patients were not seen as a rule. Most patients who were not well and not at work were seen either at home, if discharged, or in the hospital. During the visit, the patient's mental state, his work, leisure activities and social relationships were discussed. The attitudes of the relatives were explored and often observed. Questions were asked about the kind of help patients had received after discharge—whether they had attended out-patient clinics, how often they had seen their general practitioners, or whether they had been in touch with the local authority's mental health service. Later checks were made with the psychiatric social workers at the hospital, the mental welfare officers of the local authority health departments, the out-patient clinics, and the disablement resettlement officers, to ascertain how much contact these various agencies had actually had with the patient.

Refusals

Out of the 85 cases, there were two outright refusals to co-operate. These two parents, with whom close contact had been established on their sons' admission to hospital and who had then talked freely and extensively, wrote saying that their sons were doing well and they did not wish to be reminded of the painful episode. In both cases, confirmatory evidence about the patients' well-being was obtained from the general practitioner. Three parents whose sons had been in hospital throughout the survey period kept postponing the interviews, though long telephone conversations were held with two of them. In these cases, a good deal of information about the patients and their relationships with their parents was available from the hospital. Thus, the five refusals were of two kinds: those whose sons were doing well and who preferred to "forget", and those whose sons continued to be very ill and who presumably could not face further discussion of a seemingly hopeless situation.

Settled Patients living with Parents

A "settled" patient was relatively free from symptoms at follow-up and was able to work consistently. The few schizophrenic patients (6) who were able to work regularly and to adjust reasonably well to their families lived in homes bearing few of the stresses which are often associated with mental ill-health. In these families, members seemed comfortable in their social roles, which appeared to meet their emotional and intellectual needs. For example, the fathers liked their work; the parents' marriage was functioning reasonably well and neither had to turn to their children in order to fulfil frustrated needs, either by keeping the children excessively dependent on them or by pushing them beyond what they could reasonably achieve. Several of the fathers helped their sons in their search for and adjustment to work. The mothers, though they did worry about their sons' illness which was never far from their minds, tried not to show their feelings openly to the patient, because they knew that the patients would react badly to any open display of anxiety.

Although some of the fathers had moved up the social scale and their sons had not fulfilled the expectations of their early successes at school, the fathers, secure in their own careers, managed not to betray openly any disappointment or disparagement. They were content and approving if the patients could find a niche that suited them at all. Married siblings were in close contact with the family and took a lively interest in the patients. This helped to spread the load and enabled the patients to have some social contacts outside their parental home. These well-adjusted and supportive families were able to face reality rather than to deny it, and so they encouraged the patient to seek treatment when a further attack threatened. Finally, these families were able to make remarkably constructive use of any insights they gained from discussions they had had with the investigator.

All these points are illustrated in the following example. S 3 had been a clerk ever since leaving grammar school. The only boy among three children, he had always been rather close to his mother. The father gave the impression of being a thoughtful, intelligent and somewhat anxious man, who was overshadowed by his very lively and articulate wife. In the course of the talks, he realized how distant his relationship with his son had been and how little they communicated with each other. The parents also discussed what the father called the mother's overprotectiveness towards her son, without acrimony. Observing them together, their affection and consideration for each other became very clear. They reviewed with evident pleasure some aspects of their past lives; for instance, their courtship and their work together, as the mother had often helped the father in his business. They both searched for deficiencies in their attitudes and personalities which might be related to their son's illness, for example the mother's intensity and the father's self-consciousness and shyness, but they did not show a disproportionate amount of self-blame. All these strands were woven into a searching and fruitful discussion of the assets and difficulties in their family life.

On the follow-up visit 3 years later, the father told the investigator that as a result of looking at his relationship with his son, he had seen the "red light" and had made it his business to move closer to him and share more of his leisure time with him. They worked together on the family car and on the boy's motor bike. They had gone on fishing trips together. The patient, it seemed, was greatly helped not only by the closer companionship with his father but also by his relationship with his married sisters and their husbands, who invited him out and provided the only social contacts this young man was able to maintain outside his parental home. As regards work, on his return home this patient refused his old firm's offer of a travelling job and spent approximately 6 months at home doing nothing. He was in touch with the disabled resettlement officer and was eventually accepted for an industrial rehabilitation unit. While waiting for a vacancy, he started a labouring job but shortly afterwards he became ill again. His family urged him to seek treatment without delay and he made a better recovery after the second admission than after the first episode. Following his discharge, he was able to start the training course which he completed successfully. He was placed in a suitable job as a radio repairer at which he was doing well when inquiries were last made.

Unsettled Schizophrenic Patients living with Parents

"Unsettled patients" were unable to work regularly and/or continued to show serious symptoms. In considering the family organization and emotional interaction in the families of patients who remained unsettled and ill, one has to remember the social situation in which the parents found themselves. Most of these schizophrenic patients, though they were on average 25 years of age, were unable to fulfil the two crucial adult roles, those of worker and husband. Thus, in social terms, they remained dependent children.

The parents' response to this abnormal social situation appeared to cluster around two extremes; some adopted attitudes that would have been appropriate to the care of much younger children. That is to say, they became excessively protective; others reacted with hostility and rejected the patient, partly because he had frustrated their expectations and partly because he possibly reflected in some measure their own failure as parents. Neither of these parental attitudes was helpful to the patient. At times, people concerned with the treatment and rehabilitation of these patients tended to blame the unhelpful parental attitudes for the patient's continuing illness. While this may have been true in some respects, it is possible that the very unhelpful responses and internal dissents which appear to be associated with the inactive and unrecovered schizophrenic patient may have resulted from or been aggravated by the abnormal role the patient was occupying in the home.

Four groupings were apparent among the families whose schizophrenic sons showed considerable mental disturbance at follow-up, or who had not left hospital at all. These constellations can be described in psychoanalytical terms as different variants of oedipal conflicts.

PROTECTIVE MOTHERS (GROUP I)

The first family constellation that stood out clearly was one in which the mother was very protective and kept the patient closely dependent and helpless. There were five such patients. The father was excluded from the care of the patient. If the father attempted to encourage the patient towards greater activity and independence, the mother regarded him as hostile and cruel. The mother's closeness and preoccupation with the patient was usually associated with a very disturbed marital relationship.

The problems posed by these families depended on the intensity of the involvement between mother and son, the degree of the mother's own disturbance, the nature of the marital relationship and the severity of the patient's illness.

In the following example, the pathology on all these four counts was severe. S 46, a young schizophrenic of 22, discharged himself after 2 years in hospital following a row with a staff nurse. He had improved very little in hospital, but he was up and dressed and had been induced to join in the group activities of his ward. On his return home, he spent most of his time in bed doing nothing. He was confused, deluded and restless on follow-up. Once a week, his parents managed to get him to the general practitioner's surgery, where he obtained his insurance certificate and drugs, which he often did not take. The family situation was typical in general outline for this group of families. The mother had always had a very close possessive relationship with the patient, her only son among girls. This close contact was enhanced by the father's absence on war service throughout the patient's early childhood. Later, the mother found it easy to exclude the father and she never allowed him to come near to his son. When the patient broke down periodically, the mother blamed the father's lack of interest and hostility for the patient's illness, while the father blamed the mother's over-protectiveness for the final disaster. In this particular family, the mother accused the father of not taking any interest in his children, of begrudging them decent clothing, of being an incompetent worker, bringing in so little money that she had to go out to work to keep the family going, and of being spiteful and jealous towards the patient. She continually provoked the father with her accusations, which often resulted in a physical assault on her. The father's main complaint was that his wife had ruined his little business by helping herself to money whenever she felt like it, that she had always put the children first, and had put them against him from the very start so that he never had a chance. The mother freely acknowledged her spending tendencies, her desire to have the son close to her, and the satisfaction she derived from tending and feeding him, going up to his room in the evenings to read to him, and so on. She undermined any attempt by the father to encourage the patient to get up and have his meals with the family, accusing him of lack of understanding and cruelty. The father, a mild and reasonable man, resented the close involvement between mother and son, and felt completely excluded and powerless in the situation. Though intelligent, he had failed twice in business and was a railway porter at the age of 50 (it is significant that in the Army he rose quickly to the rank of Sergeant). The patient, who occasionally appeared during the investigator's visits, was confused, vague and deluded, but was well able to take in what was going on around him and to perceive the investigator's role. He had woven the visits into a phantasy of a nurse who visited his home, went up to his room, talked to him and then to his parents and made everybody feel happy. He described his feelings of not being able to function sexually, his search for maternal comfort and his despair at being cut off from other human beings in vivid, rather primitive and symbolic terms. He would point to his cigarette: "This is my comfort, my Mum". He would talk about the difficulty of "getting the parts to work again". These comments were unintelligible to his parents, until translated by the investigator.

CRITICAL AND AMBIVALENT MOTHERS (GROUP II)

There was a second cluster of eight families in which the mothers also kept the patient under close control, yet at the same time pushed him towards social achievements. The maternal attitudes were openly ambivalent and critical. The father was often benign and friendly to the patient, but was pushed aside by the mother. The mother responded to the patient's incapacity with ill-concealed disappointment, at times driving him towards performances which were almost beyond him. This was in contrast to the mothers of the first group, who went to the other extreme of making babies of their ill children. These families contained deep divisions, and in several the mother had formed a strong bond with another son who seemed to occupy the role of the leader in the home, displacing the father.

A clear example of a family situation of this kind is family S 10. This 27-year-old instrument maker had had three previous admissions and was able to return to a semi-skilled job after his key admission. After a further breakdown, he became a lorry driver's mate. The family described how the mother wore herself out looking after the patient. She got him up at 5 every morning, and if he ever felt like having a day off she insisted on his going to work. She felt that she was contributing towards his cure in many ways: she ensured that he took his tablets (stelazine); she "worked with the psychiatrist" by sending him reports before the patient's attendance at the out-patient clinic; she arranged and despatched the patient on a Butlin's holiday and so on. She maintained a permanent threat that if the patient returned to hospital, the family would not visit him or receive him back home again. The patient continued to work throughout the survey period, although he eventually returned to hospital a few months after the survey period ended.

In this family, the mother wore the trousers. The father said: "If mother says 'yes' it's yes, and if she says 'no' it's no, whatever my opinion may be." This marriage seemed to function tolerably well. He accepted his wife's drive and dominance and she appreciated the father's steadiness—he had been working as a docker for over 30 years. The patient, according to the father, "worships the ground his mother walks on", but when he had his spasms he "wants to kill her". His mother added: "He will do me in eventually." There were many stories of the patient attacking his mother, who usually appealed to the police, who in turn called in the mental welfare officer. The mother was very critical of the patient and his achievements. The father, a thoughtful man with depressive tendencies, used to stress the patient's good as well as his bad points. He considered himself the "labourer" in the family, and he saw the mother as the central figure to whom all three sons were devoted. Yet to the outside observer, the father appeared to be the important balancing force in the family. He gave the impression of being more rational than the mother and of having considerable psychological insight. For example, he thought that his wife's driving and ambitious attitude was a reaction to her deprived childhood. It was also noticeable that the patient never got out of control when the father was about. Although the mother reported that the father "bullied" the patient, this bullying seemed in the nature of quietening him down when he became upset and demanding. The patient's younger brother was clearly the mother's favourite. His achievements were highly commended. He was deeply attached to his mother and did not intend to get married for a long time; he was reported to have said: "If I get anybody like my mum, I'll be lucky." The patient led an isolated existence within the family. For instance, he never joined their decorating or gardening activities, and whenever he did attempt to do some weeding or carpentry, things went wrong.

The balance of forces which determined the functioning of this family was precarious. But the patient was able to hang on at work (probably because of his mother's insistence) until a crisis occurred, which occasionally was serious enough to warrant admission to hospital.

Hostile and Rejecting Fathers (Group III)

In a third group of six families, the conflicts centred round the father's rejection of the sick son and his hostility towards him. These paternal attitudes contained a complex mixture of disappointment and disparagement, particularly regarding the son's sexual inadequacy. The fathers also felt very jealous and competitive in relation to the son's attachment to their mothers. These fathers showed open preference for other children. In several of these families, the father was vocationally very ambitious and successful, and scathing about the schizophrenic son's lack of achievement. The father's competence and success seemed to push the patient further into inactivity. The sons, while at home with their fathers, seemed unable to contemplate work. In several families, jealousy and rivalry over the mother were barely concealed. For example, one patient arrived home one night accusing the father of not looking after his mother properly: "I'm going to look after my mum, whether you like it or not." Another patient, while talking with bitter irony about his father's achievements and handiwork at home, said, "But ah, he keeps the secrets to himself, he doesn't let one in on the act." In another family, the conflict was played out almost entirely over an old car which belonged to the patient, but which he was unable to repair without the father's help. The father told the investigator several times with great satisfaction, "You see the trouble is I can make things go; he can't."

While, in the families in Group I, the mothers openly opposed the fathers and were grossly overprotective towards their sons, in this group the fathers ruled the roost and the mothers, though feeling sympathy for the patient, were torn between their loyalties to son and to husband. In some cases, the only solution appeared to be for the patient to leave home. This was successfully accomplished in two instances. (One of them, S 27, is described on page 46.) In other cases, this solution was difficult to achieve, since there were no hostels or half-way houses in the area, and the patients were not ready to fend for themselves in lodgings. For example, S 45, a gifted music student, had never formed a good relationship with his father, who had been away for 5 years in the boy's childhood. He was a restless, striving man, suffering with chronic asthma. He had been very successful in his work and was now in a managerial job, doing accountancy jobs in his spare time.

This father had high standards for his children. The patient had never come up to his expectations and he had no sympathy whatever for his son's musical ability. He even interpreted the serious schizophrenic symptoms as an attempt to put on bohemian airs, like French artists do! All this father's hopes were now centred on the younger boy. The follow-up visit took place while the patient was in hospital. By then, after several years of recurrent disturbance, the father had made up his mind that the patient would have to find lodgings on his discharge, the ostensible reason being that he had terrified his mother before his last admission. The father felt very uneasy about this decision, and wondered aloud what the investigator would think of him for rejecting his son so completely.

ISOLATED MOTHERS AND SONS (GROUP IV)

Fourthly, one could clearly distinguish a group of widows (10) who lived alone with their sick sons and became deeply involved in their illness. These widows had no other close personal relationships, although six of them were full-time workers. The emotional involvement inherent in such a relationship, as well as the responsibility it may entail for the son, is difficult for the schizophrenic patient to contend with, as the following example shows.

S 28 was an only child who lost his father at the age of 16. He and his father had been close companions, sharing an interest in music and fishing. The son was then left with his widowed mother who had always been the disciplinarian in the family, ambitious, perfectionist and extremely capable. She had lost an outstandingly able husband with whom she had been very happy. She then pinned her hopes on her son's achievements, which were not forthcoming. The son felt oppressed by his responsibilities, dissatisfied with his achievements, and resentful of his and his mother's mutual dependence on each other. He was artistic and musical, whereas his mother was rather prosaic and practical, unable to share his interests as his father had done. He developed schizophrenia at the age of 19. He always tended to defy his mother, and now he showed strong hostility towards her and exasperation with her lack of understanding. "She feeds the stomach alright, but oh blimey, the mind—that does not exist." After a period in hospital he was discharged home, but soon was at loggerheads with his mother. He left home, could not maintain himself, came back and became physically violent towards his mother, who was very frightened of him, and so he returned to hospital. This time he stayed for over 2 years and started work from hospital in a rather uncongenial labouring job. Eventually, both he and his mother decided to try again, especially as she only lived a stone's throw from the hospital in a comfortable house. When last seen, 8 months after his discharge, the patient was still in the same job, but hanging on by a thin thread. His mother continued to be disappointed in him, complaining bitterly about his behaviour, always stressing the negative aspects, unable to see anything encouraging in her son's activities. Yet there were some hopeful signs. He was able to mix better socially and to ride difficult situations at work, and he had developed an interesting hobby which brought him into contact with other young people. But already his mother began to talk once more about attacks on her. It almost seemed as though she needed to goad her son into madness, since he could not be the sort of companion she would have liked him to be. A vicious circle was operating. A competent, efficient and lonely middle-aged widow, missing her husband badly, had fastened onto her son as a substitute who could not fulfil her hopes. The son, an immature dreamer, struggling with psychotic tendencies which were continually threatening his hold on reality, seemed to need an understanding, undemanding companion who could tolerate his immaturity and eccentricity, appreciate his modest achievements, sympathize with his artistic yet unrealistic dreams and ignore, as far as possible, his oddities. His mother could not fulfil these needs and occasionally in despair he said to her, "Can't you *feel* this?", and she would turn to the investigator in puzzlement: "I think he should get a tonic from the doctor, don't you?". These incompatible needs may well lead to renewed breakdowns.

In two instances the mothers were as disturbed as the patients, and it was difficult to know how to approach the problems of the sick couple. S 52 was the only child of a psychotic mother who had many delusions but was able to exist in the community. She worked occasionally, but mostly lived on National Assistance. The father had died when the patient was 7, and there was a long history of disturbed behaviour at school and at work. He was one of the patients who was in hospital throughout the survey period. He had been very hostile towards his mother for a long time and had destroyed much of her furniture. She continued to visit him in hospital and attended all the socials, trying to keep up a bright appearance. She discussed the possibility of treatment for herself, but felt that she did not wish to be treated separately: "I don't want to get well at the expense of Fred because he needs me, and he would not find another woman in the world who would be prepared to fall in with him." Is it possible, therefore, to keep them together? What would happen if she were to be admitted to the same mental hospital? Would it be right to deprive her of her precarious independence? Or should one leave well alone? For this patient's mother lived near the hospital, and was in touch with the kindly and understanding staff. The patient was in a very active ward and could go home for weekends if he wanted to. At first, it seemed evident to me that this mother needed active treatment, but as the years went by without her becoming appreciably worse, I began to question the wisdom of this. On the other hand, it is likely that she and her son will continue to reinforce each other's illness, unless the vicious circle is broken.

FAMILIES IN WHICH ALL MEMBERS ARE INVOLVED IN A PSYCHOTIC ILLNESS

Lastly, several patients and their families did not fit into any of these four constellations. In some instances, the investigator did not achieve a clear enough understanding of the nature of the family interaction. In other families, members were so sick and abnormal that no pattern emerged except that of chaotic relationships.

In the S 34 family, all the members were enveloped in a psychotic illness. The father, once a steady master plumber, was suffering from schizophrenia and complained about many delusions, which tortured him. He went into hospital for short periods, but usually discharged himself before he was well. His wife was a diabetic and a fierce adherent of the Plymouth Brethren. She tried to defend her religious beliefs, which he attacked. He, on the other hand, wanted her to share his delusions which she ridiculed. However, she was developing some strange beliefs herself. For example, she wondered whether she was pregnant, although she said she had not had any intercourse for 8 years. The patient developed a schizophrenic illness at the age of 24 and improved in hospital, whence he obtained a job. When he returned home, his father actively discouraged him from working and tried to draw him into his paranoid beliefs about the staff at the factory. A younger sister was very unstable, and hardly ever at work. She was said to share some of her father's delusions, and admission to a mental hospital had been arranged for her, but she only stayed for a few days. The family were living in a very dilapidated house in oppressive squalor. The curtains in the living room were drawn permanently. Debts were piling up, partly because of their very inadequate income and partly because they were quite unable to budget in a rational way. They were continually on the verge of eviction. Various social workers had attempted to give some help, but all of them were eventually beaten by the magnitude of the problems. The son, after return from the hospital, struggled to maintain a normal existence, but eventually succumbed to the abnormal environment, gave up work and was re-admitted to hospital in due course. Would it be better, one wondered, for this family to cease to exist as a unit, so as to give the son and daughter a chance of rehabilitation in a more wholesome environment?

Disturbed Families in the Not-schizophrenic Group

The interesting question arises whether similar patterns of family pathology were observed in the not-schizophrenic group. The not-schizophrenic patients showed considerable differences from the schizophrenic group in their adaptation to difficult family situations which seemed less stifling and more openly disrupted. The patients did not appear to be as vulnerable to disturbed relationships within the family. In three families, the young men were surviving fairly successfully, despite very disrupted parental marriages which led to continual unhappy strife. Two other patients were progressing well despite very hostile parental attitudes to them. Another boy, on the borders of subnormality, who had been seriously at odds with his divorced mother before his admission to hospital, returned to her after discharge. They both went out to work and lived peacably together, making few demands on each other. The young man became engaged during the survey period, with the delighted approval of his mother. Another patient, who had been badly disabled and concussed after a motor cycle accident, lived with a somewhat simple widowed father and a severely subnormal sister. He made remarkable strides in this unstimulating environment, overcoming severe physical and mental handicaps with great persistence. Indeed, the accident and his subsequent fight against his disability brought out his potential strength. He developed a much more responsible attitude towards his work and life in general than he had before his accident. In short, these not-schizophrenic patients seemed to have sufficient ego strength to cope with their unfavourable environments and to grow and mature. This was especially noticeable in the young men who were able to make a good and steady relationship with a girl. These adaptations were, however, achieved at considerable cost. Some of these patients described vividly the difficulties and anxieties they were facing. It seemed that they could have used some psychotherapeutic help to great advantage.

The family situation of the only two not-schizophrenic patients who were unable to work at all or make any kind of social adjustment is similar to that of the families of disturbed schizophrenic patients. One patient, suffering from the after-effects of a severe head injury, was the brother of S 47, whose family circumstances are discussed on page 52. There were indications that he was unstable before the accident. The other not-schizophrenic patient who made no progress at all showed many schizoid features. He described sensations which suggested a loss of reality sense and feelings of depersonalization. He had become a drug addict, mainly in order to ward off these strange feelings. His difficulties went back to his school days, and his family circumstances reminded one of the constellations found in schizophrenic families. His mother was a seductive, somewhat hysterical woman, self-centred, ambivalent and very intrusive towards the patient. She was closely attached to another son, who remained single until his middle thirties. His father seemed a well-meaning but limited man with little drive or imagination, who had not been able to make a close link with the patient and was deeply attached to his eldest daughter. The patient lived in his bedroom, where he took his meals and hardly ever talked to any member of the family. Yet he poured out his problems in a vivid articulate way to the investigator. He was re-admitted to hospital twice, on one occasion after a serious attempt at suicide. He never stayed long enough to gain any lasting benefit and his problems have remained insoluble.

PATIENTS LIVING WITH WIVES

It was reported in a previous paper that schizophrenic patients who were married or lived in lodgings made a better social adjustment than those living with their parents (Goldberg, 1966). A more detailed exploration of their social situations throws some light on how these adjustments were achieved. Only two patients in the S group went to live with wives and both their stories seem to point to similar problems. Both came from homes in which the parents lived in constant strife and where the patient had been close to his mother. One patient (S 39) became ill suddenly, on the day his wife produced twins. He made a good recovery, went straight back to his work as a carpenter and kept well for 3 years, during which time two more children were born. His mature, intelligent young wife managed everything, and shielded him from as much strain and responsibility as was possible. He hardly took any notice of or responsibility for the children. Indeed, he was in active competition with them. When the twins were being toilet-trained, he became incontinent, clearly wanting his wife to tell him when to go to the lavatory. He relapsed at a time when the youngest boy claimed an inordinate amount of attention, refusing to be in any way separated from his mother. The patient eventually recovered again, but he returned to his parents and a divorce is in progress.

The second patient (S 26) married about a year after discharge. He did not work on his return home to his deeply divided parents. His mother, practically immobilized by religious doubts and guilt, was heading for a severe depressive breakdown. Soon after her admission to a mental hospital, he began to work. He continued to do so after his marriage, although a clerical job proved too much for him and he became a lorry driver's mate. His young wife, a strong-minded devoted person, had held to him right through his illness, while she was still a student. By the time they married, she had qualified as a social worker and was the main wage-earner. There were no children when the survey ended.

Both these patients who had very severe illnesses worked while living with their wives. This seemed to support the suggestions made by Simmons and Freeman (1959) that spouses have higher expectations than parents and that the performances of married schizophrenic patients are correspondingly better than those of single patients. Similarly, Renton et al. (1963) found that only 1 of their 33 unemployed patients lived with a spouse. However, in the two cases quoted above, the patient's social adjustment seemed to depend on the ability of the wife to be reasonably independent and to function as a mother figure, rather than as a wife who needed to be supported, and as long as children did not compete with the patient's dependent needs.

Marriage has fulfilled a very different maturing function in the not-schizophrenic group. Six married after discharge from hospital, and ten had steady girlfriends. Several severely neurotic patients and some patients with adolescent behaviour problems have blossomed forth since their marriage, maturing visibly. They became able to face much more responsibility, having freed themselves from an unhealthy and difficult parental environment.

SCHIZOPHRENIC PATIENTS LIVING IN LODGINGS

Five schizophrenic patients went to live in lodgings or small hostels, or went to sea soon after discharge. All five stayed in regular work. The most instructive example was S 27, the son of a professional man, who first became ill at the age of 17 soon after leaving school, and who had been admitted to a mental hospital seven times since. His parents experienced severe marital difficulties in the past. There was a wide emotional and intellectual gulf between the patient and his father, who was a scholar with sophisticated hobbies. He felt ashamed and irritated by his garrulous son, who had sunk to the level of labouring. After his son's seventh admission, the father was near collapse himself and declared that he could not bear to have his son home again. (This situation illustrates clearly the family constellation of Group III.) It seemed likely that the patient's return would result in two psychiatric casualties in the family. When he was better, the patient was encouraged to start work from hospital at a nearby factory. There, he made friends with a work-mate, and after a few months went to lodge with him. In these working-class lodgings, 10 minutes' walk from his parents' home, he did not need to keep up sophisticated middle-class standards. He could go his own way without being prodded by his well-meaning but anxious mother. Yet he was able to remain in close touch with his home. He saw his mother twice a week, and once a week he had dinner with both parents, when the atmosphere was reasonably amicable. This solution seemed to work very well. The patient had been continuously at work for over 2 years when the survey ended; he was also on regular drug therapy (chlorpromazine), but he never saw his doctor, as his mother collected the tablets for him.

Two other schizophrenic patients were clearly escaping from very eccentric and protective mothers (Group I). Both had attended university, and were supported by a group of close and loyal ex-student friends. Both suffered a further breakdown, from which they recovered quickly, returning immediately to their usual occupation. They remained in touch with their parental homes. These young men in lodgings shared certain social characteristics. With one exception, they came from middle-class backgrounds, from families who were socially and geographically mobile. The idea of living away from home, even when not married, was culturally acceptable in these circles and was not necessarily regarded as a complete break with the family. Although four of these five families presented noticeable strains in family relationships, they all contained at least one sympathetic and understanding parent or helpful sibling. These patients were thus not wholly separated from their families, but they were sufficiently far away not to be too disturbed by the emotional tensions and involvements. At the same time, they were able to gain affection, support and friendship from the family circle when required. They still "belonged" somewhere.

In contrast, 4 schizophrenic patients who had gone to relatives in the absence of a real home (7 of the 8 parents were dead) did not do nearly as well. Though they made a good start and worked for some time, they all returned to hospital for long periods. The impression gained was that the relatives did not really want them, and looked after them only from a sense of duty. Hostel life and occasional contacts with the relatives might have been a better solution for these patients.

NOT-SCHIZOPHRENIC PATIENTS LIVING IN LODGINGS

Living in lodgings or going to residential jobs was a "therapeutic" move on the part of the 5 schizophrenic patients, all of whom had intact, though disturbing, home backgrounds. The situation was very different in the not-schizophrenic group. They were in lodgings or residential jobs either because they had no home or were rejected at home. This applied particularly to patients suffering from various forms of behaviour disorder. Although they managed to obtain employment, they changed their jobs frequently and wandered from place to place, remaining unstable and unhappy people. All had long histories of separation from their parents in early childhood, followed by experiences of rejection.

One patient (NS 72) was left in a foster-home as a small baby during the Second World War. His parents later started another family in a different part of the country and did not want to uproot him from his foster-mother. After the death of his foster-mother, the patient lived with other members of the foster-family, who did not really want him. His displacement by a black foster-baby was the last straw. He attempted suicide and was admitted to hospital. After his discharge, he was under the care of a probation officer. He lived in lodgings and hostels, feeling resentful and lonely, drifting in and out of work. He often quarrelled with the other residents; on one occasion, he inflicted grievous bodily harm on an old man and went to prison for 9 months. On leaving prison, he again attempted suicide and after two more admissions to hospital, he succeeded in killing himself. His mother, an intelligent woman, although sorry for her son, had felt unable to offer him a home. She was stretched to capacity doing full-time clerical work and looking after a schizophrenic husband. She had invested all her hopes in her youngest boy. The probation officer had been in touch with the patient for several years, but he felt that he had never been able to reach him, and that he needed more intensive psychiatric help than he could receive in the mental hospital. The hospital had labelled him an "unco-operative patient", since he was hostile and resentful, often creating disturbances on wards and in workshops. There seemed no answer to this young man's feeling of homelessness and rejection, and to his purposeless rebellion, since he always produced a situation in which people were finally driven to reject him.

Another patient (NS 79) was placed in a residential nursery during the Second World War, after his mother and father had separated. He became unstable and unmanageable at a very early age, and graduated through a series of schools for maladjusted children. His mother, who visited him through thick and thin, remarried, and he returned to his parents on leaving school. After 18 months of many changes of job and very unstable provocative behaviour, the mother finally charged him with being beyond control. Psychiatric treatment was recommended and the patient was in and out of the local mental hospital. He displayed odd and bizarre behaviour, which defeated any definite diagnosis. His charming ways enabled him to obtain employment as a shop assistant comparatively easily, but his eccentric behaviour and his pathological lying, combined with sudden depressive attacks, always led him back into the mental hospital as a place of refuge. This patient has remained an insoluble problem, haunting different hospitals. His parents were deeply concerned about him and made serious attempts to help him. Eventually, however, his stepfather, a highly successful business man, refused to have his home disorganized any longer by the continual crises, or to allow his wife to become entirely immersed in the boy's problems.

These parents were happily married, and it was clear that the patient felt the odd one out. He admired and at the same time hated his stepfather, whose success he could never match and who had carried his mother off. His feelings towards his mother were intensely ambivalent and he had blood-curdling fantasies about his natural father, who was said to be a seriously disturbed man. The stepfather was jealous of the mother's concern for her son and repelled by the boy's strange fantasies and behaviour; the mother was torn in her loyalties between her husband and the patient, and felt uneasy about her comfortable and prosperous way of life, while her son wandered from place to place. All three had some insight into their own problems. They had affection for each other, as well as strong negative feelings. However, no one had ever attempted to bring these feelings out into the open, to see whether a clearer understanding of the forces that pulled them in so many different directions could make the situation less explosive and painful, and lead to better communication between them.

These psychopaths, and others with equally severe problems in the sample, had materially comfortable homes and their parents were by no means unreasonable or without understanding or goodwill. Yet the barriers that had been erected by prolonged separations, guilt and resentment, seemed unbridgeable. The patients appeared to be lost, acting out their bewilderment and despair in hostile, irresponsible or delinquent behaviour, unable to settle anywhere or to trust anybody. In these situations, living in lodgings held no solution. The patients took their problems with them and managed to evoke the rejection they feared wherever they went. No form of traditional treatment, psychiatric or social, appeared to help them. At the same time, no intensive efforts had ever been made to tackle the problems where they had arisen and where they basically still belonged—in the nuclear family of the patient.

The tentative conclusion emerges that the therapeutic benefit of living away from the natal family may depend on earlier experiences of traumatic separations from parents, and on the extent to which the patient can still feel supported by his immediate family.

Ways of Helping

FAMILY DIAGNOSIS

How can a social worker help these families? This small study suggested that some understanding of the whole family constellation is essential before any plan for treatment can be formulated. Such an appraisal might consider three areas of family functioning.

1. The distributions of and satisfactions derived from occupational and social roles: the case examples showed how vitally important these were. The father in the S 46 family was crushed and denigrated. He did not function at a level one would have expected from his intelligence and educational background. He had failed in business and was a railway porter at the age of 50. The resulting frustrations aggravated the family tensions. At the other extreme, we observed a father who tended to put most of his energies into his job; he had climbed steadily up the social ladder, and he resented a son whose artistic bohemianism seemed to question the value of his intellectual and social achievement.

2. The nature of the interpersonal relationships, and how far mutual needs and satisfactions are met without violating the "generation barriers" (Fleck et al., 1959), or using the patient as an outward projection of the family's fears and hostilities. We saw striking examples of the violation of generation barriers in Group I, and most of the patients discussed were in part scapegoats of the family's fears and hostilities. In all the examples

quoted, communication between the members of the family was seriously disturbed. They were continually misunderstanding and misinterpreting one another's intentions and communications. Often, the investigator acted in the role of an interpreter. Conflicts were rarely handled realistically and often threatened to disrupt the whole fabric of the family.

3. In addition, a family assessment would take into consideration the family's comprehension of and outlook on the patient's illness.

If the family is considered to be functioning reasonably well, and the psychiatric assessment of the patient points to a good potential for recovery and resettlement, then the amount of support the family and the patient require after discharge will be small.

If the family is considered to be functioning well but the patient's prognosis poor, then the problem will be how to maximize the patient's chances in the community, with due regard to the possible strain and hardship that a permanently handicapped person is likely to cause his family.

If the family is considered to be seriously disturbed in any or all the three areas referred to above, the problem arises of how much these disturbances will militate against the patient's chances of successful settlement after discharge. The following questions will have to be asked.

Is it considered possible to help the family and the patient to modify any of these disturbed relationships or attitudes, or to improve the family's functioning in other respects?

If the family circumstances and patterns of functioning are considered to be relatively unalterable, can the patient be helped to learn to cope with them?

If it is not considered possible either to modify the family environment or the patient's response, can the family and the patient be helped to separate?

It follows that the length and nature of the patient's treatment in hospital will depend in part on the assessment and treatment of the family situation. In other words, it is suggested that hospital treatment should include family assessment and treatment.

TIME OF INTERVENTION

Attempts to bring about environmental changes will clearly have to start *before* the patient is discharged. Indeed, relatives are likely to be receptive to the possibility of change *on admission*—at the point of major crisis rather than at discharge. As Caplan (1964) has reminded us, in a crisis situation customary responses and defences are likely to be disturbed. A searching look at these responses may be welcomed, and attitudes are more likely to change at this point than at any other. Skilful intervention in a crisis may lead to new insight and better functioning. Thus the "breakdown" of a patient—his entry into hospital—need not necessarily be regarded as the final catastrophe, but could be used as a constructive turning point in the family's difficulties. This applies equally whether the aim is the rehabilitation of the patient into the family, or eventual separation from them.

FAMILY-ORIENTATED CASEWORK

Once a tentative assessment and a treatment aim have been established for both the patient and his family, the question arises as to which members of the family should be involved in treatment. It is clear that family-centred therapy does not mean that one must work with *all* members of the family. For example, work with the healthiest member of the family as the potentially most helpful source of support to the patient may be indicated. One might instance a young mother carrying the burden of several children and a chronically ill husband (see S 39 on page 45). On the other hand, it might be important to work with both parents together, in order to expose and work through their distorted views of each other (see S 46 on page 37). Or, one may be faced with a family situation in which separate interviews only can be tolerated and will reveal the nature of the disturbance in the family. Other considerations are involved. Is the work best carried out at home with one individual family, or will groups of several families at the hospital have greater therapeutic impact? Should these groups comprise relatives only, or relatives and patients? The answers to these questions can only be found by trying different methods in relation to defined circumstances and building up objective evidence of the differences in outcome. Systematic understanding of family functioning and of how to bring about changes are so rudimentary as yet that any kind of dogmatism is out of place. The following suggestions about methods and possible aims of family support are therefore put forward in a very tentative way.

The most challenging situation is presented by the families in Group I, where the mothers were protective and paralysing, and the fathers resented the involvement between patient and mother, while the patient was steadily deteriorating. The mothers were usually very unpopular with the hospital staff, as they continually undermined the work the latter were attempting to carry out. For instance, a mother would encourage the patient to stay in bed and rest during the weekend at home; the father would bring him back to hospital on Monday discouraged and depressed by the losing battles he was fighting complaining bitterly about his wife and his own helplessness in the situation. The investigator made some attempts to explore the problems of a few of these families in joint interviews, and to see how their contradictory views of the situation had arisen (Goldberg, 1960). Working with such families as a group has been undertaken by many others, for example

Ackerman (1961), Jackson and Weakland (1961), Laing and Esterson (1964), Satir (1964), Sheppard (1963), and Wynne (1961).

Often, the difficulties centred around the hostile relationships between the parents and the wholly negative projections each was pinning onto the other, blaming the other for the son's illness. One of the main tasks was to bring out in these family sessions, not only the recriminations and accusations, but also the good and pleasant qualities of both parents. Getting into touch again with some of the more hopeful aspects of their own as well as their spouse's personality may have helped them to tolerate a little better their own destructive drives, without having to blame them onto their partners. Gradually, such parents began to see how they were misinterpreting and misunderstanding each other, how their attitudes in turn were related to their own past experiences, as well as to the pressures of the present situation. These gains in understanding were often wiped out by the intensity of the crises during the weeks following such an exploratory discussion. Yet the investigator felt that provided such sessions could take place at frequent regular intervals, *limited* aims might be achieved. For example, one might enable the parents to co-operate better with the hospital, to make some small concessions to each other as regards the régime while the patient was at home, and to use the caseworker rather than the patient to express their despair and frustration. The patient himself may well benefit from participating in these sessions. For example, in the S 46 family, the patient, confused and deluded though he was, perceived that in the painful scenes that took place during the investigator's visits, positive attempts were made by all concerned to grapple with the problems. This was expressed in his fantasy already described, in which a nurse was visiting, seeing him and his parents, and making everyone happy. In contrast, his normal teenage sister saw only the external reality of the stormy discussions. She would announce, "Miss Goldberg is coming tonight—another row!"

The work with these and other parents could not be carried far enough to be at all certain about its effectiveness. It was clear, however, that the parents were deeply concerned over their sons, anxious to talk about their problems, and relieved that the investigator did not appear to blame them and was able to realize some of their difficulties.

Other attempts to help families in which schizophrenic patients were vegetating at home, protected by intelligent and active mothers, showed how difficult it was to offer the right kind of help at the right time. One such patient (S 47) seemed mentally alert on follow-up, in touch with reality, able to converse in a coherent and intelligible manner and clearly capable of some occupation. Yet he did not get up till lunchtime and was evasive and defensive whenever the question of work was broached. The mother, a highly intelligent commercial artist, kept the family going. She was a somewhat eccentric, strong personality who carried the main burden of two mentally ill sons. Her husband, also an artist, was less successful than his wife—he leant on her and at times drank heavily. The mother's attitude was that the patient needed patience and indulgence and she trusted in the guidance she received from spiritualist healers. The father was becoming increasingly more resentful about the situation and advocated more discipline. The parents appealed for help from various social services, but usually when a plan was made which involved letting the patient go to hospital or to occupational therapy classes, the mother would find excuses. Social workers and doctors then became exasperated and turned their backs on the situation until the next crisis evoked a fresh appeal. After the investigator had brought the situation once more to the notice of the local Mental Welfare Department, renewed attention was concentrated on this family, and a place found in a hostel, where the rule was that patients should start work within a fortnight of their admission. This time the mother let the patient go, but, faced with work, he returned home after a week. The rehabilitation plan, though theoretically correct, was put into operation too suddenly, without the necessary slow and patient spade-work which would ensure the active co-operation of patient and parents. It might well take as long as a year to get this mother to the point when she would be able to let her son go— willingly and not under pressure. This woman felt that social workers thought her odd on account of her spiritualism and were unable to appreciate her positive qualities. It seemed important, therefore, to convey to her that the helper valued her as a creative person and an excellent provider for her family, before broaching the idea that she should give up looking after her son. Conversely, one can hardly expect a patient who has not worked for 6 years and has lain in bed for most part of the day, watched over by his mother, to emancipate himself from home and go into full-time work within the course of a fortnight.

Another example illustrates the great difficulty of providing the right kind of support to a family who want to care for a mentally ill member at home. A young schizophrenic of borderline intelligence (S 21) was discharged at the request of his mother, though he had improved very little in hospital. On follow-up, he was found to be in an almost catatonic state. He took 3 hours to dress, smiled inanely, was incapable of carrying on a coherent conversation, and was totally unoccupied. His only sister was a cheerful mongol. The father was a book-keeper and owned a well-kept semi-detached house in a middle-class suburban area. As the mother was not working, their economic situation must have been very tight, though they never complained. The mother carried out her difficult task in a curiously serene manner, supported by her faith in spiritualism. She derived much satisfaction from her healing activities. The father showed more anxiety and concern. Both were very active members of the local branch of the National Society for Mentally Handicapped Children. A mental welfare officer, who was in touch with the family, secured a vacancy for the patient at a hospital for subnormal patients, as he considered that the burden of two mentally disordered children was too much for the parents. However, the mother refused the vacancy. The question arose of how far one should attempt to interfere in a situation in which the parents deliberately chose to cope with extreme difficulties.

Day hospital care or an occasional holiday admission or possibly home occupational therapy might have been helpful and acceptable measures for this family. The investigator also felt that the mother needed unobtrusive support of a sensitive kind which did not undermine her way of coping and the satisfaction she derived from her spiritualistic activities. For these endeavours seemed to make up in part for what to her must have seemed her terrible failure as a mother. It was conceivable, indeed likely, that one day her defences would crumble. At that point, the helper could come forward with more active support. However, neither the practical measures nor the kind of casework described were available, and so this family carried on without support. Possibly they were even labelled "unco-operative", since they had refused a hospital vacancy for the patient.

Enough has been said to show that the family constellation of the closely guarded schizophrenic patient poses serious difficulties to any approach. The type of help required will vary greatly, not only in relation to the needs of the patient, but also in relation to the needs of the other members of the family, and their ability to carry burdens and to modify their attitudes and expectations.

The second group of families, in which the mothers were driving their sons and provoking much hostility in them, occasionally showed certain strengths, which could be utilized to help the patient and to avoid some of the crises. For instance, in the case of S 10 (page 39), the parents' marriage was reasonably complementary and stable, they were not using the patient as a scapegoat, and the mother did not actively prevent the father from having a relationship with the patient. Indeed, the father was a potential asset. Thus it might have been possible to encourage the father to play a more constructive and positive role, not merely viewing himself as the "labourer" in the family, who only intervened when things got out of control. This might have relieved the mother of her desperate need to drive the patient towards work and health. Such a letting-up could only be achieved if one gave the mother a chance to talk about her own problems, which she had already begun to do.

Regular contact with the family would also enable one to spot and grapple with growing family tensions before they build up to serious crises of violent and disturbed behaviour. However, this family only received attention from social workers when a crisis occurred, although the mother clearly showed her need for support by sending reports to the psychiatrist at the out-patient clinic and, in her words, "working with him". The difficulty in supporting these families may well be not to upset the basic equilibrium achieved, however pathological its foundation. For example, in encouraging a more hopeful father–son relationship, one would be mindful not to challenge the mother's position of leadership in the family. Too radical an attempt to re-align relationships would probably explode the family situation beyond repair.

Work with families in Group III in which the father was rejecting the patient, or where the atmosphere in general was one of rejection, will need yet a different emphasis. In the case example given (S 45, page 40), the most helpful move for the social worker was to accept the father's plan for separa-tion as a constructive one and to help him to see that there were other ways in which he could show his concern for the sick son, for instance in assisting him to find the right sort of job. Both parents expressed great relief at the positive acceptance of their suggestions. It seemed as though the helper's acceptance of the rejection, and the recognition of incompatibility of aims and needs between the father and son, was in itself of therapeutic value. The joint task of the parent and the social worker then consisted of turning this negative piece of behaviour (rejection), which of necessity produced much guilt, into a constructive act. The investigator encouraged the father to help the son in his search for a job and lodgings. The patient also needed support in making his own way. For it was observed that such patients clung to the powerful and successful father, hoping for support and recognition, and trying to attain this in ways which only alienated the father still further.

The therapeutic value of encouraging the patient and his family to separate was not always recognized. In one family, in which the father–son conflict was very evident, the patient had returned home and seemed to be completely paralysed, either by his own hostility or possibly by the hostility surrounding him, since his slight handicap could not account for his inability to work. This young man had always lived in comparative social isolation. He had been a late and unwanted arrival in the family, and had always experienced great distance between himself and his father. He said, "I never had a father." The father had been successful in his job, rising to executive level, and he talked openly about how much more active and stronger he was than his son. The son had worked quite regularly as a costing clerk before his illness, but his job did not engage his capacities and was merely an adjunct to his main hobby, which was sailing. On his return home from hospital he refused to go back to work, although his job was open to him, maintaining that since he felt worse than before his admission, he could not possibly be considered fit for work. He led a busy existence in his bed-sitting room, playing with his tape recorder, exchanging tapes with his tape friends and keeping an intricate diary, which was a pathetic record of his failure to accomplish even the small tasks which he set himself, like dubbing his tapes. With the agility of the intelligent paranoid person, he defeated every argument one might advance in favour of a more independent and socially more useful existence. Yet underneath this denial, his problems of inadequacy were clearly visible, particularly in relation to his successful father. The patient felt his father never encouraged any of his tape-recording efforts. His childish dependence on his mother, who at least listened to his performances, was also evident. This stalemate situation posed a dilemma in after-care. The psychiatrist who treated him as an out-patient queried the necessity of getting him back to work, feeling that he and his family were accepting the present state of affairs, since nobody had complained to him about the young man's lack of occupation. The investigator, on the other hand, felt that with patient effort this young man could be helped to free himself from his paralysing feeling of inadequacy, and lead a more satisfying and useful life. She knew from interviews with the parents that they were very unhappy about the situation, although they had no idea how to alter it, and the patient gave indications that he was dissatisfied with himself. For example, he felt that he had an ungainly nose, and he sought support and help from the Samaritans who, in contrast to the psychiatrist's strict timetable, would welcome him at any time. Once more, the problem was raised, on what basis "interference" is justified, what the legitimate goals of therapy are, and what is meant by the "principle of self-determination".

This small exploration suggested that where serious antagonism between a successful father and an ineffectual son had developed over many years, the son's increased handicap brought about by his illness aroused even greater rejection and disparagement in the father. Living away from this painful competitive situation seemed the only practicable solution.

Work with lonely women in the fourth group, who make the sick son their whole life-task, will have as its aim some loosening of the bonds between them. A first step will always be a willingness to share some of the mother's burden and anxiety. These women had a great need to talk and to convince the investigator that what they were doing for their sons was helpful. Gradually, one might try to modify the mother's expectations of their sons and to stimulate other interests and activities. Several of these mothers and sons were quite isolated from kin and neighbours, and some means of reconnecting them with a social network could perhaps be found. One could search for any neighbours or relatives who were prepared to take some interest in both mother and son. If this succeeded, mother and son would begin to spread their emotional investment to other kinds of relationships, which may in turn reduce the intensity of their involvement with each other. Such experiments with good neighbours or relatives would need the continuing support of a skilled caseworker, as these odd and disturbed mother–son couples would make great demands on the tolerance of the volunteers.

The other alternative is to encourage mother and son to separate. In lodgings, a young man who has been watched over by his anxious mother could live in a more neutral atmosphere, where he could get on with life in his own peculiar and unrealistic way, without being expected to give much in return. Here, he could live in his protective shell, which nobody would threaten to penetrate. It is possible that in such a situation the relationship between the patient and his mother would improve. The mother, freed from the burden of a disturbing illness for which she may feel in part responsible, might become more relaxed, helpful and understanding in her attitude.

Another group which needs support is the wives of schizophrenic patients. It will be recalled that in the examples given, the wives had to do all the giving and organizing in these families, and received practically nothing in return from their withdrawn husbands.

Even the families whose schizophrenic sons had left home were apprehensive and puzzled. They often felt guilty about letting the patient go away, and inflicting him and his disturbed behaviour on strangers. These families appeared to welcome opportunities for talking over these problems, and needed reassurance that what they were doing was in the interest of the patient.

The needs of families whose sons or husbands are in hospital for a very long period or permanently must not be forgotten. The parents, and particularly the lonely widows who visit the patients year in, year out, need regular contact, understanding and encouragement. They need to be informed about the progress of the patient, even if they do not ask for it themselves. Group discussions might relieve their isolation. The danger in these situations is that the permanent visitors tend to be regarded as a kind of adjunct to the institution, rather than as persons with their own special needs and feelings.

At times, family support will have as its aim the consent of both patient and family to hospital treatment. On follow-up, in this small sample of 52 schizophrenic patients, 10 were completely unoccupied at home and in need of hospital treatment which they were unwilling to accept. Some were supported in this attitude by their anxious and protective parents, while in other families, parents were too frightened and incapacitated themselves to exercise any kind of influence or control. In two families, the sons were eventually admitted under a compulsory treatment order, but meanwhile the patient had deteriorated steadily for 2 years, spreading much suffering and unhappiness. The impression was gained that persistent social work contact, in collaboration with the general practitioner, might have led to earlier acceptance of treatment, and thus to some prevention of distress and deterioration.

Organization of Services

EMERGING NEEDS

This follow-up study uncovered many needs among this small group of patients and their families (Table 3).

TABLE 3.

Services received and needed by 75 Males aged 15–30
*discharged from a District Mental Hospital (1958–61)**

Services Received	Additional Services Needed	
General practitioner 37	Family support	38
Out-patient clinic 48	Intensive casework	
Occasional mental	with patient	4
health social work 28	Help with work or	
Crisis mental health	rehabilitation	16
social work 12	Help with lodgings	3
Regular mental health	Housing	1
social work 5	Psychiatric in-patient	
Help from various	or day hospital	
social agencies 16	treatment	8
	Psychotherapy	3
	No additional help	
	needed	19

* 10 patients who never left hospital were excluded.

Other investigations in Great Britain have produced similar findings (Brown, 1963; Brown *et al*, 1966; Dudgeon, 1964), although one follow-up study in Devon (Dawson, 1964) revealed a much more satisfactory state of affairs.

The needs for family support of varying intensity and emphasis are obvious from the data presented. The study also showed that more specific and timely efforts were required to help patients find suitable employment and training facilities. Needs for different kinds of day care also became apparent. The day hospital in the study area did not cater for chronically handicapped patients, had no industrial therapy and did not work in close liaison with local employment facilities. Experiments seemed to be indicated in providing various types of accommodation for patients, ranging from a hostel not too far from the hospital to specially selected lodgings or small houses, in which patients could live together. More effective measures were needed to facilitate re-admission to hospital of very ill and disturbed patients who refused treatment, and to ensure that they stayed in hospital long enough to benefit from the treatment. It is also likely that some schizophrenic patients need more careful medical or nursing surveillance in relation to drug therapy (Renton *et al.*, 1963). It is worth noting in this connection that a few patients who had had many previous admissions maintained a level of tolerable social functioning while they were on regular doses of chlorpromazine or trifluoperazine. Most other patients appeared to take their drugs irregularly, if at all.

CONTINUITY OF CARE

It will be argued that the needs revealed in this and other studies can only be met by a considerable expansion of trained personnel and supporting facilities in the community. This is probably correct. However, recruiting more trained staff and organizing hostels, day centres and workshops will not have the optimal therapeutic impact, unless hospital and community services are better integrated, and more readily accessible to the patient and his family.

There is first of all the problem of continuity of care. It has been suggested that work with the family should begin on admission. In many cases, it will have to continue long after the patient's discharge. Should the social worker function from a hospital or community base? Difficulties will arise in either case. The hospital social worker is well placed to make a family assessment on admission, and to collaborate closely with the medical and nursing staff of the hospital. Although theoretically joint-user appointments can extend the hospital social worker's functions into the sphere of after-care, the decreasing proportion of social workers now employed in hospitals and the great pressures on them, as a result of the very high turnover of patients, makes this solution impracticable.

On the other hand, evidence is accumulating that the best strategic position for the social worker, especially when dealing with schizophrenic patients, will be in the community. Over half the patients who are admitted at any one time to a hospital with a diagnosis of schizophrenia have been in hospital before. In theory, therefore, they should already be known to the local authority social workers. We also know that nowadays very few schizophrenic patients (between 10% and 15%) stay in hospital for a very long time, that is more than 2 years (Brown, Parkes and Wing, 1961). Lastly, it has been found that between 40% and 50% of schizophrenic patients admitted to hospital for the first time still show substantial social handicaps at the end of 5 years (Brown et al., 1966). This figure is appreciably higher for those patients who have been in hospital before. In other words, the bulk of socially handicapped and disturbed schizophrenic patients spend most of their lives in the community and only comparatively short though frequent episodes in hospitals. It follows that these patients and their families require a type of care which is closely related to their home base, easily accessible and continuous—at least as regards the framework of the service and the case records, for the personnel will certainly change in the course of the many years a schizophrenic patient and his family may require help (Susser, 1965).

Assuming then that the social care of the patient will be based on the local health authority, many problems still remain to be solved. One of them is the maintenance of contact between the hospital staff and the local authority worker. This is not easy, since one local health authority may serve several psychiatric hospitals. In some areas the hospitals are beginning to organize themselves into geographically determined working units. This makes it much easier for hospital and local authority staff to work together.

THE ROLE OF THE PSYCHIATRIST IN COMMUNITY CARE

This brings us to the important question of the role of the psychiatrist in community care. In most cases, psychiatric advice and consultation is desirable, and in many cases it is necessary. Three possibilities suggest themselves. The local authority may have a designated medical officer of mental health advising the domiciliary team. Second, the local authority may have a joint-user arrangement, in which the hospital psychiatrist acts as consultant to the community care team. In other areas, social workers are encouraged to refer patients to out-patient clinics for assessment and advice whenever possible. All three arrangements have advantages and disadvantages. The local authority Medical Officer of Mental Health, who usually has a public health background, may look at problems from a community and preventive angle, and thus add an important dimension to the clinically orientated casework of social workers. However, he may not be able to add specific psychiatric expertise (unless he is also a trained psychiatrist) to that of the trained social worker who, as a rule, has more experience of, and training in, social psychiatry than the average medical man.

The hospital psychiatrist will be able to advise on clinical psychiatric problems. On the other hand, he may be too patient-centred to view the sociopsychiatric problems arising in community care in the round—from the family's, the employer's or even the neighbour's angle, as well as from the patient's. This applies even more so if he were to consult in the context of an out-patient clinic. Despite these disadvantages, much can be said for the hospital psychiatrist working as a part-time consultant to the local authority team. (Croydon, Nottingham and Salford are good examples of such arrangements.) This may involve curtailing work in out-patient clinics. Would this be such a loss? Much of this work is of necessity hurried; many of the patients who require psychiatric advice are non-attenders. The psychiatrist, in his role as consultant to the community care team, may well be able to deal with a larger group of patients more effectively than working solely through direct contact. Regular consultative contacts between psychiatrists and all kinds of community care workers would enable them to learn much from each other, and to build up a common working knowledge of the patient in his social environment and of how to help him in this context.

In a recent discussion group of experienced psychiatrists and social caseworkers, in which they tried to grapple with some of the family and employment problems discussed in this paper, it became clear that neither profession had achieved a very clear understanding of these complex situations, nor had they, as yet, developed any effective treatment methods. Interesting divisions emerged: while the social workers had a more comprehensive understanding of the patterns of family interaction among their clients, they were at times very hazy about the limits that should be set to their explorations or the aims of their endeavours. The psychiatrists had a more precise idea of their patients' potentialities and of the boundaries of their intervention. They limited themselves intentionally to smaller areas of social and psychological functioning, but often closed their eyes to the family repercussions of their intervention. It seemed likely that continued discussion and evaluation on live case material would have improved the understanding and skills of this divergent, experienced and very open-minded group of experts.

THE ROLE OF THE GENERAL PRACTITIONER

What is to be the role of the general practitioner in community care? How is one to ensure that he is not left out and receives the kind of information that enables him to care adequately for the patient? As far as could be ascertained, very few patients kept in regular touch with their general practitioners, who were only called upon in emergencies. This is confirmed by other studies (Parkes, Brown and Monck, 1962). There is also some evidence arising from recent investigations of general practice (Jefferys, 1965; Rawnsley and Loudon, 1962) that general practitioners are reluctant to grapple with the problems of psychotic patients in the community. Their care is felt to be time consuming. Many doctors consider that they have not sufficient training in psychiatry to carry out this task adequately, and they also feel unsupported by the community services, which are fragmented, difficult to contact, short-staffed and rarely immediately available, unless there is an urgent crisis. No ready solutions suggest themselves. It is possible that the attachment of health visitors and, in a few instances, of social workers to general practitioners will help to integrate them into the community care team. The consultant psychiatrist to the local authority team could extend his consultative activities to interested general practitioners and help them to develop more understanding and skill in this sphere.

INTEGRATION OF SERVICES

In the last analysis, the problems of how to integrate the roles of the various specialists resolve themselves into two issues. One is training, and the other the basic structure of the health and welfare services. An integrated programme of community care will develop more easily, it is suggested, if the helping professions were to receive at least part of their training together, both at undergraduate and postgraduate level. Even when the various partners in the enterprise have learnt to collaborate with each other, they will still need a sensible framework within which to do this. This framework is bound to be complex in the realm of mental health, with its manifold aspects—medical, social and industrial. However, the tripartite division of the health services, combined with the present fragmentations of the social work services within them, is clearly inimical to a coherent development of community care for the mentally disordered, and militates against the best deployment of the scarce resources available. One cannot help deploring the comparative absence of health centres, originally envisaged in the National Health Service, where general practitioners, social workers, nurses and psychiatrists would be easily accessible to each other and to the patient. The growth of group practices, which seek closer links with nurses, health visitors and social workers are hopeful steps towards the realization of the health centre concept.

Meanwhile, many discussions and inquiries are taking place about possible ways of reorganizing the social and health services. Opportunities should be taken wherever possible to experiment with different role assignments and methods of integration, so that any new structure proposed will be based on solid experience rather than on pious hopes.

References

ACKERMAN, N. W. (1961), A Dynamic Frame for the Clinical Approach to Family Conflict, In *Exploring the Base for Family Therapy*, New York, Family Service Association of America.

BATESON, G., JACKSON, D. D., HALEY, J. and WEAKLAND, J. (1956), Towards a theory of schizophrenia, *Behavioral Science*, **1**, No. 4.

BROWN, G. W. (1963), Changing patterns of care of the schizophrenic patient, *Brit. J. Psych. Soc. Work*, **7**, No. 1, 5.

BROWN, G. W., PARKES, M. C. and WING, J. K. (1961), Admissions and re-admissions to three London mental hospitals, *J. ment. Sci.* **107**, 1070.

BROWN, G. W., BONE, B., DALISON, B. and WING, J. K. (1966), *Schizophrenia and Social Care*, Maudsley Monograph No. 17, London, Oxford University Press.

BROWN, G. W., MONCK, E. M., CARSTAIRS, G. M. and WING, J. K. (1962), Influence of family life on the course of schizophrenic illness, *Brit. J. prev. soc. Med.* **16**, 55.

CAPLAN, GERALD (1964), *Principles of Preventive Psychiatry*, London, Tavistock.

DAWSON, M. C. (1964), *Home from the Psychiatric Hospital*, published by the Devon Community Mental Health Committee.

DUDGEON, M. Y. (1964), The social needs of the discharged mental hospital patient, *Int. J. soc. Psychiat.* **10**, No. 1, 45.

FLECK, S., LIDZ, T., CORNELISON, A., SCHAFER, S. and TERRY, D. (1959), The Intrafamilial Environment of the Schizophrenic Patient, In *Individual and Familial Dynamics*, New York, Grune & Stratton.

FREEMAN, H. and SIMMONS, O. (1963), *The Mental Patient Comes Home*, New York, Wiley.

GOLDBERG, E. M. (1960), Parents and psychotic sons, *Brit. J. Psych. Soc. Work*, **5**, No. 4, 184.

GOLDBERG, E. M. (1966), Hospital work and family: a four year study of young mental hospital patients, *Brit. J. Psychiat.* **112**, 177.

GOLDBERG, E. M. and MORRISON, S. L. (1963), Schizophrenia and social class, *Brit. J. Psychiat.* **109**, No. 463 785.

JACKSON, D. D. and WEAKLAND, J. H. (1961), Conjoint family therapy, *Psychiatry* **24**, No. 2.

JEFFERYS, MARGOT (1965), *An Anatomy of Social Welfare Services*, London, Michael Joseph.

LAING, R. and ESTERSON, A. (1964), *Sanity, Madness and the Family*, London, Tavistock.

LIDZ, T. and FLECK, S. (1960), Schizophrenia, Human Integration, and the Role of the Family, In *Etiology of Schizophrenia* (ed. Don Jackson), London, Basic Books.

LIDZ, T., CORNELISON, A. R., FLECK, S. and TERRY, D. (1957), The intrafamilial environment of schizophrenic patients: II. Marital schism and marital skew, *Amer. J. Psychiat.* **114**, No. 3.

PARKES, M. C., BROWN, G. W. and MONCK, E. M. (1962), The general practitioner and the schizophrenic patient, *Brit. med. J.* **i**, 972.

RAWNSLEY, K. and LOUDON, J. B. (1962), The Attitudes of General Practitioners to Psychiatry, in *Sociology and Medicine*. Sociological Review Monograph No. 5, University of Keele.

RENTON, C. A., AFFLECK, J. W., CARSTAIRS, G. M. and FORREST, A. D. (1963), A follow-up of schizophrenic patients in Edinburgh, *Acta psychiatrica Scandinavica*, **39**, 548.

SATIR, VIRGINIA (1964), *Conjoint Family Therapy: A Guide to Theory and Technique*, Palo Alto, Science and Behavior Books.

SHEPPARD, MARJORIE (1963), Some reflections on work with the schizophrenic and his family, *Brit. J. Psych. Soc. Work*, **7**, No. 1, 13.

SIMMONS, O. G., and FREEMAN, H. E. (1959), Familial expectations and post-hospital performance of mental patients, *Human Relations*, **12**, 233.

SUSSER, M. W. (1965), Rationale for the Community Care of Mental Disorder, *Medical Care*, **3**, 52.

WYNNE, L. C., RYCKOFF, I. M., DAY, J., and HIRSCH, S. I. (1958), Pseudo-mutuality in the family relations of schizophrenics, *Psychiatry*, **21**, 205.

WYNNE, L. C. (1961), The Study of Intrafamilial Alignments and Splits in Exploratory Family Therapy, In *Exploring the Base for Family Therapy* (ed. Ackerman, N. W.) New York, Family Service Association of America.

WYNNE, L. C., and SINGER, M. T. (1963), Thought Disorder and Family Relations of Schizophrenics, *Arch. gen. Psychiat.* **9**, 191.

3. Hierarchy or Arena? The Administrative Implications of a Sociotherapeutic Regime

T. D. HUNTER

NOWHERE in the world have the complex issues associated with the organization of hospital care been satisfactorily resolved. But why is this so? What is it that complicates the administrative problems of hospitals? Does the exaggerated prestige of the doctor in modern society have the effect of distorting the organizational structure of the hospital? Is the "blocked mobility" which obtains between the different categories of hospital staff a dangerously disruptive factor? (Main and Rapoport, 1962). And are hospitals so fragmented, both horizontally and vertically, as a result of these pressures that special administrative skills are called for? In whatever direction the truth is to be found, it would be difficult to deny that, from the organizational point of view, the modern hospital is characterized by a disturbing lack of integration.

Three typical eras of hospital administration have been distinguished:

> Put briefly, an era of trustee control, emphasizing capital investment and community acceptance of hospitals, is followed by a period of control by doctors based on the increasing complexity and importance of their skills. At present, there is a trend towards domination by the administration because of the mounting complexity of hospital activities and the increasing contact with health and other agencies proliferating outside the hospital. (Perrow, 1963.)

This view of the administrative development of the hospital coincides with what we have discovered about its development as a sociomedical institution. The early hospitals were religious foundations; they had a social rather than a medical orientation. Even as it emerged from the medieval period, the hospital was "essentially an instrument of society to ameliorate suffering, to diminish poverty, to eradicate mendicity, and to help maintain public order" (Rosen, 1963). The view that hospitals should be medically, rather than socially orientated, i.e. that they should be places for the treatment of the sick and centres for the study and teaching of medicine—this view achieved acceptance only in the eighteenth and nineteenth centuries.

With the increasing complexity and sophistication of medical care in modern times, and the increased emphasis on and acceptance of hospital service, there has developed a new awareness of the social dimension of treatment, with its demand for adjunct services in addition to the usual medical and nursing care. As hospitals have had to accommodate more and more specialized functions, together with additional personnel, facilities and equipment, their organization has grown increasingly elaborate, while the cost of running them has soared.

These developments, interacting with and affected by changing trends outside the hospital, have in turn led to:

1. Greater intervention by the government in the planning and management of hospitals;
2. An increased emphasis on the over-all quality, in both human and technical terms, of hospital service and medical care; and
3. The appearance of hospital administration as a profession.

The recommended administrative structure for British hospitals—the so-called tripartite structure (Bradbeer, 1954)—is an interim solution during the present transitional phase. Based on the traditional deference of nursing staff to doctors, and on the markedly lower status *vis-à-vis* their medical counterparts of present-day lay administrative staff (Glaser, 1963), the tripartite system is essentially an oligarchic variant of classic medical dominance. It is a negative and static system, which has not produced and is incapable of producing, truly positive results. On the other hand, there is little prospect of a return to medical dominance. Under modern conditions, professional administration has become inevitable. But what pattern of administration is likely to be most appropriate, in view of the increasing trend towards professionalism among hospital staffs? Since they are mainly confined to the carrying out of certain specialized functions, existing patterns of lay administration are no more relevant to the solution of this problem than traditional patterns of medical administration, which were based on a failure to distinguish between (a) the authority of status and (b) sapiential authority, i.e. the authority of special skill and knowledge (Presthus, 1962).

All hospitals are progressively becoming less institutional and less medically orientated. But psychiatric illness, being a social rather than an individual disease, has special characteristics which are favourable to the development of these trends. The emergence of the psychosocial approach as medicine's contemporary growth point—a function performed by bacteriology 150 years ago (Vickers, 1965)—has thrust the psychiatric hospital to the forefront of a recent tendency to look upon the hospital less as a hospital than as a school of living. It is the psychiatrist who is leading the medical profession away from the medical model, and away from the authoritarian and religio-moral concept of medicine, which has held sway since the earliest times, to the contemporary concept of medicine as sociotherapy—i.e. medicine as a branch of social science (Roemer, 1960; Szasz, 1962). This means that the psychiatric hospital, which was until recently the most backward of all hospitals and the most prone to indulge in a religious or hierarchical approach to therapy and administration, is now pioneering an ambitious but exciting concept of the hospital as a "total treatment organization", which must deploy *all* its therapeutic resources, and not merely its traditional medical and nursing skills. In the development of human institutions, such leap-frogging is to be expected: growth points rarely appear where an accumulation of vested interests has produced sclerosis. The *avant-garde* role of the psychiatric hospital at the present time is directly related to its history (since the 1860's) of repression and neglect. Having been compelled to look beyond traditional formulations because of public attitudes of rejection, institutional psychiatrists came to the conclusion that the hospital was in itself a sick organization, which accommodated sick social structures as well as sick people, and which could not make a positive contribution, except by exploiting itself as a total social system and so drawing upon its deepest reserves of therapeutic potential (Jones, 1962; Clark, 1964).

This insight was not easily won. After the Second World War, it was clear that a profound change was taking place in the field of mental health, but the situation was obscured by a variety of cross-currents. Having been brought into the same system as general hospitals, the first impulse of psychiatric hospitals was to emulate their "betters" (Clark, 1956), and this impulse was in harmony with certain theoretical trends in psychiatry itself. These trends, which emphasized somatotherapy and conditioning techniques at the expense of psychodynamics, were to some extent directed at reassuring the public. They were also directed at gaining medical respectability for psychiatry, by giving it an organic rather than a functional orientation. It became a cardinal tenet of all mental health education that mental illness was the same as other illness. Moreover, the phenomenal advances in public esteem and favour which had been achieved by hospitals dealing with physical illness since the turn of the century provided an additional reason for modelling the psychiatric hospital on the acute general hospital. Simultaneously, however, and "behind the scenes", a process of interpenetration between the insights of dynamic psychiatry and the basic social sciences had been taking place (Brown, 1961; Burns and Stalker, 1961). This *rapprochement* resulted in a new orientation, which necessitated a radical redefinition of the functions of the psychiatric hospital. The view that the psychiatric hospital had its own distinctive role was vigorously proclaimed by Clark (1956) and others. These protestations were based on the pioneering work of T. F. Main and Maxwell Jones; but highly significant, too, was the American literature on the transition from custodial to therapeutic care in mental hospitals (Greenblatt, York and Brown, 1955).

In the light of this new orientation, the conventions appropriate to physical illness (and even in the physical sphere, it may well be that the orthodox conventions of sickness and cure should be regarded as oversimplifications) have little or no relevance in the mental health field. Psychiatric disorder introduces a new social dimension, so that neurosis, for example, "must always be defined as a relationship between a personality and its social setting" (Alexander, 1956). Indeed, is it society itself that is the real patient? And is this why social psychiatry has been termed a policy rather than a medical science? (Becker, 1964).

Rioch (1958) writes of "the emergence of a consistent theoretical orientation which, in a number of respects, differs from classical psychiatric theory. Whereas the early developments of modern psychiatry were concerned with the personal history and early life experiences of patients, the emerging theories lay emphasis upon current social roles and social environmental contingencies." The work of the psychiatric hospital has been revolutionized by this sociotherapeutic approach. The frame of reference is no longer the individual patient; it is the patient-in-society. Hence Open Doors, Day Hospitals, Milieu Therapy, Patient Government, and the whole cluster of concepts associated with the community care approach and with the concept of the hospital as a therapeutic community.* The overvalued intrapsychical insights of the psychoanalytical pioneers are steadily being deepened and broadened, until they achieve the status of invaluable social insights (Cummings and Cummings, 1964). While somatotherapy continues to make an important contribution to resocialization, the emphasis is placed not on the criterion of cure, but on the criterion of social competence—to what extent can the patient be helped to take his place again in the community to which he belongs?

Since it invests the administrator not merely with a supportive but actually with an integrative role, the concept of the hospital as a total treatment organization, which is prepared to make full use of the therapeutic potential of the environment, of all categories of staff, and of the patients themselves, has profound administrative repercussions. Administrative "support" may be adequate for a static régime of custodial care and symptom-suppression; sociotherapy demands something more positive, and it involves the use of non-authoritarian techniques as well as techniques devoid of the sterile bureaucratic compartmentalism, which is implicit even in "supportive", "enabling" or "co-ordinating" philosophies.

With the increasing complexity of society and the demise of charismatic leadership, as a consequence of what Weber (1947) called the "disenchantment of the world", bureaucracy became the order of the day. But conventional bureaucratic patterns are everywhere breaking down;† and they are totally out of place in the modern psychiatric hospital. The successive injection into the clinical field of sociotherapeutic innovations has had the effect of focusing attention on the problem of the over-all administration of

* I am not concerned in this paper with the distinction which Dr. Clark makes between the "therapeutic community approach" and "therapeutic communities proper".

† Over the past twenty-five years, some new orientations have emerged from organizational experiments, observations and inventions. The new orientations depart radically

the hospital. How can a unified and flexible structure be achieved, which will be capable of assisting the process of change, while at the same time providing the patient with a lucid and responsive total environment? What kind of unified structure is appropriate in the special setting of the psychiatric hospital?

In general hospitals, the industrial model of scientific management has found favour in recent years. As a religious-humane institution the hospital has been over-resistant to normal socio-economic pressures (Nokes, 1960). Accordingly, the temptation to go to the other extreme, i.e. the temptation for the hospital to produce its own variant of industrial bureaucracy, has been very strong. The essence of this solution—vertical integration within the framework of a new-style Board of Directors-cum-Management Committee—has been well expressed by Robert Moore:

> The day-to-day running of a group of hospitals is an executive task and should fairly and squarely be the responsibility of an executive officer. The board is there to take decisions on important matters outside the authority of the officer, to exercise general control, and to carry the ultimate responsibility to the Regional Board. But the practical concept should be of management by officers under the general direction of the board, instead of management by a board through a secretariat. It should be recognized that there is a fundamental distinction between the executive function, which must be a personal responsibility, and the deliberative function, which is a collective one.
>
> The vitality of hospital administration, just like that of any other organization, will be a direct reflection of the degree to which individuals are given personal responsibility and allowed to exercise personal authority. When the present position is clarified, life should become more satisfying for both officers and boards. A Board of Directors does not feel that its position is depreciated because it has a general manager exercising considerable personal authority. (McMahon, 1965.)

This concept of a business manager for the hospital has had wide acceptance in America. In this country, it is attractive to others besides lay administrators (Davies, 1962), and elements reminiscent of the American pattern are beginning to appear in British hospitals. Although, as Sir William Hart has pointed out (1965), the relationship between the permanent official and his board or committee is "more subtle than the clichés about the distinction between policy and its execution", there is considerable truth in

---

from doctrines associated with "Scientific Management" and traditional bureaucratic patterns. The central emphases in this development are as follows:

1. Wide participation in decision-making, rather than centralized decision-making.
2. The face-to-face group, rather than the individual, as the basic unit of organization.
3. Mutual confidence, rather than authority, as the integrative force in the organization.
4. The supervisor as agent for maintaining intragroup and intergroup communication, rather than as the agent of higher authority.
5. Growth of members of the organization to greater responsibility, rather than external control of the members' performance of their tasks.

H. A. Shepard (1956), *Superiors and Subordinates in Research*, Paper 12 of the Symposium on the Direction of Research Establishment, H.M.S.O., Department of Scientific and Industrial Research.

what Moore says about the need (a) to establish new relationships in the boardroom, and (b) to inject an element of dynamic management into the hospital system. But the American philosophy of patient-care differs widely from ours. When the health services are seen as part of the general business activities of the community, a business manager in the hospital may seem entirely appropriate. In this country, with its deep attachment to a "human sociology", it is correspondingly difficult to envisage a hospital director or chief executive, modelled on the managing director of a business firm. Can we accept without question the American view that the hospital is a medical factory or workshop? Is it not more likely that this concept represents a profound inversion of basic human values? (Hunter, 1963).

In spite of certain superficial resemblances, and apart altogether from the materialistic reductionism* which is implicit in the factory analogy, there is a world of difference between the factory and the hospital; sociologically speaking, they are at opposite ends of the spectrum. In the first place, industry can, to some extent, measure its work, establish priorities and make appropriate plans; the work of the hospital, consisting as it does of multiple tasks with undetermined priority (Rice, 1963), and of a series of shifting situations which do not lend themselves so readily to measurement (Brotherston, 1962), cannot be routinized and dealt with on the basis of a rigid division of labour or by means of conveyor-belt and other mass-production techniques. In the second place, hospital staffs are steadily becoming more professionalized and more resistant to the industrial model of line management, which threatens their professional independence by substituting the authority of status for the authority of knowledge and skill (Presthus, 1962).

The hospital, and above all the psychiatric hospital, may be differentiated from the factory at a still more fundamental level. The factory is an organization—an adaptation of man to his environment. The hospital, on the other hand, is an institution—an adaptation of the environment to man (Selznick, 1957). While the factory may have an over-all as well as a primary task, it is the primary task that distinguishes it as a factory (Rice, 1963). It follows that any attempt to restrict the work of the hospital to its so-called primary task of "doing something to the patients" as Hutton (1964), has tried to do, is based on an inversion of the facts.

It goes against the whole current of hospital life, where the flow—from the ward back to the administration—tends to be the opposite of the flow—from management to the factory floor—characteristic of industry. In drawing attention to this distinction, which makes vertical or authoritarian integration impractical in a hospital setting, Crockett (1960) has made an invaluable contribution. In claiming, however, that the role of the administrator is purely supportive, being in effect delegated to him by the clinician, he has

---

* I employ the term "reductionism" in the pejorative sense, i.e. as signifying a tendency to explain higher-order systems in terms of lower-order phenomena.

erred in the opposite direction. The risk of fragmentation implicit in Crockett's model is obvious and he overlooks the fundamental importance, in a dynamic culture, of over-all integration. In their study of social change in the setting of an American mental hospital, John and Elaine Cummings did not make this mistake:

> The traditional mental hospital is a granulated social system; it is crosscut horizontally by caste lines and crosscut vertically by the functional autonomy of the parts. This means that when the task of changing its operation is undertaken, the task of raising the level of integration of the system must be simultaneously undertaken. Bringing about change in each one of these social granules is beyond the power of any individual or team, and therefore, without integration and communication, any change is restricted to the granule in which it began. (1957)

If we are prepared to forget about the social context of disease, and about the sickness of society itself, if we are prepared to forget what health is all about, we can dispense with dynamic integration and allow the hospital to function as a static, closed system of highly specialized medical departments. But the primary task of "cure"—the mechanical process of removing symptoms from the patient by "doing something" to him—how often does this turn out to be a short-lived, or even an illusory, solution? Of more importance in the modern, socially orientated psychiatric hospital is the over-all task of creating a new dynamic relationship between the hospital and the community, and between the patient and society.

A sociotherapeutic régime, being the antithesis of a health-factory or industrial régime, has profound implications for the hospital's administrative structure. In particular, it necessitates:

1. The dissociation of hospital administration not only from one-man rule, or charismatic authoritarianism, but also from traditional concepts of "scientific management" or bureaucracy.
2. The fostering of rational permissiveness—i.e. the replacement of external, bureaucratic control by control from within.
3. The blurring of hard-and-fast status distinctions and the exchange of a rigid system of division of labour for a system of multi-disciplinary teams and interlocking roles.
4. The progressive dissemination of a philosophy of getting things done, instead of a philosophy of avoiding mistakes, the creation of a cadre of professional administrators and the generation of a mature atmosphere of trust, so that it will become increasingly difficult to erect administrative structures and financial procedures which are really fear-systems, or systems erected as defence mechanisms against anxiety. (Menzies, 1960.)
5. The growth of a new conception of Boards of Management and Hospital Management Committees as legitimating bodies, and as mediating structures between the hospital and the community, which exercise authority only in the special sense in which the individual patient exercises authority over his doctor. (Gouldner, 1955.)

In other words, the change of emphasis from clinical to social management of the patient has a profoundly relaxing effect on the administrative structure of the hospital. If positive (e.g. mental "health") concepts are in process of being introduced at the expense of negative, symptom-removal ones, the administrative corollary is a diffuse or open system, which allows for growth and development. Where change is inherent in an organization, too many decisions of too complex a kind require to be taken too quickly, and at too great a distance from the centre, for any other *modus operandi* to be effective or even viable (Bunker, 1965). For a finite system of line management, based on superior–subordinate relationships, and on the giving and taking of orders, there must be substituted a system of open communications and feedback. This is true of any hospital, but it is profoundly true of the psychiatric hospital. The essence of the therapeutic community approach (as distinct from the earlier total-push method of treatment, worked out by Myerson) lies in its subtle encouragement of personal growth, not only in staff, but above all in patients, who are encouraged to abandon their passive role and become the main participants in their own treatment (Clark, 1964).

The hospital administrator who aims at vertical integration is merely replacing medical by lay domination. Medical omnipotence is a myth. As Talcott Parsons has said (1960):

> In many contexts the physician is only one of a team of coequal experts in many fields. He is not even necessarily "captain" of the total team although the problem be mainly "medical". It is essentially where the problem becomes that of responsibility for the welfare of patients that his special prerogative takes precedence. . . . As part of the general process of differentiation in society, not only has medicine been becoming more specialized internally but it has been becoming at the same time a more specialized part of a larger complex of professional specialties.

But the professional administrator is faced with a similar situation. If medical omnipotence is a myth, and if it is wrong for the specialist to seek hierarchical power, it is also true that administrative omnipotence is a myth, and that it is wrong for the professional administrator to use hierarchical power primarily to restrict the activities of the specialist.

When he does not confine himself (as is the case under the present "lay" administrative régime) to a number of specialist functions, such as the finance, supply and secretarial functions, inevitably the administrator becomes involved with a wide variety of professional staff. It is all too easy for him to substitute for the growing antipathy (shared by doctors themselves) to traditional systems of medical domination, widespread misgivings about bureaucracy with its "white ants of auditors" (Clark, 1958), and its "book-keeping orientation" (Cummings, 1964). And of course, there is no doubt that the independent status of the professional would be seriously threatened by orthodox "punitive bureaucracy" as described by Gouldner (1955).

It will take a new generation of professionally trained hospital administrators to resolve this dilemma. If the clue to the future is not to be found in a simplistic system of vertical integration, deploying the various techniques of scientific management, where are we to direct our attention? Schemes of Delegation, Organization Charts, Work Study, Organization and Methods, Operations Research—all these physical techniques are in some degree essential, but the basic social techniques are absolutely vital. The administrative machine is less likely to be reduced to impotence through a badly conceived structure than through lack of motivation. And motivation is not the automatic by-product of an improved system of communications. On the contrary, it depends on the administrator's ability (a) to effect radical attitudinal changes in himself and others, and (b) to build up within, instead of superimposing upon, the hospital a unified, flexible and responsive administrative structure. Atmosphere in the hospital is all-important (Clark, 1964), and the atmosphere should be one in which the "asking of questions" is encouraged (Revans, 1964).

The elaboration of the social, as distinct from the physical, techniques of management—is this going to be the distinctive administrative contribution of the psychiatric hospital? Will it fall to the lot of the psychiatric hospital to prove the value of a genuinely integrative administrative structure which has a wide range of tolerance for personal initiative and personal growth, and which places the emphasis, not on directive techniques, but on open communications and feedback, all as part of a generally accepted learning process within the hospital (Revans, 1964)?

Ultimately, what is needed is the substitution of a new model for the traditional bureaucratic one. The false compartmentalism of the latter and, in the intensely human context of the hospital, the false dichotomy which it sets up between therapy and administration, are anathema. Based on an obsolete division of labour, organizational fragmentation is perpetuated by those interdepartmental perceptual disparities (Revans, 1964) which bedevil even the most determined attempts to make a highly differentiated system function as one. But, underneath this perceptual confusion, there do exist, at any rate in the psychiatric hospital, like some "invisible sandbank of reason", concepts of resocialization, and concepts of "whole person" therapy and of total treatment, which do in fact provide the solid basis for a unified structure.

The mistake has been to identify large-scale management with bureaucracy, and to think of bureaucracy only in monolithic terms, i.e. in terms of Weber's rational "bureaucratic" or "legal" order. There is a whole spectrum of bureaucratic forms. Gouldner has differentiated between punitive and representative bureaucracy. But even these "extremes" are only contrasting forms of Weber's legal order and do not cover the invisible seven-eighths of the iceberg. Indeed, the punitive (autocratic) and representative (oligarchic) forms are at one in their acceptance of some form of hierarchy—(whether "pyramid" or "plateau")—and it is hierarchy that is the real enemy of integration in the hospital.

A significant departure from the whole concept of hierarchy and a deliberate attempt to replace a legal by a sociological régime has been suggested by Goss (1963) who, in an effort to resolve the tensions between professionals and administrators, which are inherent in traditional organizations, has applied to the hospital situation a type of bureaucracy involving neither hierarchical authority nor specific rules. This new management pattern, which Goss terms "advisory bureaucracy", implies a system of role relationships between administrators and professionals in which the former proffer advice which the latter need not accept, but which they are obliged to "take under critical review".

A similar formulation and an explicit concept of the psychiatric hospital as a "locale or arena", where interlocking professional groups arrive at a "negotiated order" with one another and with the central administration, has been given currency in America by Anselm Strauss *et al.* (1964). It is noteworthy that the distinction which Strauss and his colleagues have drawn between hierarchy and arena closely resembles that which Burns and Stalker (1961) have drawn in the industrial field between mechanistic and organismic management systems.

Hutton (1964) has asked "Who runs a hospital?" In terms of the arena or organismic concept, the answer is that no-one does: the hospital runs itself. The administrator is the supreme non-authority at the heart of a complex of non-authorities. To the extent that he relies on conventional concepts of authority, precisely to this extent does he make it less likely that he will arrive at integrated solutions (Follett, 1949).

The arena model is equally relevant in the context of the general hospital. If the general hospital is to function with "integrated therapeutic purpose" (Brotherston, 1962), while avoiding the resistances set up by a total-push approach—it can do so only on the basis of a horizontal, or arena, as against a vertical, or line, system of management.

The hope that the tripartite system would produce integration, either through the tacit emergence of one leader or through an equal partnership of the three protagonists with the committee exercising ultimate authority, has proved illusory. The tripartite system reflects a static but insecure plateau structure; it is an oligarchic compromise, which is only partially masked by a posture of formal deference to a legally constituted committee. Only on the demise of this interim solution will it be possible to identify a genuine profession of hospital administration with a dynamic frame of reference. At present, the fragmented structure of the hospital has led to a situation in which the role of the hospital administrator has been defined in terms of certain specialized functions, instead of in terms of his central position in the total system (Stevens, 1964). This central position, however, is located, not at the apex of a pyramidal power-structure, but at the *focal* point of an arena or locale, where different professionals work together, or at least side by side, on a give-and-take basis.

Diffuse horizontal structures are more appropriate in hospital settings than finite vertical ones, because patients are not inert and extraneous material on which, factory-wise, the hospital may go to work. On the contrary, the patients are located *inside* the organization, participating directly in the arena of hospital life. Simon (1957) and Chester Barnard (1938) have shown that the clients of an organization belong to it just as much as the people who work there. It seems likely that in future, the service or consumer component in all organizations will assume increasing importance and that the organismic hospital model will have an ever wider application. Bunker (1965) has hinted at some such development; and Strauss and his colleagues (1964) are explicit:

> This characteristic feature of the modern psychiatric hospital (i.e. the hospital as a locale or arena) is also characteristic of hospitals in general. It is also becoming an increasingly prominent feature of organizations quite outside the medical field: universities are an outstanding example, as are business corporations. Sociologists have begun to recognize that older kinds of hierarchical organizational structure are being supplemented or supplanted by congeries of experts, whose ambitions are not limited to climbing the organizational ladder or to taking and giving orders.

To sum up, the modern psychiatric hospital functions as a countervailing force in so far as the dehumanizing tendencies of industrialism are concerned. For this reason, not only does it require for its own proper functioning a new pattern of administration, it also calls for the development throughout the entire social structure of new, non-directive attitudes and techniques. The psychiatric hospital, like other hospitals, is what Argyris (1965) has called a "sick organization"; but in effect it merely symbolizes the general sickness of the organizational society, the general *malaise* of a social order which has outgrown its traditional institutions. As Camus wrote in Reflections on the Guillotine (1961): "Man of the 20th Century needs laws and institutions of convalescence that will check without crushing and lead without hampering."

The modern psychiatric hospital, emerging with astonishing dynamism from all the cruelty and repression of the past, may yet provide us with a brilliant working model of just such a convalescent institution.

References

ALEXANDER, F. (1956), *Psycho-analysis and Psycho-therapy*, New York, W. W. Norton.
ARGYRIS, C. (1965), In Bravos, T.A., *Mental Hospitals*, **16**, 92.
BECKER, E. (1964), *The Revolution in Psychiatry*, Glencoe, Illinois, Free Press.
BARNARD, C. (1938), *The Functions of the Executive*, Cambridge, Mass., Harvard Univ. Press.
BRADBEER COMMITTEE (1954), *Report on the Internal Administration of Hospitals*, London, H.M.S.O.
BROTHERSTON, J. H. F. (1962), In *Towards a Measure of Medical Care*, London, Nuffield Provincial Hospitals Trust.
BROWN, J. A. C. (1961), *Freud and the Post-Freudians*, London, Penguin.
BUNKER, L. H. (1965), Management lessons from a hospital ward, *Public Administration*, **43**, 31.
BURNS, T. and STALKER, G. M. (1961), *The Management of Innovation*, London, Tavistock.
CAMUS, A. (1961), In *Resistance, Rebellion and Death*, New York, Alfred A. Knopf.

CLARK, D. H. (1956), *Lancet*, **ii**, 1005.
CLARK, D. H. (1958), *Lancet*, **i**, 805.
CLARK, D. H. (1964), *Administrative Therapy*, London, Tavistock.
CROCKETT, R. W. (1960), *Lancet*, **ii**, 359.
CUMMINGS, J. and CUMMINGS, E. (1957), In Greenblatt, Levinson and Williams, *The Patient and the Mental Hospital*, Glencoe, Illinois, Free Press.
CUMMINGS, J. and CUMMINGS E. (1964), *Ego and Milieu*, London, Tavistock.
DAVIES, J. O. F. (1962), In *Towards a Measure of Medical Care*, London, Nuffield Provincial Hospitals Trust.
FOLLETT, M. P. (1949), *Freedom and Coordination*, London, Management Publications Trust.
GLASER, W. A. (1963), In Eliot Freidson (ed.) *The Hospital in Modern Society*, Glencoe, Illinois, Free Press.
GOSS, M. (1963), In *The Hospital in Modern Society*, Glencoe, Illinois, Free Press.
GOULDNER, A. (1955), *Patterns of Industrial Bureaucracy*, London, Routledge.
GREENBLATT, M., YORK, R. H. and BROWN, E. L. (1955), *From Custodial to Therapeutic Patient Care in Mental Hospitals*, New York, Russell Sage Foundation.
HART, W. (1965), Address to the Association of Municipal Treasurers and Accountants (unpublished).
HUNTER, T. D. (1963), *Lancet*, **ii**, 933.
HUTTON, G. (1964), Who runs a hospital?, *New Society*, No. 74, 11.
JONES, M. (1962), *Social Psychiatry*, Springfield, Illinois, Thomas.
MCMAHON, R. P. (1965), *The Hospital*, **61**, 296.
MAIN, T. F. and RAPOPORT, R. N. (1962), In Welford, A. T., Argyle, M., Glass, D. V. and Morris, J. H. (eds.) *Society: Problems and Methods of Study*, London, Routledge.
MENZIES, I. E. P. (1960), *Human Relations*, **13**, 95.
NOKES, P. (1960), *Human Relations*, **13**, 141.
PARSONS, T. (1960), *Structure and Process in Modern Societies*, Glencoe, Illinois, Free Press.
PERROW, C. (1963), In *The Hospital in Modern Society*, Glencoe, Illinois, Free Press.
PRESTHUS, R. (1962), *The Organizational Society*, New York, Alfred A. Knopf.
REVANS, R. W. (1964), In *Problems and Progress in Medical Care*, London, Oxford Univ. Press.
RICE, A. K. (1963), *The Enterprise and its Environment*, London, Tavistock.
RIOCH, D. McK. (1958), In Symposium on Preventive and Social Psychiatry. Sponsored by Walter Reed Army Institute of Research and others, Washington, D.C., U.S. Govt. Printing Office.
ROEMER, M. I. (ed.) (1960), *Sigerist on the Sociology of Medicine*, New York, M.D. Publications Inc.
ROSEN, G. (1963), In *The Hospital in Modern Society*, Glencoe, Illinois, Free Press.
SELZNICK, P. (1957), *Leadership in Administration*, Evanston, Illinois, Row, Peterson.
SIMON, H. (1957), *Administrative Behaviour*, New York, Macmillan.
STEVENS, R. (1964), *Medical Care*, **2**, 208.
STRAUSS, A., SCHATZMAN, L., BUCHER, R., EHRLICH, D. and SABSHIN, M. (1964), *Psychiatric Ideologies and Institutions*, Glencoe, Illinois, Free Press.
SZASZ, T. S. (1962), *The Myth of Mental Illness*, London, Tavistock.
VICKERS, M. (1965), *Lancet*, **i**, 1021.
WEBER, M. (1947), In Gerth, H. H. and Mills, C. W. (eds.) *From Max Weber*, London, Kegan Paul, Trench, Trubner.

4. Social Therapy and Drug Treatment in Schizophrenia: a Review

DOUGLAS BENNETT

IT MUST be uncommon for clinical improvement from any form of somatic treatment to be uninfluenced at the same time by the patient's social environment. Yet social influences are rarely considered when drugs are used or their effects assessed (Sherman, 1959).

The early enthusiasm for the effect of pharmacotherapy on the populations of mental hospitals (Kramer and Pollack, 1958; Brill and Patton, 1959) has been tempered by more recent findings which emphasize the importance of the hospital environment (Shepherd, Goodman and Watt, 1961; Odegard, 1964). Odegard sampled the national figures for first admissions to all Norwegian mental hospitals in three 5-year periods; 1936–40, 1948–52, 1955–9. He showed that the discharge rate between the first two quinquennia was greater than that between the second and third. Yet it was in the interval between the second and third quinquennia that treatment with reserpine and chlorpromazine was introduced. When the discharge rates for individual hospitals were analysed, they showed a marked negative correlation between the levels of discharge in 1948–52 and those in 1955–9. In other words, Odegard believes that the pharmacotherapeutic drugs brought less benefit to patients in those hospitals with initially favourable therapeutic situations and a high discharge rate. While the condition of patients in these hospitals may have been improved, in spite of the insignificant changes in discharge rate, drug effects are not independent of changes in the social policies and condition of mental hospitals (Lewis, 1959).

When the disabilities of chronic female schizophrenic patients in three mental hospitals were examined, the proportion of patients with a similar disability varied widely (Brown and Wing, 1962). In one hospital 8% of the patients were mute; in another 24%. The amount of drugs prescribed in these three hospitals also varied widely, and could not be related to the differences in the patients' clinical and social state (Wing and Brown, 1961). Such differences were significantly related to the degree of social change and improvement in the hospital environment.

In their account of the results of treatment in schizophrenia, Kelly and Sargant (1965) claim that for two-thirds of relatively acute patients in their first admission, treatment with drugs results in a good outcome in terms of

76

social functioning. When the clinical condition of these patients is examined closely, one-third are seen to be symptom-free while another third, who appear to be functioning satisfactorily, have residual symptoms at the end of 2 years. The final third are more severely disabled; they have persistent symptoms and their social condition is one of dependence on others, either in the community or in a psychiatric hospital. The significant change, if these figures are compared with those of previous years (Harris *et al.*, 1956; Rohde and Sargant, 1961), is the reduction in the size of the group of patients with severe disabilities, and the increase in the number of patients with partial disability who are "socially independent".

In the use of drugs and social methods in the treatment of schizophrenia, one must take account both of the nature of the patient's social environment, in or out of hospital, and of his disabilities. The treatment of the schizophrenic who recovers without the development of significant disability will not be discussed here. Consideration will be given in this review only to those schizophrenic patients with a relapsing illness or severe disabilities. These patients make up at least half of all schizophrenic patients and this half presents the most difficult treatment problems. Social change, which must involve the re-organization of psychiatric hospital practices and community services, will have to be undertaken, and the part which drug therapy plays must also be reconsidered if any further advance is to be made.

The Severely Disabled Schizophrenic Patient

One-third of all patients with schizophrenia now coming to treatment for the first time develop severe disabilities. In the past such patients have accumulated in mental hospitals, and nearly three-quarters of the long-stay population in the United Kingdom is accounted for by the disease. Their primary disabilities are indicated by the chronic symptoms of schizophrenia. Secondary disabilities are often caused by institutionalization, but may also be found in patients who have never been admitted to hospital. These secondary disabilities include the patients' unhopeful attitudes to themselves and to work, as well as changes in personal habits, which have been engendered by lack of activity and stimulation in the home or the hospital. For the patient, they are as handicapping as a primary disability.

The main influence of drug treatment appears to be on primary disability, that is, on the symptoms of the patient's illness. The extent of this effect is not easily estimated. Calwell, Jacobsen and Skarbek (1964) in a short-term trial of oxypertine, assessed the results of treatment on chronic schizophrenic patients. They used the Wing rating scale, which showed a significant improvement in individual symptoms, particularly poverty of speech, although there was no significant change in the patient's basic mental state. Similar experiments have shown that while environmental factors may affect some schizophrenic symptoms, others like irritability, slowed speech and movement, hebephrenic symptoms, self-care or indifference to the environment are only affected by phenothiazine treatment (Goldberg, Klerman and Cole, 1965).

The effects of drug administration are often controlled by the use of a placebo in a double-blind experiment. The social environment in which the drug trial takes place is rarely controlled. An exception is a study of the effects of reserpine (Wing, 1956), in which behavioural changes in the treated patients were rated and compared with ratings made by a social psychologist of the behaviour of untreated patients in the same disturbed female ward (Folkard, 1959). Ratings of the mental state of the patients taking reserpine showed a significant reduction in "hostility". Observations made by the social psychologist showed no significant difference between the experimental and control groups in regard to the number of patients involved in aggressive incidents. Surprisingly, both groups improved. It was suggested that reserpine not only reduced aggression in patients receiving it, but also in patients not receiving the drug, whom the treated patients had previously provoked. These authors showed that subsequent changes in the social situation of the ward, caused by opening the ward doors or changing the staff, could result in similar alterations in the number of aggressive incidents.

A further study of relationships between the effect of tranquillizing drugs and the mental hospital ward environment has been reported (Rathod, 1958). Two groups of disturbed women patients in separate wards, three-quarters of whom were schizophrenic, were observed over a period of $3\frac{1}{2}$ years. Their behaviour and the incidence of disturbances on the wards were recorded. A control period, during which drugs had not yet taken effect, was followed by a period when one-third of the patients were taking chlorpromazine. The behaviour of patients on both wards improved. In the third period, almost half of the patients were on phenothiazine drugs, but there was no further improvement in their behaviour; instead, there was a slight deterioration. In the fourth period, an active social programme of occupation and recreation, together with staff discussions, was introduced in both wards, and at the same time the phenothiazine drugs were replaced, for all except a few patients, by placebo tablets. This was done without the knowledge of patients or staff. The social programme was accepted enthusiastically in one ward and was virtually rejected in the other. Patient behaviour continued to improve—most markedly in the ward adopting the social programme. Not only were both wards as quiet as when tranquillizers were being given, but further improvement in patient behaviour resulted from the social changes. In the last phase, nurses in the best ward were told about the placebos, and within a short time the ward showed signs of increased disturbance.

When chlorpromazine was combined with an intensive occupational therapy programme for chronic schizophrenic patients, it was found that both contributed significantly to the resulting improvement (Grygier and Waters, 1958). Occupational therapy was more effective in the long run than chlorpromazine, which altered the speed rather than the level of improvement. While the investigators assumed that drugs and occupation acted synergistically, this relationship may be more complicated. If a period of drug treatment is preceded by a phase during which patients are exposed only to the influences of the social environment, those patients improving with the *milieu* will respond poorly to drugs, and vice vera (Rashkis and Smarr, 1957). These authors showed statistically that there was an inverse curvilinear relationship between the effect of drugs and the social environment. Other models for this relationship have been described (Klerman, 1963).

The relative effect of chemotherapy and social influences for schizophrenic patients in hospital can be observed when drugs are discontinued. The results are contradictory and have been reviewed by Caffey *et al.* (1964) who undertook a controlled study in which placebos were substituted for phenothiazines in the treatment of chronic schizophrenics from sixteen Veterans Hospitals. While all patients do not relapse when drugs are discontinued, the authors found that 45% of patients on placebo relapsed within 4 months, as compared with 5% of schizophrenics on continued treatment. They do not say whether staff or patients were informed of the nature of the experiment. While all the patients had a stay of over 2 years, they are not distinguished according to the severity of their mental disabilities. Nor are the hospitals' social programmes described. However, they believe that since the relapses were evenly distributed between the sixteen hospitals, environmental factors were not important. This view would seem to contradict those studies which report considerable differences between the social condition of individual hospitals (Brown and Wing, 1962; Odegard, 1964; Jackson, 1964).

One may conclude that for severely disabled schizophrenic patients, the social environment and chemotherapy each have effects which are interrelated in a complex manner (Rashkis and Smarr, 1957; Odegard, 1964). Drugs may in some schizophrenic patients lessen primary disabilities, by reducing such symptoms as poverty of speech or social withdrawal. They may themselves produce social change in a hospital ward. If staff react favourably to improvements in patient behaviour, their assumption of more hopeful and tolerant attitudes may encourage interest and effort, which further reduce the patients' disabilities (Rathod, 1958). Similarly, a reduction in aggressive behaviour will change the social atmosphere of the ward, with benefit to non-aggressive patients (Wing, 1956; Folkard, 1959). When such improvements have been achieved, many schizophrenic patients are left with a wide range of disabilities, which are unlikely to be influenced by drug treatment (Catterson, Bennett and Freudenberg, 1963). For them, further improvement is more likely to result from change in the hospital environment and an active rehabilitation programme.

The "Middle Case" Schizophrenic Patient

The term "middle case" was used by Woodhead and Varrier-Jones (1920) to describe those patients with pulmonary tuberculosis who had a relapsing illness. A "middle case" schizophrenic is a patient who is at present living independently and working in the community, but who has persisting symptoms which are poorly controlled. These patients seem to have a greater tendency to break down under stress than other schizophrenic patients. Their social functioning is marginal; they live in the community, but they are not cured. They have difficulties in getting on with people, are often unable to make decisions and frequently cannot work under stress. Their continuing independence rests heavily on tolerant public and medical attitudes (Hopkins, 1965), and on an economic situation of full employment. They are an emotional and an economic burden to their families.

The most frequent cause of their re-admission to hospital is not, as for the chronic patient, a failure of social function, but the recurrence of acute symptoms (Freeman and Simmons, 1963). Such relapse may be occasioned either by environmental stress or by the discontinuation of medication. Pasamanick et al. (1964) undertook a double-blind controlled study, in which schizophrenic patients were treated at home under the careful supervision of public health nurses, with either a phenothiazine or a placebo. After 18 months, 83% of the patients on the drugs had remained continuously in the community, compared with 55% of those on placebos. That 17% of the patients taking phenothiazines had to be re-admitted shows that drugs alone cannot completely control symptoms. It is also evident that many schizophrenics can be cared for at home, without drugs, if they are given social support. The avoidance of hospital admission is not the only aim of treatment, and the authors note that the functioning of all too many "successful" patients was far from satisfactory. They found that families were often reluctant to look after a patient whose care imposed economic strain and caused family disorganization. Gross et al. (1961) studied the problem in another way. They separated their out-patients who were "predominantly schizophrenic" into a "control" group and a "withdrawal" group. The drugs of the patients in the "control" group were maintained, and those of the "withdrawal" group gradually decreased until they were eventually terminated over a period of 2 months. All the "withdrawal" patients then received a placebo, identical in appearance with the original tablets or capsules. Relapse was evaluated in terms of psychiatric symptoms alone. During a preliminary observation phase in which all patients were on drugs 13% relapsed, and during the experimental period 14% of the "control" subjects relapsed, compared with 57% of the "withdrawal" subjects. They noted that those patients whose families welcomed them, or who were themselves able to undertake family responsibilities, did better than the others. These studies show the importance of drugs in influencing the outcome for "independent" schizophrenic patients living in the community. They do not indicate the relative importance of such social factors as family attitudes or the patient's effect on his family in this situation.

For a study of these factors, one must turn to the work of Brown *et al.* (1962) who demonstrated the influence of the family situation on the probability of male schizophrenic patients being re-admitted to hospital. The patient's chance of re-admission within 1 year was related to ratings of his emotional relationship to, and the hours which he spent with, his closest relatives. The attitudes of families to 84 schizophrenic patients, discharged from hospitals to their own homes in the London area, was examined by Wing *et al.* (1964). Of these patients, 41% were welcomed or tolerated, but in 14% relatives showed considerable anxiety about what the patient would do next. The families of the remaining 45% were distressed by the patient's behaviour. In these cases, the patient was often violent or suicidal, noisy at night or involved his relatives in his delusions. For the "independent" schizophrenic patient, both drugs and family relationships play their part in preventing, or precipitating a relapse of the illness. Their combined effect has never been investigated.

Engelhardt *et al.* (1964), examining the effect of administering chlorpromazine and placebo to chronic schizophrenic patients under double-blind conditions, found that while chlorpromazine was effective in preventing admission, this effect diminished progressively over time. In contrast, the admission rates of patients on placebo were similar, regardless of time. They concluded that prolonged chlorpromazine administration delays, rather than prevents, hospital admission. On the other hand, Kris (1962a) suggests that if drug treatment is used together with active follow-up and rehabilitation, it can produce a significant reduction in the rate of re-admission to hospital. At present, when the "middle case" schizophrenic patient is re-admitted to hospital, his symptoms are usually rapidly controlled by the administration of phenothiazines and by his removal from a stressful environment. When the patient, after a short period of time in hospital, returns to the social environment in which he originally broke down, it is not surprising if further re-admissions follow. For the "middle case" patient who is re-admitted to hospital, an adequate assessment of his family situation, and a revaluation of his work and social capacities are essential. Family case-work and, if necessary, rehabilitation of the patient should also be undertaken (Bennett, Folkard and Nicholson, 1961).

The studies quoted seem to show that a reduction in social stress and in maintenance of drug treatment are both needed to maintain the "middle case" schizophrenic patient in health and social independence. Social stress may result in relapse, even when drugs are taken. In the absence of stress, failure to continue with the phenothiazine medication may result in breakdown or the recurrence of symptoms which disturb the family. While drugs and a reduction in social stress seem to complement each other in the treatment of the "middle case", further research may show relationships similar to those demonstrated for more handicapped patients.

Rehabilitation and Resettlement

Rehabilitation is the process of restoring a disabled schizophrenic patient to a situation in which he can make the best use of his residual capacities, in as normal a social context as possible. It should be distinguished from resettlement, which is the placement of the patient in employment. It is accepted in rehabilitation that the primary disabilities—the symptoms of the illness—may not be reducible beyond a certain minimal level. For those patients whose symptoms are not influenced by phenothiazine treatment, rehabilitation is a matter of changing attitudes and personal habits, which are the secondary handicaps. Not all schizophrenic patients suffer from fixed or stable primary disabilities. In many, symptoms fluctuate and for such patients, drugs play a part in reducing this instability. During the period on drug treatment, the patient's social and work potential must be developed. This means that patients must relearn former work and social habits, under conditions in which the expectations of performance are gradually increased. It is not enough for a patient who is going to be resettled to be able to function in the hospital setting; he must build up reserves, which will enable him to manage the greater stresses which he will experience when he returns to work. Even with adequate preparation, he may not be able to tolerate very much stress. For these reasons, it is a sensible policy to let the patient return to work while continuing to live in the hospital. He can better tolerate the extra problems of his discharge at a later date. Increasing the stress on schizophrenic patients, by activating them, is not without risk. Patients who have been free from florid symptoms for years may once again exhibit delusions or other symptoms when they are transferred to a resettlement ward or to an industrial rehabilitation unit (Stone and Eldred, 1959). While the use of phenothiazines will help to control the reactivation of such symptoms, it is not an alternative to the employment of "graded stress" in preparing the patient for resettlement (Wing, Bennett and Denham, 1964). Two carefully matched groups of chronic male schizophrenic patients from two mental hospitals in the London area attended the same industrial rehabilitation unit, while still living in hospital. Twenty-four patients from Hospital A had been socially prepared for resettlement; 4 were taking chlorpromazine; the rest were taking no drugs at all. In Hospital B, rehabilitation and preparation services had been less fully developed at the time of the experiment. Of the 21 patients attending the industrial rehabilitation unit from this hospital, only 4 were not on drugs. One patient from Hospital A who was not on phenothiazines, and 5 patients from Hospital B who were all taking drugs showed an exacerbation of their symptoms at the industrial rehabilitation unit. At the end of the follow-up year, 16 patients from Hospital A and 8 patients from Hospital B were employed. It is possible that more patients from Hospital B had an unstable relapsing form of schizophrenia, but there was no evidence of this. Nor could differences in their premorbid personality be found. When all possibilities had been considered, it seemed likely that differences in preparation and social treatment in the two hospitals accounted for the patients' differing susceptibility to relapse, and the success or failure of their resettlement. While these results might be thought to indicate the superiority of social treatment, it must be pointed out that most of the patients from Hospital A had received drug treatment during some stage of their rehabilitation. The results suggest that drugs and social therapy have separate, though interdependent, functions. They cannot replace each other completely, but must be used in a planned sequence.

After-care

Some schizophrenic patients will be resettled; others will be discharged to live as invalids in the community. Both will need various forms of social support and some will need continuing treatment with the phenothiazine drugs. Schizophrenic patients share the reported reluctance of those suffering from various medical conditions to take drugs over long periods. Such attitudes to continued treatment may be influenced by the belief that all drugs are habit-forming, or by the view that continued medication is an admission of personal inadequacy. Family, friends and workmates may encourage the patient to discontinue treatment. Families may desire to suppress memories of the patient's illness, and to this end will avoid contact with the psychiatrist (Schwartz and Schwartz, 1964). The schizophrenic patient and his family may lose interest in treatment, once they believe that he is cured; they will be unwilling to accept the fact that he needs continuing care to prevent repeated episodes of illness (Scarpitti et al., 1964). Patients themselves may refuse to take tablets without giving reasons, or they may express delusional ideas about drugs and their effects. They may deny that medication is producing improvement, or may complain of side-effects such as obesity or lassitude. They may even have objections on the grounds of conscience. Patients who have not been admitted to a mental hospital previously are significantly less likely to take their prescribed phenothiazines than those who have been in-patients (Engelhardt, Freedman and Mann, 1963). General practitioners are still poorly informed about, or have little belief in, the need for continued medication. Of eight general practitioners interviewed by Rawnsley and Loudon (1962), only four believed in physical treatment for psychiatric illness. Parkes, Brown and Monck (1962) have confirmed the known reluctance of general practitioners to prescribe major tranquillizers in adequate dosage. Psychiatrists, for their part, too readily assume that the medication is being taken as prescribed, and rarely check this by the use of a urine test (Forrest and Forrest, 1957).

Renton *et al.* (1963) concluded from their experience that there is a need for special clinics, in which all schizophrenic patients discharged from hospital can be followed-up regularly for a period of 2 years. In such a situation, the patient's urine could be tested for the presence of phenothiazines, which could be prescribed and supervised by the psychiatrist. Supportive community services could be organized by this clinic. Medication has been successfully supervised by public health nurses in the United States (Freyhan and Merkel, 1961; Scarpitti *et al.*, 1964). Such supervision does not do away with the need for the education of patients and their families, and for the instruction of general practitioners. Patients' own views and wishes must be considered. Some patients who will not take tablets will accept the phenothiazines if they are given in liquid form. None of the studies quoted claim significant therapeutic superiority for any drug (NIMH—PSC, 1964), the therapist's choice may depend therefore on the patients' acceptance or rejection of side-effects. Patients who are working complain frequently of drowsiness in the afternoon, if chlorpromazine is administered twice or thrice daily. Experience shows that they less commonly refuse, or forget to take, a single maintenance dose of 150–200 mg of chlorpromazine given in the evening. Such a dose is adequate and well tolerated. It has been suggested that those patients on phenothiazines who develop tension and depression respond well if an anti-depressant drug is added (Kris and Gerst, 1964; Kelly and Sargant, 1965). The dosages of the major tranquillizers recommended vary widely. Kelly and Sargant (1965) treated 8% of their cases with daily doses of more than 300 mg of chlorpromazine or its equivalent. Patients in the group described by Renton *et al.* (1963) took up to the equivalent of 1000 mg of chlorpromazine daily. Adelson and Epstein (1962) employed doses of up to 3000 mg of chlorpromazine or 240 mg of perphenazine daily.

If treatment with the major tranquillizers is to be continued over a period of time, it is important to know whether such treatment has any serious effect on the patient. Dinitz *et al.* (1964) found that prolonged treatment with phenothiazines had no effect on the mental functions of patients, as measured by a number of psychological performance tests. Kris (1962b) reported the condition of 31 children, born to mothers taking phenothiazines during pregnancy. There was no adverse effect on the mother, the foetus or on the early years of the child's development. A reversible or irreversible bucco-linguo-masticatory dyskinesia may result from phenothiazine medication

(Uhrbrand and Faurbye, 1960; Hunter, Earl and Thornicroft, 1964). Perphenazine is most likely to produce this undesirable effect, which occurs most commonly in elderly patients with associated organic brain lesions. Ocular and skin changes also follow the long-continued administration of phenothiazines, particularly chlorpromazine (Barsa, Newton and Saunders, 1965; Cairns, Capoore and Gregory, 1965). Visual acuity is impaired only occasionally, but the cutaneous changes are a cosmetic liability. Such complications may revive interest in the possibilities of the intermittent administration of phenothiazines, or the use of lower doses (Caffey et al., 1964).

Whatever attitudes are shown to the continuous use of tranquillizers by patients, their families or their doctors, social measures will continue to play an important part in the after-care of schizophrenic patients. Family stress may be reduced through the efforts of social workers, or by the separation of the patient from relatives with whom he does not get on. Such separation can be effected in many ways, e.g. by the relative or the patient going out to work, or by accommodating the patient in a hostel. The value of work for the schizophrenic patient's continued well-being is widely recognized. If he is too disabled to obtain open employment, some form of sheltered occupation should be found for him. Even if he is satisfactorily employed, he will still need continuing help and advice. It has been found that when a disabled schizophrenic loses his job, he may lack the initiative to find another, without help. Many will need continuing after-care for long periods. It seems evident that the best results will be obtained by the combined use of social measures and tranquillizing drugs.

Summary

In this discussion of the use of tranquillizing drugs and social methods in the treatment of schizophrenic patients, it is suggested that they should be combined to produce optimal results. Their use and relative efficacy will be influenced both by the nature and extent of the patient's disabilities, and by his social circumstances, in or out of hospital. From the patient's point of view, it is not enough to reduce or abolish symptoms. It is necessary to help him re-establish and maintain the highest degree of social functioning of which he is capable. In doing this, one cannot overlook the patient's effect on the hospital ward or his family, nor their influence on his illness.

References

ADELSON, D. and EPSTEIN, L. J. (1962), A study of phenothiazines with male and female chronically ill schizophrenic patients, J. nerv. ment. Dis. 134, 543.
BARSA, J. A., NEWTON, J. C. and SAUNDERS, J. C. (1965), Lenticular and corneal opacities, J. Am. med. Ass. 193, 10.

Bennett, D. H., Folkard, S. and Nicholson, A. K. (1961), Resettlement unit in a mental hospital, *Lancet*, **ii**, 539.

Brill, H. and Patton, R. E. (1959), Analysis of population reduction in New York State mental hospitals during the first four years of large-scale therapy with psychotropic drugs, *Am. J. Psychiat.* **116**, 495.

Brown, G. W. and Wing, J. K. (1962), A comparative clinical and social survey of three mental hospitals, *Sociol. Rev. Monog.* **5**, 145.

Brown, G. W., Monck, E. M., Carstairs, G. M. and Wing, J. K. (1962), The influence of family life on the course of schizophrenic illness *Brit. J. prev. soc. Med.* **16**, 55.

Caffey, E. M., Diamond, L. S., Frank, T. V., Grasberger, J. C., Herman, L., Klett, C. J. and Rothstein, C. (1964), Discontinuation or reduction of chemotherapy in chronic schizophrenics, *J. chron. Dis.* **17**, 347.

Cairns, R. J., Capoore, H. S. and Gregory, I. D. R. (1965), Oculocutaneous changes after years on high doses of chlorpromazine, *Lancet*, **i**, 239.

Calwell, W. P. K., Jacobsen, M. and Skarbek, A. (1964), A comparative study of oxypertine and trifluorperazine in chronic schizophrenics—a new application of the Wing rating scale, *Brit. J. Psychiat.* **110**, 520.

Catterson, A. G., Bennett, D. H. and Freudenberg, R. K. (1963), A survey of long stay schizophrenic patients, *Brit. J. Psychiat.* **109**, 750.

Dinitz, S., Scarpitti, F. R., Albini, J. L., Lefton, M. and Pasamanick, B. (1964), *An Experimental Study in the Prevention of Hospitalization of Schizophrenics: Thirty Months of Experience*. Mimeographed.

Engelhardt, D., Freedman, N. and Mann, D. (1963), The influence of previous hospitalization on the clinical course of psychopharmacologically treated schizophrenic outpatients, *Comp. Psychiat.* **4**, 337.

Engelhardt, D. M., Freedman, N., Rosen, B., Mann, D. and Margolis, R. (1964), Phenothiazines in the prevention of psychiatric hospitalization, *Arch. gen. Psychiat.* **11**, 162.

Folkard, M. S. (1959), A sociological contribution to the understanding of aggression and its treatment, *Netherne Monog.* No. 1.

Forrest, F. M. and Forrest, I. S. (1957), A simple test for the detection of chlorpromazine in urine, *Am. J. Psychiat.* **113**, 931.

Freeman, H. E. and Simmons, O. G. (1963), *The Mental Patient comes Home*, New York, Wiley.

Freyhan, F. A. and Merkel, J. (1961), Clinical and Social Aspects of Compensatory Drug Treatment, In *Mental Patients in Transition*, p. 302 (ed. Greenblatt, M. *et al.*), Springfield, Ill., Thomas.

Goldberg, S. C., Klerman, G. L. and Cole, J. C. (1965), Change in schizophrenic psychopathology and ward behaviour as a function of phenothiazine treatment, *Brit. J. Psychiat.* **111**, 120.

Gross, M., Mitchman, I. L., Reeves, W. P., Lawrence, J. L. and Newell, P. C. (1961), Discontinuation of treatment with ataractic drugs, *Recent Advances in Biological Psychiatry*, **3**, 44.

Grygier, P. and Waters, M. A. (1958), Chlorpromazine used with an intensive occupational therapy program, *Arch. Neurol. & Psychiat.* **79**, 697.

Harris, A., Norris, V., Linker, I. and Shepherd, M. (1956), Schizophrenia: a prognostic and social study, *Brit. J. prev. soc. Med.* **10**, 107.

Hopkins, J. H. S. (1965), Letter: the discharged schizophrenic, *Brit. med. J.* **i**, 383.

Hunter, R., Earl, C. J. and Thornicroft, S. (1964), An apparently irreversible syndrome of abnormal movements following phenothiazine medication, *Proc. roy. Soc. Med.* **57**, 758.

Jackson, J. (1964), Chapter 3. Toward the Comparative Study of Mental Hospitals: Characteristics of the Treatment Environment, p. 35, In *The Psychiatric Hospital as a Social System*, Springfield, Ill., Thomas.

Kelly, D. H. W. and Sargant, W. (1965), Present treatment of schizophrenia—a controlled follow-up study, *Brit. med. J.* **i**, 147.

Klerman, G. L. (1963), Assessing the influence of the hospital milieu upon the effectiveness of psychiatric drug therapy: problems of conceptualization and of research methodology, *J. nerv. ment. Dis.* **137**, 143.

KRAMER, M. and POLLACK, E. S. (1958), Problems in the interpretation of trends in the population movement of the public mental hospitals, *Am. J. pub. Health*, **48**, 1003.

KRIS, E. B. (1962a), Five years' experience with the use of drugs and psychotherapy in a community aftercare clinic, Suppl. *Am. J. pub. Health*, **52**, 9.

KRIS, E. B. (1962b), Children born to mothers maintained on pharmacotherapy during pregnancy and postpartum, *Recent Advances in Biological Psychiatry*, **4**, 180, New York, Plenum Press.

KRIS, E. B. and GERST, D. (1964), Combined perphenazine—amitriptylline as adjuvant therapy in psychiatric aftercare, *Amer. J. Psychiat.* **121**, 498.

LEWIS, A. J. (1959), The impact of psychotropic drugs on the structure, function and future of psychiatric services (a) In the hospitals, *Neuropsychopharmacology*, 207–212. Proc. First Int. Cong. Neuropsychopharmacology, Rome, 1958 (Bradley *et al.*, eds.), Amsterdam, Elsevier, 1959.

NIMH—PSC, COLLABORATIVE STUDY GROUP (1964), Phenothiazine treatment in acute schizophrenia, *Arch. gen. Psychiat.* **10**, 246.

ODEGARD, O. (1964), Pattern of discharge from Norwegian psychiatric hospitals before and after the introduction of the psychotropic drugs, *Am. J. Psychiat.* **120**, 772.

PARKES, C. M., BROWN, G. W. and MONCK, E. M. (1962), The general practitioner and the schizophrenic patient, *Brit. med. J.* **i**, 972.

PASAMANICK, B., SCARPITTI, F. R., LEFTON, M., DINITZ, S., WERNERT, J. J. and McPHEETERS, H. (1964), Home versus hospital care for schizophrenics, *J. Am. med. Ass.* **187**, 177.

RASHKIS, H. A. and SMARR, E. R. (1957), Drug and milieu effects with chronic schizophrenics, *Arch. Neurol. Psychiat.* **78**, 89.

RATHOD, N. H. (1958), Tranquillizers and patients' environment, *Lancet*, **i**, 611.

RAWNSLEY, K. and LOUDON, J. B. (1962), The attitudes of general practitioners to psychiatry, *Sociol. Rev. Monog.* **5**, 49.

RENTON, C. A., AFFLECK, J. W., CARSTAIRS, G. M. and FORREST, A. D. (1963). A follow-up of schizophrenic patients in Edinburgh, *Arch. psychiat. Scand.* **39**, 548.

ROHDE, P. and SARGANT, W. (1961), Treatment of schizophrenic in general hospitals, *Brit. med. J.* **ii**, 67.

SCARPITTI, F. R., LEFTON, M., DINITZ, S. and PASAMANICK, B. (1964), Problems in a home case study for schizophrenics, *Arch. gen. Psychiat.* **10**, 143.

SCHWARTZ, M. S. and SCHWARTZ, C. G. (1964), *Social Approaches to Mental Patient Care*, New York, Columbia University Press.

SHEPHERD, M., GOODMAN, N. and WATT, D. C. (1961), Application of hospital statistics in the evaluation of pharmacotherapy in a psychiatric population, *Compr. Psychiat.* **2**, 11.

SHERMAN, L. (1959), The significant variables in psychopharmaceutic research, *Am. J. Psychiat.* **116**, 208.

STONE, A. A. and ELDRED, S. H. (1959), Delusion formation during the activation of chronic schizophrenic patients, *Arch. gen. Psychiat.* **1**, 177.

UHRBRAND, L. and FAURBYE, A. (1960), Reversible and irreversible dyskinesia after treatment with perphenazine, chlorpromazine, reserpine and electroconvulsive therapy, *Psychopharmacologica*, **1**, 408.

WING, L. (1956), The use of reserpine in chronic psychiatric patients: a controlled trial, *J. ment. Sci.* **102**, 530.

WING, J. K. and BROWN, G. W. (1961), Social treatment of schizophrenia: a comparative study of three mental hospitals, *J. ment. Sci.* **107**, 847.

WING, J. K., BENNETT, D. H. and DENHAM, J. (1964), *The Industrial Rehabilitation of Long-stay Schizophrenic Patients. A Study of 45 Patients in an Industrial Rehabilitation Unit*, M.R.C. Memo No. 42, London, H.M.S.O.

WING, J. K., MONCK, E. M., BROWN, G. W. and CARSTAIRS, G. M. (1964), Morbidity in the community of schizophrenic patients discharged from London mental hospitals in 1959, *Brit. J. Psychiat.* **110**, 10.

WOODHEAD, G. and VARRIER-JONES, P. C. (1920), *Industrial Colonies and Village Settlements for the Consumptive*, Cambridge, Cambridge Univ. Press.

5. Epidemiology and Mental Disorder: a Review*

MICHAEL SHEPHERD and BRIAN COOPER

THOUGH it is now fashionable to speak of the epidemiology of mental illness, this conjunction of terms appeared in the literature only rarely before 1949, when it was chosen as the title of a conference organized by the Milbank Memorial Fund to explore common ground between psychiatrists and public health workers (Milbank Memorial Fund, 1950). Since then a spate of publications, especially in North America, the Scandinavian countries, and the United Kingdom, has signalized the confluence of two medical disciplines. The number of these investigations is now so large, and their nature so varied, that it is advisable to demarcate the boundaries of psychiatric epidemiology. In Britain this task has been made easier by the cataloguing of current research projects by the M.R.C. Committee on the Epidemiology of Mental Disorder (Rawnsley, 1963), itself only some 4 years old. Just over 100 projects are listed, of which approximately one-third are focused on the psychological and social aspects of mental illness, either causal or concomitant; about one-quarter, which includes genetic studies, are concerned with the incidence or prevalence of different forms of psychiatric morbidity; one-sixth concentrate on prognostic or follow-up studies, and almost as many on primarily administrative issues; the remaining small miscellany comprises studies of diagnosis, vital statistics, and the evaluation of therapeutic procedures.

These topics can be taken as representative of the modern view of the scope of the epidemiological method in psychiatry; they fit well, for example, into the outline sketched by Lin in his recent W.H.O. monograph (Lin and Standley, 1962). At the same time, it is apparent that to call the majority of such studies "epidemiological" is, in one sense, to do little more than attach new labels to old bottles: their objectives have been among the legitimate goals of psychiatric research for over a century. Clearly, some understanding of the evolution of psychiatric epidemiology is necessary if its present status and, still more important, its future prospects are to be assessed.

Historical Development

Many of our current notions on psychiatric epidemiology were in circulation before 1914, the year in which Goldberger published the first of a series

* Reprinted from the *Journal of Neurology, Neurosurgery and Psychiatry* (1964) **27**, 277.

of papers which were to demonstrate beyond argument the professional epidemiologist's contribution to the study of mental illness. There were several well-documented accounts of the so-called psychic epidemics. The development of intelligence testing and the early studies of suicide had established the value of the ecologist's method; and the older psychiatrists, as Lewis has pointed out, were familiar with such basic epidemiological themes as the relationship between mental disorder and migration, isolation, occupation, and socio-economic change (Lewis, 1962).

In view of these promising trends, it is of more than historical interest to examine the reasons for the relative neglect of the mass aspects of mental disorder in the earlier part of this century. How well the concepts of epidemiology had been established is clear from Frost's masterly review, published in 1927, which summed up the thinking of his day (Frost, 1927). Epidemiology, he wrote, being

> essentially a collective science, its progress is largely dependent upon that which has been made in other fields. Since the description of the distribution of any disease in a population obviously requires that the disease must be recognized when it occurs, the development of epidemiology must follow and be limited by clinical diagnosis, and by the rather complex machinery required for the systematic collection of morbidity and mortality statistics. Epidemiology must also draw upon statistical methods and theory, because even the simplest quantitative descriptions must be stated statistically; and more minute descriptions, involving perhaps the demonstration of complex associations, may require the application of quite elaborate statistical technique. Moreover, quantitative epidemiological descriptions, in terms of frequencies of disease in different population groups, require, as part of their data, more or less detailed statistics of population, implying the prior development of demography.

Unfortunately, Frost's vision was partially blinkered by the conventions of his day, for he goes on:

> usage has extended the meaning of epidemiology beyond its original limits, to denote not merely the doctrine of epidemics, but a science of broader scope in relation to the mass phenomena of diseases in their usual or endemic as well as their epidemic occurrences. Although it is clear from current usage that the definition of epidemiology has been extended beyond its original sense, it is not clear just how far it has been extended. It is certain that its scope is not usually limited to the diseases in which epidemics are characteristic, since it is entirely in conformity with good usage to speak of the epidemiology of tuberculosis; and it seems customary also to apply the term to the mass phenomena of such non-infectious diseases as scurvy, but not to the so-called constitutional diseases, such as arteriosclerosis and nephritis . . .
> In this sense epidemiology may be defined as the science of the mass phenomena of infectious diseases, or as the natural history of the infectious diseases.

Inasmuch as this definition would exclude most mental illness from the purview of the epidemiologists, their disregard of psychiatry—with some rare and distinguished exceptions—could be attributed to the state of development of their subject. The failure of their leading psychiatric contemporaries to interest themselves in the mass phenomena of mental illness, on the other hand, can be more readily explained in terms of professional priorities. Many psychiatrists were preoccupied with a set of biological and phenomenological concepts, hoping to establish a scientific nosology with, in Adolf Meyer's words, "the psychological facts in their patients as mere symptoms of more or less hypothetical diseases back of them" (Meyer, 1912). Yet to the more discerning epidemiologists these "psychological facts" were inseparably part of the mass phenomena of mental disorder; to Greenwood, for example, they figured prominently among his procatarctic factors of disease, and he wrote of them with characteristic hard-headedness:

> It is my business to point out that while a fairly consistent description of the aetiology of such crowd-diseases . . . can be provided by means of the hypothesis that the psychological element in the mixture of interactions expressed in bodily illness is the determinant, methods which have ignored that element have led to no consistent account of the facts at all. For this severely practical reason I hold that practical epidemiologists cannot afford to neglect psychology. *What* psychology they should study is not for me to say (Greenwood, 1935).

Thirty years later, it is easier to appreciate that for the epidemiologist, concerned primarily with the study of populations, a meaningful psychology must extend beyond the individual organism. Unfortunately such a psychology was lacking a generation ago. Meyerian commonsense psychology, shaped by its originator's interest in the social sciences and construing mental illness as "the reaction of a personality (conceived as made up of constitutional endowment plus experience) to a situation in the social environment" (Leighton, 1951), might have provided an acceptable theoretical system had it not been for the clumsiness of most psychobiological formulations. At the same time, attempts to frame a theory of group behaviour based on instinctual propensities (Trotter, 1942) became submerged by the growing influence of Freudian psychology, and were to remain neglected until the contemporary renewal of interest arising from comparative ethology. In his discussion of group psychology Freud gave lucid expression to the latent antithesis between his own outlook and that of the social psychologist:

> Group psychology is . . . concerned with the individual man as a member of a race, of a nation, or as a component part of a crowd of people who have been organized into a group at some particular time for some particular purpose. When once natural continuity has been severed in this way, if a breach is thus made between things which are by nature interconnected, it is easy to regard the phenomena which appear under these special conditions as being expressions of a special instinct ("herd instinct", "group mind"), which does not come to light in any other situations. But we may perhaps venture to object that it seems difficult to attribute to the factor of number a significance so great as to make it capable by itself of arousing in our mental life a new instinct that is otherwise not brought into play. Our expectation is therefore directed towards two other possibilities, that the social instinct may not be a primitive one and insusceptible of dissection, and that it may be possible to discover the beginnings of its development in a narrower circle, such as that of the family. (Freud, 1955.)

While this point of view does not preclude an interest in the mass phenomena of disease, the emphasis of so authoritative a theorist tended to produce a concentration on individual psychopathology at the expense of a psychology of social involvement. Indeed, as one sympathetic critic has observed: "With certain exceptions, social pyschology and psychoanalysis do not contradict each other—they no longer speak the same language" (Brown, 1961). Linguistic difficulties can be expected to impair communication. It is therefore not surprising that misunderstandings arose between epidemiologists and depth psychologists over questions of mutual interest. Psychodynamic embellishments, for example, lent a baroque façade to the severe outlines of the notion of accident proneness; and psychoanalysts have tended to show so little regard for the ecological approach to suicide that as late as the mid-1930's one of their most prominent representatives could claim that " . . . statistical data on suicide as they are compiled today deserve little if any credence" (Zilboorg, 1936).

But if the growth of epidemiological psychiatry between the wars was retarded by these circumstances, a few investigators were able to anticipate the subsequent renaissance. Far-sighted workers in the public health field, like Greenwood and Wilson, initiated collaborative studies with psychiatrists. Some psychiatrists—E. O. Lewis in Britain, Brugger in Germany, Rosanoff in the United States—affirmed their concern with public health aspects of their work by conducting large-scale community surveys (Lewis, 1929; Brugger, 1931; and Rosanoff, 1917); while others were led to the same field of study by an interest in genetics (Strömgren, 1950). In America statisticians like Malzberg and Pollock made use of data compiled in mental hospitals (Malzberg, 1940; Pollock, 1925), and sociologists of the Chicago school began to study the urban ecology of mental illness (Faris and Dunham, 1939; Robinson, 1950). Scattered, uncoordinated, and deriving inspiration from several disciplines, these studies paved the way for the rapid expansion which was to follow the Second World War.

The rapidity of this expansion owed something to the unprecedented interest taken in the mental health of both the military and civil populations during the conflict. Its chief impulse, however, came from the post-war renewal of interest in the psychosocial components of morbidity and the emergence as a separate discipline of social, or "comprehensive", medicine. Epidemiological methods are fundamental to the aims of social medicine, which stands or falls by the ecological approach to illness—and especially to non-infectious, chronic illness where mental diseases take their natural place among Ryle's "diseases of prevalence, which also have their epidemiologies and their correlations with social and occupational conditions, and must eventually be considered to be in greater or less degree preventable" (Ryle, 1948). Already in 1944 the Goodenough Report had underlined the importance of social medicine for British psychiatry; and what we now term social psychiatry has flourished to the point of pre-eminence in this country. The working assumption of the social psychiatrist is contained in Morris Ginsberg's statement that: "Though the individual consists largely of his social relations, there is a core of individuality in each person which is uniquely his own and which is in the last resort unshareable and uncommunicable" (Ginsberg, 1956). It is an assumption which harmonizes not only with the undogmatic eclecticism of British psychiatry but also with the philosophy of the National Health Service in a welfare state where the conflicting claims of the citizen and his society constitute a basic political issue.

Problems of Method

An historical perspective, then, however limited in scope, can elucidate some of the reasons for the recent upsurge of interest in epidemiological psychiatry. It also helps to account for the comparatively meagre success so far attained. But this relative failure cannot be fully understood without reference to the factors which limit the application of epidemiological methods to mental disease. The limitations spring partly from a lack of basic information which time and effort can be expected to supply; but over and above these remediable deficiencies are more intractable problems; for convenience these may be subsumed under two main headings, the causation of mental illness, and the classification and measurement of psychiatric disorders.

The Causation of Mental Illness

To some modern epidemiologists, there are no *a priori* grounds for regarding mental illness as qualitatively different from other types of morbidity, so that the same tools which have proved so efficacious in the study of organic disease can be readily adapted to that of psychiatric disorder. Thus Reid comments that " ... many mental illnesses are as much 'crowd diseases' as is typhoid fever", and again: "Although these (epidemiological) models were designed to fit the behaviour of infectious disease, there is no reason why some appropriate forms should not apply to the aspects of crowd behaviour, such as the dissemination of psychological disorders in human populations" (Reid, 1960).

This viewpoint overlooks some important aspects of psychiatric disorder, which are discussed in a report of the W.H.O. Expert Committee on Mental Health (W.H.O., 1960), and can be summarized as follows: first, there are individual factors in the causes and manifestations of many psychiatric diseases which, because they belong to the sphere of values, cannot be fully quantified. Secondly, the aetiology of mental disorder is essentially multifactorial in nature. Thirdly, there are considerable social and cultural differences in what is considered psychically abnormal in different surroundings, and in the way such abnormality is treated. Finally, human character and behaviour deviations show infinite variation, ranging from severe psychosis to mild personality disorders which many would regard as outside the boundaries of psychiatry.

In practice, mental illness is rarely infective, but it is often communicable. The extensive literature on mass outbreaks of irrational behaviour, extending from the so-called psychic epidemics to the more sophisticated modern studies of "socially shared psychopathology" (Gruenberg, 1957), testifies to the interest taken by many workers in the nature of this communication. Penrose has made a spirited attempt to retain the classical triad of host, environment, and agent in his mathematical model of crowd behaviour, with the morbid or exaggerated idea in the role of noxious agent (Penrose, 1952). For most workers, however, the causes of abnormal group behaviour are to be sought in the reactions of more or less predisposed individuals to particular sets of physical, psychological, or social circumstances. On this point there is agreement between attempted explanations otherwise as far apart in time and spirit as Hecker's "sympathy" or "imitation" (Hecker, 1859), Durkheim's "collective disposition" (Durkheim, 1951), and Kräupl and Taylor's "pluralistic emotions" (Taylor, Kräupl and Hunter, 1958).

This emphasis on host–environment interaction is carried over in the epidemiological approach to the large mass of non-infectious and non-communicable psychiatric illness even when a physical agent like alcohol can be identified. Traditionally the study of factors pertaining to the host has been the domain of genetics, with a large contribution from epidemiology. Recent developments in genetics, to which reference is made later in this article, have brought the two disciplines still closer and if, as Böök has recently asserted, the geneticist must now " . . . ask the question 'what does the gene do to this individual' in the same sense as the virologist inquires about the effect of a specific virus" (Böök, 1961), then the prospects of collaboration are closer still.

For the moment the epidemiologist's primary concern is with the influence brought to bear on the phenotype at different epochs of the life span. In the earliest paranatal phases of development the influences are dominantly physical; as the organism undergoes "psychosocial evolution", to borrow Medawar's phrase, so the social environment becomes increasingly important and the epidemiologist turns naturally to his colleagues in the social sciences for help. From them he has already received, and made good use of, such conceptual tools as class, mobility, isolation, and kinship; and when the delineation of social systems assumes primary importance, as with some forms of delinquent behaviour, the contribution of the social scientist becomes crucial. Unfortunately, however, the social sciences are still handicapped by what T. H. Marshall terms "a relative shortage of apparatus", which makes it difficult to " . . . provide schemes of analysis by which complicated problems are reduced to simple formulae" (Marshall, 1963). Until these formulae become available the epidemiological study of social and interpersonal events, and the subject's perception of them, will remain gravely handicapped.

CLASSIFICATION OF PSYCHIATRIC DISORDERS

The epidemiologist must identify his cases before he can count them, and he should be able to define and classify what he identifies. The nature of most psychiatric disorders, however, is so ill-defined as to preclude an aetiological classification. Within the major functional psychoses diagnostic practices have been shown to differ widely (Kreitman, 1961). Variation is even more pronounced among the minor disorders, where the inadequacy of current systems of classification is most exposed. Estimates of the amount of neurotic illness dealt with by general practitioners, for example, have varied widely (Kessel and Shepherd, 1962) and Crombie has pointed out that the International Classification of Disease does scant justice to the psychiatric case-load in general practice, whose importance he has indicated by proposing a fivefold subdivision of total morbidity into (i) an illness, all or nearly all organic; (ii) an illness, mainly organic, but with some emotional content; (iii) an illness with emotional and organic components in equal proportion; (iv) a mainly emotional illness but with some organic content; and (v) an illness all or nearly all emotional (Crombie, 1963).

Along with the task of classifying declared morbidity goes that of identifying and classifying mentally ill persons who do not seek medical or social care. This ill-defined zone of disability is populated not only by individuals who exhibit psychological symptoms, anomalies of behaviour, and deviant personality traits, but also by those who fail to meet the "social-cultural expectations" (Zubin, 1963) of their social group, and so demand assessment within a particular social context. The principal case-finding instruments available today are psychiatric and structured interviews, psychological screening tests and scales, and ratings of social adjustment to family, peers, work, and community (Blum, 1962). For none of these methods is there at present adequate information as to reliability, validity, stability over time, or the importance of cultural factors in determining the accepted norm.

Uncertainties of diagnosis are closely linked to the problem of measurement. Mortality rates cannot often be applied usefully to psychiatric disorders, though when they are relevant, as in the case of suicide and of general paresis, they have been employed to good effect. Traditionally, the morbidity statistics for mental illness have been derived from mental hospital records, and first admission rates have provided a valuable guide to the incidence of major psychotic illness. Outside hospital practice, the records of industrial sickness absence and of general practice consultations have made it possible to use spells of sickness and doctor–patient contacts as indices of morbidity. By and large, however, the chronic, fluctuating course of much minor psychiatric disability places a heavy strain on the customary units of measurement. Duration may be difficult to determine, and operational measures such as "episodes" of illness are not easily defined. The definition of illness proposed by Hinkle and Wolff, for example, as "any symptom or syndrome that the American medical profession at the present time generally accept as evidence of ill-health" (Hinkle and Wolff, 1957), can be commended more on patriotic than on scientific grounds. More complex indices such as the "lifetime prevalence rate" are correspondingly less precise. The epidemiologist is thus seriously handicapped in his efforts to measure the rates of specific disease groups or reactions, and in the past he has tended to use global estimates of mental disorder, often lumped together with the rates for suicide, juvenile delinquency, crime and divorce, as catch-all indices of mental ill health. The case remains unproven for bringing together such disparate items on a linear scale to estimate the sickness of a society.

Applications of the Epidemiological Method to Psychiatry

This chequered background helps to explain why it is more informative to dwell on the uses rather than the achievements of the epidemiological method in psychiatry. Morris has suggested that there are seven uses for epidemiology, namely, for historical study, for community diagnosis, for study of the working of health services, for estimating the individual risks of acquiring disease, for completing the clinical picture, for identifying syndromes, and for establishing the causes of illness (Morris, 1957). These several uses are, as he admits, no more than variations on a single theme, the "study of the health and disease of populations and groups in relation to their environment and ways of living". The spectrum of these seven variations passes from scientific analysis to public health action; each in turn can now be considered in relation to mental illness, the connections being illustrated with relevant examples.

AETIOLOGICAL STUDIES

The primary scientific business of epidemiology is to do with the aetiology of disease, and its techniques are especially useful in assessing the relative importance of multiple causes. After nearly 50 years the studies of pellagra by Goldberger and his associates remain the most convincing demonstration of the value of this method applied to a neuro-psychiatric condition; or, to be more precise, of the method in the right hands, for it is not always recalled that the Thompson Commission, working at the same time on the same problem with the same methods, reached radically different conclusions (Siler, Garrison, and MacNeal, 1917). Goldberger himself summed up the essence of his work as follows when he pointed out that to suggest a faulty diet as the root cause of pellagra was also to draw four inferences. "These are", he wrote, "first that a difference in diet as between pellagrins and non-pellagrins be demonstrable; second, that the disease must be curable by a proper diet; third, that it must be preventable by such a diet, and, fourth, that it may be experimentally produced by diet" (Goldberger, 1927). The establishment of these four postulates, and the coincident eradication of a major scourge, constitute one of the most remarkable achievements in modern medicine, whose details unfortunately still lie buried in the archives of the U.S. Public Health Reports, and merit much wider publicity. From the original accounts it is clear that although he was dealing with a condition in which the deficiency of a physical factor was both a necessary and sufficient cause, Goldberger was also alert to not only the massive socio-economic role of poverty in pellagra but also to the more subtle part played by psychological factors. Thus, in his first paper he suggested that, contrary to popular belief, pellagra was unlikely to be a communicable disease because of the exemption of nurses and attendants in mental hospitals where the disease was rife among the inmates. He commented drily: "The writer from personal ob-servation has found that although the nurses and attendants may apparently receive the same food, there is nevertheless a difference in that the nurses have the privilege, which they exercise, of selecting the best and greatest variety for themselves. Moreover, it must not be overlooked that nurses and attendants have opportunities for supplementing their institutional dietary that inmates as a rule have not" (Goldberger, 1914). Again, on the appearance of deficiency symptoms among some residents of S. Carolinian villages with adequate food supply, Goldberger wrote as follows: "A great variety of causes may operate to bring about individual peculiarities of taste with respect to food. They may have their origin in the seemingly inherent human prejudice against the new untried food or dish; they may date from some disagreeable experience associated with a particular food; they may arise as the result of ill-advised, self-imposed or professionally directed dietary restrictions in the treatment of digestive disturbances, kidney disease, etc.; they may originate as a fad; and in the insane they may arise because of some delusion such as the fear of poisoning, etc." (Goldberger, Wheeler and Sydenstricker, 1920).

All subsequent experimental studies, including the recent work on the inborn metabolic error of Hartnup's disease (Hersov and Rodnight, 1960), have served to confirm and elaborate on the broad picture of pellagra as defined epidemiologically. To be sure, the disease lent itself to this approach: it was well described clinically; the proximate causes were concurrent; and individual variation was relatively small. Goldberger himself was aware of these advantages and correspondingly cautious about the prospects of epidemiological research in other, more obscure, mental illnesses. Declining an offer to undertake research into schizophrenia, for example, he wrote: " . . . in five or more years I could probably find out nothing. Much work will be needed on the physiology of the central nervous system and on many collateral problems before dementia praecox can be understood" (Parsons, 1943). Time has proved him right. A recent review of the epidemiological contributions to our knowledge of psychiatric aetiology suggests that the volume of work is more impressive than its results (Milbank Memorial Fund, 1961).

The quest for causes has, in general, been directed towards the establishment of associations between significant events in the life history and the subsequent appearance of mental illness. These events can be subdivided chronologically into those with effects which are delayed in time, and those which are close enough to the outbreak of illness to be regarded as proximate or precipitant. The latter group has lent itself to population studies most conveniently in times of upheaval. Rawnsley, for example, has assessed the mental health of the Tristan da Cunha community evacuated to this country after the volcanic eruption in 1961 and has been able to compare his findings with those of a Norwegian expedition which visited Tristan in 1937–8 (Rawnsley and Loudon, 1964). The outstanding feature described by the Norwegians had been an outbreak of hysterical spells among the women of the island; the 19 survivors with a history of these "spells" were shown 25 years later to exhibit higher recent medical consultation rates and, in particular, to suffer from a form of psychogenic headache, which, in turn, proved to be significantly more often present among the wives of the island's leaders. Table 1 represents Rawnsley's attempt to relate the two indices of morbidity, i.e., an earlier hysterical "spell" and a psychogenic headache, to the social factor of status: though the numbers are too small to be conclusive they suggest strongly that the paired associations are independent of the remaining variable.

For the study of proximal precipitants under more normal conditions Gordon has emphasized the value of analysing infrequently occurring, single events, by analogy with point epidemics, and has exemplified his argument with the psychoses after childbirth (Thomas and Gordon, 1959). His

TABLE 1.

Relationship between Psychogenic Headache, Hysterical Cases (1937), and Social Position in the Tristan da Cunha Community

	Leaders' Wives		Controls	
	1937 Cases	Non-cases	1937 Cases	Non-cases
Psychogenic headache	9	5	2	4
Other symptoms	1	8	1	16

suggestion has been followed up by Paffenbarger, who, by examining area hospital records over an 18-year period, identified a group of women whose first mental illness had occurred in relation to childbearing; 125 post-partum psychoses were detected, comprising a first-attack rate of 0.7 per 1000 live births (Paffenbarger, 1961). A control group was derived from women of the same race whose deliveries immediately preceded or followed those of the index subjects. The two groups were compared in respect of age, parity, age at marriage, social class, period of gestation, birth weights, and the somatic complications of pregnancy and parturition. The small numbers involved limited detailed comparison, but there was a definite tendency for the frequency of recorded somatic complications to differentiate between the two groups. To test the specificity of these findings, Paffenbarger went on to make identical comparisons with two other index groups, namely, mothers who had developed late post-partum haemorrhage, and mothers whose infants had developed hypertrophic pyloric stenosis. In neither were the differences of the same order as those found with the psychotic mothers.

Essentially the same method of retrospective analysis of hospital records has been employed by Pasamanick and his co-workers to examine the significance of much earlier events in the individual life history. They collected information about the complications of labour recorded on birth certificates or hospital records, and compared the data obtained with those relating to infants selected from the same batch of birth certificates and matched for a number of relevant variables. The logic of this procedure, in the authors' own words, runs as follows:

> (1) Since prematurity and complications of pregnancy are associated with foetal and neonatal death, usually on the basis of injury to the brain, there must remain a fraction so injured who do not die. (2) Depending upon the degree and location of the damage, the survivors may develop a series of disorders. These extend from cerebral palsy, epilepsy, and mental deficiency through all types of lesser degrees of damage sufficient to disorganize behavioural development and lower thresholds to stress. (3) Further, these abnormalities of pregnancy are associated with certain life experiences, usually socio-economically determined, and consequently (4) they themselves and their resulting neuro-psychiatric disorders are found in greater aggregation in the lower strata of our society. (Knobloch and Pasamanick, 1960a.)

The use made of this method is illustrated most clearly by reference to mental subnormality, one stage along their "continuum of reproductive casualty". Their retrospective studies had suggested a significant association between subnormality and not only such physical features as prematurity, maternal complications of pregnancy and neonatal-abnormalities, but also socio-economic status, race, and season of birth. To assess the individual importance of these several factors the authors then resorted to a prospective study, following up 500 premature babies and a control group of full-term infants matched for hospital of birth as well as for socio-economic circumstances (Knobloch and Pasamanick, 1960b). At 40 weeks the premature infants exhibited a higher incidence of neurological abnormalities and a lower development quotient on the Gesell development examination. These findings were confirmed when 300 of the children were re-examined more than 2 years later, but in addition it was then noted that whereas at 40 weeks the development quotients of white and coloured control children were virtually identical the groups had diverged by the age of 3 years. Table 2 shows that whereas the white children then exhibited an improvement of their adaptive and language skills, the opposite was true of the negroes. The sharpest decline was recorded for the children whose mothers had received the poorest education. These differences, which were not evident in other fields of behaviour, are attributed by the authors to sociocultural factors.

TABLE 2.

Comparison of Developmental Quotients at 40 Weeks and 3 Years of Age in Full-term Infants by Race (Baltimore, Maryland, 1952–3)

Age at examination	Developmental Quotients			
	40 Weeks		3 Years	
Race	White	Non-white	White	Non-white
No. of cases	(223)	(269)	(77)	(82)
Field of behaviour general				
(adaptive)	105·4	104·5	110·9	97·4
Gross motor	114·7	113·4	113·7	112·5
Fine motor	97·6	99·2	100·7	98·6
Language	102·5	102·9	106·0	90·1
Personal-social	108·6	106·5	110·5	106·8

Longitudinal studies of this kind, in which a cohort of normal subjects is followed up in order to define variations of development, and so to assess the significance of deviant behaviour, represent an epidemiological technique of increasing importance. Other examples include the study by Douglas of a national sample of British children born during 1 week in 1946 (Douglas and Mulligan, 1961), and Mangus and Dager's survey of factors related to personality change in the second decade of life (Mangus and Dager, 1959). The information provided is especially valuable for child psychiatry which has long suffered from the lack of normative data against which to evaluate supposed disorders of behaviour. These studies, however, are slow to mature and can be usefully supplemented by cross-sectional surveys. In the Buckinghamshire Child Health Survey, for example, data have been collected about a 10% sample of all school-children between the ages of 5 and 15 in an English county (Shepherd, Oppenheim and Mitchell, 1966). Figure 1 shows the reported frequency distribution, by age and sex, of bedwetting, a common cause of referral to child guidance clinics. There stands out a small but persistent group of daily bedwetters up to the age of 10–11, most of whom were receiving no medical attention, and were not regarded as presenting psychiatric problems.

As an aid to the study of human development, epidemiology helps to assess the impact of life experiences on innate characteristics. The newer technical advances have now made possible the extension of epidemiological research into the field of genetics proper. In mongolism, for example, Cohen, Lilienfeld and Sigler have pointed out that the newly discovered chromosomal abnormalities have already made it necessary to estimate (1) the chromosomal constitution of a representative sample of phenotypically normal subjects; (2) the comparative incidence of mongolism, in order to examine the effect on non-disjunction of external events like ionizing radiation; (3) the possible association between trisomy and translocation and maternal age; and (4) the relationship between mongolism, leukaemia, and ionizing radiation (Cohen, Lilienfeld and Sigler, 1963). All these questions are open to a form of epidemiological study which can be expected to proliferate in the wake of other cytogenetic discoveries.

ILLNESS-EXPECTANCY STUDIES

Estimating the individual expectation of psychiatric illness has also been a joint concern of genetics and epidemiology. Some of the outstanding early investigations of mental disorder in communities were inspired by a primary interest in genetics, and indeed Fremming, whose longitudinal study of mental illness on the island of Bornholm is a model of its kind, wrote of survey methods that "the most important purpose of such research is to provide reliable figures for the expectation of hereditary mental diseases in the general population" (Fremming, 1951).

The classical contribution of epidemiology in this sphere, however, has been the concept of accident proneness. The origin of this term can be traced back to 1919 when Greenwood and Woods, in their report to the Industrial Fatigue Research Board, suggested that the observed frequency distributions of accidents in a group of factories fitted best mathematically with the hypothesis of initially unequal liabilities to accidents rather than to pure chance or to a bias in the direction of individuals who had already sustained at least one accident (Greenwood and Woods, 1919). Further work tended to substantiate this notion of "accident liability", but in 1926 Farmer and Chambers transmuted a statistical into a psychological concept, defining "accident proneness" as "a personal idiosyncrasy predisposing the

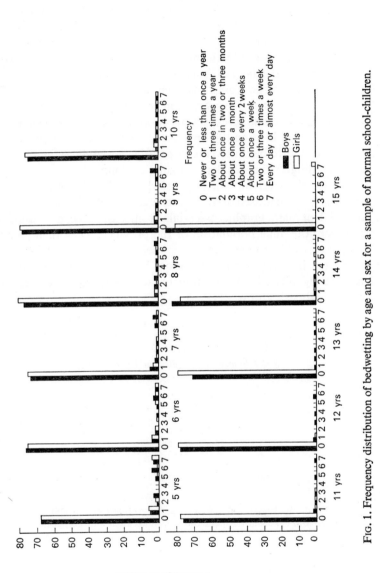

FIG. 1. Frequency distribution of bedwetting by age and sex for a sample of normal school-children.

individual who possesses it in a marked degree to a relatively high accident rate" (Farmer and Chambers, 1926). Though the evidence has never established a dichotomy between individuals who are and are not accident-prone, nonetheless, as Adelstein has commented, the concept "was seized upon as the open sesame to all accident problems" by many subsequent workers who were impressed by the more speculative assumptions of psychosomatic medicine (Adelstein, 1952). That a more rigorous application of the concept may still prove rewarding has been demonstrated recently by Smart and Schmidt (1962). Basing their work on the suggestion that patients with psychosomatic illnesses tend to experience morbid tension, and seek release by physical action which is often ill-considered, they argued that such patients would therefore tend to be involved comparatively frequently in all forms of accidents, including traffic accidents. From a group of 271 male hospital patients in Ontario with an unequivocal diagnosis of peptic ulcer, they ascertained that 135 possessed driving licences, and that this subgroup did not differ in social or demographic essentials from either the remaining ulcer patients or from the male population of the province. They then compared the age-adjusted traffic-accident rates for the 135 index cases with those of male car drivers in the general population. Table 3 shows that this group experienced a significantly higher rate of accidents than average, and so constituted a high-risk group.

TABLE 3.

Traffic Accidents of Male Peptic Ulcer Patients and Expected Accidents
1 January 1956—30 June 1959

Year	Observed	Expected	Pooled x^2	P
1956	12	8·382		
1957	10	8·440		
1958	11	7·856		
1959 (6 months)	6	3·632		
Totals	39	28·310	4·0366	$<0·05$

The pooled x^2 had one degree of freedom. An x^2 of $5·1066$ ($P < 0·025$) was obtained by using the observed and expected frequencies of both accident and non-accident drivers in the sample.

COMPLETING THE CLINICAL PICTURE

In the use of epidemiological techniques as aids to the completion, or extension, of the clinical picture of mental disease, perhaps the most interesting development in this country has been the new look taken at the general practitioner under the National Health Service. The crude statistics of the age–sex distribution of neurotic illness as obtained from hospital data and from general practice (Fig. 2) indicate the dimensions of the problem of neuroses in the community (Kessel and Shepherd, 1962).

Study of the nature of the clinical and social phenomena exhibited by these patients (only a small minority of whom are ever referred to a psychiatrist) constitutes a major task for the future. So does their outcome, for whereas prognostic studies of the major forms of psychiatric illness are well-established, our knowledge of the natural history of the minor disorders

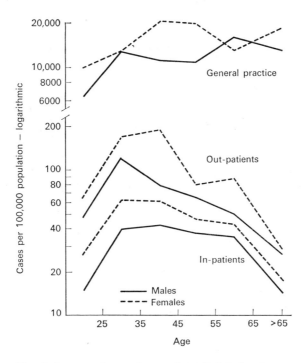

FIG. 2. Age prevalence of neurosis studied during 1 year.

is still in its infancy. Meanwhile evidence is accumulating to suggest that psychological and social factors can affect the outcome of some established physical disease whose course is known to differ widely from case to case (Querido, 1959). Recently, for example, Rutter has conducted an anterospective study of a sample comprising 80 cases of established peptic ulceration followed up for six months after their discharge from hospital in-patient care (Rutter, 1963). During their stay in hospital observations were made on the patients' physical condition and radiological status by a physician; at the same time the psychosocial variables were assessed independently by the psychiatrist and psychiatric social worker. After 6 months the patients were re-examined by all three observers independently. Surprisingly, outcome could not be correlated with any of the somatic or social factors but Tables 4 and 5 show that affective features present at the initial psychiatric examination were significantly related to the patient's state after 6 months, whether this was assessed either by the presence of ulcer pain or by incapacity for work.

TABLE 4.

Association between Anxiety at Interview and Pain at Follow-up

Pain	Anxiety			Total
	None (A)	Mild (B)	Moderate or Severe (C)	
	No.	No.	No.	No.
None	22 (57·9%)	12 (50·0%)	5 (31·3%)	38
I	12 (31·6%)	6 (25·0%)	1 (6·3%)	19
II	4 (10·5%)	6 (25·0%)	10 (62·5%)	20
Total	38	24	16	77

$x^2 = 13·358$, $p. < 0·001$, $c. = 0·38$ (2 $d.f.$, combining groups B and C for calculation of chi-square).

TABLE 5.

Association between Anxiety at Interview and Work Incapacity at Follow-up

Work Incapacity	Anxiety		
	None	Present	Total
None	31	17	48
Present	4	11	15
Total	35	28	63
Not applicable	9	12	17

$x^2 = 6·532$, 2 $d.f.$, $p. < 0·02$.

Extending the clinical picture to include the sub-clinical or "incipient" cases with declared illness raises particular difficulties in psychiatry. How important this problem can be is well shown in the sphere of mental subnormality when intelligence test results are compared with clinical findings. In the study of Stockholm children cited by Penrose, for example, a group of 300 children, excluded from ordinary schools on the ground of feeble-mindedness, was examined with a modified version of the Binet–Simon test (Penrose,

1949). A sample of the normal school population was similarly examined. It was shown that the distribution of intelligence scores was quite continuous, with no indication of a natural boundary between the normal and the defective children. There was a close correlation (about $+ 0.8$) between the test scores and the clinical diagnosis of feeble-mindedness, but the correspondence was by no means perfect; had the ascertainment of mental deficiency been made on test scores rather than on clinical examination, a somewhat different group would have been selected as abnormal.

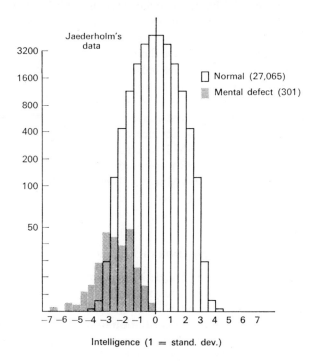

FIG. 3. Distribution of intelligence (Pearson and Jaederholm, 1931).

The clinical picture can also be extended by comparisons between mental illness in different environments as by the description of the so-called exotic psychiatric disorders (Arieti and Meth, 1959). The possibilities of this approach have been explored by Murphy in his careful study of the urban distribution of mental illness in Singapore (Murphy, 1955). By relating the rates of mental hospital admission to areas of residence in terms of defined census tracts, he was able to show, in accordance with expectation, that positive relationships existed, some tracts being associated with much higher rates than others. Unlike his predecessors working in the Occident, however, Murphy did not find the highest rates of illness in the densely populated lower class slum districts. Again, when the residential areas were classified by cultural and ethnic characteristics, it emerged that, contrary to findings elsewhere, geographic mobility correlated positively with manic-depressive disorder, and negatively with schizophrenia. The key to these discrepancies, Murphy suggested, lay in the special sociocultural features of Singapore which distinguish it from the pattern of most western cities. Emphasizing the importance of the supportive culture which exists in the Singapore slum areas, he commented: "There is a tendency in the West to think of the slums as being populated by people who have no ambition and have made no effort to get out of them; in Singapore one might say that a considerable proportion of the slum dwellers are there precisely because they have ambition—at least the ambition to leave their native land in search of something better." With regard to the unexpected distribution of the functional psychoses, he suggested that the association found in other societies between high rates of schizophrenia and lack of cultural support is understandably absent in Singapore, because "what causes or at least is linked to the rise in the schizophrenia rate is not the absence of cultural support but the efforts of both society and the individual to regain or retain such support". In Singapore, where the stranger must contend with an attitude of *laissez-faire* indifference, "the evidence", says Murphy, "suggests that an affective type of breakdown may be encouraged when the individual lacks the support of a surrounding culture and is not led to make an effort to assimilate".

DELINEATION OF SYNDROMES

A W.H.O. expert committee (W.H.O., 1960) has recommended that this method be employed in all prevalence surveys on the grounds that symptoms constitute the most easily standardized and measurable units of observation, and that knowledge of their distribution in populations, independent of the charting of formal illness, leaves the way open for new discoveries. There is, however, an understandable reluctance on the part of clinically trained psychiatrists to revert to purely symptomatic levels of description perhaps for the reason that Lewis has advanced: "It is humiliating because it throws us back to the infancy of medicine" (Lewis, 1961).

The recording of enumerated symptoms has proved most valuable so far in screening techniques, employed mainly where large numbers have to be examined rapidly, as in induction procedures (Brodman *et al.*, 1954). The use of a similar technique in an area prevalence survey has been described by MacMillan (MacMillan, 1957). A more promising field for the mapping of new syndromes, however, is that of child psychiatry, where an established nosology is still lacking and the clinician relies less on symptoms than on signs of morbidity, particularly on disturbances of behaviour. Case identification is here more difficult in that it may depend, not so much on the observation of intrinsically abnormal behaviour, as on exaggeration of normal traits or the persistence of certain kinds of behaviour beyond the appropriate stage of development. To this extent, pathological disturbance may be equated with deviation from the norm, and the significance of any observed item of behaviour cannot be assessed without some knowledge of its frequency by individual age groups. Thus in a current British research project, the Buckinghamshire Child Health Survey, information has been gathered on a sample of 6000 normal school-children, and also on child guidance clinic attenders with known psychiatric disturbance (Shepherd, Oppenheim and Mitchell, 1966). The data, collected from questionnaires completed by parents and teachers, cover the occurrence and frequency of most commonly recognized symptoms, and also provide for the rating of various characteristics on a simple three-point scale. In this way, a picture is being built up of behavioural norms for this population, and the significance of the least common characteristics tested by comparison with the child guidance sample. Observed clustering of symptoms or uncommon characteristics can then provide a basis for the delineation of syndromes or abnormal patterns of behaviour.

COMMUNITY DIAGNOSIS

With this type of study epidemiology enters the realm of public health and medical administration. Though its more immediate concern is likely to be with the planning of health services, the diagnosis of health and disease in whole communities has prevention as its ultimate goal. In this context, the survey of mental deficiency carried out over thirty years ago by E. O. Lewis can still be regarded as a model (Lewis, 1929). He took six geographical areas of England and Wales, each with a population of about 100,000, and of widely differing type; three were urban and three rural, and they included a metropolitan suburb, a mining area, and a northern cotton town. Lewis was able to show that they were representative of the country as a whole in respect of such characteristics as social class and occupation, incidence of treated mental disorder, and ascertained mental deficiency. He then carried out in each area a survey of adult mental deficiency based on the reports of all available medical and social agencies, together with a screening of all school-children. This latter, the most important part of the investigation, was carried out in three stages. First, the teachers in each school were asked to pick out the children of each age whose school work and general performance were poorest; about 15% of the whole school population was sorted out on this basis, so that there was no possibility of any significant number of retarded children being missed. Secondly, all these children were then submitted to group intelligence tests, which were supervised and scored by Lewis's assistants. Thirdly, all children whose scores on the group tests suggested a degree of mental retardation were examined individually by Lewis, using both intelligence tests and medical inspection. In the infants' departments, where group tests were inapplicable, 6% of the most backward children were examined individually. By these methods Lewis obtained a total prevalence rate for the six areas surveyed of 8·57 per 1000, a figure which still commands substantial agreement.

Where sufficient knowledge has been established a psychiatric condition, like any other, can be identified by screening procedures, and prophylactic measures can be introduced by the public health authorities. In the case of phenyleketonuria, for example, it has already proved possible for 124 British local health authorities at the request of the Ministry of Health to undertake the routine screening of infants aged 4–6 weeks and so to identify 39 cases from more than 650,000 tests; the possibility of treating these early cases with low phenylalanine diets then opens the way to preventive action (Medical Research Council, 1963). Unfortunately few psychiatric disorders are sufficiently well defined for large-scale, rational prophylactic or therapeutic measures to be feasible and most community studies have been concerned chiefly with the prevalence of mental ill health. The results of these surveys are least equivocal when the patient's condition is clearly identified by contact with a medical or social agency.

In Britain the National Health Service has led to so wide a coverage of the population by general practitioners that the extent of such conspicuous morbidity can be estimated from their returns. The amount of illness is not inconsiderable. A study of our own, for example, has recently shown that the reported one-year period prevalence rate for adult psychiatric illness reported by some eighty practitioners in the London area was as high as 140 per 1000 (Shepherd et al., 1964). These estimates, however, represent only a fraction of the reported rates of medically inconspicuous morbidity. Here the investigator is compelled to employ an operational definition of mental ill health and to examine whole populations or samples of them by questionnaire or interviews: often he undertakes a large, extensive survey supplemented by a smaller intensive study. For the purpose some workers adopt a pragmatic approach with reliance on the subjects' reports, supplemented by direct questioning. In a study of a new housing estate, for example, Martin et al. interviewed a sample of 750 families at home, using a check-list of symptoms: 22% of the adults admitted to "nerves", 17% to "depression", 12% to sleeplessness, and almost as many to undue irritability (Martin, Brotherston and Chave, 1957). Other workers assume that there is a scale along which mental health or personality can be placed and measured; the authors of the mid-town Manhattan project (Srole et al., 1962), for example, quote with approval the view . . . "that an emotional adjustment exists on a quantitative continuum and that trained psychiatrists or psychologists are able to place an individual in his position on this continuum . . . " (Wittson and Hunt, 1951). On either assumption the results are disconcerting. The families on the housing estate exhibited at least one symptom in 35% of cases; of the mid-town residents only 18·5% were deemed mentally "well". It must be concluded either that mental ill health approaches the rule or that the criteria by which it is assessed are inadequate. At present the operational criteria of individual investigators differ so widely as to render comparative studies in place or time more useful than attempts to chase the chimera of "true" prevalence.

Comparison between the prevalence rates of mental ill health in more than one area usually goes with a search for ecological correlates, ranging from relatively simple factors like overcrowding to complex indices of social structure like those employed by Leighton in N. America (Leighton, 1959) and Loudon in S. Wales. Comparisons over time are harder to come by but the results of Essen-Möller's forthcoming second survey of the overt and latent mental disability in south Sweden should be of particular interest (Essen-Möller, 1961). Mention must also be made of the large anterospective study of Wilner and his colleagues who examined the effect of the quality of housing on mental and physical health by a three-year follow-up of 300 families moved from slum to superior accommodation with a control group of 300 slum families; they succeeded in demonstrating that determination and half a million dollars can prove the obvious, but their work stands as a monument to the practical use of epidemiology in social research (Wilner *et al.*, 1962).

Historical Studies

As a means of demonstrating changes in the character or distribution of illness the use of the historical method in psychiatry has been limited until recent years. With the help of this method it is possible to analyse time trends to determine, above all, whether the amount of mental illness has altered and whether it has been affected by therapeutic or other measures. Anecdotal studies like those of Haeser (1882) and Hecker (1859) on the dancing manias of the Middle Ages are descriptively important but their value is much enhanced when reliable statistics are also available. Hare, for example, from a study of contemporary records and clinical descriptions, was able to plot the spread of general paresis across Europe, and to adduce a certain amount of evidence supporting the hypothesis of a neurotropic strain of spirochaete originating in northern France at the end of the fifteenth century (Hare, 1959). He was also able to make use of statistical data to examine more recent trends, thereby demonstrating a steady decline in the prevalence of general paresis which has long antedated modern methods of treatment.

To the long-standing controversy on the putative increase of mental disorder, Goldhamer and Marshall made a useful contribution by comparing mental hospital admission rates in Massachusetts over an interval of 100 years (Goldhamer and Marshall, 1953). They found that the nineteenth and twentieth century age-specific rates were radically different; in the earlier period there was a relatively high concentration in the 20–50 age group, whereas in the more recent period the majority of patients admitted were in their fifties and sixties. On the evidence they suggest that while a large part of the seeming increase was due to a growing tendency to admit to hospital patients with mental disorders associated with the senium, some of the increment might be attributed to a true rise in the incidence of these conditions, especially cerebral arteriosclerosis.

In a different field, Halliday has studied the patterns in the incidence and distribution of certain "psychosomatic" disorders over the first half of this century (Halliday, 1949). He found evidence of a marked increase in the incidence of peptic ulcer among males, but not among females, so that the sex ratio for this group of disorders had changed considerably during the period under review. Conversely, for diabetes there had been a marked increase among females, but not among males. Over a period of 50 years the male/female ratio for deaths ascribed to this disease had fallen from 2 to 0·5. Halliday postulated that such striking changes in the sex distribution of disease must be associated with some corresponding changes of male and female psychosocial roles in our society.

Studies of Health Services in Action

The perspective obtained from historical studies can be of service in the assessment of current health services and the prediction of future needs. The present debate on the future of British mental hospitals, for example, has been largely inspired by the recorded fall in mental hospital residents over the past decade. According to one prediction the need for beds will have fallen about 40% by 1975, largely because of an anticipated run-down of the population of chronic hospital inmates (Maclay, 1963). As this decline has coincided approximately with the introduction of tranquillizing drugs, some workers have claimed a causal association between the two events. That this is not necessarily so has been shown by the static picture obtained from individual institutions which had enjoyed the benefits of a major programme of administrative reform, with favourable consequences for the bed state, before the advent of tranquillizers (Shepherd, Goodman and Watt, 1961). Such figures suggest that the social concomitants of drug therapy play an important part in affecting the flow of patients from hospital.

Attempts to examine directly the workings of the mental health services in action have been surprisingly few. Recently, however, Lawrence has made an operational study of the emergency procedures in London by concentrating on the social determinants of admission to a metropolitan observation ward (Lawrence, 1963). She was able to obtain relevant information about not only a group of patients but also a sample of the 20% of people who were referred to the mental welfare department without further action being taken. Her findings indicate that however important the medical aspects of the case both the breakdown in tolerance which initiated referral and the decision of the D.A.O. to take action were also affected strongly by social and administrative pressures and by the attitudes and beliefs of contiguous figures in the immediate environment.

Future Prospects

No survey, however brief, of the past and present status of psychiatric epidemiology can be complete without some reference to its future. At a recent American conference devoted to the future of psychiatry hopes were pinned to the development of giant electronic digital computers "permitting the posing of questions and obtaining of answers which were never dreamed of in the past" (Pasamanick, 1962). It would seem to be more realistic to recognize that the questions are already with us and that most of the answers are more likely to come from human than from mechanical brains. Nor is it necessary to accept the complementary American prophecy of "the continued application of human ignorance and error to research method and analysis and interpretation of data", provided the clinical and the social investigator can be imbued with a viewpoint which was clearly outlined by Sir James Spence:

> His main task is to place the phenomena (of disease) in temporal and in quantitative relationships with each other. This leads him to know the course of a disease as it may be expected commonly to occur. His next task is to determine the variation from that course, and to find correlations between these variations and aetiological factors or alternative treatments. When possible he uses statistics to express these variations. He uses statistical estimates of variations also in designing the extent of his study. If the disease under study is one which varies little in its course he limits his number of examples. . . . He thus comes to know disease as a predictable sequence of events, and the knowledge gained becomes the basis, the only basis, by which the underlying process of disease in the living patient can be rationally interpreted (Spence, 1954).

Spence was talking here about clinical science but his summary of its logic might be transposed verbatim to what is now being called clinical epidemiology. This discipline can and should supplement and expand the psychiatrist's traditional concern with the individual patient. "Psychiatry", as Odegaard has insisted, "is forced to study groups and populations because it deals with individuals, not in spite of that fact" (Odegaard, 1962).

Acknowledgements

The authors would like to acknowledge the sources of several tables and figures in the text. They are: Professor K. Rawnsley (Table 1), *Pediatrics*

(Table 2), the Editor and publishers of the *Journal of Psychosomatic Research* (Tables 3, 4 and 5), of the *Journal of Mental Science* (Fig. 2), and of *Annals of Eugenics* (Fig. 3).

References

ADELSTEIN, A. M. (1952), *J. roy. stat. Soc. A.* **115**, 354.
ARIETI, S. and METH, J. M. (1959), In *American Handbook of Psychiatry* (edited by S. Arieti), **1**, New York, Basic Books.
BLUM, R. H. (1962), *Milbank mem. Fd. Quart.* **40**, 253.
BÖÖK, J. A. (1961), In *Causes of Mental Disorders: A Review of Epidemiological Knowledge, 1959*, New York, Millbank Memorial Fund.
BRODMAN, K., ERDMANN, A. J., LORGE, I., DEUTSCHBERGER, J. and WOLFF, H. G. (1954), *Amer. J. Psychiat.* **111**, 37.
BROWN, J. A. C. (1961), *Freud and the Post-Freudians*, p. 124, London, Penguin Books.
BRUGGER, C. (1931), *Z. ges. Neurol. Psychiat.* **133**, 352.
COHEN, B. H., LILIENFELD, A. M. and SIGLER, A. T. (1963), *Amer. J. publ. Hlth.* **53**, 223.
CROMBIE, D. L. (1963), *Lancet*, **i**, 1205.
DOUGLAS, J. W. B. and MULLIGAN, D. G. (1961), *Proc. roy. Soc. Med.* **54**, 885.
DURKHEIM, E. (1951), *Suicide: a Study in Sociology*. Translated by J. A. Spaulding and G. Simpson, Glencoe, Illinois, Free Press.
ESSEN-MÖLLER, E. (1961), In *Comparative Epidemiology of the Mental Disorders* (Proc. 49th A.M. Amer. Psychopathogical Ass.), edited by P. H. Hoch and J. Zubin, p. 1, New York, Grune & Stratton.
FARIS, R. E. L. and DUNHAM, H. W. (1939), *Mental Disorders in Urban Areas: an Ecological Study of Schizophrenia and other Psychoses*. Chicago, University of Chicago Press.
FARMER, E. and CHAMBERS, E. G. (1926), *Industr. Fatigue Res. Bd.* Rep. No. 38, London, H.M.S.O.
FREMMING, K. H. (1951), *The Expectation of Mental Infirmity in a Sample of the Danish Population* (*Occasional Papers on Eugenics*, no. 7), p. 12, London, Cassell.
FREUD, S. (1955), Group Psychology and the Analysis of the Ego. In *Complete Psychological Works*, **18**, 69, London, Hogarth Press.
FROST, W. H. (1927), In *Public Health and Preventive Medicine*, **2**, 163, London, Nelson.
GINSBERG, M. (1956), In *On the Diversity of Morals*, p. 157, London, Heinemann.
GOLDBERGER, J. (1914), *Publ. Hlth. Rep.* (*Wash.*), **29**, 1683.
GOLDBERGER, J. (1927), *De Lamar Lectures*, p. 128, New York, Williams & Wilkins.
GOLDBERGER, J., WHEELER, G. A. and SYDENSTRICKER, E. (1920), *Publ. Hlth. Rep. Wash.* **35**, 2673.
GOLDHAMER, H. and MARSHALL, A. (1953), *Psychosis and Civilization* (2nd ed.), Glencoe, Illinois, Free Press.
GREENWOOD, M. (1935), *Epidemics and Crowd-Diseases*, p. 133, London, Williams & Norgate.
GREENWOOD, M. and WOODS, H. M. (1919), Industrial Fatigue Research Board Report, No. 4, London, H.M.S.O.
GRUENBERG, E. M. (1957), In *Explorations in Social Psychiatry* (edited by A. H. Leighton, J. A. Clausen, and R. N. Wilson), London, Tavistock.
HAESER, H. (1882), *Lehrbuch der Geschichte der Medicin* (3rd ed.), Jena, Fischer.
HALLIDAY, J. L. (1949), *Psychosocial Medicine*, London, Heinemann.
HARE, E. H. (1959), *J. ment. Sci.* **105**, 594.
HECKER, J. F. C. (1859), *The Epidemics of the Middle Ages*, Translated by B. G. Babington (3rd ed.), London, Trubner.
HERSOV, L. A. and RODNIGHT, R. (1960), *J. Neurol. Neurosurg. Psychiat.* **23**, 40.
HINKLE, L. E. and WOLFF, H. G. (1957), In *Explorations in Social Psychiatry* (edited by A. H. Leighton, J. A. Clausen and R. N. Wilson), London, Tavistock.
KESSEL, N. and SHEPHERD, M. (1962), *J. ment. Sci.* **108**, 159.

KNOBLOCH, H. and PASAMANICK, B. (1960a). In *Mental Retardation*. Proceedings of the 1st international conference on Mental Retardation (edited by P. W. Bowman and H. V. Mautner), New York, Grune & Stratton.

KNOBLOCH, H. and PASAMANICK, B. (1960b), *Pediatrics*, **26**, 210.

KREITMAN, N. (1961), *J. ment. Sci.* **107**, 876.

LAWRENCE, A. R. LE V. (1963), Ph.D. Thesis, University of London.

LEIGHTON, A. H. (1951), *Bull. Johns Hopk. Hosp.* **89**, 73.

LEIGHTON, A. H. (1959), *My Name is Legion*, New York, Basic Books.

LEWIS, A. J. (1961), In *Comparative Epidemiology of the Mental Disorders* (edited by P. H. Hoch and J. Zubin), p. 229 (Proc. 49th A.M. Amer. Psychopathological Ass.), New York, Grune & Stratton.

LEWIS, A. J. (1962), *Yale J. biol. Med.* **35**, 62.

LEWIS, E. O. (1929), Board of Education and Board of Control Mental Deficiency Committee Report, pt. 4, London, H.M.S.O.

LIN, T.-Y. and STANDLEY, C. C. (1962), The Scope of Epidemiology in Psychiatry. Public Health Papers, No. 16, Geneva, W.H.O.

MACLAY, W. S. (1963), *Amer. J. Psychiat.* **120**, 209.

MACMILLAN, A. M. (1957), *Psychol. Rep.* **111**, 325. Monograph suppl. 7, Southern Universities Press.

MALZBERG, B. (1940), *Social and Biological Aspects of Mental Disease*, Utica, New York, State Hospital Press.

MANGUS, A. R. and DAGER, E. Z. (1959), In *Epidemiology of Mental Disorder* (edited by B. Pasamanick). *Amer. Ass. adv. Sci. Publ.*, no. 60, Washington, D.C.

MARSHALL, T. H. (1963), In *Sociology at the Crossroads and other Essays*, p. 41, London, Heinemann.

MARTIN, F. M., BROTHERSTON, J. H. F. and CHAVE, S. P. W. (1957), *Brit. J. prev. soc. Med.* **11**, 196.

MEDICAL RESEARCH COUNCIL (1963), *Brit. med. J.* **2**, 1691.

MEYER, A. (1912), *J. Amer. med. Ass.* **58**, 911.

MILBANK MEMORIAL FUND (1950), *Epidemiology of Mental Disorder*, New York.

MILBANK MEMORIAL FUND (1961), *Causes of Mental Disorders: a Review of Epidemiological Knowledge*, 1959, New York.

MORRIS, J. N. (1957), *Uses of Epidemiology*, Edinburgh, Livingstone.

MURPHY, H. B. M. (1955), Unpublished manuscript.

ODEGAARD, O. (1962), *Proc. roy. Soc. Med.* **55**, 831.

PAFFENBARGER, R. S. (1961), *J. chron. Dis.* **13**, 161.

PARSONS, R. P. (1943), *Trail of Light*. Indianapolis, Bobbs-Merrill.

PASAMANICK, B. (1962), In *The Future of Psychiatry* (Proc. 51st meeting Amer. Psychopathological Ass. 1961) (edited by R. H. Hoch and J. Zubin), New York, Grune & Stratton.

PEARSON, K. and JAEDERHOLM, G. A. (1931), On the inheritance of mental disease, *Ann. Eugen. (Lond.)*, **4**, 362.

PENROSE, L. S. (1949), *The Biology of Mental Defect*, London, Sidgwick & Jackson.

PENROSE, L. S. (1952), *On the Objective Study of Crowd Behaviour*, London, Lewis.

POLLOCK, H. M. (1925), *State Hosp. Quart.* **10**, 1934.

QUERIDO, A. (1959), *Brit. J. prev. soc. Med.* **13**, 33.

RAWNSLEY, K. (1963), M.R.C. Committee on the Epidemiology of Psychiatric Illness. Unpublished.

RAWNSLEY, K. and LOUDON, J. B. (1964), *Brit. J. Psychiat.* **110**, 830.

REID, D. D. (1960), Epidemiological Methods in the Study of Mental Disorders. Public Health Papers No. 2, pp. 8 and 15, Geneva, W.H.O.

ROBINSON, W. S. (1950), *Amer. sociol. Rev.* **15**, 351.

ROSANOFF, A. (1917), *Psychiat. Bull.* **2**, 109.

RUTTER, M. (1963), *J. psychosom. Res.* **7**, 45.

RYLE, J. A. (1948), *Changing Disciplines*, London, Oxford University Press.

SHEPHERD, M., COOPER, B., BROWN, A. C. and KALTON, G. (1964), *Brit. med. J.* **ii**, 1359.

SHEPHERD, M., GOODMAN, N. and WATT, D. C. (1961), *Comprehens. Psychiat.* **2**, 11.

SHEPHERD, M., OPPENHEIM, A. N. and MITCHELL, S. (1966), *Proc. roy. soc. med.* **59**, 379.
SILER, J. F., GARRISON, P. E. and MACNEAL, W. J. (1917), Third Report of the Robert M. Thompson Pellagra Commission of the New York Postgraduate Medical School and Hospital, New York.
SMART, R. G. and SCHMIDT, W. S. (1962), *J. psychosom. Res.* **6**, 191.
SPENCE, J. (1954), *Lect. sci. Basis Med.* **2**, 5.
SROLE, L., LANGNER, T. S., MICHAEL, S. T., OPLER, M. K. and RENNIE, T. A. C. (1962), *Mental Health in the Metropolis: the Midtown Manhattan Study*, New York, McGraw-Hill.
STRÖMGREN, E. (1950), *Congrès International de Psychiatrie: VI. Psychiatrie Sociale*, p. 155, Hermann, Paris.
TAYLOR, F., KRÄUPL and HUNTER, R. C. A. (1958), *Psychiat. Quart.* **32**, 821.
THOMAS, C. L. and GORDON, J. E. (1959), *Amer. J. med. Sci.* **238**, 363.
TROTTER, W. (1942), *Instincts of the Herd in Peace and War* (2nd ed.), London, Scientific Book Club.
WILNER, D. M., WALKLEY, R. P., PINKERTON, T. C. and TAYBACK, M. (1962), *The Housing Environment and Family Life*, Baltimore, Johns Hopkins Press.
WITTSON, C. L. and HUNT, W. A. (1951), *Amer. J. Psychiat.* **107**, 582.
WORLD HEALTH ORGANIZATION (1960), Eighth Report of the Expert Committee on Mental Health. *Wld. Hlth. Org. techn. Rep. Ser.* no. 185.
ZILBOORG, G. (1963), *Amer. J. Psychiat.* **92**, 1347.
ZUBIN, J. (1963), Unpublished manuscript.

6. Alcoholism in Britain*

M. M. GLATT

IN AUGUST 1964, London was the host city for the Tenth European Institute on the Prevention and Treatment of Alcoholism. Had such a congress taken place in England only 10 years earlier—in itself something which no one could have imagined at the time—all that visitors from abroad could have been told was that there was one small alcoholic unit working under the National Health Service, that there was not one special ward or out-patient clinic anywhere in the country devoted entirely to the treatment of alcoholics, and that apart from the old-established Society for the Study of Addiction, a few nursing homes, and some temperance organizations, virtually no one cared about the alcoholic (Pullar-Strecker, 1952; Dent, 1952; Rees and Glatt, 1954; Pullar-Strecker, 1955; Glatt, 1955a). In fact, visitors from abroad were often told by official agencies that there was no alcoholic problem in the country. A pamphlet on *Health Education* published by the Ministry of Education in 1956 spoke of " . . . a welcome and continuing reduction in the heavy drinking which at times in the 18th and 19th centuries caused great harm to our society. . . ."

It is certainly strange that it was probably the success of the campaign against drunkenness waged in the earlier part of the century which was largely responsible for the lack of interest in the problem of alcoholism by the State, and the professional and general public alike. Yet inebriety had been common in England already in the Middle Ages, and the origins of the licensing system go back longer than 400 years. Widespread drunkenness was at its height in the first half of the 18th (as a consequence of the arrival of cheaply produced gin) and even more so in the 19th century, during the era of free trade in beer, when gin palaces and ale houses vied with each other in attracting customers (Wilson, 1940; Glatt, 1958a). These conditions were depicted by Hogarth and later by Cruickshank. Whereas numerous well-meaning efforts over centuries by social reformers, including the temperance societies, Churches, legislators and (very rarely) also by doctors, had failed to extricate the country from the tight grip of drunkenness, legislative action taken by Lloyd George during the First World War succeeded almost over-night, through heavy taxation and cutting down on the facilities and times

---

* The first section is largely based on a review (1960) prepared for the Joint Committee of the British Medical Association and the Magistrates Association.

for drinking. Since then, a number of factors acting in combination, such as social changes, educational influences, and competing interests, have prevented drunkenness from becoming a widespread menace once again. By the middle of the 20th century, leading medical journals in the country had almost written off alcoholism as a problem in this country and were hardly publishing anything on it. Drunkenness convictions—200,000 at the turn of the century—had fallen to less than 50,000; reported deaths from "alcoholism" from 3000 in 1901 to 34 in 1954; reported deaths from liver cirrhosis from over 4000 in 1901 to about 800 in the years 1944–8—and all this despite a population increase of 25% (Glatt, 1958a). The tentative estimates of the World Health Organization's Alcoholism Subcommittee in 1951 showed England and Wales to have the lowest proportionate number of alcoholics out of eleven countries listed (W.H.O., 1951).

Recent Developments and Statistics

All this and (probably most important) the fact that the sight of drunken men, formerly so familiar, had become a rarity, explains to some extent the attitude of complacency of the State and the public, which could not be shaken by warnings of a few dedicated individuals such as Drs. J. Y. Dent, H. Pullar-Strecker and Lincoln Williams. Yet drunkenness is, of course, not synonymous with alcoholism, which is a very complex condition. There are no reliable figures available regarding the extent of alcoholism in this country,* but all the indirect indices point to an increase of the problem over the past 10–15 years. None of these indices by itself could be considered to show an increase of the problem, but when they all point more or less in the same direction, they can be taken to show the general trend.

1. *Convictions for public drunkenness* have risen steadily from a low figure of 20,000 in 1945 to 48,000 in 1950, 54,000 in 1955, 68,000 in 1960, and 84,000 in 1962—the highest figure since an isolated peak in 1920.† Stated in number per 10,000 of population aged 15 years and over, there has been an increase from 7·09 in 1945 to 23·26 in 1962. This rise took place in men only, whose proved offences increased from 16,000 in 1945 to 79,000 in 1962, whereas the figure in women remained more or less stationary (4300 in 1945, 4800 in 1962). One must, of course, remember that only a proportion of drunken people come under observation, fewer are arrested, and still fewer are convicted. Women, with their tendency to secret drinking at home, are less likely to get drunk in public than men. The changing attitudes of the police over the years and in varying localities represent another factor complicating the interpretation of such data.

* When referring to alcoholism in the paper, it is understood in the sense defined by the World Health Organization's Alcoholism Subcommittee Second Report in 1952.
† Public drunkenness convictions in 1963 and 1964 fell to 83,000 and 77,000 respectively.

One important aspect of drunkenness convictions is that of the steady rise of *youthful drunkenness*. The number of offences proved against persons under 21 in England and Wales rose from 3500 in 1954 to 9400 in 1962 (9300 in 1964). Excessive drinking amongst youngsters is responsible to a large extent for their frequent appearance in court for offences including crimes of violence, theft and hooliganism. Quite apart from this connection between heavy drinking and delinquency, speculations about the possible relationships between today's excessive juvenile drinking and the possible development of alcoholism 10 or 15 years later must give rise to grave misgivings.*

2. *Convictions for driving or being in charge of a vehicle* whilst under the influence of drink in England and Wales have risen steadily from approximately 3900 in 1955 to over 8000 in 1963. Such figures naturally underestimate vastly the real number of heavily drinking drivers and their contribution to traffic accidents. For example, quite a few of our alcoholic patients have admitted having been involved in accidents whilst under the influence, without having been convicted or, occasionally, even charged with it (Glatt, 1964a). Alcohol, even in small amounts, has been found to impair driving performance, judgement, etc. (Drew, Colquhoun and Long, 1958). In line with recent findings in Sweden (Andreasson, 1962) and Canada (Schmidt, Smart and Popham, 1962), it has also been our experience that alcoholics contribute much more than their fair share to traffic accidents caused by drinking drivers. Whilst no reliable estimate can be given, the proportion of 10% of alcoholics among drunken drivers in England is not likely to be an overestimate. Moreover, it has been found that serious and fatal injuries are more likely with high blood alcohol levels, and these are naturally not uncommon in alcoholics. Recent urine tests among a sample of alcoholic patients on admission to the unit at St. Bernard's Hospital showed levels corresponding to a blood alcohol level of over 150 mg per 100 ml in almost 50% of those patients who had taken drink shortly before admission (Glatt, 1964b). Just as youthful heavy drinking is linked with the big social problem of juvenile delinquency, so alcoholism is also closely involved in that of safety on the roads.

3. *Admissions to mental hospitals* in England and Wales for "alcoholism", which amounted to over 450 in 1952, stood at nearly 1900 in 1960; for "alcoholic psychosis" the increase was from 200 in 1952 to 600 in 1960. Together, alcoholism and alcoholic psychosis made up 1·1% of the total of admissions to psychiatric hospitals in 1952, as against 2·2% in 1960 and

---

* The increase of youthful drunkenness illustrates the need for health education to counteract factors such as the glamorizing of drinking by some forms of advertising, social pressures to drink, the desire of some youngsters to acquire status by lavish spending and delinquent behaviour, and the failure to find a constructive way of spending leisure-time and an outlet for energy, whilst at the same time having more money in their pockets.

3·6% in 1961 (when there were nearly 2800 admissions for alcoholism and alcoholic psychosis—a rate of 0·6 per 1000 of the total population of 46 million). The increase affected both men and women; in 1955, nearly 800 men were admitted for alcoholism and alcoholic psychosis as against 2150 in 1961; 270 women in 1955 against 610 in 1961. There are, of course, other alcoholics who are admitted not into psychiatric hospitals but to general hospitals because of physical complications, such as haematemesis, cardio-myopathy, injuries, etc. Rise of admission rates for alcoholism to hospitals does not necessarily mean an increase of alcoholism rates in the population; to some extent at least, it must be connected with the formation of specialized units in psychiatric hospitals (Warlingham Park Hospital being the first in 1952 (Glatt, 1955a and 1955c)), and with the gradual emergence and accept-ance of the illness concept of alcoholism. Similar considerations hold good for the increase of admission rates for alcoholic women, who nowadays are certainly more prepared to come forward than a few years ago, but they do not seem to explain the rise of admission rates for alcoholic psychosis. The latter might have been expected to necessitate hospital admission in former years, independent of the provision of specialized units and changing attitudes. One is left with the impression that whilst factors other than a rise in alco-holism rates may have contributed considerably to the increasing admission rates, by themselves, they may not explain the whole story.

4. *Mortality from liver cirrhosis* is often employed as an index of alcoholism prevalence, despite all theoretical objections. In the U.K., factors other than alcoholism are certainly responsible for the great majority of cases of liver cirrhosis; recent estimates on the contribution of alcoholism to death from cirrhosis vary between 5% and 25%. According to figures published by the Ministry of Health, alcoholism contributed more than 15% to liver cirrhosis mortality in the period 1932–6; during 1952–6 it was less than 10%—and then more often amongst men than amongst women. In relation to such statistics, one has also to remember that in England, doctors are often reluctant to mention alcoholism as a cause of death, and the family of the deceased will often play down his drinking habits a great deal. On the other hand, the connection between alcoholism and liver cirrhosis in Britain is also illustrated by the finding of a high Standard Mortality Rate amongst groups with a presumably high alcohol consumption, such as publicans (S.M.R. 925, as against an average S.M.R. of 100), barmen and publicans' wives (S.M.R. approximately 500) (Registrar General's Decennial Sup-plement, 1951).

Keeping the possible limitations in mind, the statistics show an increase of deaths from liver cirrhosis from approximately 820 in 1948 to 1260 in 1957 and 1320 in 1963; in men, from 500 in 1948 to 670 in 1957 and 700 in 1963; in women, from 310 in 1948 to 540 in 1957 and 620 in 1963. The rates of such deaths per million living males rose rather irregularly from 27·1 in

1950 to 33·0 in 1961; per million living females, there was a more steady rise from 19·4 in 1950 to 27·0 in 1961 (Registrar General's Annual Statistical Reviews).

5. *Alcohol consumption* per head in the U.K. has shown a marked increase as regards wines and, to a lesser extent, spirits, whereas beer consumption has remained at a fairly steady level. Wine consumption rose from 0·23 gallons in 1950 to 0·53 gallons per head in 1961; spirit consumption from 0·2 gallons in 1950 to 0·3 gallons in 1961. Beer consumption has not changed a great deal from its 1954 level of 80·0 litres per head. These trends may be also illustrated by the total consumption figures of intoxicants in the U.K. There was a rise in consumption of imported wines, from 15·4 million gallons in 1938 and 17·1 in 1959, to 22·2 in 1962 and 26·2 in 1964; of spirits, from 10 million proof gallons in 1938, to 13·90 in 1959, 15·85 in 1962 and 18·36 in 1964; and of beer, from 25 million bulk barrels in 1938, to 26·06 in 1959, 28·56 in 1962 and 30·00 in 1964.*

Throughout the centuries, beer or ale had been the drink of the common man in England. Britain (at that time still including Eire) led the world in beer drinking in 1914, whereas in 1963 Britain's beer consumption (19·3 gallons per head per year) was fifth in the world, following that of Belgium, West Germany, Australia and New Zealand. The change in drinking habits in England was well described by Lord Cohen (1964):

> Spirit drinking is becoming more popular. The cocktail party has superseded the tea party, commercial transactions are conducted too often at meals whose preliminaries are numerous "short drinks", dinner in high places finishes more often with brandy than with port, and the English workman is gradually becoming attuned, as did his Scottish drinking counterpart two centuries ago, to a tot of whisky.

Recent years have seen in this country the emergence of what has been called the "expense account alcoholic"—the executive and traveller who is encouraged by accepted practices, during his work, to imbibe more than finally turns out to have been good for him.

All other factors being equal, heavy spirit consumption (average content of absolute alcohol: 40%) carries a greater risk of leading to alcoholism than wine (15%), and even more so than beer (5%). However, by themselves, these figures do not tell us anything about the proportion of heavy drinkers among all consumers of alcohol, i.e. about the size of the population that is mainly at risk. If the increase of consumption were rather uniform throughout the population, the rising alcohol consumption might possibly be considered a "problem of alcohol" rather than a problem of "alcoholism".

6. *The national drink bill in the U.K.* (*Great Britain and Northern Ireland*). The rising alcohol consumption is reflected in the figures showing the yearly

---

* The 1962 figures show that wine drinking had reached a new peak; and spirit consumption had reached its highest level for 40 years, equivalent to four bottles a year for each adult (Report of Commissioners of H.M. Customs and Excise, 1963).

personal expenditure on alcoholic drinks (although the increase in taxation, etc., has to be taken into consideration). These have risen steadily from £680 million in 1946 to £906 million in 1956 and £1316 million in 1964. Beer expenditure increased from £550 million in 1956 to £760 million in 1964, and expenditure on spirits, wines, etc., from £360 million in 1956 to £556 million in 1964. Of the total of Britain's consumer expenditure in 1964 of £21,000 million, alcoholic drink contributed £1316 million, and tobacco £1344 million. Between 1963 and 1964 drink expenditure increased by over 11% as against a rise of 7% of total consumer expenditure. Alcoholic drink took 1s. 3d. out of each pound spent in 1962, and tobacco 1s. 4d. as against 5s. 7d. spent on food. Whatever else might be said about drinking and smoking, drinkers and smokers between them more than finance the National Health Service (which costs the State about £1000 million per year). Revenue from taxation of alcoholic liquors in 1963 amounted to £481 million (as against just over £400 million in 1950), i.e. approximately 18% of the total revenue, but is still less than revenue from tobacco taxation—tobacco duty amounting to approximately £900 million, or nearly one-third of the total revenue.

7. *The number of alcoholics.* Although statements are often made about the number of alcoholics in England and Wales, no reliable figures are, in fact, available as no comprehensive field surveys have been carried out. Using as a basis the Jellinek Formula (which has as its foundation the percentage contribution of alcoholism to the total number of deaths from cirrhosis of the liver), the Alcoholism Subcommittee of W.H.O. in 1951 estimated the number of "chronic alcoholics" (i.e. those with mental or physical complications) as 86,000—a figure which Jellinek regarded as "probably reliable". In the U.S.A. at the time, 1 alcoholic in 4 was said to develop the complications of "chronic alcoholism". The assumption that a similar ratio might hold good in England brought a total estimate of alcoholics in England and Wales to about 350,000; Jellinek regarded this figure as "hardly better than a guess" (W.H.O., 1951).

Several years later in 1956, Parr tried to estimate the number of alcoholics known to general practitioners in this country by means of a questionnaire, which was sent out to the Members of the Research Register of the College of General Practitioners (Parr, 1957). The replies showed that the incidence of alcoholism in general practice amounted to roughly one-tenth of the W.H.O. estimate—110 per 100,000 adults, as against 1100 per 100,000. However, such low figures cannot be regarded as representing more than the "top of the iceberg". Unfortunately, alcoholics and doctors tend very often to go out of each other's way. For example, a great proportion of alcoholic patients seen at the Alcoholic Unit at Warlingham Park between 1952 and 1957 stated that although they had shown clear features of alcoholism for 10–15 years, they hardly ever consulted their family doctor about it. They did not tell him about their drinking, and they were not asked about it. In fact, referrals often came from other sources although, if more recent experience at St. Bernard's Hospital is a pointer, matters have begun to change. Doctors in this country generally receive little teaching in their student days about the early features of alcoholism, and they all too often equate "alcoholism" with its complications—a viewpoint which obviously militates against early diagnosis. This valuable survey, therefore, highlights the great need for proper undergraduate and postgraduate medical education in this field. It shows that there exist at least 35,000 fairly advanced alcoholics who—in the terms of the W.H.O. definition used—"require treatment". But it cannot be employed as an index of the number of alcoholics in this country (Glatt, 1957b).

More recently, between 1960 and 1963, an attempt was made to obtain some information about the prevalence of alcoholism by the Steering Group on Alcoholism formed by the Joseph Rowntree Social Service Trust. The field work was undertaken by two agencies—health visitors and probation officers—in five English towns. These officers attempted to estimate the incidence of alcoholism in families observed by them over a certain period. The probation officers' inquiry alone indicated a total of over 10,000 obvious alcoholics, but of course one has to remember that both probation officers and health visitors see only certain segments of the population. From an analysis of their findings and of the smaller practices in Parr's G.P. survey, Prys Williams concluded that the number of obvious alcoholics in England and Wales was at least 70,000, while earlier-stage alcoholics numbered at least 200,000 (Steering Group, 1965; Prys Williams and Glatt, 1966).

Summarizing this part of the discussion, it can be estimated (even in the absence of comprehensive field studies) that the number of alcoholics in this country amounts to several hundred thousands, and that there are indications that the problem is on the increase. Taking into consideration that alcoholism, perhaps more than any other illness, closely affects the lives of relatives as well, it seems that 1 million people in this country may be more or less directly affected by alcoholism.

8. *Alcoholism in industry.* Little attention has been paid to the possibility of an alcoholic problem in British industry, and no extensive studies have been carried out there. An attempt made by an industrialist in 1957 to get some information met with indifference, and elicited only negative replies from his business colleagues, hardly anyone of whom knew any alcoholics in their concerns and factories (A Managing Director, *B.J.A.*, 1957). However, several minor investigations among our own patients indicate that the problem of alcoholism in British industry cannot be insignificant. Thus, of 200 male alcoholics seen at Warlingham Park between 1952 and 1956, more than 50 % had begun to lose time off work due to their drinking habits, on the

average 10 years before hospital admission, and had first lost a job 7 years before admission (Glatt, 1957a). Of a sample of male alcoholics seen in 1964 at the unit at St. Bernard's Hospital, 75% had been drinking to excess for more than 5 years, and 50% had realized for at least 5 years that their work capacity had deteriorated and that they needed help (Glatt and Hills, 1964). They did not do so, mainly because of their fear of getting the sack. As at Warlingham Park Hospital, most of these men were in age-groups between 30 and 45, i.e. in their potentially most productive time of life. They came from all social classes, often showing marked socio-occupational decline. Of the St. Bernard's sample of 40 men, none had originally been an unskilled labourer (class V), but one-third were doing unskilled labouring jobs before admission to the hospital. At both hospitals, alcoholics came from all social classes, but classes I and II predominated, and naturally even more so in private practice, where half the alcoholic patients were people such as company directors, managers, etc.

The influence on factory production, etc., is clear even from such small samples. In 1962, of a total working population in the U.K. of over 25 million people, nearly one-third (9 million) were employed in manufacturing industries. Assuming as minimum estimates the proportion of alcoholics among these 9 million (who are generally at an age where alcoholism is a risk) as 1%, we would get a figure of 90,000. Or, if one were to assume that two-thirds of the 9 million were drinkers, and 2% of them might become alcoholics—again a conservative estimate—the figure would be 120,000. Clearly, there is an urgent need for research and for a planned educational programme in relation to alcoholism in industry.

9. *Scotland and Northern Ireland.* The present exposition is mainly concerned with conditions in England, but a few figures relating to other parts of the U.K. may be of some interest. (Some of the preceding statistics have, of course, included Scotland and Northern Ireland.) No field studies have been carried out, but the problem of alcoholism, at least in Scotland, is generally assumed to be greater proportionately than in England. To some extent, this is probably connected with the fact that the national drink in Scotland is whisky, in contrast to beer in England, and that the *per capita* consumption of spirits has always been higher in Scotland than in England (Tongue, 1955). The late Dr. A. A. McDougall, a Scottish psychiatrist specially interested in alcoholism, estimated the number of "addictive drinkers" in Scotland approximately 10 years ago as between 20,000 and 25,000, out of a total population of 5 million. The death rates from alcoholism in 1954 in Scotland were $0 \cdot 6$ for men and $0 \cdot 2$ for women (as against $0 \cdot 1$ for both sexes in England) per 100,000 of population (*Brit. Med. J.*, 1956). The death rate from liver cirrhosis in Scotland (1957) was $4 \cdot 7$ per 100,000 compared, for example, with $2 \cdot 6$ in England and Wales (1956), $2 \cdot 3$ in Northern Ireland (1957), $2 \cdot 1$ in Eire (1957) and $10 \cdot 7$ in the U.S.A. (1956) (*Demographic*

Yearbook, United Nations, 1958).* Convictions for offences against the Intoxicating Liquor Laws (i.e. chiefly for drunkenness) have always been proportionately much more frequent in Scotland than in England and Wales; e.g. per 100,000 of population in 1948, 140 in Scotland, as against 76 in England and Wales, and in 1954, 233 as against 126 (*Demographic Yearbook*, United Nations, 1958). Drunkenness convictions in Scotland (Craigie, 1963), after showing a decrease in the past (e.g. from 17,000 in 1938 to 7000 in 1948) have again gradually climbed up: 8000 in 1950, 12,300 in 1955, 13,500 in 1960, 15,000 in 1962. The increase has affected only men. The figure for women has remained fairly stationary over the past 10 years, amounting to over 900 per year (in 1962 about one-tenth of the figure for male convictions). Admissions to psychiatric hospitals (Craigie, 1963) for alcoholism in Scotland increased from 630 in 1956 to 990 in 1960 and 1495 in 1962; among men, from 610 in 1956 to approximately 1240 in 1962; in women, from 120 to 260. Whereas in 1956 alcoholism accounted for approximately one-eighth of total male admissions to psychiatric hospitals, its proportion has risen to nearly one-fifth (18·7%). The corresponding proportion in England and Wales is just above 1 in 20. In women, the corresponding increase was from 2·2% to 3·1% in Scotland.

As far as alcoholism in Ireland is concerned, one might expect it to be proportionately higher than in England, both from the high rates found among Irish Americans, as well as from the relatively high proportion of Irish admissions to alcoholic units in England (Sullivan and Glatt, 1956). A table compiled by Phillipson (1964), comparing admissions for alcoholism and alcoholic psychoses to psychiatric hospitals in England and Wales, Scotland, Northern Ireland and the Republic of Ireland, shows for 1962 approximately 730 alcoholic admissions in Northern Ireland and 785 in the Republic (approximately 3700 in England and Wales and 1500 in Scotland). This gives rates per 1000 of total population of 0·522 (N. Ireland), 0·280 (Republic), 0·08 (England and Wales) and 0·299 (Scotland) respectively, amounting to a percentage of total admissions to psychiatric hospitals of 11 (N. Ireland), 5·4 (Republic), 5·3 and 0·6 (for men and women in England and Wales), and 18·7 and 3·1 (for men and women in Scotland) respectively. For Northern Ireland, studies among general practitioners carried out in recent years by Grant and Boyd (1962) gave an alcoholism rate of 191 per 100,000 adults in rural Northern Ireland. This compares with Parr's findings (1957) in England and Wales of 110 per 100,000 adults and of 240 per 100,000 in Scotland.

All in all, these scattered observations confirm the general impression that alcoholism is more prevalent in Scotland, Northern Ireland and the Republic

---

* Deaths from liver cirrhosis in Scotland between 1952 and 1961 increased in males from 100 to 134 (per 100,000 population, from 4 to 5) and in females from 66 to 100 (per 100,000 population, from 2 to 4).

of Ireland than in England. However, the lack of interest and of planned treatment programmes seems to have been just as much in evidence. Whereas Alcoholics Anonymous has been active in all parts of the U.K. (including Scotland) and in Eire for nearly 20 years, it was only in 1964 that the first alcoholic units were started in Scotland and Northern Ireland. However, certain institutions, such as Crichton Royal Hospital in Dumfries, have been treating alcoholics for years (McAdam, 1964) and recently, the Standing Medical Advisory Committee of the Scottish Health Services Council has appointed a Subcommittee on Alcoholism. The fact that, with the assistance of the International Council on Alcohol and Alcoholism, international congresses on alcoholism have recently taken place in Dublin and Cardiff (1965), as well as in London (1964), bears witness to the increase of interest in the problem in many parts of the British Isles.

Social Distribution

The admission rate to psychiatric hospitals in England and Wales for alcoholics is much greater for the higher social classes. A similar anomalous social distribution was also found among male alcoholics admitted to Warlingham Park and among members of A.A. (Glatt, 1955a, 1961b), and also among male admissions to psychiatric hospitals in Scotland in 1961 (Morrison, 1964). Does this mean that alcoholism in Great Britain is largely an affliction of the middle class, or merely that for some reason or other, alcoholics belonging to other social strata are less likely to look for help to hospitals and A.A.? In favour of a real difference in prevalence among the various social classes is a comparison with the different mortality rates from liver cirrhosis. Such mortality rates are considerably higher for classes I and, to a lesser extent, II, than for classes III, IV and V, as Brooke (1959) has shown for the years 1949–53.

On the other hand, among samples of homeless alcoholics (Glatt and Whiteley, 1956) seen at a London reception centre (a place for people without any means and usually harbouring a considerable proportion of excessive drinkers), or admitted to a London observation ward, the majority were found to be working in unskilled labouring jobs (class V). Unlike the often highly educated and intelligent male alcoholics seen at Warlingham Park or among A.A. members, they were usually of average or low intelligence. Another difference was that whereas among the male alcoholics seen at Warlingham Park only about one-third were psychopaths (Glatt, 1961a) (another third were "psychoneurotics" and the rest fairly "normal" or average types of personalities), the homeless alcoholics were in the majority psychopathic. Finally, in contrast to the Warlingham Park male alcoholics, the great majority of the homeless alcoholics were unmarried.

Our later findings in observation wards in London, at St. Bernard's Hospital and at the St. Marylebone and Paddington out-patient clinics for alcoholics (Glatt, 1961c) bore out the impression that alcoholism is by no means uncommon among classes III–V. Of special interest is the contrast in the social class distribution between the male alcoholics admitted in 1952–7 to the unit at Warlingham Park and those admitted in later years to the unit at St. Bernard's Hospital. At the time, Warlingham Park, having the only special unit in the country, admitted alcoholics from all parts of England. These patients, as a rule, had some degree of insight and of motivation to do something about their alcoholism. In contrast, male alcoholics at St. Bernard's during the first few years were admitted only from the local catchment area, but often quite independent of any "motivation", and through having got into trouble because of intoxication, or because of associated psychiatric disorders, such as D.T.s or auditory hallucinations. It was also interesting that, as a rule, among alcoholics seen at the St. Marylebone Out-patient Clinic in the period 1958–60, those belonging to classes I–III had been referred by their general practitioners, and those from class V by probation officers, Common Lodging Houses (housing the homeless who still have little means left), prisons, etc. Naturally, class V is also preponderant among down-and-out crude spirit drinkers found in bombed-out areas, in London and other large cities.

These studies show that male alcoholics are found at every level of English society, even if the liver cirrhosis mortality rates may indicate a heavier affliction of the upper middle class (perhaps associated with their relatively greater consumption of the more expensive spirits (Hulton Readership Survey, 1954)). This consideration clearly points to the urgent need for more intensive education in this field, especially among the working class, where apparently the concept of alcoholism as an illness that could and should be treated is even less known than in the middle class.

Among alcoholic women, all social classes were represented in the alcoholic units of Warlingham Park and St. Bernard's hospitals, although women alcoholics belonging to class I in general fight shy of such public units and prefer private nursing homes, relatively more so than male alcoholics.

Social class distribution among male and female alcoholic prisoners has been investigated by Parr (1962), Epps (1957) and Woodside (1961), who all found a strong preponderance of class V. From a study of offences of drunkenness in the London area in 1957, Parr (1962) calculated the total number of "habitual drunkards" coming before the courts annually as 4500. Approximately one-fifth of the offences were attributable to "habitual offenders", having more than one offence of drunkenness on record. Parr also calculated that the annual total of 67,000 drunkenness offences in England (in 1957) would be accounted for by 54,000 once-only and 4500 habitual offenders.

Among the prison population, heavy drinkers form a considerable proportion. A recent inquiry carried out by Cooper and Maule (1963) among recently discharged male prisoners found that 56% were heavy drinkers. Of the alcoholic prisoners, 54% were in social classes IV and V, as compared with only 29% for the population of England and Wales as a whole (1951 census), and with 4% among members of A.A. Of the heavily drinking ex-prisoners, 32% were divorced or separated and only 14% married, as compared with 3% of divorced or separated and 78% married among all males in the general population aged 20–64. The marriage breakdown rate, i.e. the proportion of marriages that ended in divorce or separation (whether legal or not)—known to be high among alcoholics—was found by these authors to be 70% among the heavy drinker ex-prisoners. This compared with 50% of non-drinking prisoners, 6% among male and female alcoholics at St. Bernard's Hospital, and only 4% among the male population of the country as a whole.

In samples of alcoholics drawn from various sections of the population (alcoholic unit, homeless alcoholics, out-patient clinic) and studied by us approximately 10 years ago, 30–40% had been before the courts or in prison, though mainly for petty crimes only (Glatt, 1958b). In view of the prevalence of a history of problem drinking among people appearing before courts or arriving in prison, it is gratifying to note that in recent years there has been an increasing tendency to refer such people to psychiatrists interested in alcoholism or, where indicated, to special hostels or units, and that A.A. has been allowed to establish groups in certain prisons. But this, of course, is only a beginning.

Types of Alcoholism

It has been estimated that in this country "less than 5% of major mental disorder is directly and solely due to alcohol" (Stafford-Clark, 1952). No systematic statistics have recently been published, but in personal observation over the past 14 years in psychiatric hospitals and alcoholic units, the present author has come occasionally across withdrawal convulsions, D.T.s, alcoholic dementia, auditory hallucinations and Korsakoff's syndrome, though Wernicke's disease seems very rare. A small proportion of alcoholics seen in alcoholic units and out-patient clinics are periodic drinkers; possibly 20% show evidence of mild peripheral neuritis; 75% when tested by a battery of liver function tests showed evidence of (usually reversible) impaired liver function (Kay, Murfitt and Glatt, 1959). Among a sample of female alcoholics observed a few years ago at St. Bernard's Hospital, 15% had a history of D.T.s, 13% showed evidence of peripheral neuritis; Korsakoff's syndrome occurred only once (Judge and Glatt, 1961). However, alcoholics with definite physical complications will be sent relatively more frequently to general hospitals.

It is not unlikely that, as in the U.S.A., the great majority of alcoholics in Britain are those in relatively early phases. The fact that only about 1 out of

10 alcoholics in this country is known to his general practitioner and that roughly only 1 alcoholic out of 100 has joined A.A., both seem to point in this direction. Of course, one has to remember that unless the public is made to realize, through education, that alcoholism is an illness, learns to recognize its early features, and is made aware that it can be successfully treated, early alcoholics will not come forward for treatment.

The great majority of alcoholics seen in alcoholic units are those without mental or physical complications. As in the U.S.A., it seems that it is only a minority who show the complications denoting "chronic alcoholism".

Almost all the published work in Great Britain on alcoholism until very recently has dealt with the "loss of control" (Jellinek's gamma) alcoholic. This is the type who is usually seen at A.A. meetings, or presenting himself voluntarily for treatment at alcoholic units. This type, for example, was predominant at Warlingham Park, but even there 15% denied the occurrence of "loss of control" (Glatt, 1961b). Much smaller was the proportion of "loss of control" among down-and-out drinkers, among alcoholics coming from prison, and also among people such as publicans and their wives, barmen and merchant seamen (Rose and Glatt, 1961), i.e. individuals whose occupations frequently expose and tempt them to excessive drinking (Glatt, 1961c). Such drinkers occasionally developed mental and physical complications of "chronic alcoholism", despite the absence of "loss of control". Possibly, alcoholism with physical complications, despite the absence of compulsive drinking and "loss of control", might be the most common variety seen in general hospitals. Thus, Brigden (1957) showed that of 13 (beer or spirit) drinkers suffering from "alcoholic cardiomyopathy" and admitted to general hospitals, 4 were engaged in the liquor trade. The excessive drinking pattern seen in some of the alcoholics among the groups mentioned above resembled often the "inability to abstain" (Jellinek's delta) variety or also "non-addictive" alcoholism (Glatt, 1961c).

It is interesting to speculate about the possible connection in this country between the type of alcoholic drink preferred and the predominant variety of alcoholism amongst certain social groups. Inquiries carried out a few years ago by the Hulton Research team (1954) have shown that spirit drinking is relatively more common among the higher income brackets and beer drinking more among the lower income groups. The type of alcoholic predominant at Warlingham Park was usually a middle-class, "loss of control" spirit drinker, whereas beer or cider were the favourite drinks among the down-and-outs and amongst some of the "occupational" alcoholics. This would conform to some extent to the statement by the World Health Organization Committee (1955) that "loss of control" alcoholism was more frequent in spirit-drinking countries and the "inability to abstain" (which seems to be a less misleading term than "inability to stop") type in some of the predominantly beer-drinking groups. Aetiologically, psychogenic factors, e.g. emotional conflicts, seemed more prevalent in our "loss of control" addicts, whereas environmental social factors, e.g. easy access or lack of taboo on heavy drinking in the social group, seemed to have played a relatively bigger role in inducing, or at least facilitating, heavy drinking among the other types of alcoholics (Glatt, 1961c). To some extent, this distinction reminds one of Jellinek's discussion (1957) of the different emphasis (in regard to aetiology) put by some French and American writers on alcoholism. The French, with the "inability to abstain" type common in France, stress social factors; the Americans, with spirit drinking and "loss of control" predominating in the U.S.A., stress the aetiological significance of personality factors.

Although other varieties of alcoholism than the gamma type have found more attention in Britain than previously during the past few years or so, this cannot be taken as demonstrating an increase of such other forms of alcoholism. Rather, it illustrates the greater interest taken in these other varieties since the publication of Jellinek's last book on *The Disease Concept of Alcoholism* (1960). It also may reflect the fact that members of other than the upper social strata come under greater medical attention now, and these may contain a relatively higher proportion of Jellinek's delta type or of "non-addictive" alcoholics. Parr (1962) has suggested that heavy weekend beer drinking may be the commonest form of excessive drinking among social groups IV and V. On the basis of the difference in popularity of alcoholic drinks, it might also be expected that in Scotland, not only should alcoholism be more prevalent than in England, but also that gamma alcoholism should be relatively more, and delta alcoholism less, common. But it is not yet known whether or not this is so.

Voluntary Organizations

In the absence of any planned state programme, it was left until recently to a few voluntary societies and organizations to call attention to the problem of alcoholism. In the last few years, along with the establishment of alcoholic units under the National Health Service, there has also been a welcome increase in the interest shown by voluntary organizations. Of course, National Health Service facilities and those provided by voluntary societies often work hand in hand, and some specialists are active in both. Among the voluntary organizations, some concentrate mainly on matters of education, and others on treatment and rehabilitation.

1. EDUCATION

(a) *The Society for the Study of Addiction* (formerly, Society for the Study of Inebriety) is a scientific body whose objects are the systematic study of addiction to alcohol and to other drugs. It was founded in 1884, and has both medical and lay members, many of them outside Great Britain. It actively supports research and, with the help of a grant from the Brewers' Society, has financed work on biochemical aspects of alcoholism by McLeod at the Burden Institute in Bristol (McLeod, 1953, 1955, 1957), and research by Camps at the London Hospital, St. Bernard's Hospital, etc., on the importance of hypoglycaemia. Its *Proceedings* were first published in 1884, and replaced in 1903 by the *British Journal of Inebriety*, later renamed the *British Journal of Addiction*.

(b) *The National Council on Alcoholism*, established in 1962, bases its programme on the model of the very successful National Committee on Alcoholism in the U.S.A. It is a voluntary agency, consisting of both professional and lay members. It recognizes alcoholism as a treatable illness, a public health problem and a public responsibility. It is concerned with alcoholism, not with social drinking; its approach is scientific and non-controversial, and it is not allied to any temperance movement. The council aims to make its concepts widely known by means of the formation of local councils, each having as its chief activity, an information centre on alcoholism. Seven information centres have so far been opened in London, Liverpool, Gloucestershire, Cardiff, Glasgow, Brighton (since closed) and Leeds (since closed). The Liverpool centre, opened in July 1963, dealt in its first year with over 400 people. Twenty-seven per cent came voluntarily, 27% were introduced by relatives, and 46% were sent by religious bodies, the social services, the police, or by their doctors. The National Council undertook a public appeal for £750,000 in September 1964. Its first executive director was a recovered alcoholic.

(c) *The Camberwell Council on Alcoholism.* The C.C.A. (Camberwell is a district in South London) was set up as an experiment in 1962; its prime mover and chairman being the (then) local medical officer of health, Dr. M. D. Chalke. Its objects are to find out more about the impact of alcohol on the community and, by joint effort, to help in the solution of some of its problems. It aims not only at discussion, but also at positive action. It started the publication of its *Bulletin on Alcoholism* in June 1963. During its first year, it carried out a study of the homeless, rough-living surgical-spirit drinking alcoholic, and in 1965 it held an information and discussion week. With the help of a voluntary organization (Helping Hands) a half-way house has been opened, which eventually should house sixteen alcoholics during rehabilitation (St. Giles House).

(d) *Steering Group on Alcoholism*, formed by the *Joseph Rowntree Social Service Trust*. Established in 1956, this body was chiefly interested in the social aspects of alcoholism. It carried out surveys, (e.g. on alcoholism prevalence in certain English cities), and published a file of treatment facilities in the country sent out to general practitioners who indicated their interest.

Some of its members took a leading part in the formation of the National Council on Alcoholism.*

(e) *Helping Hands Organization.* Formed recently by Mr. B. Richards, a retired businessman, the organization intends to support rehabilitation houses for alcoholics and similar institutions, such as St. Giles House, Camberwell.

(f) Certain *temperance societies*, such as the Church of England Temperance Society, have taken a very active part in the problem of rehabilitating alcoholics. The Temperance Council of the Christian Churches, which is formed by temperance societies of all different shades and opinions, has arranged several successful conferences on alcoholism and publishes regularly its *Focus on Drink and Gambling*. There has long been a split in the British temperance movement between the more conciliatory "suasionists" and the prohibitionistic "suppressionists". The latter are mainly represented by The United Kingdom Alliance, which publishes two highly informative (though naturally biased) journals—the *Alliance News* and the *Research Student*. On the other side of the fence, a magazine (*A Monthly Bulletin*), often carrying interesting news on alcohol problems and alcoholism, is also published by the brewing industries.

2. TREATMENT AND REHABILITATION

(a) *Spelthorne St. Mary* is a branch house of the Anglican Community of St. Mary the Virgin, Wantage, and is devoted to the treatment and rehabilitation of female alcoholics and drug addicts. Its work was begun in 1879. The staff consists of Wantage Sisters and includes a number of state registered nurses, as well as a physician at present, and treatment is carried out with the help of visiting psychiatrists. The average number of patients is 45–50; the average stay 6 months. Occupational therapy is an essential part of the treatment, but a great deal seems to depend on the spiritual atmosphere and family spirit. The aim at Spelthorne is rehabilitation of the whole personality (*Church Times*, 1964).

(b) The *Reginald Carter Foundation* was started by the Church of England Temperance Society in 1956 as an out-patient centre for alcoholics, but it also functions as a permanent "open house". About 100 people are being treated there, at a cost of £6000 a year.

(c) The *Harry Lloyd Foundation Clinic* was, like the Carter Clinic, founded a few years ago in London by the Church of England Temperance Society to give out-patient treatment to alcoholics.

(d) *St. Luke's House and St. Mary's House.* Alcoholic rehabilitation centres for male and female alcoholics were started in 1961 by the West London Mission. They function mainly as half-way hostels for alcoholics who have already received treatment and are homeless. Preliminary reviews

---

* This Steering Group was disbanded in 1965.

show 20–30% of satisfactory discharges from the centres (Ingram-Smith, 1965).

(e) *Regent Street Clinic*, situated in the heart of London, and run by a probation officer, aims to help mainly in cases where the alcoholic still has a family and where both husband and wife can attend the clinic. Unlike (d), it is non-residential.

(f) *Royal London Discharged Prisoners' Aid Society* assists people who are in prison or have just left it including, naturally, many alcoholics.

(g) Organizations such as the *Salvation Army* and the *Church Army* have helped many alcoholics who needed a place where they could recover from a bout of intoxication, or which they could use as a temporary basis during rehabilitation. Their hostels and centres (the Church Army catering more for the educated type of individual) have often been of help in cases for whom hospital admission could not be secured.

(h) Last, but certainly not least in importance, is the work of *Alcoholics Anonymous*. The first European group was started in Dublin in 1946, the first English group in London 1 year later. The British A.A. may now have approximately 5000 members, and there are groups in England, Scotland, Wales and Ireland. In England alone, there are now over 150 groups, including a number functioning in hospitals and a few recently started in prison. A.A. works in close contact with individual doctors, with voluntary organizations, and with the N.H.S. alcoholic units, and has been increasingly accepted as a valuable ally by the medical profession in the U.K. In recent years, a number of Alanon Family Groups have also been established, one of the first of which was started by wives of ex-patients of Warlingham Park Hospital.

Apart from these organizations, there exist a number of *private nursing homes*, catering to a major or minor extent for alcoholics. By-and-large, most of them rely on mixtures of psychotherapy and drug therapy, sometimes working closely with A.A. Compared to the work of the N.H.S. units described later on, the emphasis in some of these nursing homes is more on drug therapy (such as apomorphine by injection, following the method of the late J. Y. Dent), and where psychotherapy is employed, it is individual rather than group. The method generally used for sobering-up and detoxication is more or less identical with that described below.

The Alcoholic Unit in the National Health Service*

Following, to some extent, proposals expressed a year earlier by a joint committee of the British Medical Association and the Magistrates Association (*Brit. Med. J.* 1961; *Brit. J. Addict.* 1961), a memorandum of the Ministry

* This section is based on a paper read at the Tenth European Institute on the Prevention and Treatment of Alcoholism, London, August 1964.

of Health in January 1962 recommended that hospital treatment for alcoholism should, as far as possible, be given in special regional units (*Brit.
J. Addict*. 1962). This memorandum constituted a clear reversal of the former
official policy and practice of scattering alcoholics haphazardly into numerous
local hospitals (*Brit.J.Addict*. 1961, 1962; Glatt, 1955c). Thus, by 1960, only
two hospitals had special units established for the treatment of alcoholism,
and of just over 2000 alcoholics admitted in 1959, more than half were
scattered throughout 100 different psychiatric hospitals, the numbers admitted to each hospital varying from one to nineteen (Phillipson, 1964).
During the past few years, ten new alcoholic units have been established in
England, one in Scotland, and one in Northern Ireland. It is intended to
describe here the functioning of such units and their possible contribution
to the management and prophylaxis of alcoholism. This is mainly on the
basis of personal experience at a variety of centres, rather than on a systematic
review of the literature.

The Term "Alcoholic Unit"

Clearly, a hospital treatment centre can be no more than one part of an
integrated service for alcoholics. A comprehensive service catering for
alcoholics of all types and in all phases of their addiction must provide out-
patient and community services, half-way houses and hostels, as well as in-
patient facilities. This whole integrated complex of facilities should be
regarded as the "unit", rather than the in-patient facility by itself, and should
be the responsibility of one medical director, thus allowing transfer of the
patient from one facility to another, which may often become necessary. This
unit should, of course, work in close contact with general practitioners,
Alcoholics Anonymous, and other voluntary and official agencies, especially
the local medical officer of health, and should also have easy access to
general hospitals, for patients requiring sobering-up and detoxication only.

Views differ as to the best place for the alcoholic in-patient facility. Should
it be independent, or attached to a general or psychiatric hospital? Alcoholics
are often reluctant to enter psychiatric hospitals, and therapists who use an
exclusively or predominantly physical approach may feel that the best site
would be the general hospital. On the other hand, the "therapeutic community" atmosphere may often be difficult to achieve in the general hospital
(although this has been done, for example, by Hudolin in Yugoslavia
(Hudolin, 1964)). To a large extent, alcoholism is a mental health problem,
and medically it is the psychiatrist who is, or should be, particularly interested. The psychiatric hospital can provide the suitable atmosphere and the
comprehensive treatment now generally favoured, including occupational
therapy, recreational facilities, etc. Our experience over the past 14 years
has shown that the majority of alcoholics admitted in the past to such units

situated in psychiatric hospitals found the experience very rewarding, once they had overcome the initial shock (Glatt, 1955a). In many ways, alcoholics proved to be of great help to non-alcoholic hospital patients (e.g. as organizers of patients' committees, editors of hospital journals), and they themselves benefited from participating in the activities of the whole hospital community. The stigma, unfortunately still attached to psychiatric hospital admission (as it is, of course, also to the diagnosis of alcoholism itself), is gradually decreasing.

Special centres for alcoholics only, situated in separated blocks in a progressive psychiatric hospital, provided with their own entrance and given a special name, different from the main hospital, might therefore appear a feasible method. Being least expensive to establish, such centres are also not too difficult to realize. On the other hand, experience in private nursing homes in this country and in centres abroad, such as Kalksburg in Austria (Tuchmann, 1964), has shown that homes situated independently from any hospital could perhaps serve the purpose just as well.

Very often, the question is debated as to whether in-patient or out-patient therapy is preferable for the alcoholic. To a large extent, this question seems to be academic, as there will always be a need for both. In this country at present, with a stigma attached to the term "alcoholism", with the lack of training in this field for medical students, and with the lack of understanding and information among the general public, a great many alcoholics, when first seen, are in need of at least a preliminary period of in-patient treatment. With the decrease of the stigma, with better medical training, and with increasing education of the general public, it can be confidently expected that patients will present themselves at an earlier stage, so that in time, extramural services will become progressively more important. Therefore, the shift of emphasis within the integrated complex of the alcoholic unit may be progressively towards its extramural components, but there will always be a demand and need for in-patient facilities as well.

The Therapeutic Community; Staff Attitudes, Atmosphere, Community Living

In the hands of different therapists, many forms of treatment have led to success with alcoholics. This may be partly explained by the hypothesis that most of these therapies bring about some disruption or breakdown of the original personality, so that the ground becomes clear for the development of new, healthier attitudes (Williams, 1956). But one could also argue that an important common factor may be the basic attitude of the therapist towards the alcoholic patient (Glatt, 1965b). Many alcoholics are very sensitive and emotionally insecure; having experienced rejection in the past, they expect it again and are on the lookout for it. To some extent, they may provoke it themselves by their own over-compensatory grandiose, aggressive attitude. The alcoholic will react to imagined or real censure or pressure by the staff, by excessive use of such defence mechanisms as denial, rationalizations and projections; and his reactions, in turn, may become motivations for hostile actions or further drinking. A "holier-than-thou" attitude alienates the alcoholic patient; an accepting, understanding attitude will go a long way towards winning his confidence. Once the alcoholic patient feels "accepted" by the therapist, he will often be found an extremely co-operative and rewarding patient. An accepting attitude may very often be a much more important therapeutic factor than the special tools which the therapist prefers to use. The all-important, permissive "atmosphere" will largely depend on informed, understanding attitudes of all members of the staff of the unit.

It is necessary for staff members not merely to pay lip service to the disease concept of alcoholism, but also to accept it emotionally. This task will be made easier if staff are encouraged to keep an open mind, to watch the gradually changing attitudes of alcoholic patients, to attend the group meetings regularly, and occasionally to attend open meetings of A.A., etc. Staff members will have to learn to look at alcoholism as a relapsing illness and not see it as a personal affront, or a personal failure, if ex-patients relapse. One has to become aware of the paradoxical situation in which the alcoholic often finds himself, i.e. that he knows quite well that he cannot really go on living (and drinking) the way he does, but that he cannot visualize, either, being able to live without drink. Even voluntary patients do not really want, initially, to give up drinking. What they do want is to get out of the mess into which drink has got them, or to learn to drink and to reap its "benefits" without getting into a mess. Thus, the average alcoholic is very ambivalent in his attitude to therapy; one part within him says "yes" to it; the other part says "no". This aspect partly explains some of the emotional difficulties confronting the would-be therapist of alcoholics. The non-alcoholic looks at the problem from the perspective of what alcohol has done *to* the alcoholic. The latter, for a very long time at least, considers mainly what alcohol has been doing *for* him, and how—admittedly temporarily (but yet immediately)—it has brought relief and has helped him to adjust. Points such as these often make it difficult for therapists and nursing staff to accept the alcoholic emotionally as a sick man, and may have to be discussed in regular staff meetings again and again. Without a knowledgeable, understanding staff, alcoholic units cannot possibly succeed. There is, therefore, an urgent need for adequate under- and postgraduate training in this field for medical, nursing and other professional staff. This is a training which may well be best provided in such centres themselves.

The atmosphere will also largely depend on the attitudes of the patients themselves. Whatever were originally the most important reasons for his heavy drinking, the alcoholic feels himself gradually more and more isolated from society. In a community formed exclusively by alcoholics, on the other hand, he no longer feels judged and rejected. They all have undergone similar disastrous experiences like himself; they all speak the same language; and in such a community, perhaps for the first time for many years, he gets the feeling of belonging. He gets encouragement and the opportunity to participate actively in a large range of occupational, recreational and psycho-therapeutic group activities. Meeting other alcoholics, who have behaved as "badly" in the past as he has done himself, diminishes the often enormous guilt feelings (which have often been motivations for further drinking). By helping others, he regains his self-respect and self-confidence. Hearing other alcoholics speak freely in the group meetings of their problems and seeing that they allow their defences to come down, he may find courage to do likewise ("Jan", 1963).

The running of the group and of its affairs can be largely left to the patients, who can be given a large degree of autonomy and thrive on it. They choose their own group leaders and their own committees; they organize their own work routine, including distribution of daily chores in looking after their ward, and are encouraged to develop initiative and a feeling of responsibility, and to practice self-discipline, etc. On the other hand, the nursing personnel have opportunity to observe patients' reactions to difficulties, to authority and to "sibling" figures, as well as to the inevitable problems arising in interpersonal relationships from living together at close range, and to bring these problems up at group discussions.

In a community and in groups formed exclusively by alcoholics, they find it easy to identify with each other and to accept voluntarily a group code. Under these circumstances, it will be found that alcoholics in such units do not very frequently present the problems of management and of lack of discipline which are so often found when they are dumped haphazardly into places where they neither find other alcoholics nor a staff experienced in handling, and willing to accept them.

COMPREHENSIVE TREATMENT: THE NEED FOR TEAMWORK

It seems likely that a number of factors, e.g. psychological, sociological, and pharmacological, in dynamic interaction, enter into the causation of alcoholism. In turn, alcoholism brings about mental, physical, social, and other changes. It is thus a complex psycho-somato-social disorder, so that, on theoretical grounds alone, it would seem highly unlikely that one form of therapy should invariably be the best for every alcoholic. Rather, it would seem that after the evaluation of the factors present in the individual case, a combination of several out of the available forms of therapy should be selected, according to the needs of the patient concerned. From the therapeutic aspect, the question should not be, "Is alcoholism a symptom or a disease?", nor whether one should follow "Freud or Pavlov?". As a general rule, one might say that it is often just as dangerous to neglect the importance of pre-alcoholic personality factors altogether (e.g. by relying totally on physical therapies) as, on the other hand, to concentrate one's whole interest on the psychological study and therapy of emotional conflicts, to the complete exclusion of the investigation and treatment of the drinking behaviour and of complications arising secondarily from it. Rather than approaching an individual case with preconceived ideas, epitomized by questions such as "Symptom or disease?", therapeutic techniques should be of sufficient range and flexibility to be adjusted to the varying needs at different stages.

As a sufferer from a complex illness of multifactorial origin, the alcoholic requires help from many different sources. Treatment and rehabilitation must be the concern of a whole team of helpers—family doctor, psychiatrist, nurse, social worker, clergyman, welfare agencies, the alcoholic's family, boss and fellow employees, fellow alcoholics, etc. Often, indeed, the agency first approached may not be the most suitable one to help the alcoholic concerned, who should be transferred to the member of the team best qualified to help—not in order to shift the problem, but to share it. In the unit, the work of the various team members should be co-ordinated, e.g. by regular staff meetings, quite apart from the opportunity given to the staff to attend the patients' group psychotherapy meetings, and thereby to gain insight into the emotional problems and difficulties of alcoholics.

TREATMENT PROGRAMME IN THE IN-PATIENT CENTRE

Acute phase

It must be clearly understood that the sobering up and detoxication processes are only initial phases in the over-all therapeutic programme and must always be followed up by a long-term rehabilitation programme. This point should be made quite clear to the practitioner and to patients before it is agreed to admit them. Otherwise, all that one achieves is to render the alcoholic physically fit to resume drinking after discharge with renewed vigour and fervour. The fact that the main purpose of his admission to the centre is long-term rehabilitation, and not merely sobering up, should be impressed on the patient before admission, and he should be urged to present himself for admission in as sober a state as possible. Even so, it will be found that the great majority will have been drinking heavily right up to the time of admission. Thus, among approximately 100 women alcoholics admitted between April 1964 and December 1965 to the unit at St. Bernard's Hospital, the alcohol content in the urine was above 100 mg per 100 ml in almost 75% (67 out of 92) and between 200 and 500 mg per 100 ml in just over 50% (48 out of 92).

Therefore, treatment will generally have to start with sobering-up and detoxication. Sudden complete withdrawal is the method of choice, except in very sick or old people. There is, however, in a small minority of very heavy drinkers, the risk (as yet not widely appreciated) of epileptiform withdrawal convulsions (Isbell *et al.*, 1955; Glatt, 1955b). Generally, the danger is chiefly within the first 24–36 hours, but exceptionally we have seen them as late as the seventh day after withdrawal. Since we started the prophylactic administration of anticonvulsants (Glatt and Lumb, 1955) in all but very mild cases, their occurrence became much less frequent, although such medication cannot be relied upon to prevent them with absolute certainty. It has to be remembered that a proportion of alcoholics also habitually take barbiturates to excess, without necessarily admitting it. In any such case of doubt, phenobarbitone would therefore be preferable to hydantoinates as a prophylactic anticonvulsant.

Another withdrawal manifestation, which may occur about 3–5 days after sudden complete withdrawal, and occasionally also after very rapid decrease (relative withdrawal), is delirium tremens (Isbell *et al.*, 1955; Glatt, 1958c). The great majority of our cases seemed to be caused by sudden withdrawal, although others could certainly not be explained on this basis. However, in the type of alcoholic patient seen in this country, the management of the acute phase generally presents few problems. In recent years, our routine medical treatment has included as tranquillizing agents either chlordiazepoxide (Librium) or the French–Swedish preparation chlormethiazole (Heminevrin), both of which seem quite satisfactory. (A double-blind controlled trial carried out by us in 1963 showed statistically significantly better results with Heminevrin than with the placebo (Glatt, George and Frisch, 1965).) The possibility of the development of dependency must, however, be kept in mind. Vitamins, especially of the B group, are given parenterally in high doses and later orally, and, where hypnotics seem necessary, nonbarbiturates are given for a few days after admission. As mentioned above, approximately 25% of alcoholics also take barbiturates to excess (Glatt, 1961b). These are chiefly those belonging to the middle class, who tend to be of the "loss of control" type. Therefore, since 1954, we have not given barbiturates to alcoholics, except to those who were also dependent on these drugs. As many alcoholics also tend to abuse stimulating drugs, such as the amphetamines and phenmetrazine, these drugs have not been employed either. No drug with either a sedative or stimulating effect on the C.N.S. can be said to be completely free from the risk of leading to dependency in alcoholics. This also holds good for the non-barbiturate hypnotics, and we have come across habitual abuse of glutethimide (Doriden), methypyrlone (Noludar), and dichloralphenazone (Welldorm), although they seem to carry a somewhat lesser risk than the barbiturates. Drinamyl, a combination of a barbiturate and an amphetamine, carries a great risk of leading to dependence in alcoholics, who have abused it in this manner for many years before it was recently "discovered" and abused by teenagers. In the case of tranquillizers, however, the only one which in our experience has led to physical dependence so far has been meprobamate.

The unit arrangement offers a very good opportunity to carry out a comprehensive form of long-term therapy, including physical, psychological and social methods of treatment, and a close collaboration with A.A. This comprehensive form of treatment has, over more than 12 years, proved itself to be a feasible and very popular method at Warlingham Park and at St. Bernard's Hospital.

1. *Physical methods*

Of the physical methods, the sensitizing drugs (Disulfiram, Antabuse) and the somewhat milder citrated calcium carbimide (Abstem) (Glatt, 1959) have proved to be very valuable in suitable cases, and also particularly in the out-patient clinic. One often hears the view expressed that disulfiram is useless because the alcoholic can always discontinue it. This is certainly true, but then no treatment in alcoholism is of any value unless, in the course of one's contact with the patient, one can win his co-operation. The alcoholic who sees in disulfiram a drug with which his doctor or his wife try to "fence" him in, will most certainly try to fight back and stop taking it. If, however, he can learn to regard such drugs as an ally to that part within himself that wants to cope with the drinking problem, he may benefit a great deal. Formerly, a great drawback in starting disulfiram administration was the unpredictability of the strength of the test reaction; however, for many years, we have abandoned the test reaction as superfluous anyway; standing instruction is given in the risks involved. Occasionally, we have also employed apomorphine, emetine aversion and (recently) electrical techniques of aversion therapy. In our experience, which of course differs from that of some other observers, the main value of such techniques is to tide the alcoholic over the first few months, which for him are the most difficult ones. Once he has got over the first six months, the going becomes progressively easier and the risk of a relapse much smaller (Glatt, 1961a).

2. *Psychotherapy*

Among psychotherapeutic methods, group psychotherapy (Glatt, 1958a) seems to be of special value for many alcoholics who, whatever may have been the main original reason for their illness, later on feel isolated and rejected. Our own groups are dynamically orientated, in this way differing from the inspirational-repressive approach of A.A. meetings. Group and A.A. meetings can be a very good complement to each other, provided that patients clearly understand the difference between the essentially uncovering, searching group technique, and the repressive, faith-centred approach of A.A. In our experience, mixed groups and purely male groups work well; female groups can work but are more "sticky", as they too readily degenerate into mutual admiration societies. What approach the therapist adopts will depend not only on his personal leanings and training, but also on the composition of the group. Where there are several psychopaths in the group, the doctor's approach may often have to be more active, in order to prevent a "take-over bid by the psychopaths".

Group psychotherapy has proved to be most helpful in hospital practice, as well as with out-patients. In our set-up, groups have also been run by psychiatric social workers (chiefly for relatives) (Flintoff, 1963), the hospital chaplain (spiritual problems being often very prominent in alcoholics), and the charge nurses (whose groups deal largely with administrative problems). We have also found out-patient groups valuable—attended both by alcoholics and their relatives—as they help towards better appreciation of each other's difficulties.

3. *Social Therapy* (Flintoff, 1963; Forrest and Glatt, 1956)

This includes items such as work with the alcoholic's family, help with living conditions and with the work situation, etc. To a large extent, this will be the responsibility of the psychiatric social worker, who naturally is a very important member of the therapeutic team—in particular as the intermediary between hospital and the family, the social services, the local authority Health Department, and mental welfare officers (who themselves are well placed to carry out some social work on behalf of the unit), and in maintaining contact with ex-patients after discharge.

Without the inclusion of his family into the therapeutic programme, treatment cannot be regarded as complete. (As already mentioned, Alanon, organized by the families of alcoholics, may be very helpful in this respect.) Special emphasis on "family therapy" is laid by Dr. M. Evans (1965), at the Alcoholic Unit at Whitchurch Hospital near Cardiff. Another distinctive feature of the work of this unit is its close collaboration with the Medical Officer of Health for Cardiff—the so-called "Cardiff Plan", providing for a very successful collaboration of hospital unit and local authority in looking after alcoholics and their families. It is clear that in the rehabilitation of alcoholics, as also of drug addicts, a much more active role than hitherto is essential on the part of local authorities, in close collaboration with hospital units.

4. *After-care*

This is the most important phase of the over-all programme. The alcoholic will need support for a long time and should be strongly encouraged to maintain contact with the staff of the unit.

The important role of the psychiatric social worker is well known, and by her groups with the relatives she can do a great deal to alter the human environment, by influencing the attitude of the alcoholic's family (Flintoff, 1963). Apart from the usual means of after-care, certain additional methods have proved very helpful (Glatt, 1955a, 1961b). These include regular reunion meetings, attended both by ex-patients and patients who are at the time in hospital; a regular monthly magazine, edited and written by ex-patients and patients, which gives ex-patients the feeling that even after discharge they still "belong" and are not forgotten. The proud "old school tie" feeling is quite common and in marked contrast to the doubt and suspicion often present on admission. There is also continuous assistance given by a committee, formed by recovered ex-patients. In fact, the opportunity to mobilize enthusiastic ex-patients as voluntary helpers is one of the great assets of the unit (Glatt, 1962).

As stated above, special out-patient clinics and half-way houses are integral parts of a comprehensive alcoholic unit. Half-way houses, in the form of day-and-night or weekend hostels, would often circumvent the need for hospitalization and can greatly shorten the length of stay in hospital. The in-patient facilities, by allowing regular attendance of out-patients and day-patients, also serve at the same time the functions of a day-and-night hostel. Naturally, such half-way houses are needed especially for such people as the homeless or unemployed, for a temporary period after leaving hospital, or after having been first seen in the out-patient clinic. There may be a case for special hostels for down-and-out alcoholics and for ex-prisoners, aiming at a more comprehensive programme of resocialization and re-education. Experience has shown that alcoholics do not mix well with other (non-alcoholic) hostel inmates, and that there is, therefore, a need for half-way houses limited to alcoholics. At present, some of our female ex-patients go to St. Mary's House. The Middlesex County Council had agreed in 1963 to establish a half-way house (30 beds) to work in conjunction with St. Bernard's in-patient facility, but this never materialized, as Middlesex was absorbed in 1965 into the Greater London Council.

There is no longer any need to stress the great contribution which A.A. can make to the work of the alcoholic unit, in the hospital, the out-patient clinic, the half-way house, in after-care, etc. A.A. groups have been active, at Warlingham Park Hospital for example, for more than 14 years (Glatt, 1955a), and hospital patients have gone regularly to the meetings of outside A.A. groups. In turn, many discharged patients have, after leaving hospital, taken an active part in the work of A.A., and have been instrumental in starting many new groups in various parts of the country. The patients here, within 6 months of the establishment of the unit, also started, with the help of the General Service Office of A.A., an A.A. group in Croydon, which has been going strong ever since, and has played host to many successive generations of Warlingham Park alcoholic in-patients.

Problems arising in a Hospital Treatment Centre

In a therapeutic community formed by alcoholics, and when alcoholics feel accepted by an understanding staff, many of the difficulties often described in management are rare. However, a number of problems are bound to occur from time to time.

1. *Relapses*

The long-term aim of treatment should be contented sobriety. However, in many cases, one will have to be satisfied with a much more limited goal, and it must be remembered that alcoholism is essentially a relapsing illness. Treatment has not necessarily been in vain when an ex-patient relapses after a period of sobriety. It matters a great deal to the alcoholic, and possibly even more to his family, that instead of previous almost continuous drunkenness, he has now been able to keep sober and at work for several months, and the atmosphere at home has then been a happy one. A relapse should be regarded as a challenge to the therapist to resume, and perhaps intensify, his endeavours, in co-operation with the alcoholic. Many alcoholics only achieve final success after a number of relapses. It is important, above all, that the nursing staff should understand this concept of alcoholism as a relapsing condition, and should not become too easily despondent about the news that an ex-patient who seemed to be doing so well in hospital has relapsed since discharge.

Naturally, difficult problems arise in regard to how long one is to persevere with patients who drink repeatedly when allowed out of hospital for a day or weekend; and as to when and how often one should re-admit ex-patients who have relapsed. Our guiding principle here has been the impression gained by the hospital staff as to the patient's sincerity of "trying" whilst in hospital, and the way in which he has attempted to stay sober after discharge. If a patient has really tried to co-operate whilst in hospital, and if he has made genuine attempts after discharge, it has been our policy to re-admit him. If he shows no evidence of trying, and if he seemed to look at the hospital as no more than an operational basis from which to embark sooner or later on fresh drinking excursions, he has been put on a "blacklist". The majority of those on the blacklist have been psychopaths who, after an initial attempt at co-operation and at identification with the non-psychopathic majority, failed to stay the course, often discharging themselves prematurely. The average length of stay has been 2–3 months, but where there is a half-way house, one should be able to shorten this considerably. During their stay, patients are encouraged to leave hospital to spend weekends at home, in order not to lose touch with the outside world, and also to have an opportunity to test their newly gained insight in reality situations, outside the sheltered hospital atmosphere.

2. *Psychopathic alcoholics*

Contrary to the views of many people, the great majority of alcoholics are not basically psychopaths, even though many of them behave as if they were whilst, and as long as, they are drinking heavily. The question as to whether psychopaths should be admitted to such a unit is a difficult one. A few psychopaths can be carried by a "good" group, but if there are more than a sprinkling, they will prove a disrupting element and lead to many administrative difficulties, taxing the morale of the staff and patients alike. Therefore, no more than a few psychopaths should be admitted at any one time. Possibly, the establishment of a special centre for "alcoholic psychopaths", under similar conditions, but with a much less permissive atmosphere and longer duration of stay, might be worth a try.

3. *Compulsory admissions*

All other factors being equal, patients admitted voluntarily ("informally" in this country) will do better than those compelled to enter a hospital centre. But the general view that one can only treat alcoholics who want to give up drinking from the start is almost certainly wrong, particularly in respect of those with basically a fairly good personality. As we have seen in a number of cases, compulsorily admitted alcoholics may do quite well, in spite of a strong initial refusal to co-operate, if they are treated in a therapeutic community alongside other alcoholics. Under such circumstances, the motivation to do something about their drinking problem, although completely lacking at the time of admission, may gradually be induced. The argument that it should be left to the alcoholic himself to decide whether to ask for treatment or not is not a realistic one, seeing that such a man is a slave to his compulsion and not really master of his decisions. It is interesting that almost all our recovered ex-patients, when looking back on their past, confess that although they themselves would have strongly objected to a compulsory admission at the time, in retrospect, it would have been best if such a thing could have happened to them years before they finally entered hospital. It must also be added that the great majority of our patients over the past decade were really voluntary in name only. Many came in such a sorry mental or physical state, often pushed along by the threat of wives leaving them, or of being sacked from their jobs, that they were hardly any longer in a state to say "no" to hospital admission. In cases of compulsory admission, patients should remain for at least 1 month or so, in order to give them a chance to get over the initial adjustment and emotional difficulties and to make good contact with other patients.

4. *Mixed units*

In our experience, a unit composed of both sexes is best, although there is no difficulty in running an exclusively male unit. As shown in the example of the female alcoholic and addiction centre run by Anglican Sisters at Spelthorne St. Mary in Surrey, an exclusively female unit is also quite feasible. In the case of a mixed unit, the risks arising out of heterosexual "acting-out" must, however, be kept in mind. Although latent homosexuality may be an important aetiological factor in some cases of alcoholism, it is mainly in heterosexual relations that difficulty may arise within alcoholic units. This is the more so since so many marriages of alcoholics are on the verge of a break-up, and it is easy for these people to believe that they have now encountered the perfect, understanding partner in a group member of the opposite sex. Pairing-off should be actively discouraged and the group encouraged to discuss such matters freely.

5. *Drug addicts*

So far, this country has no special units for the treatment of drug addicts. Many alcoholics are also addicted to other drugs, and there is no great difficulty in treating middle-aged people dependent on drugs such as hypnotics and stimulants alongside alcoholics in the same units, although preferably there should be separate discussion groups for addicts in addition to the ones which they may have together with alcoholics. However, the type of youngster who in recent years has begun to abuse Drinamyl ("purple hearts") or marihuana seems to present, in many respects, a quite different problem. This may be partly because of the marked difference in age and in the psychopathology involved. In youngsters, apart from often very marked underlying personality defects, factors such as the search for "kicks", "experimenting", wanting to be "with-it", boredom, etc., may frequently be at the back of abuse of drugs. Addicts to the opiates and its synthetic substitutes, and to cocaine, would seem to require a much less permissive and more prolonged in-patient régime than is usually necessary for alcoholics (Glatt, 1965a).

Alcoholic Units as Centres of Training and Research

Apart from the main therapeutic purpose of alcoholic units, they also function well as centres for the training and education of professional staff—medical students, doctors, nurses, psychatric social workers, clergymen, probation officers, etc., and for research in this field. Hitherto, there has been very little special training of professional workers in this field. Whatever training there has been has centred largely on the bodily and mental complications of alcoholism, which are late events and occur in a small minority of alcoholics only. It has largely neglected the teaching of the essential and early phases. The result, unfortunately, is that many practitioners think of a possible diagnosis of alcoholism only when the condition has reached a very late phase, at a time when the patient may have been an alcoholic for a period of 10–15 years. For years, he may already have been suffering from alcoholic amnesias, been losing time from his job, have made life a nightmare for his family, and been in the habit of driving his car with his ability markedly impaired by his drinking (Glatt, 1961b). The aim should be early, rather than late, and sometimes unfortunately too late, diagnosis. By spending short periods in alcoholic centres, getting to know alcoholics (and thus freeing themselves from the misconceptions as to what, and who, is an alcoholic), attending group sessions, etc., professional workers will be likely to learn much more about the condition. An additional method, which has proved very helpful, is the participation of recovered alcoholics at lectures, discussions and meetings with groups of doctors, students and other organizations (Glatt, 1962). Recovered alcoholics who are prepared to talk freely and to answer any questions put to them by the audience relating to their own past experiences, provide vivid demonstrations of the fact that many alcoholics want to, and can, make a come-back.

As already pointed out, alcoholic units cannot be expected to succeed without the presence of well-informed and understanding medical and nursing staff; just drafting people into this work means courting failure and disappointment. The training of such personnel is probably best carried out in existing alcoholic units.

The contribution of alcoholic units to the task of prevention is not limited to the field of education only. Such units can also be excellent centres for research into many aspects of the problem. Alcoholics who are treated in these centres often develop a great interest and an almost missionary spirit to help others and are only too willing and anxious to co-operate with research projects. How much opportunity for research is inherent here may perhaps be illustrated by two sets of figures obtained at Warlingham Park, keeping in mind that staff was very limited and that there were no extra personnel available for research. Study of the "drinking histories" (Glatt, 1961b) of male alcoholic patients at Warlingham Park, showed that the hypothetical average male alcoholic had become a regular drinker in his mid-twenties, and entered the prodromal phase in his early thirties and the crucial phase in his mid-thirties, without seeking advice from a doctor until he almost reached the age of 40, i.e. 10 years after the appearance of pro-dromal signs. The hypothetical average female alcoholic patient here was a few years older than her male counterpart; heavy drinking started in her early thirties, prodromal signs appeared first in her late thirties, much more rapidly followed by obvious evidence of alcoholism than in the male. Both among men and women approximately 25% gave a history of suicidal attempts, which were more common among the predominantly younger psychopaths (approximately 33%) than among the older non-psychopathic alcoholics (21%). Habituation to drugs, generally to barbiturates, and often also to amphetamines, was common in the history of both the men (25%) and the women (28%). However, these patients cannot be regarded as a representative cross-section of alcoholics in this country. They were, in the great majority, middle-class and "loss of control" (gamma) alcoholics (86%); whereas alcoholics of the working class, who may often be of the "inability to abstain" type (delta) or non-addictive, inveterate drinkers, as yet do not very often apply voluntarily for help. However, conditions in this respect have begun to improve in recent years.

The treatment results (Glatt, 1961a) obtained at Warlingham Park on a follow-up of at least 2 years after leaving hospital showed about one-third recovered, one-third improved, and one-third not improved. Naturally, one has to keep in mind the difficulties in comparing results obtained by different observers, since so much depends on the composition of the case material. One-third of our patients could be classified as psychopaths, results among whom were very bad, whereas among the non-psychopaths, the results were much better, to a statistically highly significant degree. Statistical evaluation of the results separately for psychopaths and non-psychopaths showed further that men did better than women and, largely because of the greater prevalence of these factors among non-psychopaths, older age, high intelligence, sus-tained marriage relationships, and better occupational status were further indicators of a favourable prognosis (Glatt, 1961b).

An interesting finding during the study of drinking histories has been the recognition of the importance of alcoholism as a common cause of "impaired" and drunken driving (Glatt, 1964a). Over 50% of alcoholic car drivers admitted court appearances for a charge of drunken driving, and the great majority of alcoholic car drivers admitted having habitually driven in an alcohol-impaired condition for many years. What was particularly interesting was the finding that this had first occurred quite early in their drinking career, on the average in the late twenties or early thirties in men, i.e. in the pre-alcoholic or prodromal phase. The finding that recurrent alcohol-impaired driving is a common prodromal symptom in alcoholism seems to be important prophylactically, both for the early recognition of alcoholism and for diminishing the considerable risk stemming from one of the important sources of traffic accidents (Glatt, 1964a).

Conclusion

There is some evidence that at long last alcoholism, so long a neglected problem in this country, is again attracting attention from the State and the medical profession. It is an important public health problem, affecting all social classes, and is an important community liability and responsibility. The National Health Service, local authorities, and voluntary organizations have to co-operate in providing a comprehensive programme of prevention and rehabilitation. The alcoholic unit, viewed as an integrated complex of in- and out-patient facilities, and of hostels, etc., can make a valuable contribution to the management and prevention of alcoholism, and the rehabilitation of alcoholics. The opportunity given in such centres, through methods such as community living and group therapy, to make use of the readiness of alcoholics to identify with each other and to mobilize the help of recovered ex-patients as voluntary assistants, and to work in very close co-operation with A.A. for mutual benefit, can be regarded as a special therapeutic asset. The unit also provides excellent opportunities for the training of the professional undergraduate and post-graduate, for the education of the lay public, and for research into the various aspects of this complex disorder.

References

ANDREASSON, R. (1962), In *Alcohol and Road Traffic*, Proc. 3rd Internat. Conf., London.
BRIGDEN, W. W. (1957), *Lancet*, **ii**, 1243.
Brit. J. Addict. (1961), **57**, 131.
Brit. J. Addict. (1962), **58**, 103.
Brit. Med. J. (1956), Annot. **i**, 1350.
Brit. Med. J. (1961), **i**, 190.
BROOKE, E. M. (1959), *J. Ment. Sci.* **105**, 893.
Church Times (1964), June 26.
LORD COHEN OF BIRKENHEAD (1964), 10th European Institute Prevention and Treatment of Alcoholism, London.
COOPER, J. and MAULE, H. G. (1963), Annual Meeting, British Association (New Society, Sept. 19).
CRAIGIE, H. B. (1963), Personal communication.
DENT, J. Y. (1952), *Brit. J. Addict.* **49**, 33.
DREW, G. C., COLQUHOUN, W. P. and LONG, H. A. (1958), *Brit. Med. J.* **ii**, 993.
EPPS, P. (1957), *Lancet*, **ii**, 182.
EVANS, M. (1965), 11th European Institute Prevention and Treatment of Alcoholism, Oslo.
FLINTOFF, W. P. (1963), *Brit. J. Addict.* **59**, 81.
FORREST, C. and GLATT, M. M. (1956), *Case Conference*, **2**, 19.
GLATT, M. M. (1955a), *Brit. J. Addict.* **52**, 55.
GLATT, M. M. (1955b), *Brit. Med. J.* **ii**, 738.

GLATT, M. M. (1955c), *Lancet*, **i**, 1318.
GLATT, M. M. (1957a), *Brit. J. Addict.* **54**, 21.
GLATT, M. M. (1957b), *Brit. J. Addict.* **54**, 47.
GLATT, M. M. (1958a), *Brit. J. Addict.* **55**, 51.
GLATT, M. M. (1958b), *Brit. J. Delinq.* **9**, 84.
GLATT, M. M. (1958c), *Lancet*, **ii**, 1015.
GLATT, M. M. (1959), *J. Ment. Sci.* **105**, 476.
GLATT, M. M. (1961a), *Acta Psychiat. Scand.* **37**, 143.
GLATT, M. M. (1961b), *Acta Psychiat. Scand.* **37**, 1, 88.
GLATT, M. M. (1961c), *Med. World*, **55**, 111.
GLATT, M. M. (1961d), *Brit. J. Clin. Pract.* **15**, 153.
GLATT, M. M. (1962), *Brit. J. Addict.* **58**, 13.
GLATT, M. M. (1964a), *Lancet*, **i**, 161.
GLATT, M. M. (1964b) 27th Internat. Congr. Alcohol and Alcoholism, Frankfurt a.M.
GLATT, M. M. (1965a), *Lancet*, **ii**, 171.
GLATT, M. M. (1965b), *J. Irish Med. Assoc.* **57**, 67.
GLATT, M. M. and HILLS, D. R. (1964) 1st Internat. Congr. Social Psychiatry (*Brit. J. Addict.* **61**, 71).
GLATT, M. M. and LUMB, I. (1955), *Pharm. J.* **175**, 392.
GLATT, M. M. and WHITELEY, J. S. (1956), *Mschr. Psychiat. Neurol.* **132.**
GLATT, M. M., GEORGE, H. R., and FRISCH, E. P. (1965), *Brit. Med. J.* **ii**, 401.
GRANT, A. P. and BOYD, M. W. T. (1962), *Brit. J. Addict.* **58**, 39.
Health Education (1956), Min. Educ. Pamphlet No. 31, London, H.M.S.O.
HUDOLIN, W. (1964), 27th Internat. Congr. Alcohol and Alcoholism (*Brit. J. Addict.* **61**, 29).
Hulton Readership Survey (1954), London.
INGRAM-SMITH, N. (1965), *Brit. J. Addict.* **60.**
ISBELL, H. *et al.* (1955), *Quart. J. Stud. Alc.* **16**, 1.
"JAN" (1963), *Brit. J. Addict.* **59**, 93.
JELLINEK, E. M. (1957), *World Health*, **10**, 4.
JELLINEK, E. M. (1960), *The Disease Concept of Alcoholism*, New Haven, Connecticut, Hillhouse Press.
JUDGE, C. and GLATT, M. M. (1961), *Med. J. Austral.* **48**, 590.
KAY, W. W., MURFITT, K. and GLATT, M. M. (1959), *J. Ment. Sci.* **105**, 748.
A MANAGING DIRECTOR (1957), *Brit. J. Addict.* **54**, 5.
McADAM, W. (1964), 10th European Institute Prevention and Treatment of Alcoholism, London.
McLEOD, L. O. (1953), *Brit. J. Addict.* **50**, 39.
McLEOD, L. O. (1955), *Brit J. Addict.* **52**, 93.
McLEOD, L. O. (1957), *Brit. J. Addict.* **53**, 139.
MORRISON, S. L. (1964), *Health Bulletin*, **22.**
PARR, D. (1957), *Brit. J. Addict.* **54**, 25.
PARR, D. (1962), *Brit. J. Criminol.* **3**, 272.
PHILLIPSON, R. (1964), Health Congress of Royal Soc. of Health, London, Royal Soc. of Health.
PRYS WILLIAMS, G. and GLATT, M. M. (1966), *Brit. J. Addict.* **61**, 257.
PULLAR-STRECKER, H. (1952), *Brit. J. Addict.* **49**, 21.
PULLAR-STRECKER, H. (1955) *Lancet*, **i**, 1072.
REES, T. P. and GLATT, M. M. (1954), *Ment. Health (London)*, **14**, 11.
REGISTRAR GENERAL, *Annual Statist. Reviews*, London, H.M.S.O.
REGISTRAR GENERAL, *Decennial Suppl., England and Wales* (1951), Occupat. Mortal., Pt. II, Vol. **2** (Tables), London, H.M.S.O.
54th Rep. Commissioners H.M. Customs and Excise for year ending March 31, 1963, Cmnd. 2216, London, H.M.S.O.
ROSE, H. K. and GLATT, M. M. (1961), *J. Ment. Sci.* **107**, 18.
SCHMIDT, W. S., SMART, R. G. and POPHAM, R. E. (1962), In *Alcohol and Road Traffic*, Proc. 3rd Internat. Conf., London.
STAFFORD-CLARK, D. (1952), *Psychiatry Today*, London, Penguin.

STEERING GROUP ON ALCOHOLISM, JOSEPH ROWNTREE SOCIAL SERVICE TRUST. Report prepared by G. Prys Williams, London, 1965.

SULLIVAN, J. D. and GLATT, M. M. (1956), *J. Irish Med. Assoc.* **39,** 146.

TONGUE, A. (1955), *Alcohol Production and Consumption in Great Britain and Northern Ireland.*

TUCHMANN, E. (1964), 1st Internat. Congr. Social Psychiatry (*Brit. J. Addict.* **61,** 59).

UNITED NATIONS (1958), *Demographic Yearbook*, New York.

WILLIAMS, LINCOLN (1956), *Alcoholism*, Edinburgh and London, E. and S. Livingstone.

WILSON, G. B. (1940), *Alcohol and the Nation*, London, Nicholson & Watson.

WOODSIDE, M. (1961), *Brit. J. Criminol.* **1,** 221.

WORLD HEALTH ORGANIZATION EXPERT COMMITTEE ON MENTAL HEALTH, (1951), *Techn. Rep. Ser.* **42,** 8.

WORLD HEALTH ORGANIZATION EXPERT COMMITTEE ON MENTAL HEALTH, (1955), *Alcohol and Alcoholism, Techn. Rep. Ser.* **94,** 8.

7. Industrial and Social Rehabilitation

Donal F. Early

The prospect of discharge for the patient who has spent more than 2 years in a psychiatric hospital is still poor. The majority of hospitals were, and still are, kept in a state of permanent shortage of money. Staff is, therefore, always less than is required. The development of industrial therapy within the hospital has introduced an element of realism into patients' activities, and provided that the aim of fitting the patient for work in open industry or in the nearest equivalent under sheltered conditions is ruthlessly pursued, the possibility of industrial departments stagnating and becoming poor quality occupational therapy departments is avoided.

In Bristol, the system of industrial rehabilitation which we established in 1960 remains basically unchanged. The hospital Industrial Therapy Department leads to the Industrial Therapy Organization Factory, which, in turn leads to open industry or to sheltered industry.

The Industrial Therapy Department in hospital which, between 1958 and 1964, provided employment for between 300 and 400 patients is beginning to show a fall in numbers, although production and earning capacity have remained fairly constant. It is anticipated that this department will eventually be reduced to between 200 and 250 patients. The initial problem of the long-term patient has been largely dealt with and the future of the more ill patients who remain is more doubtful; their progress is likely to be much slower than the progress of those who were treated initially. However, a considerable number of patients with long-standing illness are still being admitted, and a smaller number of patients with recent illness whose remission makes it difficult for them to adjust to industrial life can benefit by training in the industrial therapy departments.

The Industrial Therapy Organization continues to offer training facilities to hospital patients, as well as to others from the hospitals for sub-normals, and to patients referred from the local authority, out-patient departments, general practitioners, Ministry of Labour and the National Assistance Board. The organization's activities have become more diversified and to the original contract factory is now added a 5-minute car wash, a petrol filling station, a sheltered workshop and the group placement scheme. In 5 years, about 120 patients have been placed in open employment and presently there are 21 employees in the car wash, 25 in the sheltered workshop, 2 in the

149

petrol filling station and 52 in the group placement scheme. In all, I.T.O. has under its supervision 183 people at the present time.

Financial independence does not, in itself, fit a patient to live in the open community. Nine wage-earning patients still remain in hospital.

It is the statutory responsibility of the local authority to provide care for patients discharged from hospital. In 6 years since the Mental Health Act, local authorities have generally made little progress in the matter of hostel provision or in providing an adequate service to help sustain and to maintain schizophrenics in the community. Local authorities in many cases tend to blame hospital medical staff and regional hospital boards for their failure to inform local authorities of patients' needs and for their failure to support local authorities when they provide services which they consider to be appropriate. Such criticism is undoubtedly valid in many cases. However, few local authorities have been able adequately to increase their staff to deal with a potentially very large problem, and many have adopted policies without prior consultation with the hospital psychiatric services. Some local authorities have built or acquired hostels, only to be left with large numbers of unoccupied beds and with the conviction that the problem has been wrongly represented to them. Others have hostels which they cannot staff. In Bristol, the local authority decided in July 1961 to build or to acquire two hostels for discharged psychiatric patients which would be unsupervised as far as nursing care was concerned. These were to house approximately 15 people each. The authority also planned two hostels of up to 30 beds each for patients recovering from psychiatric illness or stabilized with continuing symptoms. In August 1964, the authority opened a hostel with 14 beds (10 male and 4 female). There has always been a number of wage-earning patients living in hospital, whom the hospital psychiatrist considered suitable for this hostel but who, for one reason or another, were not considered suitable by the local authority. It appeared, therefore, that wage-earning patients would have to be discharged to the community prematurely, with the resultant risk of rapid relapse or remain in hospital.

One of the points of agreement with the Ministry of Labour when the group placement scheme was established was that patients chosen for such groups should have a reasonable hope, within the foreseeable future, of being discharged from hospital. With this particular point in mind, the Bristol Industrial Therapy Housing Association was formed in 1963. In the autumn of 1964 this association bought an hotel in one of the residential districts of Bristol. This operation was financed by a loan of £10,000 on generous terms from the Transport and General Workers Union. With this money, the hostel was renovated, central heating was installed and the previous rather primitive conditions were modernized. In March 1965, the hotel opened to its first guests and there are now 19 residents, who were previously in-patients in hospital and 2 ex-patients as housekeepers. Patients who had been considered unsuitable for the local authority hostel are living in the hotel and going to work from there and have been for the past 9 months. A nursing sister from the hospital resigned from the nursing service and became manageress of the hotel, which is run on non-institutional lines. The maintenance cost per guest is comparable to that charged in student guest houses in the city.

The Housing Association has also taken over from the Housing Department of the local authority the tenancy of six houses, which were built close to the hospital on land acquired from the Ministry of Health (Early, 1960). These houses have taken an unconscionable time to materialize, but are now in occupation. A male nurse and his wife occupy one of these six houses, which are built in a row of three pairs. His wife acts as supervisor to ensure the smooth management of the houses, and already 23 patients have been discharged from hospital and are in residence. It is too early yet to say what degree of independence they will be able to attain individually or in groups as a result of their present living conditions. The overhead costs of running the houses will, like the hotel, be covered completely by income from residents. There is no other source of income.

The problem of staffing schemes for both domestic and industrial rehabilitation is, and will remain, a vital one. It may be that specially trained industrial therapists and/or occupational therapists with a training modified to suit modern needs would be the best solution. However, such trained workers do not exist, certainly not in the numbers in which they are required. There may be a good case for specially trained hostel wardens. Again, such people do not exist and local authorities have shown little indication that they are willing or able to avail themselves of training courses for such wardens. It has been argued that 2 months (the length of time proposed by the National Association for Mental Health for their course for wardens of hostels for mentally disordered adults) is too long and that the course is too expensive (£95 per person for tuition and full maintenance). From within the hospital service, the problem of development becomes painfully obvious. There is no source of continuing and qualified help, except from the nursing profession. Once it has been established that a nurse's duty lies wherever a patient requires help, there need be no further difficulty in a nurse accepting the wide variety of duties which social and economic rehabilitation demand. In every psychiatric hospital there is a reservoir of enthusiasm and of ability which, with careful selection, can cover all facets of patient activity. Our economic development has depended upon in-service industrial training of nurses, who now not only supervise patients in the hospital therapy departments but also in the Industrial Therapy Organization Factory, in the car wash, in the sheltered workshop and who also supervise groups of patients working in open industry (sheltered placement groups). In a similar way, the manageress of our hotel is a retired nursing sister who lives in quarters in the hotel with her son (a student nurse) and the supervision of the council house tenants is by a male nurse's wife, helped by him.

Some of the factors militating against the successful social rehabilitation of long-stay patients are becoming clearer. Behaviour which is likely to be classified as "eccentric" will be accepted in a society which has been prepared for it. Less positive symptoms, such as the lack of volition, isolation, poverty of ideation and flatness of affect, render social integration difficult. Many patients are deficient in the most elementary skills with common measures, e.g. money, weight. It is becoming obvious that a more efficient preparation for discharge will be necessary before patients will have a reasonable chance of living successfully in the community. Industrial training is useful, but in many cases will not be enough and patients will need social training, in a wider sense, in hospital before discharge. Shortage of staff could here again excuse inactivity. In the continuing impecunious state of the hospitals, no finance for development is likely, and here again unless the talents of the nursing profession can be utilized and developed, little progress is likely to take place. In Glenside Hospital in September 1964, a schoolmaster who had qualified as a nurse was appointed to organize a Department of Group Activities, with the emphasis on extramural orientation of patients in preparation for discharge. No attempt is made to form a stereotyped organization based on leadership in the generally accepted sense. The emphasis is laid on opportunities being offered to patients to make their own decisions. With this male nurse, a sister was also appointed. The progress in the first year has been encouraging and the department is in the process of being expanded. With the more intensive training of the in-patient population, it is possible that many of the remaining patients who appear to have little chance of industrial or social rehabilitation may make progress. Evidence is accumulating that even the most withdrawn patients can, if treated intensively, make considerable progress.

Unless the hospital organization is sufficiently realistic to enable the local authority to accept the validity of the hospital criteria of suitability for discharge, and unless the local authority is realistically geared to accept hospital discharges, little progress will be made. It will require a degree of mutual confidence and co-operation which does not universally obtain at present to prevent disintegration of what should be an integrated service before, during and after admission to hospital.

It may be argued that the services statutorily divided as they are will prove inadequate to cope with new developments.

Reference

EARLY, D. F. (1960), *Lancet*, ii, 754.

8. Rationale for the Community Care of Mental Disorder*

M. W. Susser

THROUGH the centuries, medical thinkers have tried to apply to mental disorder the conceptual model of organic disease. They have searched for hidden causes, and described clinical entities, their outcome and treatment. In trying to develop a deterministic view of mental disorder they have had to compete with folk-concepts of witchcraft, religious personifications of evil, and philosophies which took the world as given and human behaviour as manifestly purposeful. Their struggle is won: determinism in psychiatry is now common to all schools, so that a mentally disordered patient is generally regarded as having an illness for which a cause might be found.† Even such problems as crime, amoral behaviour and marital discord are sometimes subsumed to medicine under the head of psychopathology. The current dominance in British society of this medical interpretation of mental disorder has much to do with the transformation in the care of mental patients.

To conceive of mental disorder as illness carried wide social implications. Sickness is more than a matter of disease and disturbed functioning. The sick person has a special status or social position in relation to others, and an implicit social role, a "sick role".[2, 3] This status absolves him from most social responsibilities, except that of seeking his recovery, and entitles him to the help of his fellows. The grounds on which an individual is given these privileges do not depend only on the presence of disease; some diseases, for instance malnutrition, or bronchitis, entitle sufferers to sick privileges in one society and not in another. The behaviour of a person with disease is thus prescribed by society, and sickness and disease can be dissociated.

The rules for according the sick role are implicit in the values and attitudes of each society.[4] In conformity with these values mental disorders may be accepted as supernatural or rejected as aberration. In Ghana, spontaneous confessions of witchcraft by depressives are taken at face-value,[5] while in middle-class Sussex hypochondria in depressives is badly tolerated.[6] Traditional means of dealing with mental disorder contribute to the current social norm and cannot be ignored in the treatment of mental disorder.

---

* Reprinted from *Medical Care*, 3, 52.
† Some recent writers have put forward new grounds to question the medical concept of mental disorder.[1]

In a society which interprets mental disorder as illness, the mentally disordered person can be accorded the socially privileged position of the sick. In England the Mental Health Act of 1959 framed the laws relating to the management of mental disorder on the medical model. Patients are referred to psychiatric agencies as sick persons, with the expectation that they will receive medical treatment and improve. The function of the agencies is primarily to bring about recovery or improvement, and only incidentally is it custodial. The patient may not always voluntarily seek aid as in the "ideal type" of the sick role, but the convenient assumption is made that he would if his disease did not prevent him from recognizing his need. (So far has the concept permeated medical thought that some do not distinguish the custodial and disciplinary work of mental institutions from therapy.)

The legal adoption of the medical model of psychopathology has in itself affected the career of the mentally sick person. Many patients who formerly might have been confined for long periods are allowed to live free from constraint in the community, as can be deduced from the great reduction in the average duration of stay in mental hospitals.[7] The change cannot be ascribed to drugs alone, for it began before their introduction,[8] and in some countries where drugs are much used comparable changes have not been reported. Functional psychosis now often presents as a series of acute episodes with quiescent intermissions, rather than as a chronic deteriorating condition; in Salford, 6 recurrences present for each new case of schizophrenia, and 2–3 for each of depressive psychosis.[9]

It may be supposed that the altered career of mental patients in society has had an influence on their behaviour independent of the underlying pathological processes. We do not know to what extent external circumstances precipitate acute episodes, but they are certainly important in phases of remission, and in less severe forms of mental illness. Studies are available to show that the status and roles of the patient in the family, at work and elsewhere influence the level of his performance in the community. In mental hospitals, for example, characteristic reactions to the social situation have been described: "institutional neurosis" is a form of adaptation in the old-time hospital to the system of authority, the administrative structure and the allocation of roles in the structure.[10, 11, 12]

Separating reactions to social situations from the symptoms of disease is especially difficult with mental disorder, because the diagnosis of both reaction and disease usually rests on their resultant in observed behaviour, without the anchor of organic pathology. The rationale for treating mental disorder in the community, however, depends on the distinction between them. Situations in the community, no less than those in the hospital, elicit characteristic responses, although these are likely to conform more closely to the norms of behaviour in the community. The community mental health service tries to extend the number of situations in which relatively normal social roles can be learned or resumed by the patient. To this end it devises institutions and groups which can provide controlled experience, tolerance, and approbation throughout the process of learning.

This experience is voluntary by preference, but sometimes compulsory. Admission to hospital, considered in these terms, can be one form of situational change, and is properly a part of the facilities for community care. It administers a situational shock, which forces the patient to recast, or at least to review, his perception of himself, and the order of his relations with others. These others, too, must review their perception of the patient and their relations with him. Responses to the shock are various,[10] but in assessing the effect of hospital admission they must be weighed together with the influence of drugs and electroconvulsive therapy. Indeed, there are meagre grounds for attributing long-term effects to any specific treatment.

Critical readers may ask what is the practical contribution to therapy of this theoretical position. Many psychiatrists are gloomy about the outcome of psychiatric illness. They are more pessimistic than is usual with doctors accustomed to applying the medical model of the sick role in their work; most physicians have little difficulty in maintaining the optimism and belief in themselves necessary to the effective performance of the doctor's role. A comparison of the actual results of psychiatrists and physicians on medical wards leads one to think that the more optimistic outlook of the physicians is perhaps related to action effective in the short term and to a lack of feedback from their discharged patients, many of whom die off and are silent. In Scotland, only about 50% of patients discharged 2 years before from acute medical wards had achieved lasting improvement, about 25% never worked again, and another 25% were dead.[13] For rough comparison one might take a follow-up study of schizophrenic patients in London, discharged from hospital 1 year before. Of these patients 25% maintained a good work adjustment, 25% maintained good work adjustment but were re-admitted, and about 50% maintained only irregular work.[14]

The significant difference here between psychiatry and internal medicine is that the majority of patients with chronic mental disorders survive for many years, and the survival rates continuously improve. As their number in the community grows, the theory of the sick role has increasing practical implications. It can guide us in exploring situations which extend, alter, or otherwise manipulate the social roles available to the patient. Much of what is done in community care must be empirical, just as with other treatment. Nevertheless it is probably fair to say that recent studies have given as many leads about *milieu* therapy as about drug therapy; and I shall discuss some of these in what follows. Psychiatrists can add considerably to their range of treatments by devising social situations to exploit this new knowledge. The work of a psychiatric agency seldom needs to be viewed as a caretaking operation, except in the case of rapidly progressive organic diseases.

The Mutability of Situations

The factors which influence the social performance of mental patients can be grouped in two categories. Some relate to the general features of long-continued sickness, and many of these are hypothetical or derived from direct observation. Others relate to the specific features of mental disorder, and most of these have been demonstrated in special studies and measured observations.

GENERAL FACTORS

Although in industrial societies the bed-ridden patient has long existed, the chronic ambulant patient is a recent phenomenon. The ambulant sick role, because it does not fit the stereotype of the past, presents society with a problem of adaptation.[15] The patient is neither obviously ill nor well, and his condition is not temporary but permanent. This permanent state of semi-dependence makes possible a prolonged escape from many everyday responsibilities. Any chronic ambulant patient may meet with suspicion from relatives and others who resent his exemption or suffer by it. "If he is sick, why doesn't he improve with treatment?"

We are faced with a further dilemma, not peculiar to psychiatry, in accommodating families and the wider society to the chronic ambulant sick role. In many disorders, including schizophrenia, the best treatment is often to keep the patient active rather than inactive and resting. We present families with a conflict when they are asked to regard a mental disorder as disease, and yet to deny the patient the usual exemptions from social obligations conferred by the sick role.

The precise threshold at which chronic disease leads to the outright assumption of the sick role depends not only on the patient's physiological and psychological function but also on his social and family relations. The nuclear family, for instance, draws on relatively meagre human resources and is not well suited to cope with sickness.[16] Should a parent fall sick, substitutes are not easily found, and the family is deprived of important adult roles and services. The loss of the paternal breadwinner may cripple the family economically, and the loss of a mother threatens it with break-up. At the emotional level the demands set up by the dependence of a sick parent conflict with the similar demands of dependent children, so that there is overlap and competition in the performance of the sick role and the child's role.

The capacity of the family to support a dependent member is not constant, but fluctuates with the progress of its cycle of development. During the phase of expansion and child-rearing this capacity is diminished. Supportive capacity also varies with the type of social network of which the nuclear family is a component part. Networks are founded on the formal obligations between kin, and on the material resources of that society.[15, 17, 18] They may be close-knit and contained in a small area, or loose-knit and dispersed, according to the migration and mobility engendered by occupation and marriage. A close-knit network may compensate in supportive strength for poor material resources.

SPECIFIC FACTORS

Within this general setting of chronic sickness a number of factors special to mental disorder have been demonstrated.

1. *Accommodation of family roles*

In each family the accustomed organization of roles, continually adjusted as children grow and achieve new statuses, creates a balanced system of relationships. The adaptation to change occasioned by growth, bereavement, or sickness may be more or less successful.

When one of the family members suffers from mental disorder, special problems of adaptation arise. In the case of mental illness in a husband or wife, the spouse must find a means of accommodating to disordered behaviour. Sometimes accommodation occurs only at the cost of generating neurosis in the healthy spouse.[19, 20] When husband or wife has come to terms with psychosis in the spouse by an adjustment of conjugal roles, any added strain may tilt accommodation into declared sickness, to end perhaps with extrusion of the sick member from the family.[21, 22]

The degree of acceptance or hostility shown to the patient can be taken as a reflection of the accommodation of family roles. Hostile relatives reduce the patient's chance of survival in the community.[23] Trained social workers and good family doctors can probably reduce hostility if they act early enough. The duration of face-to-face contact in the household may be a significant element in the level of hostility; the shorter the contact between schizophrenic patients and their families the better the results.[23] Contact can be shortened by ensuring employment or attendance at day centres, and by providing alternative residence. Results in hostels and lodgings are better than in hostile homes, or in common lodging-houses and other refuges for the "down and out".[24] Removal of the patient from everyday relationships, to hospital if necessary, can relieve acute domestic tension built up in the preceding phase of illness; it allows time on all sides for cooling off, and for reorientation of attitudes. This creates a malleable situation in which behaviour changes can sometimes be brought about, in the family chiefly by social workers and family doctors, and in the patient chiefly by psychiatrists.

The return of the extruded member after prolonged absence may lead to difficulties in re-allocation of family roles, as the analogy of returning prisoners-of-war illustrates.[25] In the absence of fathers taken prisoner during the Second World War, their families had of necessity rearranged the roles of parents and children. The father's return disturbed existing relations. Wife and children were older and had grown unaccustomed to an authoritative male, and the resumption of family roles by the father often proved a painful process. This sometimes led to the break-up of families, but the husbands and wives who had spent time in special rehabilitation centres made the transition more successfully. Trained social workers should be able to give equivalent help to families upon the return of the long-separated patient.

At discharge from hospital, therefore, readjustment of roles within the family is a factor to be considered with the duration of the patient's hospital stay. The difficulties of adjustment are related to the composition of the family to which the patient returns. Parental families offer patients discharged from hospital a better chance of survival in the community than do conjugal families.[24, 26]

2. *Social performance and expectations*

Accommodation may permit the patient to remain in the family, however, without requiring of him a high level of social performance. Thus, in one study, patients who returned to parental families were found to maintain a much poorer level of social performance than those who returned to conjugal families.[27] This result was followed up by an attempt to devise measures of the expectations of family members about the performance of particular domestic roles, on the hypothesis that the behaviour of patients might be reciprocal with these expectations.[26, 28, 29] The level of expectations was found to be connected with the formal status and roles of the patient. Wives expect more of husbands (who must fulfil demands as spouse, breadwinner, and father) than do mothers of sons (who can remain socially dependent).

This proved a difficult hypothesis to explore further, because the level of expectation is likely to be modified by the feed-back from actual performance. Where roles are demanding, expectations are high; when performance is poor, expectations are likely to be lowered. Such homeostatic adjustment of expectations in relation to performance could explain the high expectations found with good performance, since on retesting after an interval, a fall in expectations was associated with a decline in performance. Nevertheless, the main tenor of this work does suggest that mental patients respond to high expectations in carrying out their roles. In therapeutic groups such as day centres and hostels, skilled leadership can allow the discipline necessary to maintain high levels to co-exist with the growth of individual responsibility.

3. *Kin support*

The amount of effective social support available to patients influences both their admission to hospital and the duration of their stay. Kin may be altogether lacking or dispersed, or available and ineffective, or available and effective, according to the stage of the family cycle, the type of social network, social mobility, and material resources.[15, 30] Lack of support from kin is a major factor in admission among the subnormal.[31, 32, 33]

Among other mental patients, marital status gives some measure of *available* support. In mental hospitals those who are single, separated or divorced and widowed are over-represented.[34, 35, 36] The divorced are over-represented because of a high rate of mental disorder among them, but the single and widowed (and widowed men in particular) are over-represented because of a higher admission rate than other patients.[8]

The visiting of patients in hospital by relatives can be taken as an indication of *effective* support. Visiting of schizophrenic patients was correlated (until recently) with their chances of discharge from hospital.[37] Now that discharge rates are so high, this correlation has disappeared. In different communities where the interest in patients shown by relatives is much the same, however, their willingness to offer accommodation has been found to vary.[38] This can be ascribed to the better resources of some communities than others in housing, finance, and the supportive strength of the family network.[4, 15, 17, 18, 39] Residence in hostels, foster homes or supervised lodgings can overcome such difficulties.

4. *Employment and occupation*

Mental patients who obtain regular work on leaving the hospital tend to settle successfully in the community. In both psychotic and high-grade subnormal patients who are out of hospital, this correlation holds seemingly independent of clinical condition;[14, 31, 40, 41] it accords with the importance attached to occupational roles in industrial societies.

The chances of achieving regular employment can be improved by keeping a job open during admission.[14, 41] Jobs are more likely to be kept open for salaried workers than for wage earners, and this probably contributes to the marked disparity in employment success between higher social classes and lower, and between white-collar and manual workers.[14, 42] Similar disparities between the social classes have been shown to exist among patients discharged from general hospitals.[13] Although most jobs rated high on the social scale make greater intellectual demands than manual jobs, there may be more tolerance in exacting these demands and more room for deviations from work routine.

The return to work requires study from within the work organization in order to expand the opportunities available to mental patients. The conditions most favourable to the integration of mental patients could be defined by such studies; these conditions relate to foremen and men on the shop floor as well as to the patient's functional capacity. The effects of the patient's dysfunction on production lines and incentive bonuses, and the effects on workmates of his aberrant behaviour or merely of his reputation for it, must all be significant in the recruitment and assimilation of mental patients to work groups.

Employment chances are also improved in the case of schizophrenic patients who have had a lengthy stay in hospital and in the case of subnormals, by a period in a rehabilitation or industrial training centre.[43, 44] Psychological studies give some leads about the kind of stimuli to which mental patients in training respond. For instance, although schizophrenic patients function well in an aura of approval, checks and admonitions seem better to break through their retardation and withdrawal than competitive incentives and rewards.[45] This is quite contrary to results with severely subnormal patients, who respond well to incentives and rewards.[43] Subnormal patients can learn to carry out some simple tasks at the same speed as normal workers, although it takes them longer to learn. Moreover, they are capable of transferring their learned abilities from one task to another, and the period of training for subsequent tasks is reduced.[46] A surprising number of severely subnormal patients have been placed in open industry.

Probably the same generalizations apply to women workers as for men. In the case of housewives, the equivalent correlation for success after discharge must be with the performance of household tasks. One study shows that women who return from hospital and have to perform household tasks do better than those who do not.[47]

Co-ordinated work between psychiatrists and social workers, in hospital and out, is called for to help patients make the best use of opportunities for employment.

5. *Social work after the patient's discharge from hospital*

One preliminary result suggests that early follow-up by social workers improves the immediate prognosis for discharged patients, as measured by return to hospital.[48] It is difficult to eliminate the effects of selection on such results. In another study significant benefit was not demonstrated,[49] but taken together with other studies which show the importance of preparing jobs for the patient's discharge and arranging for the supervision of his medication, this preliminary finding seems to indicate the value of co-ordinated work on the part of the mental hospital and the various social services in the community.

6. *Accommodation to specific disorders*

Although many characteristics are common to social roles in all types of mental disorder, each type has special problems. For instance, the anguish of periodic depression, the origins of which are explicable only in terms of the patient's inaccessible private world, seems to confuse communication and relationships in a less provocative way than do the more continuous but apparently painless private incongruities of thought and of affect in schizophrenia. In both these functional psychoses, however, interpretations of illness can help families to accommodate to the personal difficulties of relationships and to the social difficulties of aberrant conduct. The difficulties of the functional psychoses contrast with those of personality disorders, in which unpredictable deviant conduct strains accommodation because it appears to be wilfully amoral.

Accommodation seems particularly difficult to achieve in deteriorative organic disorders. Senile dementia makes heavy physical and psychological demands on relatives,[6] and the asymmetry of the felt obligations of husband, wife and children to the dependent old person can create a growing focus of familial conflict. Severe subnormality simulates deterioration because the gap continuously widens between the timetable for normal development and the child's actual progress, but it differs in that it places equal obligations on both parents. It, too, may be a focus of conflict, which may exaggerate tendencies to behaviour disturbance in a subnormal child.[50, 51, 52] A folk-lore of hereditary stigma attaches to subnormality, and attendant shame, guilt and anxiety may colour the attitudes of parents; moreover, both may not equally accept the prospect of a permanently dependent child which cannot fulfil many normal parental hopes. In these organic disorders, when kin are no longer effective because of strain or loss, the patient usually needs supervised care in a substitute home more than any strictly medical treatment.

High-grade subnormality without brain disorder also causes special problems.[53] This condition presents as educational retardation and social deviance during pubescence and adolescence. When educational retardation is its main expression, strain is minimal, for the retardation is in part a product of the family culture and congruent with it. Prolongation of the sheltered educational environment of schools and day centres then gives time for maturation.

When social deviance (delinquency in boys and promiscuity in girls) is superadded, the patient has usually suffered personality damage from derangement of family function and structure. In such cases a substitute home is essential to buy time during a prolonged "adolescent" phase of social dependence. These young people have been deprived of normal learning experience within the family, but it has so far proved difficult to devise a *milieu* capable of repairing this. Fostering them in families may yield better results than placing them with groups in hostels.

7. *Transitional states*

Some evidence suggests that certain social crises which impose on an individual an adjustment of status and roles can lead to continuing emotional disturbance. These include school entry, transfer from one school to another, the separation of children from families, migration, maternity, bereavement, and retirement.[54, 55, 56, 57, 58] Such social transitions can serve both to define vulnerable individuals and to bring them needed help. The hypothesis of stressful transitions thus points to the possibility of preventive mental health.

The hopes of prevention are also raised by the implication of studies of prenatal environment, and of genetics, but these are not within the scope of this paper.

Facilities for Community Care

A variety of situations and facilities is required to realize the potential therapeutic value of accumulated knowledge. In England the Mental Health Act faced local health authorities with the task of developing psychiatric services for patients outside mental hospitals. The inventiveness of hospital psychiatrists in extending their work in the community provided a starting point, and the experience of public health in dealing with tuberculosis as a chronic ambulant sickness provided a model for development.[59, 60] We have discussed our own experiences in Salford in annual reports[9, 48, 62, 63] dealing with the past five years. In outline the facilities include social work, day centres, psychotherapeutic clubs, and hostels.

The functions of these institutions and the extensions of the therapeutic situation which they provide can be considered under two heads:

1. To socialize mentally disordered individuals, whether they are retarded in development or whether they have lost the ability to fulfil everyday social functions because of mental illness. To socialize means, broadly, to inculcate the values of a culture as they are expressed in the norms and sanctions attached to its multiple social roles. The aim of therapy is to stimulate awareness of these norms and responsiveness to them, and to nurture aspirations to assume roles functional in the community and attainable by the patient. Such roles need not be conformist.

2. To provide social support for persons dependent because of mental disorder, particularly when they lack effective kin. This support includes residential care, and "minding" to relieve family tension and strain.

Social Work

Social work is carried out by a variety of workers with appointments in hospitals and other agencies, but chiefly by mental welfare officers. The mental welfare officer has evolved from the official of the past, who acted only according to legally prescribed responsibilities, into a social worker who assumes many voluntary responsibilities according to his professional judgement. The social worker guides individuals and families through the complexities of social agencies in the modern industrial state to the agency appropriate to their needs. In the course of this exploration, he advises about those personal problems which emerge or for which his help is solicited. In counselling, his field of operation is not so much intrapsychic as inter-personal, and he is concerned with the field of social relations. The mental welfare officer is the executive agent of services for community care. If community care is to be effective, therefore, he must be able to work in collaboration with the psychiatrists and general practitioners responsible for the medical care of the patient, as well as with his colleagues in the public health team.

Day Centres

Although young subnormal children and their families can benefit from nurseries for normal children, special centres must cater for those whose physique outgrows that of their peers in playing age, for those with physical handicaps, and for those with behaviour disturbances. Indeed, at some stage most subnormal children must be provided for in day training centres which substitute for schools. Treatment in these centres can be ruled more by the individual needs of a particular child than by the group needs of an age-set. The problems of disturbed subnormal children are difficult to distinguish from those of psychotic children, even when differential diagnosis is possible, and experiment and research has still to define the best environment for each. Education and training of older subnormal persons is continued in adult centres, where they learn a modicum of reading and reckoning, and domestic, social and industrial skills. In most sectors of community care trained staff is not available. In this sector, however, suitably trained staff in the persons of nursery, infant and remedial teachers is available, but barriers of finance and administration often prevent its recruitment.

Other day centres cater mainly for mentally ill patients. In their case, although strict segregation from normal patients need not be maintained, and they must also learn to adjust to work routines, formal education is replaced by education about personal and social problems through group discussion and informal exchanges.

SUPERVISED LODGINGS

Hostels, foster homes, small households of patients and pre-arranged lodgings can all serve patients who are partially dependent because of their mental disorder but do not require hospital treatment. Such patients have often remained in hospitals merely because they required a substitute home, and not for any special treatment. Some patients need a substitute home because no effective kin are available, or because of a failure of accommodation within the home. Other patients require support when they first resume social relations in the community after discharge from hospital. Hostel residence enables the patient to maintain some roles within the community while yet being given support.[61] With such support many patients are capable of obtaining and keeping jobs when they have long been disabled, non-productive and socially dependent. The stay of patients in hostels is often short, but may have to be long-term or even permanent. These experiments present many difficulties, and we have still much to learn about the organization of therapeutic group living.[62]

SOCIAL CLUBS

Therapeutic clubs provide a setting in which patients can learn or relearn the proprieties of social intercourse, gain support from personal relationships, and develop self-confidence from the exercise of social activities.[63] They can also assume responsibilities by running the club.

Conclusion

The proper use of all these facilities requires an adequate assessment of the mental patient. This takes into account the demands he makes on his family in terms of physical organization, of psychological resilience, and of social resources, including the support available from kin. It places equal emphasis on the demands which families make on the patient, and considers the patient and his family as an interacting system within a particular culture. Moreover, in industrial societies complete assessment cannot ignore the patient's associations outside the family. Almost everyone has some such associations, whether for work or for leisure, whether to obtain services or to fulfil the obligations of citizenship.

These manifold functional associations are more or less discrete.[64] The ways in which the needs of a patient are perceived by a particular medical agency tend to be limited by this discrete quality of functional associations in our society, a quality exaggerated by the self-sufficiency of large organizations. In the hospital the patient is totally encapsulated and he tends to be seen in terms of the restricted roles of a person dependent on the hospital for all his needs; in the public health service he tends to be seen as a person with disordered relations with his family, with other supportive institutions, or with the law; in industry he is seen as a worker with observable effects on productivity.

Each of these frames of reference is accurate in itself, but insufficient and biased in relation to the set of references encompassed by the patient's life. The psychiatric observer's conscious effort to attain a frame of reference adequate to the whole range of the patient's interactions through time is eased by free access to each observation point. Inco-ordination of psychiatric services obstructs free access, and for this reason presents a fundamental defect in a system of medical care.[65] The administrative structure of the psychiatric services of the first half of this century evolved around the custodial functions required by the laws concerned with mental disorder; the role of mental patient was almost entirely confined to the mental hospital, and the flow between hospital and community was a mere trickle. That structure cannot sustain the rising flood of patients passing between hospital and community of recent years; hence the current drive towards co-ordination and continuity of care. Co-ordination eliminates the unhelpful alternative of hospital or community, expands the range of therapeutic situations, and allows the best use to be made of available facilities. The mental hospital can then be an institution which not only serves the community but also interacts with it.

Further advances require fresh observations, opportune measurement and continuous analysis; sociological interpretations need the support of thorough clinical psychiatry and psychology. This is a time for experimental research with services and their flexible development. We may safely say that in a rapidly changing world this time stretches into the predictable future.

Acknowledgement

Many of the ideas in this paper have been developed in discussion with Dr. Zena Stein; she also drew my attention to relevant literature, and read and criticized the paper.

References

1. SZAZ, T. (1962), *The Myth of Mental Illness*, London, Secker & Warburg.
2. SIGERIST, H. E. (1960), *The Sociology of Medicine*, New York, M.D. Publications (Ed. Roemer, M. I.).
3. PARSONS, T. (1951), *The Social System*, Illinois, Glencoe Press.
4. EATON, J. N. and WEILL, R. J. (1955), *Culture and Mental Disorder*, Illinois, Glencoe Press.
5. FIELD, M. (1961), *Search for Security*, London, Faber & Faber.
6. SAINSBURY, P. and GRAD, J. (1963), Mental illness and the family, *Lancet*, 544–547.
7. GENERAL REGISTER OFFICE. The Registrar General's Statistical Review of England and Wales, 1959—Supplement on Mental Health, London, H.M.S.O., 1962.

8. SHEPHERD, M. (1957), *A Study of the Major Psychoses in an English County:* Maudsley Monographs, London, Chapman & Hall.
9. STEIN, Z. A. (1964), Preliminary Results of the Survey of Mental Sickness in Salford, in Susser, M. W., *Report on the Salford Mental Health Services for 1963*, City of Salford Health Department.
10. STANTON, A. H. and SCHWARTZ, M. H. (1954), *The Mental Hospital*, New York, Basic Books.
11. GOFFMAN, E. (1957), Characteristics of Total Institutions, in *Symposium on Preventive and Social Psychiatry*, Walter Reed Army Institute of Research, Washington.
12. WING, J. K. and BROWN, G. W. (1961), *J. ment. Sci.*, **107**, 847.
13. FERGUSON, T. and McPHAIL, A. V. (1963), *Hospital and Community*, London, Oxford University Press.
14. MONCK, E. M. (1963), Employment experiences of 127 discharged schizophrenic men in London, *Brit. J. prev. soc. Med.*, **17**, 101.
15. SUSSER, M. W. and WATSON, W. (1962), *Sociology in Medicine*, London, Oxford University Press.
16. FOX, R. C. and PARSONS, T. (1952), Illness, therapy and the modern urban American family, *J. Social Issues*, **13**, 31.
17. TOWNSEND, P. (1957), *The Family Life of Old People*, London, Routledge & Kegan Paul.
18. BOTT, E. (1957), *Family and Social Network*, London, Tavistock.
19. POND, D., RYLE, A. and HAMILTON, M. (1963), Marriage and neurosis in a working class population, *Brit. J. Psychiat.*, **109**, 592.
20. KREITMAN, N. (1964), The patient's spouse, *Brit. J. Psychiat.*, **110**, 159.
21. SCHWARTZ, C. G. (1957), Perspectives on deviance—wives' definitions of their husband's mental illness, *Psychiatry*, **20**, 275.
22. SIMPSON, H., MESSINGER, S. L. and TOWNE, R. D. (1962), Family processes and becoming a mental patient, *Amer. J. of Soc.*, **68**, I, 88.
23. BROWN, G. W., MONCK, E. M., CARSTAIRS, C. M. and WING, J. K. (1962), The influence of family life on the course of schizophrenic illness, *Brit. J. prev. soc. Med.*, **16**, 55.
24. BROWN, G. W., CARSTAIRS, G. M. and TOPPING, G. (1958), Post-hospital adjustment of chronic mental patients, *Lancet*, **ii**, 685.
25. CURLE, A. and TRIST, E. L. (1947), Transitional communities and social reconnection, *Human Relations*, **I**, 42, 240.
26. FREEMAN, H. E. and SIMMONS, O. G. (1963), *The Mental Patient Comes Home*, London, J. Wiley & Sons.
27. DAVIS, J. A., FREEMAN, H. E. and SIMMONS, O. G. (1957), Rehospitalization and performance level among former mental patients, *Social Problems*, **5**, 37.
28. DINITZ, S., LEFTON, M., ANGRIST, S. and PASAMANICK, B. (1961), Social and psychological factors in the rehospitalization of female patients, *Arch. of Gen. Psychiat.*, **4**, 363.
29. DINITZ, S., LEFTON, M., ANGRIST, S. and PASAMANICK, B., (1961) Psychiatric and social attributes as predictors of case outcome in mental hospitalization, *Social Problems*, **8**, 322.
30. STEIN, Z. A. and SUSSER, M. W. (1960), Estimating hostel needs for backward citizens, *Lancet*, **ii**, 486.
31. STEIN, Z. A. and SUSSER, M. W. (1960), The families of dull children, classification for predicting careers, *Brit. J. prev. soc. Med.*, **14**, 83.
32. SAENGER, G. (1960), Factors influencing the Institutionalization of Mentally Retarded Individuals in New York City. *A Report to the New York State Interdepartmental Health Resources Board.*
33. LEESON, J. E. (1963), The place of the hospital in the care of the mentally subnormal. *Brit. med. J.*, **i**, 713.
34. NORRIS, V. (1959), *Mental Illness in London*, London, Chapman & Hall.
35. LOWE, C. R. and McKEOWN, T. (1950), The care of the chronic sick, Part 2, social and demographic data, *Brit. J. prev. soc. Med.*, **4**, 61.
36. ABEL-SMITH, B. and TITMUSS, R. M. (1956), *The Cost of the National Health Service in England and Wales*, Cambridge University Press.

37. BROWN, G. W. (1959), Social factors influencing length of stay of schizophrenic patients, *Brit. med. J.*, **ii**, 1300.
38. RAWNSLEY, K., LOUDON, J. B. and MILES, H. L. (1962), Attitudes of relatives to patients in mental hospitals, *Brit. J. prev. soc. Med.*, **16**, 1.
39. WILMOT, P. and YOUNG, M. (1960), *Family and Class in a London Suburb*, London, Routledge & Kegan Paul.
40. CHARLES, D. C. (1953), Ability and accomplishment of persons earlier judged mentally deficient, *Genet. Psychol. Monogr.*, **47**, 3.
41. COHEN, L. (1955), Vocational planning and mental illness, *Personnel and Guidance J.*, **34**, 28.
42. COOPER, B. (1961), Social class and prognosis in schizophrenia, Parts 1 and 2, *Brit. J. prev. soc. Med.*, **15**, 17.
43. O'CONNOR, N. and TIZARD, J. (1956), *The Social Problem of Mental Deficiency*, Oxford, Pergamon Press.
44. WING, J. K. and GIDDENS, R. G. T. (1959), Industrial rehabilitation of male chronic schizophrenic patients, *Lancet*, **ii**, 503.
45. WINDER, C. L. (1960), Some Psychological Studies of Schizophrenics in *Etiology of Schizophrenia* (ed. Jackson, D. D.), New York, Basic Books.
46. CLARKE, A. D. B. (1960), Laboratory and Workshop Studies of Imbecile Learning Processes, *Proceedings of the London Conference on the Scientific Study of Mental Deficiency*, **1**, 89.
47. DINITZ, S., ANGRIST, S., LEFTON, M. and PASAMANICK, B. (1962), Instrumental role expectations and post-hospital performance of female mental patients, *Social Forces*, **40**, 3, 248.
48. SUSSER, M. W. (1963), *A Report on the Mental Health Services of the City of Salford for 1962*, City of Salford Health Department.
49. MEYERS, H. J. and BORGOTTA, S. F. (1959), *An Enquiry into Mental Patient Rehabilitation*, New York, Russell Sage Foundation.
50. TIZARD, J. and GRAD, J. (1961), *The Mentally Handicapped and their Families*, Oxford University Press.
51. ADAMS, M. (1956), Social work with mental defectives, Part I, *Case Conference*, **3**, 4.
52. ADAMS, M. (1957), Social work with mental defectives, Part II, *Case Conference*, **4**, 1.
53. STEIN, Z. A. and SUSSER, M. W. (1963), The social distribution of mental retardation, *Amer. J. Mental Defic.*, **67**, 811.
54. TYHURST, J. S. (1957), The Role of Transition States—Including Disasters in Mental Illness, *Symposium on Preventive and Social Psychiatry*, Walter Reed Army Institute of Research, Washington.
55. CAPLAN, G. (1961), *An Approach to Community Mental Health*, London, Tavistock.
56. HERSOV, L. A. (1960), Persistent non-attendance at school, *Child Psychol. Psychiat.*, **1**, 130.
57. BOWLBY, J. (1952), *Maternal Care and Mental Health*, W.H.O., Monograph Series, **2**.
58. PARKES, M. (1964), Recent bereavement as a cause of mental illness, *Brit. J. Psychiat.*, **110**, 198.
59. WRIGHT, S. L. (1963), The adult psychiatric patient in the community, *Public Health*, **77**, 4.
60. MAY, A. R. and GREGORY, E. (1963), An experiment in district psychiatry, *Public Health*, **78**, 1.
61. CLARKE, D. H. and COOPER, L. W. (1960), Psychiatric half-way hostel, *Lancet*, **i**, 588.
62. SUSSER, M. W. (1964), Group Problems of Community Care, in *Report of the Mental Health Services of the City of Salford for 1963*, City of Salford Health Department.
63. KUSHLICK, A. (1962), in *A Report on the Mental Health Services of the City of Salford for 1961*, City of Salford Health Department.
64. GLUCKMAN, M. (1955), *Custom and Conflict in Africa*, Oxford, Blackwell.
65. SUSSER, M. W. (1962), Changing roles and co-ordination in mental health services, *The Sociological Review Monograph*, **5** (ed. Halmos, P.), University of Keele.

9. Advisory Mechanisms of the National Health Service

T. M. CUTHBERT

Structure of the Service

The National Health Service is in effect a very large business organization, having an annual turnover of over £1000 million, of which at least £100 million is spent on mental health. At its head, instead of a Chairman of the Board, it has a political figure, a Minister of Health, who is answerable to the whole country (the shareholders) through their elected representatives in Parliament.

The aspect of the hospital branch of the Health Service most prominently displayed to public view is that concerned with its executive functions, where the chain of command runs from the Minister through the Ministry of Health (one branch of the Civil Service) to his agents, the fifteen regional boards, and from them to over 300 hospital management committees and on to the individual hospitals.

In the family doctor branch of the service, the direction of control is similar and runs from the Minister and the Ministry to local executive councils, and thence to the family doctor.

The third branch of the service, that which is concerned with preventive medicine and public health, encompasses a wealth of community medical services, e.g. maternity, child welfare, school medical and dental, immunization, ambulance, health visitor, geriatric nursing, home help; in fact all forms of pre- and after-care services, as well as services for handicapped persons of all varieties. These are administered by the local health authorities, acting in respect of the National Health Service as the Minister's agents, and here the line of communication is Minister, Ministry and County Council or County Borough Council to Local Health Department.

In each of these branches of the Health Service, there are facilities at every level for consultation and for obtaining advice. This advice can be transmitted upwards through the line of communication to the Ministry, or sometimes directly from the periphery to the Ministry. In either case, it is a function of the Health Ministry (sometimes called the Department) through its senior officials, medical and lay, to keep the Minister informed on the working of the whole service and to brief him on any matter concerning his department which may be raised in Parliament, or about which he should, in the interest of the nation's health, make an announcement.

Functions of the Service

Because of the ever-changing needs of medicine and of the necessity to deploy its available resources to the greatest effect, the Health Service must, like any progressive business organization, continuously re-examine its own structure and the functioning of each part of its organization. It must also anticipate and evaluate such things as the effects of changing social patterns of living and working, and new therapeutic methods and resources. It must assess the results of research and determine professional manpower requirements at all levels and it must ensure the efficiency with which available financial resources are utilized. Moreover, it must maintain, despite its size, a reasonable degree of flexibility.

While much information and advice is, in fact, fed back to the Ministry through the peripheral local advisory machinery and through the regional offices of the Ministry of Health, much of this is, of necessity, related to local or regional requirements. Although this can be collated within the Ministry, the resultant composite information still requires to be expertly evaluated. Of the numerous possible decisions, those which are most appropriate to the overall picture have to be selected and, having been selected, may have to be justified—sometimes because they are expensive or unpopular, or because the reason for them is not understood.

The Advisory Mechanisms of the National Health Service

In Relation to the Minister

Action should always be based on knowledge and the National Health Service has, from its very beginning, possessed a built-in central arrangement for the provision at the highest level of all—the Minister himself—of the most competent advice available within the United Kingdom. This is the establishment known as the Central Health Services Council and the Standing Advisory Committees.

The Central Council

Under the National Health Service Act, 1946, it is "the duty of the Minister to promote the establishment of a comprehensive Health Service . . . designed to secure improvement in the physical and mental health of the people . . . and the prevention, diagnosis and treatment of illness. . . ." This is the whole purpose of the Act and after stating this in section 1, the Act immediately proceeds in the next section to provide an essential tool ready to the Minister's hand: "there shall be constituted . . . a Council, to be called the Central Health Services Council" ("The Central Council"), whose duty it shall be "to advise the Minister upon such general matters relating to the Services provided under the Act . . . as the Council think fit, and upon any question referred to them by him relating to those services."

It will be seen that the Council has a duty to advise the Minister. This is responsible advice about which the Council does not have to wait to be consulted—it can and often does take the initiative.

Moreover, the constitution and membership of the Council are so arranged that it always has amongst its members the Presidents of the great medical colleges (physicians, surgeons, obstetricians and gynaecologists), the President of the statutory body responsible for medical training and professional conduct (General Medical Council), the Chairman of the Society of Medical Officers of Health (Preventive and Public Health) and the Chairman of the Council of the Association which represents over 70% of British doctors.

Additionally, the Minister appoints 35 members who are known to be experienced in different fields within the Health Service. Thus, there are 15 persons practising medicine, of whom 2 must have special knowledge of mental illness and mental subnormality; 5 (not doctors) must have experience in hospital management; 5 (also not doctors) experience in local government; 3 are to be dental practitioners; 2 are persons experienced in aspects of the mental health services; 2 are registered nurses and 1 a certified midwife; and there are 2 registered pharmacists. The constitution of the Council may only be varied by the Minister after he has consulted the Council itself.

THE STANDING COMMITTEES

The Act gives the Minister power to constitute what are in effect committees (but not subcommittees of the Central Council) with more specialized functions, but first he must consult the Central Council itself. These Standing Committees have the duty of advising both the Minister and the Central Council on those aspects of the Health Service for which they are by statutory order appointed. The Standing Committees thus expand the field of expertise available to the Minister and enable the Council itself to obtain specialized experience in depth, on a wider variety of subjects than would otherwise be possible.

The composition of any Standing Advisory Committee is determined by the Minister, firstly by consulting the Council and appointing such of its members as appear to the Council to have appropriate experience in the work of the Committee and who the Council, in effect, nominate. The other members are appointed after consultation by the Minister with certain organizations in the field of each committee's work, and which are "recognized" by him as being representative of that field. These organizations may nominate certain of their members for appointment by the Minister. The size of each committee is fixed by statutory order and although each may invite the attendance of outside experts to discuss particular items, none may co-opt. The Standing Committees may form subcommittees for special purposes and these may co-opt.

Both the Central Council and the Standing Advisory Committees appoint their own Chairmen and Vice-chairmen. The Ministry must, however, appoint the secretary to each committee, though the Council and the committees may, if they so wish, appoint from amongst their members someone to act as a joint secretary; in practice, this right is never exercised.

INTENTIONS OF THE ACT REGARDING "ADVICE"

It is abundantly clear that the intention of the Act is to provide the Minister, and through him his Department and the whole service, with an authoritative advisory machine whose views, formulated on the basis of a multidisciplinary membership, should never be partisan and should always derive from the best experience and knowledge available at any given time.

Another intention, re-affirmed by the Council itself in its first report to the Minister, is that all those selected to serve on the Central Council or the Advisory Committees (or any of their sub- or special committees) shall do so as individual experts in a personal capacity to the Minister himself. None is regarded in any sense as a representative of the body which may have nominated him or of any organization to which he may belong. This principle is, in fact, applied throughout the whole of the Health Service and membership of boards and management committees, etc., is always on a personal basis and never a representative one.

While such a principle may appear to be somewhat undemocratic, it is in line with long-established constitutional practice, as it helps to ensure that the member's loyalty is not in conflict, and that his or her advice will be of an impartial as well as an expert nature.

THE ANNUAL REPORT

It is, therefore, the intention that the Minister shall have impartial and expert advice and, while he is not bound to act on that advice, it is intended that he shall not conceal the fact that advice of a particular type has been rendered to him. He must lay before Parliament annually a report by the Council of its work and of the work and advice tendered also by the Standing

Committees. The Minister may only withhold publication of all or part of the report if he is satisfied, after consulting the Council itself, that publication would be contrary to the public interest.

Each report of the Central Council, preceded by a statement on it by the Minister, is ordered to be published by the House of Commons. These annual publications, which are always informative and well written, contain many detailed reports on all sorts of current problems.

INTER-RELATIONSHIP OF COUNCIL AND COMMITTEES

The relationship of the Standing Advisory Committees to the Central Health Services Council is complex, and it must be realized that these committees are statutory bodies in their own rights and that they have, therefore, duties and powers (in an advisory sense) which are very real. This relationship is dealt with in more detail in Appendix 1 to this chapter.

MISCELLANEOUS INFORMATION

Three other points require briefly to be made.

1. The Council and the Advisory Committees are composed of members whose tenure of office is limited by regulation to a period of 3 years, after which a member may be re-appointed for a further period of 3 years. Thus, there is opportunity for constant renewal of membership and for ensuring that advice is always kept up to date.

The only exception to this rule is provided by the 6 *ex officio* members of the Central Council, who are members by virtue of their professional high offices, and of which 5 change annually.

2. The advisory machinery here described relates to England and Wales; it is mirrored north of the Border by a Scottish Central Health Services Council and Scottish Standing Advisory Committees. In fact, whenever possible, Joint Committees between the two advisory structures are formed and Anglo-Scottish Joint Committees play a large part in overcoming any tendency to the development of divergent policies.

3. Immediately on their formation, both Central Health Services Councils affirmed their intentions not to concern themselves with matters for which existing machinery was already in operation. Thus, matters properly the concern of Whitley Councils (Salaries and Conditions of Service) and of Appeals Tribunals continue to be regarded as being outside the sphere of the advisory machinery.

The very real success of this interesting experiment in what might perhaps be called Statutory Co-operation is in large measure due to the quality of the men and women at the top, both in the Department—the medical and lay Civil Servants, and to the Chairmen and Vice-chairmen of the Central Council itself.

Functioning of Advisory Mechanisms

GENERAL

Ministers themselves invariably express their appreciation of the help and advice which they receive, though the annual reports do occasionally reveal instances of ministerial disinclination to act on advice tendered.

A case in point occurred very early in the life of the Council, when a sharp division of opinion arose on the composition of the membership of certain Advisory Committees. One part of the Council held that certain committees should be purely technical in function and, therefore, entirely composed of professional members; the remainder of the Council held that even a purely technical committee should contain at least a small lay component. On a vote, the latter opinion prevailed by a narrow margin and in consequence, advice was tendered to the Minister in accordance with the majority view. The Minister, however, was unable to accept this recommendation, holding that he must be able to look to certain committees for purely technical advice and to others for more general advice affecting the service as a whole. This was a most statesmanlike decision, the wisdom of which has been amply demonstrated by the quality of the proceedings of the Technical Advisory Committees (Medical, Dental, Pharmaceutical and Ophthalmic) over the years.

The remaining Advisory Committees (Nursing, Maternity and Midwifery, Mental Health, Cancer and Radiotherapy) are concerned with the development of particular services in all their aspects and are, therefore, logically composed of both professional and lay members. For example, the Standing Mental Health Advisory Committee in 1964 was made up of a Professor of psychological medicine (Chairman); a senior consultant psychiatrist; two aldermen, both experienced in the mental health services of their local authorities, and a senior male psychiatric nurse—all these were also members of the Central Council. In addition, the Minister had appointed, after consultation with various "recognized" organizations—one male and one female psychiatric nurse—both of some seniority; two medical officers of health; a child psychiatrist; a Professor of psychological medicine (vice-chairman); two senior consultant psychiatrists; one psychiatric social worker (tutor); a Professor of child health holding a personal chair; a general practitioner with interest and experience in mental health, and a senior consultant psychiatrist (at present President of the Royal Medico-Psychological Association).

VOLUME OF WORK

The volume of work discharged by the Council and Committees during the first 17 years of the National Health Service was colossal. It is only possible here to highlight some of the major achievements and a few of the more interesting activities, though the work of one Advisory Committee (Mental Health) is outlined in greater detail. It must not be forgotten, however, that the ordinary work of the parent committee continues *pari passu* with the work of the subcommittees, and that this routine activity is also directed towards the tendering of advice. Indeed, in the first annual report, it is recorded that the Minister remitted thirty separate items for consideration by the Council and the committees, which themselves originated more than a dozen other matters on which they submitted advice to the Minister. Many important reports have been produced by the Advisory Committees themselves, e.g. Selection of Maternity Cases for Admission to Hospital.

FREQUENCY OF MEETINGS

Meetings of Council and committees take place quarterly, or more frequently if required. The Council meets regularly, but some Advisory Committees only meet relatively infrequently. This tends to occur in those Advisory Committees which delegate most of their technical work to subcommittees (e.g. Cancer and Radiotherapy with its three special subcommittees) and in the year following the completion by an Advisory Committee of a major report. Such a year occurred in 1958 when no less than seven major reports were before the Council.

It must not be forgotten that the tasks of obtaining information and of collating reports imposes much work on the various sections of the Department and all this takes time. Nonetheless, it is a little surprising that an Advisory Committee concerned with so large a field as mental health should have found nothing to occupy its attention during the year 1964. Other committees with more circumscribed fields, having put their houses in order in the early years and now only holding watching briefs, can perhaps afford to rest on their laurels, but mental health is a vast and expanding field and much remains to be done in it.

In general, the Standing Mental Health Advisory Committee has not produced the same volume of work as have some of the other committees in particular the Nursing Advisory Committee, which is also a mixed professional and lay committee.

The Work of the Advisory Mechanisms

POLITICAL FACTORS

It is impossible in any national service to avoid political issues, and while the advisory machinery never concerns itself with politics, its advice to the Minister must, from time to time, raise political issues. The reverse situation sometimes occurs as, for example, in the development of exfoliative cytology. Advice tendered by the committees suggested a natural and progressive development of the required facilities, but outside and political pressures resulted in a more rapid development of this service. Fluoridation of water supplies is an example of the Council's advice needing the political authority of the Minister before it could hope to become effective, and the extreme care with which the whole subject was investigated technically before the Minister could act with confidence and safety is well demonstrated in the Annual Reports of the Council.

THEMES AND CRISES

While the scope of the advisory machinery is almost limitless, its work is always directed to the one end—that of tendering the best possible advice to the Minister. Certain matters recur so frequently as to become almost themes while others are sudden, urgent and vitally important, but once dealt with, do not recur. As examples of the former, may be cited the various shortages of professional staffs to which reference is constantly being made: nurses, particularly psychiatric nurses, midwives, physiotherapists, occupational therapists, medical social workers, dentists, doctors of all grades, and pharmacists. Committees are constantly reviewing these shortages and suggesting ways in which the various services might be rendered with greater efficiency in the use of manpower. But they are always concerned to ensure that there shall be no lowering of professional standards.

There have been several occasions on which the need for guidance has been urgent as, for example, in the winter of 1949 when the bed situation in hospitals, due to mounting waiting lists, necessitated the development of a clear admission policy. This was worked out on the basis of immediate priorities and long-term action by the Standing Medical Advisory Committee, to which the Council referred the matter. But not all the advice was found to be universally acceptable, notably the recommendation that a Bed Bureau should be established in each area with a senior medical officer able ultimately to order the admission of an emergency. Nor was that in which teaching hospitals were invited to accept a reasonable number of chronic sick patients. These make interesting reading today, when complaints on these very aspects of the Service are still far from uncommon. The thalido-mide crisis was also speedily dealt with and ultimately, the advice tendered led to the formation of new procedures for ensuring the safety of drugs.

TECHNICAL MEMORANDA

Probably the most satisfactory aspect of the activities of the advisory machine is to be found in the various memoranda of advice; these are always well summarized in the annual reports, and some are also issued as health memoranda to hospital authorities and to local authorities. Several have been documents in the great tradition of the British humanists—notably, Reception and Welfare of Hospital In-patients, 1952—"The Patients' Charter"; Visiting of Children in Hospital, 1954; Human Relations in Obstetrics, 1960; Visiting of Patients in Psychiatric and other Longstay Hospitals, 1961; and the Field of Work of the Family Doctor, 1963.

The publication at intervals since 1956 by the Standing Medical Advisory Committee of technical information, particularly the series of memoranda on preventive and social aspects of medicine, issued to family doctors and others concerned and, through medical schools, to senior students, has been greatly appreciated. Each paper is short and informative and deals with a particular disease or disability, on which clinicians may have special opportunities for direct preventive action.

Within the Technical Committees, communication between members is facilitated by a common language—that of medicine, and this does enable factual information to be understood by all and scientific deductions to be made and translated into realistic advice. A disadvantage inherent in the composition of the multi-disciplinary type of committee is shown in the difficulty sometimes experienced in holding the interest of the whole com-mittee all the time, especially when the matter before it is largely of a sectional nature, often expressed in an alien jargon or based on an unfamiliar ethic.

There is also a tendency for this type of committee to produce compromise recommendations, which frequently make its reports unacceptable to the progressively minded. Regrettably, these also have a tendency subsequently to appear in Ministry memoranda, in the form of somewhat banal statements and in platitudinous advice. A paradoxical achievement is the education of the Ministry's lay staff and this is not without value, even though it does tend to produce occasionally rather unrealistic formulations.

THE MENTAL HEALTH ADVISORY COMMITTEE 1949–63

All the Standing Advisory Committees commenced their activities with a rush of remits, necessitating additional meetings in the first 2 years, and mental health immediately involved itself, in addition to the Report on the Care of the Aged, in a detailed consideration of:

Prevention and After-care Services,

Arrangements for the After-care of Psychiatric "Casualties" from the Armed Forces, and

Problems arising from the Shortage of Psychiatric Social Workers—a discussion arising out of the interim report of the Mackintosh Committee (appointed by the Minister in 1948).

Other matters before this committee in 1949 included:

Boarding-out and Family Care—techniques desirable in themselves, but especially so as a means of relieving over-crowding in mental hospitals.

The Use by the Courts of certain Provisions in the Criminal Justices Act 1948, relating to Services provided under the National Health Service Act.

Employment of Lay Psychotherapists.

Establishment of Psychiatric In-patient Units in Undergraduate Teaching Hospitals.

The Supply of Nurses in Psychiatric Hospitals.

This last remit is a good example of a theme in advisory committee work, as in 1949 the Mental Health Committee gave preliminary consideration to the problem, and in the following year, this subject occupied most of its energies. It was felt that serious shortages of all grades of nursing staff (especially female) were evident, and that there was little chance of any solution to this problem within the next few years, largely because of the insufficient intake of students and their high wastage rate. In considering this whole situation, the committee had to observe the principle that pay and conditions of service were outside its purview. Nevertheless, it made six main recommendations to the Minister, the last of which concerned enrolled assistant (mental) nurses; and on that, it made seven subsidiary recommendations.

These main recommendations now make rather quaint reading:

The need for bold departure from tradition;

Experiments in selection of student nurse entrants;

Job analysis to determine such shortened period of training as would contain only the essentials of what a mental nurse should know for the efficient discharge of her duties;

Encouragement of experimental schemes for double qualification;

Abolition of the nursing assistant grade except when a student, having passed the Preliminary Examinations of the General Nursing Council and having completed the course of training, had failed to pass the Final R.M.N. Examination; apart from this, nursing assistants should not be employed in psychiatric hospitals, and if any were, then the proportion of nursing assistants should not exceed a fixed proportion of the total nursing staff.

Two years later, the committee somewhat modified its previous advice to the Minister, because the continuing serious shortage of nurses and wastage of students were still necessitating the employment of nursing assistants—a policy which would clearly have to continue in the foreseeable future. The provision of systematic instruction to fit this grade for its tasks was thus unavoidable. The committee also advised that the pay differential between psychiatric and other nurses should be increased and the incremental periods for qualified staff should be reduced in number, in order to arrest the decline in recruitment of male nurses.

In 1953, the Council accepted a report from the Nursing Committee on the position of the enrolled assistant nurse in the National Health Service, noting that the opinion formulated in relation to the enrolled assistant nurse in the psychiatric field, was at variance with the opinions of the Standing Mental Health Advisory Committee, and inviting both committees to consult together. It is interesting to observe that the Council was concerned particularly about the status of the enrolled assistant nurse relative to other grades, notably that of student nurse; the problems of this relationship are not yet resolved, despite a circular letter from the General Nursing Council to the appropriate training schools in 1964.

The Council also gave consideration to the training of mental nurses, in the light of the difficulties being experienced by many psychiatric hospitals in recruiting and retaining students, particularly at a time when new techniques and treatments were calling for higher standards of nursing; it felt strongly that while it should be open to psychiatric nurses to widen their experience in nursing by taking general training, the basic qualification in mental nursing should be quite adequate to fit the psychiatric nurse for promotion to higher posts in the psychiatric field, without any further need for additional qualification in general nursing. Any weakness in general nursing experience should be made up by reciprocal secondment schemes with local general hospitals (this view was known to be acceptable to the Standing Nursing Advisory Committee) and combined training schemes should be encouraged experimentally, as should postgraduate schemes of training in other fields of nursing: all these have been effected.

During the next year, however, the differences of opinion between the Standing Mental Health and the Standing Nursing Advisory Committees on the question of establishing a grade of enrolled assistant nurse in psychiatric hospitals was finally dealt with by the Council itself, which set up a Working Party, after the two committees had failed to agree in joint discussions. This ultimately resulted in the Minister being advised by the Council that an urgent need existed in psychiatric hospitals, which could be met by a sub-ordinate nursing grade, and that the nursing assistant properly experienced and supervised could fulfil this role. The Council thought that there was much to be said in favour of a statutory roll of assistant nurses, but that at that time, the response to training and the limited facilities for this made it unlikely that psychiatric hospital nursing needs could be met entirely by such a grade. The Council advised, however, that nursing assistants should be given a practical training along the lines already laid down, and that these recommendations should be given a trial over the period of the next 3 years.

During this period, the Mental Health Advisory Committee produced (1957) a paper on the Employment of Ward Orderlies in Psychiatric Hospitals as a contribution to the staffing of these hospitals, and this was accepted by the Council.

In 1962, the Standing Nursing Advisory Committee, jointly with the Standing Mental Health Advisory Committee, considered the employment of state enrolled nurses in psychiatric hospitals. At that time, psychiatric hos-pitals were not training pupil nurses, as they were unable to meet the re-quirements of the syllabus, and in consequence, only a very few state enrolled nurses were employed in these hospitals. The General Nursing Council was considering revision and extension of the syllabus for pupils on the lines of a common basic training, plus additional training in optional specialties (including psychiatry), and this would permit psychiatric hospitals to secure the General Nursing Council's approval as Pupil Training Schools and thus make available a supply of specially trained state enrolled nurses. The Standing Nursing Committee endorsed these new proposals and in similar manner, the Standing Mental Health Advisory Committee also endorsed them but required safeguards, e.g. that the proportion of state enrolled nurses in relation to other staffs should not be excessive, that experienced existing nursing assistants should be eligible for enrolment, and that there would still be a useful place for nursing assistants who did not wish to train for the roll. The Council accepted this combined advice (together with the Mental Health Committee's reservations) and this policy is now in full operation.

The Mental Health Advisory Committee was much concerned with other staffing shortages and, in particular, it gave much consideration to the de-velopment of Regional In-Service Training Schemes for Clinical Psychologists. It continued to give advice that such schemes should be fostered and de-veloped, calling for reports periodically on the progress made in the regions. In this way, it followed a pattern of activity which almost amounted to executive action, as the recurring advisory pressures did result in executive action and regional training schemes were developed.

In like manner, the Committee kept under review the whole question of Medical Staffing of Psychiatric Hospitals and Units, calling for information on the numbers of consultants, senior registrars and registrars, and reporting to the Council that if psychiatric hospitals were to continue satisfactorily to change their character, by more effectively discharging their primary purpose of treating patients and restoring as many of them as possible to the community, more and better doctors would be required. The committee noted that existing establishments (in 1954) were short by 20%. Information obtained by the committee suggested that certain shortcomings within the service itself might be causally related to this situation. The committee reviewed in detail such matters as housing, training arrangements, lack of extramural activities, unsuitable senior registrar appointments, inadequate medical libraries—all of which were thought to be implicated in the poor response to recruitment, and universities were reminded that medical education requirements were changing and that some were still without chairs of psychiatry. The need for a career grade short of consultant status was recognized as being particularly desirable in these hospitals. Advice to the Minister closely followed these conclusions and he at once recognized the special need for the provision of accommodation in remote hospitals and the need to increase the senior registrar establishments, but the plea for increased registrar establishments did not receive the support of the Council or of the Standing Medical Advisory Committee.

Already in 1950, the Standing Mental Health Advisory Committee had given some thought to the needs of training psychiatrists and it tendered advice to the effect that boards of governors should give high priority to the provision of in-patient psychiatric units for both sexes in or near the teaching hospitals; such units should be of 60-bed size (though 20 beds would enable a start to be made), and should contain facilities for occupational therapy.

In 1962, the Council was again considering recommendations made by the Mental Health Committee, after consideration of a paper prepared by the Department on Beds for Psychiatry in Teaching Hospitals. The Committee advised that the need for improving and extending the teaching of psychiatry was increasingly evident from: (1) the shortages of suitable psychiatrists available for existing posts, (2) the increased demand arising out of the provisions of the Mental Health Act, whereby any hospital could admit and treat mentally ill patients, and (3) the greater understanding of social factors in the causation and treatment of mental illness.

Other matters which were considered by this Committee resulting in advice to the Minister, and which have born fruit, include:

Arrangements for Treatment of Psychiatric "Casualties" from the Armed Forces and assistance to the Ministry of Labour in connection with the Psychiatric Examination of Recruits for National Service;
Development of Psychiatric Day Hospitals;
Some Problems of Management of certain High-grade Subnormal Persons;
Industrial Occupational (therapeutic) Schemes;

Provision for the Treatment of Alcoholism;
Retention of Psychiatric Records;
Education of the Public in Mental Health;
The Visiting of Patients in Psychiatric Hospitals—a particularly helpful and
    successful memorandum.

A valuable study undertaken by the committee in 1962–3 reviewed the need for In-patient Accommodation for Mentally Ill and Seriously Maladjusted Children. The Committee found that in 1963, there were eighteen in-patient units of this type, providing 370 beds (about 8 per million of the population) and that these units were of very varied type and function. There was little doubt that, as experience with other services had shown, the extent of the need would only emerge as the provision of services improved and clearly, there was an urgent need for expansion of units for children. The committee was of the opinion that, for assessment and short-term treatment, 20–25 beds per million of the population would be required, and for long-term hospital care, 25 beds per region should be provided initially. The figures for adolescents were assessed at 20–25 beds per million, as a minimum to be provided over the next few years. The committee also advised that the development of in-patient facilities should go hand-in-hand with the expansion of out-patient diagnostic services, and that educational facilities should be available, through close liaison with local education authorities; location of units would have to be determined by accessibility to a main centre of population and to neurological and paediatric facilities, schools for maladjusted children, and child guidance or child psychiatric centres. This advice was issued to hospital authorities in H.M. Circular (64) 4.

The Committee has also produced a series of papers incorporating advice on matters having a direct bearing on the provision and development of services to patients. For example, in 1949, while the Standing Medical Advisory Committee was studying the problems of treatment of the elderly chronic sick, the Mental Health Committee was also considering a remit from the Minister on the provision which should be made for persons suffering from (mental) infirmity due to old age. The resultant joint advice tendered by the Council contained, *inter alia*, the recommendation that Hospital Geriatric Services should be developed at general and teaching hospitals, and that each unit should contain a psychiatric observation section and a long-stay annexe for patients suffering from mental infirmity arising from old age who did not need treatment in mental hospitals. While progress has been made in this direction, the facilities so far developed are nothing like as comprehensive as present conditions demand or as was originally envisaged. This is a matter about which the Committee should constantly be importuning the Minister.

Consideration of the subject of Psychiatry and the General Practitioner in 1956 led the Committee to the conclusions that there was still too great a tendency to regard psychiatric illness as a matter primarily for the hospital and specialist services, and that there were many patients who need not be treated in hospital if their family doctors would undertake their treatment. Also, that no useful advice could be given to the Minister at that time because it was rather for the profession itself to stimulate the interest of its members. In 1960, however, the committee approved a departmental paper (published in the series on Social and Preventive Medicine) on the Part of the Family Doctor in the Mental Health Service. This dealt with the function of the family doctor as holding the balance between hospital and community care, and stated that for services in curative and preventive psychiatry the family doctor, the psychiatrist and the many social agencies should each contribute: "the results are proportionate to the efficiency of the team rather than to the expertise of any one member of it".

The paper went on to emphasize the role of the family doctor in the recognition of all forms of mental disorder, including the field of child psychiatry, and his experience in the disposal of each case to the most appropriate agency; it stressed that his particular role lay in the provision and management of the after-care period.

Another series of papers having a profound effect on the development of therapeutic services available to patients were:

Co-ordination of the Functions of Mental Hospitals and Local Authorities;
Care and After-care of the Mentally Disordered;
The After-care of Patients discharged from Mental Hospitals;
Hospital Services for the Mentally Ill;
Improving the Performance of existing Mental Hospitals.

The subcommittee appointed by the Standing Mental Health Committee in 1959 to report on the Training of Staff of Training Centres for the Mentally Subnormal produced a most comprehensive series of recommendations, and these were passed to the Council with the backing of the parent committee in 1961. This report was published in full by the Stationery Office in 1962 after the Council had advised that it be implemented in stages, after discussions with all the interested bodies.

The committee also discussed and, where appropriate, tendered advice on many current issues, for example, the Mackintosh Report on Psychiatric Social Work, the Report of the Royal Commission on the Law relating to Mental Illness and Mental Deficiency, and the ensuing Mental Health Bill, and the Report of the Working Party on Social Workers (Younghusband).

FUTURE BUSINESS

Underlying much of the recent work of this committee has been the assumption by the Ministry that there will inevitably be a considerable run-down in the numbers of beds occupied by the mentally ill and arising from this, as well as for other good reasons, future psychiatric practice should be extensively developed in the new district general hospitals. It has already been shown that there are grave dangers in relying too greatly on this assumption and in pursuing this course of action too vigorously. Warnings to this effect have already been sounded by the Advisory Committee, which will have to remain alert to the dangers of inadequate bed provision, of the development of two standards of psychiatric practice, of the neglect of the therapeutic needs of the medium and longer-stay patients, and of delay by local authorities in providing community and after-care services, which do not appear to be developing as smoothly as was envisaged. The reaction of the community to the demands made on it to develop care must continue to be assessed, and advice will be needed on the support required if care is to be undertaken extensively.

There is a grave danger also that the rising tide of geriatric patients will be allowed to swamp the services of existing psychiatric hospitals as, clearly, there will be little place for such patients in the new psychiatric units. The urgent problem of providing accommodation elsewhere than in psychiatric hospitals for the elderly with some degree of mental enfeeblement has not yet been resolutely tackled.

While techniques of management for psychotic and neurotic patients in the community are now well established, little progress is being made in providing facilities to meet the challenge of psychopathy—surely a major social problem today. More concern might also be shown over the slow progress in the development of forensic psychiatry.

A serious drop in the morale of psychiatric nurses is a distinct possibility if changes in psychiatric practice take place too drastically or too suddenly, or if the load placed on them continues to increase. There is no reason why some of their special skills should not be incorporated in the training programmes of other branches of nursing, to the benefit of the service as a whole. Geriatric practice would be almost revolutionized if those nursing the elderly were taught the appropriate skills in handling patients who were suffering from organically determined confusion and restlessness.

Finally, the development and expansion of all the medical, educational, social welfare and other services which are taking place make it unrealistic to assume that a sufficient number of workers of good intelligence and sound personality will be found to staff the whole of the growing mental health services, especially when other professions and expanding government departments and industrial and commercial enterprises are "fishing in the same waters". Shortening of the working week appears to be a continuing national policy and the Mental Health Committee will, no doubt, therefore be giving earnest consideration to the steps which may have to be taken to economize and rationalize professional manpower, particularly in the hospital branch of this service.

Conclusion

The advisory mechanisms are elaborate; their formation represents an honest attempt to provide the Minister with up-to-date, impartial and authoritative advice in accordance with sound constitutional practice. These mechanisms do provide him with this, and with the support which he requires in operating and in developing the service.

The Council and the committees also produce valuable reports, especially on technical matters, and some of the documents issued by the Ministry as a result of their deliberations restate the central position of the patient as a human being with needs and rights. These reports and memoranda constantly serve as correctives to the undoubted tendency towards mechanization, inherent in any large organization.

Certain weaknesses are apparent in the advisory mechanisms. In particular, the tendency, resulting from the very nature of many of the committees, for compromise advice to be formulated occasionally, and for this to become somewhat platitudinous.

Again, while the composition of the Council ensures its technical competence, the very eminence of many of its members and of those who serve it from the Department does result sometimes in somewhat unrealistic advice being tendered.

The advisory machinery might well add to its undoubted usefulness if it could somehow be adapted to provide a better platform for the discussion of the many current difficulties which beset the whole service, and which are often of a very practical nature. Indeed advice on the day-to-day working of the service at all levels might become a truly prophylactic function of the whole advisory apparatus.

Appendix 1

RELATIONSHIP BETWEEN
CENTRAL COUNCIL AND STANDING COMMITTEES
(From the Annual Report 1949, page 3)

The Council's relation to the Standing Advisory Committees is one which has no exact parallel:

(a) These Committees are independent statutory bodies which derive their authority direct from section 2 (3) of the Act and which may submit advice direct to the Minister. If they do submit such advice, they must, however, send copies of their reports to the Council which may express its views thereon. The Committees normally receive remits direct from the Minister and when they do so, they send their reports direct to the Minister. Where such reports concern only the service with which that particular Standing Advisory Committee is concerned, it has been our (the Council's) normal practice merely to record that we have no comments to express on the report; where a report raises wider issues, however, we have expressed a view thereon and forwarded it to the Minister. In two cases we have suggested to the Minister that reports should be referred back to Standing Advisory Committees for further consideration. The Minister has undertaken not to act, except in emergency, on the report of any Standing Advisory Committee before the Council has had an opportunity to express its views thereon.

(b) The Standing Advisory Committees can also act as if they were Committees of the Council and the Council can remit matters to them; if it does so, the report must be sent back to the Council. The Committee may also, of its own volition, decide to send a particular report to the Council rather than to the Minister if it feels that the Council may wish to consider the implications of the report in a field wider than that with which the Committee is concerned.

(c) The Council is also charged by section 2 (5) of the Act to make an annual report to the Minister, not only on its own proceedings, but also on those of the Standing Advisory Committees, i.e. the Committees do not make their own annual reports.

In view of the foregoing, it has been accepted that the Council should act as a pivot for all the Committees, that it should ensure that similar procedures are adopted throughout, and that there is due co-ordination between the work of the Committees, so that the central advisory system of the National Health Service works as a whole and not as a number of disjointed parts offering unrelated advice to the Minister.

10. Mental Health Services in Northern Ireland*

Alex. T. Elder

THE Mental Health Service in Northern Ireland does not differ fundamentally from that provided in England and Wales. But a brief description of the administrative machinery and of certain terminology in use which is particular to Northern Ireland will be helpful. In England and Wales, the term "mental subnormality" is in use, and in Scotland, "mental deficiency". In Northern Ireland, a person suffering from arrested or incomplete development of mind (whether arising from inherent causes or induced by disease or injury), which renders him socially inefficient to such an extent that he requires supervision, training or control in his own interests or in the interests of other persons, is known as "a person requiring special care". This category covers both subnormality and severe subnormality.

By the Health Services Act (Northern Ireland) 1948, an autonomous corporate body was created, called the Northern Ireland Hospitals Authority, with ownership of all health service hospitals. All aspects of the Mental Health Services are administered through a statutory mental health services committee, and this responsibility also covers hospital services for the mentally subnormal. The Ministry of Health and Local Government was given the duty of co-ordinating the health services, including the prevention of mental subnormality, and the care, supervision, training, and occupation of the mentally subnormal. As from January 1965, this duty was vested in a newly created Ministry of Health and Social Services.

There are in Northern Ireland (population 1,448,000) six long-term hospitals for the mentally ill, with a total bed complement of 6162. This provision of 4·2 beds per 1000 of population is rather unevenly divided at the moment throughout the province, because most of the permanent psychiatric hospitals date back to last century, and population trends have altered considerably in the interval. Figure 1 illustrates the location of the six hospitals, with their bed complement and the approximate population served in each catchment area. Figure 1 also shows the position of the principal village community centre for the mentally subnormal. This will have a final complement of 1000 places, though there are also many other smaller centres scattered throughout Northern Ireland, such as the 400-bed unit based on Armagh.

---

* Based on a paper read before the Mental Health Section, Royal Society of Health, at its Annual Congress, 1964.

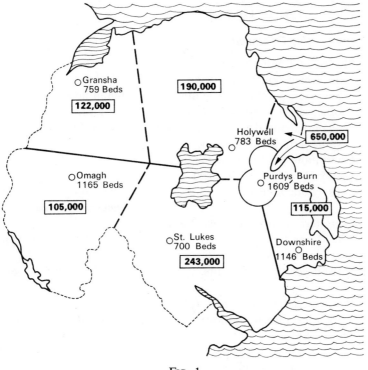

FIG. 1.

A later study by Mulligan, Robinson and Casement (1964) suggests a future division into five "clinical" areas, i.e., Greater Belfast (population 685,000), Londonderry and Omagh (230,770), Coleraine and Antrim–Ballymena (223,487), Lurgan and Newry (303,949), and Downpatrick with North-east Down (136,007).

Classification of Services provided

The following, for brevity and clarity, is a deliberate simplification, although it is by no means an over-simplification. The classification of diagnostic and treatment centres presents many difficulties.

TYPE OF UNIT	LOCATION
A. *Diagnostic, Out-patient and Treatment*	
(i) Diagnostic and assessment clinics	In the community. Possibly extramural hospital facilities or general or mental hospital
(ii) Out-patient clinics for adults and children	
(iii) Special child psychiatry units	
(iv) Mother and baby units (puerperal)	

Type of Unit	Location
B. *Diagnostic plus Treatment*	
(i) Short-stay (under 3 months) Treatment units for psycho-neuroses, psychosomatic illness, other acute temporary states, alcoholic and drug addiction, plus short-term rehabilitation.	Mental hospitals or units, in or attached to general hospitals
(ii) Continuing treatment or medium-stay (3 months to 2 years) Psychotic illness.	Mental hospital or units in general hospitals
(iii) Long-term treatment (over 2 years) (a) Long-term sick under 65 years of age.	Mental hospital, hospitals for long-stay
(b) Psychogeriatric units.	Units in mental or general hospitals
(iv) Psychogeriatric assessment (plus long-term rehabilitation)	Units in general hospitals or in mental hospitals
(v) Special units Forensic psychiatry.	Special hospitals in Gt. Britain
Units for child offenders.	*Ad hoc*
C. *After-care*	
(i) Convalescent units (plus rehabilitation)	Determined by geography (seaside or country)
(ii) After-care assessment villas plus rehabilitation (schizophrenia)	Hospital or extramural
(iii) Domiciliary after-care	
(iv) After-care services to prisons, and borstals (plus rehabilitation)	In the community
D. *Day Hospitals*	Attached to hospitals or *ad hoc* in the community
E. *Care of Mentally Subnormal*	
(a) Training centres	*Ad hoc*
(b) Long-stay and continuing care	
(c) Working villages plus rehabilitation hostels, and sheltered workshops	In or associated with village communities

TYPE OF UNIT	LOCATION

F. *University Teaching Facilities*

Research units	*Ad hoc*
Clinical psychology	Patient beds are associated
Post-graduate teaching	with a university Depart-
(general practitioner, nurses,	ment of Mental Health
ancillary professional workers)	

Some of these categories can be calculated on a local basis, some best on a regional basis, and only a few at national level. It will be seen that the overall position in Northern Ireland differs very little from the general assessment of 4 beds per 1000 of population, initially quoted by the Ministry of Health, London. Based on a study made by the General Register Office, a forecast has been made that the present proportion of 2500 beds per million of population may be reduced by half over the next 15 years. This, in fact, agreed with the forecast of Tooth and Brooke (1961) (PEP, 1963) though doubts were raised by others (Jones, 1963a). The Northern Ireland Hospitals Authority (1962) drew attention to the distinction which must be drawn between total admissions and actual numbers of patients on the register. It stated that the number of admissions to psychiatric and special care hospitals increased from 6054 in 1961 to 6687 in 1962, but also point out that there was a fall of 194 in the total numbers of patients in residence at 31 December 1962, compared with 31 December 1961. Though it has been shown (Fig. 1) that the present disposition of mental hospital beds throughout Northern Ireland is somewhat uneven, the view of the Nuffield Provincial Hospital Surveyors (1945) that "in the re-organization of hospital services after the war a real effort should be made to re-integrate the two services— mental and physical" was accepted. This policy of integration has been proceeding for some years now, and in several areas, integration of hospital management committees and administration has already been accomplished. By this means, it is possible to effect a better balance of beds in each of the areas, though the establishment of acute psychiatric wings in general hos- pitals—either new ones or by extensions to existing ones—is of necessity a somewhat slow process. An overall calculation of the specific needs of Northern Ireland was made by several workers in the last few years (Mulligan, 1963; Elder, 1964), and these studies suggest that local needs can be met by planning bed or place ratios of the order shown in Table 1.

It is realized that this overall estimate of 3·28 hospital beds per 1000 of population does not agree with the assessment originally made by Tooth and Brooke. Examined in detail, however, the measure of disagreement lies in the estimates of requirements for the long-term psychiatric sick up to 65 years of age, and also in the requirements for the psychogeriatric group. It is held

TABLE 1.

Hospital and Local Authority Services

Short-term sick	0·34
Continuing care	0·60
Long-term sick	
under 65 years of age	1·70
over 65 years of age	0·64 to 1·0 varying with the area

3·28 to 3·64 beds per 1000 of population

Subnormal persons of all ages requiring places in day centres	0·86	Places per
Subnormal requiring full-time institutional care	2·0	1000 of
Educationally subnormal all categories—education authorities	2·25	population
Places in the community for total subnormality of *all* categories including the educationally subnormal	5·50	

(Mulligan's (1964) later assessment would put the requirements for Northern Ireland even higher, e.g.

Short-term and continuing care	1·08
Long-stay under 65 years	1·90
Long-stay over 65 years	1·1)

in Northern Ireland that community care services, however well developed, can have little effect on the hospital needs for the long-term age-groups up to 65 years. Local authority services may help in lowering some hospital bed needs for age-groups over 65 years, but only if local authorities are provided with additional assistance by way of professional staff of various types.

The Calculation of the Specific Needs

(a) SHORT-TERM ILLNESSES

The Northern Ireland Regional Hospitals Council, established with the help of the Nuffield Provincial Hospitals Trust, assessed the hospital requirements in 1945 at 240 beds for a (then) population of 1,200,000, or 0·2 beds per 1000 of population. Today, this position is not materially different from what it was in 1945. Other short-term requirements for conditions such as alcoholism and drug addiction were variously assessed, through the co-operation of all the mental hospitals and the Northern Ireland Ministry of Home Affairs. It has been possible to get total figures for Northern Ireland, which suggest a level of about 0·05 beds per 1000 for the treatment of alcohol and drug addiction, based on an average length of stay of 4 weeks for alcoholism and 8 weeks for drug addiction. But there are difficulties in such an assessment. First of all, it is based on user requirements, and not on need. Some psychiatrists say that drug addiction really requires anything up to 6 months for long-term treatment, while chronic alcoholism needs a stay of about a third longer than patients are usually prepared to accept.

Alcohol addiction in Northern Ireland now accounts for over 800 admissions per annum, of which one-third are first admissions. These numbers rose from around 700 in 1962 to 819 in 1964 and in addition, 19 patients were admitted suffering from alcoholic psychosis. Bed requirements can be based only on total admissions, plus re-admissions. A more correct assessment, therefore, would be $0 \cdot 05$ to $0 \cdot 15$ beds per 1000 of population (average $0 \cdot 1$). For short-term treatment, of up to 3 months, of the neuroses, alcohol and drug addiction, and assessment of psychosomatic manifestations, the Northern Ireland total requirements of $0 \cdot 3$ beds per 1000 of population differed very little from Tooth and Brooke's assessment of $0 \cdot 34$ beds per 1000 of population. It was therefore regarded as confirming the findings of Tooth and Brooke for this particular category of patient.

(b) MEDIUM-STAY PATIENTS

In this category a different picture emerged. Proportionately fewer of these are informal admissions and the average length of stay varies from 3 months to 2 years. This category has been called the "continuing treatment" group; Tooth and Brooke assess the need at $0 \cdot 53$ per 1000 of population. Mulligan (1963), working on requirements for the County Armagh Mental Health Service, recorded a need for 120 beds for a catchment area of 200,000 population or $0 \cdot 6$ beds per 1000.

The real difficulty here lies in the future of treatment for the schizophrenic. Kathleen Jones (1963b), quoting an American report, states that "short of an unexpected and near miraculous breakthrough (i.e., in psychotropic drugs), we may have many years of unrewarding basic research ahead of us—indeed if such a cure is possible". One of the greatest difficulties in assessing the need for beds for the treatment of schizophrenia lies in the number of re-admissions, which are now numerous. It may well be that some form of assessment and rehabilitation unit which is within the hospital but allows a patient more or less the amenities of the community during the period of his assessment, would prevent premature discharge. In so doing, it might not only act as an additional safeguard to the public, but also as a brake on the re-admission rate.

The Influence of the Day Hospital on Short- and Medium-stay Treatment

Farndale (1963), who has collected more factual data than any other present-day writer on the subject, states that it is doubtful whether day hospitals have produced a corresponding reduction in the number of in-patient beds, although to the extent that many day patients would otherwise have been in-patients, beds are being saved. It seems clear that some day hospitals are creating a new clientele and may be increasing the demand for psychiatric treatment. If they lead to an additional demand, this may negative some of the potential savings. It is doubtful whether in the short term there will be any savings in money, as day treatment is not always cheaper than in-treatment.

The experience of Dr. R. W. Whiteley, Consultant Psychiatrist in charge of the Clifton Street Day Hospital, Belfast, seems to bear this out (1963). He has found it necessary to divide his clientele into an assessment clinic, comparable to an out-patient department, and a day treatment hospital with some rehabilitation services attached. This Belfast day hospital has clearly proved to be an aid to general practitioners and a convenience to the public, because it is situated in the centre of the city and many miles from the nearest psychiatric wards. The population catchment area is approximately 250,000 persons and attendances in 1963 were of the order of 2013, of which 1522 were re-attendances at the out-patient department. Attendances of day patients coming for *treatment* totalled 8079 (males 2262, females 5817). The conditions treated were mainly neuroses, schizophrenia and endogenous depression. Only $4 \cdot 5\%$ of these patients in 1963 had to be admitted subsequently to the psychiatric wards.

It cannot be said that the existence of day hospitals in the catchment area of the main Belfast mental hospital has affected the in-patient admission rate. Admissions fell from 1724 in 1962 to 1534 in 1963 and had one ceased the evaluation at this point, a false conclusion might have been drawn, because admissions rose again in 1964 to 1774. The present trend upwards has been reflected in other mental hospitals. Some of it is unquestionably due to an increased turnover, with an increase in the number of re-admissions. These accounted for 50% of all admissions to the Belfast hospital in 1964. At the same time, it is estimated that $20–25\%$ of patients attending the day hospitals might have become in-patients if the day hospital had not existed. Gibson (1965) has drawn attention to the value of a fully developed psychiatric in-patient research and out-patient unit at the large Belfast City Hospital and showed that such a unit, when properly used, could reduce the need for a myriad of day hospitals scattered throughout the city. It would appear that when one takes into account the value of day centres which may be provided by local health authorities, there is an outstanding need for the setting up of some form of Area Liaison Committee to correlate the work of hospitals and local authorities in this field of community mental health supervision, so as to avoid duplication and overlapping of services. Whether for geographical or other reasons, a day hospital may reasonably be set up at the centre of a catchment area, as defined by the location of general practitioners and convenience to the public. Planning for the Northern Ireland day hospitals includes the following:

(a) an out-patient facility;
(b) a treatment facility, to include convulsive therapy, test rooms and rooms for individual clinical and psycho-analysis;
(c) a recreational facility; including a quiet room;
(d) occupational therapy, giving a wide range of coverage of arts and crafts;
(e) domestic facilities;
(f) administrative facilities;
(g) some facility for mothers to bring children;
(h) possibly some small overnight accommodation.

A useful report, produced in 1964 by the patients' committee of the Day Hospital, Clifton Street, Belfast, recommended that the best type of premises for a day hospital would be an old private house, inconspicuously sited in grounds which could be used for gardening and recreation.

> The hospital should be limited to 50 patient places, as being conducive to a happy, friendly atmosphere. Nurses and staff should wear ordinary clothes and mix with the patients as much as possible and there should be provision for games and sports, and discussion rooms, as well as the more orthodox and accepted provision for occupational therapy.

Long-term Sick

Provision for this category has given a good deal of difficulty, but a clearer picture emerged when these were separated into a younger age-group of long-term sick and a psychogeriatric group, with a borderline of 65 years of age. Mulligan gave the total need for a population of 200,000 as 600 beds, 350 of which would be for those under 65 years of age. Recently (1963), with the help of the Northern Ireland Hospitals Authority's Statistical Branch, records of discharges were started from two of the largest mental hospitals, serving a total combined population of 320,000. Using the usual punch-card system and international classification of psychiatric illness, a method already employed by Kidd and Meenan (1959), with international code numbers 300 to 320 (but excluding the psychogeriatric) it was found that on 31 December 1963 there were 315 males and 321 females who could not be discharged in the foreseeable future, i.e. had been resident already for anything from 2 to 5 years. Thus, a population of 320,000 required 546 beds for this category, or $1 \cdot 7$ beds per 1000 of population. The younger long-stay group required 40% of the total accommodation. By the same process of assessment, it was found that the psychogeriatric group produced a requirement which could vary in the separate areas between $0 \cdot 6$ beds per 1000 and $1 \cdot 3$. The primary consideration is the provision of beds for the elderly, whether these be physical ailments in geriatric wards or psychogeriatric cases, or a combination. One has, therefore, to consider the needs of each area comprehensively and to decide what is required, whether at a general hospital, or separately, or at a mental hospital, or at combined hospitals. The total requirement for the geriatric groups is rising, and it would seem that, in the not too distant future, a figure of 5 beds per 1000 of population, depending on the contribution of the local health and welfare authorities, would not be unrealistic for this long-term group with mental and/or physical deterioration.

The Mentally Subnormal

Applying the Wood Committee's findings (1929) to Northern Ireland, the Nuffield Surveyors considered there would be, in a population of 1,200,000, just over 10,000 mentally subnormal persons, of whom 3000 would benefit from institutional care, and of these 560 would be children. It is interesting to compare the final assessment in a present population of 1,448,000, and thanks are due to the Ministry of Health and Social Services for the table of statistics (Table 2) which shows the position as it was at 31 December 1962. At that time there was no waiting list.

TABLE 2.

Subnormal persons requiring supervision in the community	2702 ⎫	
Subnormal persons under guardianship	10 ⎭	2712[a]
Subnormal persons in institutional care in Northern Ireland	1843 ⎫	
Subnormal persons in institutional care outside Northern Ireland	50 ⎭	1893
To effect a proper comparison with the Wood Committee forecast, the numbers of pupils in the care of the education committee should be added as follows:		
Number of educationally subnormal pupils in		
special schools	774 ⎫	
special classes (primary)	1529 ⎬	3144
(secondary)	841 ⎭	
		7749

[a] These figures include 105 persons in welfare authority homes.

The largest centre for the subnormal (or "special care cases") is mostly centred in a village community, 17 miles north of Belfast in a rural area, and 2 miles from the town of Antrim. This community, known as Muckamore Abbey Hospital, has a present complement of 700 places, which is being extended soon to 1000 places (1963). It is built on a villa system and Table 3 shows the gradings in separate villas. The plans of the next stage will include villas for male and female geriatric patients and for male and female "difficult" cases. The latter, though envisaging security precautions, should not be confused with the maximum security units recognized in forensic psychiatry.

TABLE 3.

Classification of Villas

Medium-grade amenable males in the older age group
Medium-grade amenable male patients
Unit for maladjusted male patients
Low-grade ambulant older boys
Medium-grade amenable older boys
Higher-grade amenable adult females
Medium-grade amenable females
Disturbed adult females
Amenable boys and girls
Low and medium-grade maladjusted children
Children's cot and chair unit and nursing unit

Muckamore House Extension	Amenable females in the older age group
Muckamore House Sick Hospital	Teachers College
	Cot and chair children, and sick and physically handicapped patients

The whole residential concept is that of a community in itself, with a "school" for suitable children, workshops, recreation centre, garden and eventually a swimming pool. Hostels for suitable cases transferred from Muckamore for training pending employment have been established, as also have sheltered workshops, administered in association with the national insurance schemes. All these units have worked in association with the basic village community, from which the young people emerge, and it should be noted that this whole system is operated by the Northern Ireland Hospitals Authority. For special care services, the province is divided into three administrative areas. In addition to residential provision, there are twenty-four schools or occupation centres in the community, and a specialized Teachers Training College.

Cases requiring Maximum Security Care—Forensic Psychiatry

Warren (1963), dealing with adolescent patients whose instability of behaviour is so marked that it can be described as psychopathic, states that their number is "relatively small, although individual cases can give rise to much anxiety to all concerned". Heaton-Ward (1963) deplored the too ready use of the term "psychopath" as a diagnosis and sometimes as a means of "dismissing the problem created by the persistently anti-social". He went on to say that he regarded true psychopathy as a relatively rare condition. The Northern Ireland findings certainly agreed with this, and if one interprets the words used in legislation—"abnormally aggressive and seriously irresponsible conduct"—in the strict sense in which it is recognized in forensic psychiatry, the number of places required on a local population basis does not seem to justify special provision. Use is therefore made of suitable accommodation in Great Britain, to which the relatively few cases arising in Northern Ireland are transferred as the occasion requires. This is therefore one aspect of the mental health service which would appear to be better dealt with on a large regional basis, if not on a national basis (Snell, 1963).

Borstals and Child Delinquency

The same need for suitable premises to allow for proper classification of residents, and their separate consideration in treatment and after-care, exists in this service. Consultant psychiatrists attend at the approved schools and borstals and provide specialist advice to the authorities and treatment for the trainees referred to them. It is doubtful whether the class of child usually seen by child guidance clinics is that from which the delinquent derives. Certain problem families are well enough known to the health visiting service of the local authorities. Preventive action has its psychiatric and psychological elements, but there is a gap in supervision and care which needs to be closed. A good deal of research remains to be done in this field, if one is thinking in terms of a comprehensive service.

Post-graduate Teaching

The fulfilment of preventive psychiatry, development of after-care services and a possible reduction in hospital beds will be achieved only with the full development of post-graduate research and teaching, in which the general practitioner, as well as the medical officer of health, can play his full part. If any doubts exist about the reduction of hospital beds on any other than a very long-term basis, it is simply on account of the determination of what reasonable steps any local health authority may be asked to undertake by way of "nursing home" or hostel provision.

Each catchment area of approximately 250,000 population would require at least two clinical psychologists. This objective is slowly but progressively being achieved in Northern Ireland, training being provided by the University Department of Psychiatry in Belfast, which estimates that each clinical psychologist can deal with 200–250 patients per annum, on the basis of 60% of this work being of diagnostic content, and 40% for treatment purposes.

General Consideration

The problem of defining hospital requirements should be looked at in a versatile way. For instance, it is a wonderful opportunity to plan a new combined general hospital for general ill-health and mental ill-health within any area. At the same time, some areas are already well served by mental health services but not so well served by general beds. Perhaps in some areas the general beds could be erected in the grounds of an existing mental hospital, thus accomplishing the same object. There are examples of both methods in Northern Ireland.

Flexibility in planning, and close co-operation with architects is very important (Baker, Davies and Sivadon, 1959). Many problems remain to be assessed. For example, ought a psychogeriatric assessment unit to be sited with the long-stay wards, or lie contiguous to short-term psychiatric care and assessment units? It is not suggested that these psychogeriatric bed needs, of say 30 beds per population of 200,000 persons, need be an additional load on the calculation. Also, how far should accommodation for "special" cases of subnormality coupled with a second (physical) handicap be sited locally at day centres, or centralized?

It should also be noted how rehabilitation services enter all phases of the planning. These services can be active or passive, vocational or occupational, and can affect all ages, all categories and be exceedingly diversified. Extra-mural and community care services should help to reduce short-term illnesses and re-admission rates, but can have little effect on the need for beds for continuing care and long-term illness.

In the geriatric and psychogeriatric sections, local authorities could play a more vital part if hostels existed, along the lines of American nursing homes, with a small nucleus of nursing staff trained in general and psychiatric nursing, a visiting general practitioner, and a panel of consultants, including geriatrician and psychiatrist, available for domiciliary visits when required. The expense of this must be weighed against the social value to the community, but is worthy of further examination and trial.

The hospital service is geared for certain undertakings and, unless the local authorities are to have appropriate staff and equipment on the one hand, and can do certain tasks less expensively on the other, there would seem to be a natural limit to their effectiveness in this field.

Lastly, although there are child guidance services, there remain the problems of the early detection of delinquency, and the prevention of wrong-doing, in which field a good deal of research remains to be carried out.

All this adds up to the need for the closest liaison between hospitals, local authorities and various centralized government services. Area liaison committees for mental health services would clearly be a useful first step in planning any area development.

References

BAKER, A., DAVIES, R. L. and SIVADON, P. (1959), *Psychiatric Services and Architecture*, W.H.O. Public Health Papers No. 1.

EASTERN SPECIAL CARE MANAGEMENT COMMITTEE (Northern Ireland Hospitals Authority) (1963), Descriptive brochure.

ELDER, A. T. (1964), *A Comprehensive Mental Health Service*, Papers of Royal Society of Health Congress, Torquay.

FARNDALE, W. A. J. (1963), *Day Hospitals*, 13th International Hospital Congress, Paris.

GIBSON, JOHN (1965), *Comprehensive Psychiatry at the General Hospital*, Papers of Royal Society of Health Congress, Eastbourne.

HEATON-WARD, W. A. (1963), Psychopathic disorder, *Lancet*, **i**, 121.

JONES, KATHLEEN (1963a), *The Community and Mental Health*, World Fed. for Mental Health, 16th Annual Meeting, Amsterdam.

JONES, KATHLEEN (1963b), Administrative problems in the Mental Health Service, *Pub. Hlth.* **78**, (1) 11.

KIDD, C. B. and MEENAN, J. C. (1959), Urinary incontinence in longstay mental patients, *Ulster Med. J.*, **28**, 201.

KNOX, S. J. (1963), *An Introduction to the Northern Ireland Mental Health Act 1961*, Northern Ireland Association for Mental Health.

MULLIGAN, J. A. S. (1963), County Armagh Mental Health Services, Personal communication.

MULLIGAN, J. A. S., ROBINSON, C. B. and CASEMENT, E. (1964), *A Survey of Psychiatric Services in Northern Ireland Hospitals*, A Report to the Northern Ireland Hospitals Authority.

NORTHERN IRELAND HOSPITALS AUTHORITY (1962), 15th Annual Report, p. 70.

POLITICAL AND ECONOMIC PLANNING BROADSHEET (1963), *Psychiatric Services in 1975*, **29**, 468.

RED BOOK (1946), *Plan for the Hospital Services of Northern Ireland*, Northern Ireland Regional Hospitals Council.

SNELL, H. K. (1963), The new prison at Grendon Underwood. *Medico-Legal Jnl.* **31** (iv), 175.

TOOTH, E. C. and BROOKE, EILEEN (1961), Trends in the Mental Hospital population and their effect on future planning, *Lancet*. **i**, 710.

WARREN, W. (1963), Mental ill-health in adolescence, *Pub. Hlth.* **77** (2), 82.

WHITELEY, R. W. (1963), Psychiatric problems of a day hospital in Belfast, Personal communication.

SECTION B
THE INTERNATIONAL SCENE

11. A Comparative Study of Facilities for the Retarded in the Soviet Union, United States and United Kingdom

MICHAEL CRAFT

THE child in the U.S.S.R. is the prize possession of the state—the Soviet's great hope for the future. In theory at least, all men are born endowed with equal potentialities in the U.S.S.R., and it is up to the state to provide education and, later, work opportunities, commensurate with the need of each. Recent publications have described how the state provides for the needs of the retarded (Alt and Alt, 1959; Kety, 1962; Field, 1964).

Any comparison of facilities provided by different societies must first start with an appreciation of their underlying philosophies. The English-speaking reader will be well aware of society's attitudes to the retarded in Britain and America, with the steady disappearance of feelings based on stigmata of degeneration, fears of the criminal retarded and emphasis on undue reproduction. Both in the U.K. and the U.S.A., society lays emphasis on merit and intellectual ability, and particularly in Britain, most children are educationally streamed so that those of high intelligence obtain education of high calibre. The marked contribution of genetic inheritance to intelligence is recognized, together with the right of the better provided family to make better than average provision for its children. From the above publications, it seems that the U.S.S.R. disagrees with both these last two Western tenets. The assumption that children are genetically endowed with markedly different intellectual potentialities and the use of tests of intelligence to stream educational groups was decreed against in the famous Central Council resolution of 1936, which argued against the pedagogics (Wortis, 1950). As Sirkina (1948) points out, natural endowment has some influence, but mainly provides the raw material, to be shaped by environmental influences into the final form. As Giliarowski, Solovieva and Vinokurova (1936) enthusiastically put it, in the U.S.S.R. there are boundless possibilities of environmental changes designed to bring out the best in each citizen.

As in Britain and the U.S.A., Soviet psychiatric facilities for children can be divided into three types: out-patient, day and residential, and follow the familiar Western pattern of diagnosis, investigation and treatment. Whilst the quality and availability of medical services varies between outback, prairie and city in the U.S.S.R., much as in the U.S.A., the arrangement of services also differs. In the U.S.A., the private group practice of specialists may be the first diagnostic port of call, whereas in Britain, the state-paid family doctor should be first to see the backward child. In the U.S.S.R., it will probably be the doctor in charge of the local village dispensary. Referral onwards to out-patient facilities might include the neuropsychiatric diagnostic facilities in area dispensaries, similar departments in paediatric or university defectology clinics, or mother and baby units. In cities, there are also mental health and psychological guidance centres.

TABLE 1.

	Soviet Union (1961)	U.S.A. (1961)	England and Wales (1963)
Total population	216,100,000	183,742,000	47,022,700
Non-psychiatric hospital beds	1,637,600	895,892	262,527
Psychiatric beds	207,800	775,108	209,575[a]
Percentage psychiatric beds of all beds	11·2%	46·4%	44·4%
Psychiatric beds per 1000 population, 1961	0·96	4·22	4·45 (1963)
Psychiatric beds per 1000 pop. planned for capital cities	2·0	N.K.	2·4 (1972)
Psychiatric beds per 1000 pop. planned for whole nation	1·3–1·5	N.A.	2·6 (1972)
Doctors per 100,000 pop.	197	141	118·7[b]
Psychiatrists per 100,000 pop.	8·4	6·4	4·8[c]
Public psychiatric beds per individual psychiatrist	27·4	183·9	93·3
Total hospital staff ratio to patients	1 to 1	1 to 4	N.K.

[a] Psychiatric beds in regional hospitals, teaching hospitals and the three special hospitals.
[b] Estimated 55,800 active doctors in England and Wales (31.12.63).
[c] Based on 2274 psychiatrists in N.H.S.

Day facilities include day hospitals in large centres, for the Soviet Union was the first European country to start these (Craft, 1959). In addition, there are night sanatoria, play groups, and day nurseries. These last amounted to 4 million places by 1951 (Wortis, 1950) and include care both for children of working mothers and for handicapped children. The U.S.S.R. is said to be a country in which children are the only privileged class (Kety, 1962) and in which all adults are expected to show care for, interest in, and love for children. The official line is that no effort should be spared to aid parents to keep their young children at home, and the variety of types of day and night care for children is remarked upon by visitors. Physical chastisement appears to be deplored, and recent observers remark upon its absence, even after provocation of adults by children.

Residential placements under the Health Ministries include sanatoria for children with neurosis, psychiatric beds in general hospitals, and hospitals and colonies for groups who are epileptic, or who show disturbed behaviour, such as the Gorky colonies (Makarenko, 1950), and other colonies for long-term neuropsychiatrically handicapped children. These last provided 1,251,000 beds in 1950 (Wortis, 1950), but this particular figure exemplifies the difficulties in comparing information between the U.S.S.R. and other countries, since criteria are so different. Field (1964), after a very careful discussion on statistical comparisons between the U.S.S.R. and the U.S.A., gives the figures in Table 1, with British figures kindly furnished by the Ministry of Health.

As Field (1964) comments, figures do not tell the whole story, for the terms used do not mean the same thing in different countries, even when carefully translated. In the U.S.S.R., statistics are often ambiguous and, as will be shown, almost all retarded children there are regarded as an educational, not a health problem. The difficulties of comparing mental health statistics in different countries have been discussed in detail recently by Rapoport (1960), Alt and Alt (1959), Field (1964) and Wortis (1950).

Diagnosis

It is perhaps easiest to compare international practice by following the history of the regarded in the Soviet Union through the seven ages of man.

Free diagnostic facilities are available for infants in the U.S.S.R. at factory or district clinics; a district serves a population of 4000, and, in theory, is staffed by seven doctors. A neuropsychiatric specialist will serve four districts, or 16,000 people; to him are referred the most damaged children. The clinic has all standard diagnostic equipment available, and the child may stay for from 2 weeks to 6 months. The central figure in this investigation is the neurologist, who is usually neurophysiologically trained and firmly reared along Pavlovian principles. He may be a university teacher, and he will have access to full diagnostic facilities for investigation. An electroencephalogram is an important aspect of these investigations. Due to the strong bias upon organicity in the U.S.S.R., and the scant regard for genetic endowment, diagnostic emphasis is likely to be placed upon slighter evidence of neurological impairment than in the U.K. The idiot* group of children apparently remains the responsibility of the Health Ministry in the U.S.S.R., as in the U.K. and in most North American states.

As far as possible, all Soviet children are given at least a year's trial at school, and this would include most of the imbecile group* which, both in

---

* Since the old terms are internationally used and accurately defined (idiots I.Q. 0—19; imbeciles I.Q. 20–49) they are used here in preference to the new terms of subnormal and severely subnormal, which lack adequate definition.

the U.K. and the U.S.A. would be excluded and placed in training centres or hospitals. Once U.S.S.R. children are in the education system, tremendous efforts are made to provide the child with maximum educational stimulus and help. This imbecile group remains the responsibility of the Education Ministry.

Those children who are obviously not learning as fast as the general group are placed in a special remedial class of 10–15 under a specially trained teacher, speech instructor and psychologist, often aided by brighter pupils, who apparently act partly as leaders and even as pupil teachers, gaining much prestige in doing so. Due to this detailed and individual tuition, it is said that a number of retardates return to the general classes. Others transfer to the district special schools, which are run in urban areas predominantly on a day basis and in rural areas mainly on a boarding basis. This group of children seems to include most of our imbecile group, and a proportion of those we would call educationally subnormal. Statistical comparisons between the U.S.S.R. and U.K. are hard to make, for the complete rejection of the I.Q. tests by the U.S.S.R. and the retention of this group of children firmly under the wings of the Ministry of Education means that they merge almost imperceptibly into the main child population, so that figures are not divided into identifiable streams. In British comprehensive schools, even the non-graded special educational stream is the subject of special ministerial returns, and as such, distinguishable from the rest of the school, but in the U.S.S.R., statistics are simply not available for the number needing special education. The members of the American President's Panel on Retardation toured various districts of the U.S.S.R. over a period of 3 weeks and tried hard to obtain figures (Kety, 1962). Their best approximation was to compare the U.S.A. figure of 5 million retardates (3% of relevant population) with the Soviet view that just under 1% of their child population were retardates. The Soviets took the view that this was a reflection of their ways of life (!) but in their report the Americans suggested it might also be due to differing ways of caring for backward children.

In Britain, public health doctors take the main responsibility for diagnosis and resultant streaming, at least in the subnormal grades, but in the U.S.S.R. this is the function of the "defectologist". This person is a specially qualified teacher, often a graduate of 5 years' tuition in the State Institute of Defectology. He is paid 50% more during his undergraduate years and 25% more in his postgraduate years than colleagues in standard classes. There is further reward for research and for extra projects with retarded children during holidays. A defectologist thus gets paid a similar salary to a physician; it is a high-status post and there is no shortage of applicants. The U.S.S.R. position is very different from the comparatively low pay, duration of training, status and working conditions for those teaching markedly retarded children in Britain.

In the U.S.A., the situation varies from state to state, but since there is a strong tendency to group retarded children into large colonial schools, the salary of teachers is apt to vary with the affluence of the state and the determination of the colony superintendent.

Education

The Soviet defectologist teaches groups of ten to fifteen children, in a day or boarding school of some 200 children. The total staff of all types around the school may amount to half the total children and, as mentioned earlier, every adult is expected to be constructive in his attitude to the children on campus. For a 200-place school of standard size, there is likely to be a staff of twenty teachers and sixty leisure-time and night staff. Discipline is firm, but verbal; the Panel (Kety, 1962) report that the children seemed remarkably happy, and it was rare to see a child smacked. Since most Soviet doctors (75%) were women, it was perhaps easier for them to show affection for children, although medical influence upon campus children was minor, the major influence being that of the defectologist. Admission and discharge of children and their transfer between streams was primarily an educational matter, with important decisions being taken by a team of four, consisting of defectologist, neurophysiologist, psychologist and teacher.

Actual day-time care seems to follow a similar pattern in the U.S.S.R. as here, with a planned sequence of meal followed by quiet formal tuition, then activity by way of games before the next meal; followed by afternoon class, games and meal, then evening television, and a quiet period before sleep. Prior to 1962, children left school at 16, but because of the many failures in shop and factory this was raised to 18, with better results. The last 3 years of school now include a gradually widening range of manual skill tasks, so that the school-leaver will be already prepared for the production line or commune employment that may lie ahead of him. In the U.S.S.R., as in Britain, the main employment lying ahead of retardates consists of labouring, bench work and repetitive factory work.

Diagnosis in the U.S.A. seems to be shared between general hospital clinics staffed by paediatricians, and local group practices. Because provision for the retarded is a state responsibility in the U.S.A., and the fifty states vary greatly in provisions, it is extremely difficult to make meaningful generalizations. The likely differences between Alaska and California are obvious, but the difference in provision between Nebraska and nearby Wyoming is also extreme. Nebraska is very active in research, day and residential provision, due to interested people locally; the needs of the retarded in Wyoming, on the other hand, do not have a high priority.

Connecticut has two old-established state training schools, of which South-bury with its Yale connections is world famous. The provision of beds (or residential school places) reaches over 2 per 1000 state population, and it becomes clear to the visitor that this is achieved by teaching many of the moron group in hospital colonies. In Britain, these would be called educationally subnormal, and in special schools, in the U.S.S.R. these, together with the next duller group, the imbeciles, are also in school. It is fair to say that whilst Connecticut, even by United States standards, makes unduly generous provision for the retarded now, further new units of 100–200 beds are being constructed near the large centres of population to provide training for children nearer their parents. The total number of places, and thus children labelled as retarded, will in the future be yet higher. Compare this situation with a Mid-West state, where state aid, facilities, teachers and doctors are noteworthy mainly by their absence, and it can be seen that generalizations can be quite unreal.

Late Diagnosis

Some of the imbecile and retarded group in the U.S.S.R. do not manage to respond either to intensive individual tuition or to specially graded sets of educational instruction, and on the advice of the team or school doctor are referred once more to the clinic or the dispensary. These are two different entities. The first is the in-patient unit for investigation, often attached to a university or to a department of a larger hospital institute, and staffed by a neurophysiologist with his team of assistants, and other specialists. This dispensary is likely to be an area mental health centre, also staffed by a neurophysiologist but with a more psychiatric bent, whose main job and interest it is to look after the mental health, neurological and psychiatric behaviour problems of the district. There may be a few beds attached to the dispensary for emergency use, but work here is more at an out-patient and supportive level. The dispensary doctor may refer new cases to a clinic for detailed laboratory investigation by the neurophysiologist, and would then send a detailed account of the local situation, with the main events leading up to the referral. In its turn, the university clinic sends a full account of the investigations back, with a commentary, usually containing a pronounced organic view. It is the job of the area dispensary neuropsychiatrist to interpret the findings to the special school, to whom he hands over the child's care, and to visit the child in an advisory capacity, as and when required. During adolescence, when further behaviour problems may arise, the dispensary doctor is in a privileged position to organize field work, social services and even to bring pressure on local factory executives.

Work, At School and After

Soviet parents, like those elsewhere, display a distressing tendency to protect their slower children, and to do for them things they should do themselves. The special school lays much emphasis on self-help. The children are expected to make their own beds, dress themselves, often with help from each other, and to help about the residential school with small tasks. The Soviet defectologists seem to be as keen on the residential school method for older children as the U.K. government is keen on day classes. Soviet teachers point out that teaching needs to be consistent and continuous, and that the day child may advance three steps by day, but slip back one or two at night. At school, picture sequences are used to show the child how he does his job; when he has mastered it, a flap goes down—with a picture of praise showing him what is behind. Self-competition does more to encourage a game than interclass competition, which is discouraged, for Soviet defectologists feel the latter tends to result in advancing the bright and causing apathy in the dull.

After the retardate leaves school, the local factory or commune is expected to help in job placement. Work is a man's right, according to Rubinstein (1946), paraphrasing the relevant article of the Soviet constitution, and this applies to all community misfits, whether it be the imbecile, the physically handicapped, or the ex-convict. All are expected to work in their home district. Suitable jobs at their working ability must be found, comrade workers have a duty to take an interest in, if not supervise them, and some thought is given to a change of job if the first does not appear to suit them.

Chronic Brain Damage and Residential Placement

Chronic brain damage is the main Soviet category used for the entity of subnormality. Few of the defective or subnormal are in an institution in the U.S.S.R. Field (1964) notes that the Soviet Union has only, in proportion to the population, 15% of the number of general psychiatric beds of the U.S.A. although, annually, nine times as many admissions take place as in the U.S.A. As far as Field could decide, and he notes that comparisons of U.S.S.R., U.S.A. and U.K. statistics give rise to many errors, per 100 psychiatric beds, $3 \cdot 4$–$3 \cdot 9$% are occupied by oligophrenic patients in the U.S.S.R. and in the U.S.A. $0 \cdot 84$–$1 \cdot 90$% (dependent on year). There appear to be fewer total retardates in U.S.S.R. general psychiatric hospitals than in either the U.S.A. or the U.K., in proportion to the population. Reasons for this may be:

1. The greater number of Soviet retardates carried and working in the community.

2. With fewer neuropsychiatric colonies in the U.S.S.R., more sub-normals are living and possibly working in the community, so that when they become disturbed, they are more likely to be admitted to a general psychiatric hospital.
3. The great destruction of accommodation in the U.S.S.R. between 1939 and 1945 obliged the U.S.S.R., like Holland, to place emphasis on the partly disabled remaining in the community (Querido, 1956).

Comparisons between the U.S.S.R. and the U.K.

Both countries have welfare state facilities, affording paid leave to working pregnant mothers, free maternity care and confinement (where necessary in hospital), as well as expert attention to mother and child in the neonatal period. In both countries, neonatal mortality and morbidity are low, and children as a group are increasing in height and weight, compared with past generations.

It is at the stage of diagnosis that differences in care start. Britain at present appears to have both fewer doctors and fewer psychiatrists in relation to population than the U.S.S.R. In both countries, the local or family doctor is asked to see the child first. In Britain, he may well refer a severely handicapped child, functioning at idiot level, to the local paediatrician, who has primarily a medical interest. In the U.S.S.R., the child will be referred either to a dispensary or a clinic. At the latter, a neurophysiologist will initiate investigations, usually as leader of a team of experts, consisting of biochemist, speech therapist and psychologist. The interview is to elicit any signs of past cortical or biochemical damage, and utilizing Pavlovian lines of inquiry where feasible, to assess present function and point out future possibilities. The two medical experts will naturally show a bias in their diagnostic formulation, the one to biochemical and possibly abnormal genetic endowments, the other to any possible environmental damage to the brain.

The difference between the U.S.S.R. and the U.K. becomes most marked at the school age of 5 and onwards. It seems that far more imbecile children are both afforded a chance of state schooling in the U.S.S.R., and are per-sisted with, than in the U.K., to judge from the literature and reports of Western visitors. To some extent, inspection by visitors is admissible evidence here, for mongol children are usually imbeciles, and visitors to the U.S.S.R. have remarked how commonly they are seen in the special classes. In the U.S.S.R., most trainable children or imbeciles are an educational responsi-bility, whereas in the United Kingdom most such children are excluded from school and placed in local health authority training centres. In logistical terms, this means that less than 1 % of Soviet children appear to be a health responsibility (day or residential); up to 2% may be in the U.K.; whereas some 3% may be in the U.S.A. (Kety, 1962). This bias in health or educational training is also demonstrated in the liability to institutionalization. In the U.S.A. and U.K., the residential, trainable child is found in hospital, cared for by nurses. In the U.S.S.R., he is usually found in boarding schools, taught by defectological teachers, firmly returned to his family and community each holiday time, and at the termination of his training at 18. Until recently, the lack of community work training provisions for the retarded in the U.K. and U.S.A. influenced up to a third of hospital admissions being adolescent in age-group. In most states in the U.K., as in the U.S.A., where admissions were referred through the court, the hospital had to accept, resulting in gross overcrowding of many provincial hospitals.

Although one or two educational authorities in Britain, such as Birmingham and Monmouthshire, have placed social training classes for imbeciles under Burnham-paid teachers of the Education Department, most British local authorities formally exclude imbeciles from school, and transfer them to a local authority day training centre under the mental health division. Here the child is exposed, in a pleasant, amiable and happy way, to simple manual skills, and music and movement tuition by occupational supervisors. Until recently, most British supervisors have been untrained, and many of them have been housewives. However well meaning they may be, their lack of training is in marked contrast to that received by teachers of the retarded in the U.S.S.R. In the latter country, such children are seen as an educational challenge, due to be exposed (in American terms) to a high-powered diagnostic team, a battery of experts, and total push educational stimuli. It is fair to point out that, despite the use of American terms, such experts are rarely available for the American imbecile, who is unlikely to have the financial resources for the care of experts.

In the U.S.S.R., the child failing to keep up with the normal schooling pattern is, in theory, first assessed by the team of specialists noted earlier, then placed in small remedial classes under well-qualified teachers, and later, if he fails to return to the normal stream, placed in a special (often residential) school, and taught by defectologists. These teachers have a 5-year course, geared to their eventual subjects, and are specially paid. As a result, classes for such children are small and well organized; they have short lessons suited to the expected short attention-span, and a suitable alternation of physical and mental stimulation. Each child's endeavours are compared—often on a visual chart—with its past achievements. No interpersonal competition is expected. All available sensory channels—tactile, visual, auditory and vibratory—are used to stream knowledge and information, and at regular intervals, the child is reviewed by the panel of disciplines, comprising the school's specialists.

In the Soviet Union, the results in adolescence are said to be youngsters who have good relationships with their parents and—more importantly—

their parent community, the latter being required to provide employment for them on departure from school.

In Britain, the leaving age from a junior training centre is optional, but prescribed in law for the educationally subnormal schooling system as 16. In the Soviet Union, the child from both avenues moves on at the age of 15 to the pre-employment, or manual stage, prior to school leaving at 18. In these last 2 or 3 years, he is introduced to the various factory, manual or repetitive skills which he will be expected to demonstrate when he returns to his parent community and local factory.

Work

The difference between post-school practice in the U.S.S.R. and U.K. seems to be the availability of jobs to the mentally handicapped school-leaver. In Britain, whilst there are certain provisions of doubtful use in the Disabled Persons Register and in local authority sheltered workshops, the possibility of suitable jobs will vary with the zeal of the social worker and the prevailing climate of employment. In the U.S.S.R., each man has a right to a job, and if he is somewhat handicapped, then in theory at least, the local commune or factory is expected to find a suitable job for him. In practice, of course, this is interfered with by the application of government norms, the deployment of labour, and various local issues of personality which seem to be as important in the U.S.S.R. as in the U.K. It seems as if in the U.S.S.R., as in other countries, there are pressure groups which to some extent cut across governmental policy.

In the U.S.A., employment prospects for the retarded adult are much more haphazard, and depend on the affluence of the state and its employment level. In the more industrial cities, the liability for automation to throw the retarded out of work is to some extent offset by sheltered workshops run by city authorities, often aided by philanthropy. In Southern and Mid-Western states, there continue to be strong tendencies to institutionalize social problems in large and distant colonies.

In neither the U.S.S.R. nor the U.K. are there eugenic policies which militate against the mentally handicapped in society. In both countries, they can marry and procreate, except that in the U.S.S.R. the unwanted child can be legally aborted at parental request. It is said that this prevents unnecessary suffering to both the unwanted child and rejecting parent.

It seems that current policy in all three countries emphasizes continued community care of mentally handicapped adults, although for obvious reasons this is more difficult to achieve in the more materialistic and less family-centred parts of the U.S.A., than under the social welfare provisions in the U.K. and U.S.S.R. The high proportion of unemployed on the general American scene also adds to the problem of placing the retarded American adult. In the U.S.S.R., even if he is convicted, the retardate is returned to his community and factory, there to live down his past mistakes. Often he is on parole, or under the guardianship of a shop steward. At all events, the need for institutionalization is said to be about a third of that in this country and the U.S.A., and is handled in suitable colonies for the most neurophysiologically damaged person (Field, 1964; Kety, 1962).

Older Age Groups

As in Britain, the U.S.S.R. finds facilities necessary in the later ages of man, for those handicapped persons whose parents die and whose relatives are not prepared to aid. In both countries, these facilities can be residential neuropsychiatric colonies, although in Britain, small welfare homes or mental health hostels are increasingly advocated, whereas in the Soviet Union, the already considerable grant given to parents caring for unstable or handicapped dullards may be substantially increased where relatives or friends come to help. These considerable grants are initiated by the dispensing neuropsychiatrist, and make a difference to the ease of finding alternative lodgings for the handicapped. In the U.S.A., provisions vary tremendously from state to state, at least two having no legal provisions at all. Since Federal aid applies primarily to capital programmes, there is little onus on the state to act. As might be expected, in general the wealthier the state, the more facilities appear to be available.

Summary

Care of the retarded, both in prevention and in treatment, is described as currently practised in the U.S.S.R. Using this description, comparisons are made between the U.S.S.R. and the U.K., with an occasional comment on American practice, and the major differences noted. In the U.S.S.R., diagnosis follows a neurophysiological bent, and retarded children are said to comprise only 1 % of the population. It seems probable that different fractions are covered in each country by the term.

In training, the main differences appear to be in the care of the imbecile group. In the U.K., this group is in the care of local authority mental health departments, under partially trained or untrained staff. In the U.S.S.R., such children are seen as an educational challenge, and receive the undivided attentions of defectologists—a highly trained and plentiful teacher-group. The age of leaving school in Britain is now 16, and in the U.S.S.R. 18, but in the latter, this includes 2–3 years' manual training to factory requirements.

The final difference between the U.S.S.R. and the U.K. is seen in job placement. In the former, the retardate has work as a state right; in the latter, a niche has to be found, often from a benevolent employer, by an overworked social worker. Since in the former country the retardate was seen to have community rights, while in the latter, until quite recently, he was accepted into the community on sufferance, this might be one reason behind the marked difference in rates of institutionalization.

References

ALT, H. and ALT, E. (1959), *Russia's Children*, New York. Quoted by Field (see below).
CRAFT, M. J. (1959), *Amer. J. Psychiat.* **116**, 257.
FIELD, M. G. (1964), *Review of Soviet Medical Sciences*, **1**, 1.
GILIAROWSKI, V. A., SOLOVIEVA, Z. A. and VINOKUROVA, A. I. (1936), *Problems of Psychoneurology of Children and Adolescents*, Moscow and Leningrad.
KETY, S. S. (Chairman) (1962), *Report of the Mission to the U.S.S.R.*, President's Panel on Mental Retardation, Washington, U.S. Department of Health, Education and Welfare.
KIRMAN, B. (1962), Some Impressions of Soviet Psychology. Unpublished.
KLINE, N. S. (1960), *Annals of the New York Academy of Sciences*, **84**, 4.
KRATTER, F. E. (1965), Survey of the Mental Health Services in the U.S.A., with Special Emphasis on Mental Retardation. Unpublished paper, Brockhall Hospital, Lancashire.
LURIA, A. R. (1963), *The Mentally Retarded Child*, Oxford, Pergamon Press.
MAKARENKO, A. (1950), *The Road to Life*, Moscow, Foreign House Publishing Co.
DEPARTMENT OF NATIONAL HEALTH AND WELFARE (1964), Mental retardation in the Soviet Union, *Canada's Mental Health*. Supp. 42, Ottawa.
QUERIDO, A. (1956), In *Elements of a Community Mental Health Programme*, New York, Millbank Memorial Fund.
RAPOPORT, R. N. (1960), In Kline, N. S., *Annals of the New York Academy of Sciences*, **84**.
RUBINSTEIN, S. L. (1946), *Foundations of General Psychology*, Moscow.
SIRKINA, B. E. (1948), How to develop the abilities of children, *Semia i Shkola*, **2**, 22–5.
TIZARD, J. (1958), *Lancet*, **ii**, 1325.
WORTIS, J. (1950), *Soviet Psychiatry*, Baltimore, Williams & Wilkins.

12. Mental Health Services in a Developing Country of South-East Asia (Sarawak)

K. E. Schmidt

THE present account describes our approach to the mental health situation in Sarawak, a developing country of South-East Asia. The measures being undertaken now can at the best be described as highly experimental, but a decision had to be made whether to improve only the institutional care that was already being carried out, helped by the opening of the new Sarawak Mental Hospital in June 1958, or whether the aim should be seen as providing some sort of mental health service for at least the most accessible parts of the country. This, in fact, has been increasingly the aim since 1958.

The Country

Sarawak is a country of the size of England and Scotland, and is the most western of the three previously British territories of northern Borneo. In 1963 it became a State in the Federation of Malaysia. The Indonesian part of Borneo, called Kalimantan, covers the much greater part of this—the third largest island in the world. Sarawak, once the land of the White Rajahs, is thinly populated by approximately three-quarters of a million people, constituting one of the most astonishing multiracial societies imaginable. The rivers are still the main arteries of communication; they all flow from the mountains in the interior of the island towards the China Sea in the north, which offers a marine trunk-communication route.

Initially, the views of several of the ethnic groups in the country on mental illness will be summarized, to give a picture of the soil on which this service was built, as part of the Government Medical Service.

Ethnic Grouping and Examples of Views on Mental Illness

The three main ethnic groups are: firstly, the indigenous peoples or natives of Sarawak, as they proudly call themselves (Iban or Sea-Dayak and others); secondly, the Chinese; and thirdly, the Malay. The Malay, whilst having absorbed a great amount of blood from both indigenous groups (by marriage

213

and conversion to Islam) and from the Chinese (by adoption of Chinese children), remain, as do the Chinese, culturally apart.

The Chinese

There were 229,000 Chinese in Sarawak in 1960, according to the Census of that year. It is not possible at this stage to give an account of Chinese views on mental illness, owing to many difficulties. These are that the Chinese themselves are divided into several fairly closely-knit communities, which have no unifying language, and indeed often little contact. It was impossible to find any single group amongst them which could be identified culturally, and yet be somewhat representative of the Chinese in Sarawak on the whole in its views. Many of the Chinese have adopted the Christian religion; their degree of acculturation with Western ideas is very variable, though considerable, and no unifying concepts could be enucleated as regards their ideas on mental illness. There are eight different groups, e.g. Hokkien, each with their own language. Apart from groups converted to Christianity by the Anglican, Roman Catholic and Methodist missions, often working in close proximity, there are many Buddhists and agnostics. The few who live traditional Chinese lives are old people. The middle generation is uncertain which way to turn, and poorly definable superstitions are rife. This generation has few clear concepts, and little knowledge of Chinese culture, whereas the young generation has none. They are very much like the present generation elsewhere. They study hard to get on, and they like the Beatles and other pop singers. The Chinese are, however, very active in trade, agriculture, industry and politics. In their restless economic strivings, they appear to have little time to think much about Chinese views on mental illness, and accept what Western medicine has to offer. There are Chinese medicine men who treat mental illness. The total number of patients treated by them is but small, and the writer was unable to detect much uniformity of views and methods amongst them. Further, most of the Chinese are first- or second-generation immigrants from the mainland. Those elderly Chinese who were interviewed said that the cause of mental illness was: firstly, imposition by the spirits as punishment for evil thoughts or deeds; secondly, evil charming, usually believed to have been carried out by the Malay; and thirdly, encountering and being molested by a soul from a grave. Traditional cure is usually effected by healers, who fall into a trance and scribble Chinese characters on a piece of paper, which are then in turn interpreted. Prayers and drinking of water are carried out and the patient may be admitted for some time to a Buddhist temple as a boarder. Violent cases, however, have often been chained to temple walls. As with the other ethnic groups, these practices have quickly fallen into disuse with the arrival of Western methods of treatment during the last few years.

The Malay

The following remarks do not represent a study of the views of the Malay on mental illness, but are intended to show some of the problems and difficulties of this subject. The Malays live near the sea coast of Sarawak, mainly in fishing villages, on stilts on the tidal river banks. The 1960 Census assessed them as the third largest ethnic group with 129,000 people. According to T. Harrisson (personal communication) almost all of them are pagan natives of Sarawak converted to Islam. Those interviewed in the course of this investigation traced their ancestry to Sumatra, Java, Malaya and the Sulu Islands of the Philippines. However, all have a way of life which is different from the indigenous people of Sarawak. All embrace Islam, and "Malay" therefore means "Mohammedan" in the present context. They also have a different feeling-tone, and mostly look different and dress differently. It may very well be that they are a cultural rather than an ethnic group. Individual Malays are often accused today by their Chinese or Iban neighbours of spell casting, if cases of mental illness occur. Likewise, a Malay healer (*dukun*) will often be consulted prior to such patients being presented to the government health services or private practitioners.

Those Malays who were asked about the views held by their community on the causes of mental illness quoted the following, in order of frequency:

(a) Too intense religious studies and other preoccupations.
(b) Disobedience to certain Muslim rites, e.g. when on a pilgrimage to Mecca, looking up at the ceiling on entering the Kasbah, which Muslims are forbidden to do.
(c) Economic failure, loss of money.
(d) Loss of love-object, death of a beloved relative.
(e) Pent-up emotions, e.g. frustration, which may lead to running amok.
(f) Charming by spells from others.

The Iban or Sea-Dayak

This group, the strongest of the native peoples of Sarawak, is also numerically the largest of all ethnic groups in the country. According to the 1960 Census, it comprised 237,000 people. These are the true natives of Sarawak— the famous head-hunters of old. They have considerable force of character and are faithful, hospitable friends.

We have investigated their views on mental illness in detail (Schmidt, 1964). They live in longhouses by the riverside, which are erected on stilts, and each family occupies a room. All rooms open to the communal verandah. Their idea of community life is one of a balance between the individual and the group, and between the group and its physical and spiritual environment; this balance is regulated by their laws.

They believe in a deity called *petara* ("almighty god") but there are many minor ones, most of these being spiritual heroes. Their world is also populated by many spirits, some of whom are departed ancestors; these may assume the shape of animals. The balance between the Iban and his environment is also regulated by many taboos.

Their views on the causation of mental illness have a rich variety. The commonest is the violation of a family taboo, such as not to eat cobra meat. Such an act makes the soul of a person vulnerable to a spirit, who may carry it away. Evil spirits in the form of animals may mislead a person into the jungle, and there confuse him and rob him of his mind. Another commonly accepted cause of mental illness is the failure of a person to carry out a request made by a spirit in a dream, such as to hold a feast in his honour. It is also believed that casting of a spell by another man may turn a person insane, as may trespassing under offerings to the spirits, or walking under women's clothing. Frustration in love, laziness, social disgrace and economic failure are other recognized causes, as are contact with a promiscuous woman, anaemia, and retained placenta.

Though there is also a wide variety of clinical conditions, the writer was unable to relate them to the above causes in a one-to-one causal relationship. There are no less than eighteen descriptive terms, and they cover almost the whole range of clinical states contained in any Western textbook of psychiatry—from violent behaviour to withdrawal, from mania to depression and from autistic talk to muteness. At the same time, dementia, feeble-mindedness and delirium are clearly delineated.

The Bidayu or Land-Dayak

This group comprises about 57,000 people. Many of their longhouse communities in the mountains of western Sarawak have been broken up into villages, which are situated in the more fertile valleys. They are a peaceful people, though at one time they were also keen collectors of heads.

They recognize two categories of mental illness; one refers to those kinds of abnormality which show decrease in psychomotor activity, and the other denotes all those which show an increase.

They recognize that insanity may be inherited, or that it may be secondary to physical illness. Other recognized causes are loss of a love-object, infliction by evil spirits, spell casting by evil men, entrance of noxious fumes into the head and insect stings.

Since, as with the Iban, supernatural agencies are believed to have great influence on the day-to-day lives of the Bidayu, those agencies have means by which they communicate with man. Animals, especially certain birds, pigs, dogs and ant-eaters, are thus believed to be favoured as messengers. But also the way a tree will grow, unusual knots in vines and phenomena such as thunder, lightning, rainbow and whirlwind may indicate intentions, feelings or movements of spirits.

The spirits may inflict mental illness if man trespasses on sacred places, or cuts trees which are believed to be the abode of spirits, if he eats food which has been reserved as offering to the deities, or if he breaks taboos, especially those given to celebrants of rites. Mental abnormality is treated by a native healer, as well as physical illness. He has special abilities to communicate with the spirits, and is able to catch the soul of a mentally sick patient, which is thought of as having gone astray.

There are a variety of healing ceremonies which the native healer conducts, such as the imposition of taboos for 7 days, or sprinkling certain prepared waters over the patient, the calling back of a soul which has gone astray, spraying the patient with saliva, or the application of salves. All these ceremonies are aimed at re-integration of the individual into the group. (For further details see Nissom and Schmidt, 1965.)

The Murut

These people form more or less one ethnic group, together with the Kelabit. They are mountain people, living on both sides of the ridges which separate Malaysian Borneo from Kalimantan. They also live in longhouses, and are excellent rice farmers and cattle breeders (Harrisson, 1959). They view the human personality as consisting of body, mind (which includes planning ability) and soul (or spirit). Spirits may be good or bad, and there are many which cannot be traced to stem from departed humans. Spirits may assume animal shape, or enter a living person and govern his actions. As with the other ethnic groups, taboos play a great role in Murut life. The Murut believe in a god called *mangai*, who may assume the shape of a certain bird, and from its flight, omens will be read.

Their principal native healers have the task of driving out the foreign spirit, who has taken possession of the patient. The ceremony he conducts is family centred. There are others who merely dispense medicine. As with the other ethnic groups, supernatural forces are thought of as being the causes of mental abnormality, often in punishment for broken taboos. A few examples will be quoted. The commonest kind is characterized by tormenting hallucinations of beings waiting to kill the patient. It is assumed that water has been drunk from a sacred well, which is the abode of powerful spirits. Tree insanity is due to trespassing under trees which are the abode of spirits. The condition finds its expression mostly in aggressive acts and sleeplessness. (For details, see Schmidt, 1965.)

There are many other ethnic groups in Sarawak and it can be expected that investigation of their "systems of psychiatry" would yield a similarly rich structure, as presented in the above accounts.

Setting up a Mental Health Service

It is against this background of vastly different thinking about mental illness of the various cultures, that our attempt at setting up a mental health service in Sarawak must be viewed (Schmidt, 1963).

The Sarawak Mental Hospital

In a previous communication (Schmidt, 1961), the author reported on the management of schizophrenia in Sarawak Mental Hospital. The present account reports on further developments. This new mental hospital, opened in 1958, is situated 7 miles south of Kuching, the capital. Its capacity is up to 350 beds. There were 330 in-patients in 1958 which have been reduced to 250 at present. Our team tries to care for the mental health of the country with 1 psychiatric bed per 2500 of the population. This relationship stands in contrast to Western countries, where there is usually 1 psychiatric bed for 300 of the population. We were indeed fortunate that the psychiatric revolution of the middle fifties enabled us to overcome this discrepancy. The hospital has been planned in such a way that an extension to 600 or even 1200 beds was possible, and indeed envisaged. However, between the planning of the hospital in 1954 and its realization in 1958, psychiatry has taken on a "new look".

Since 1953, in the world at large, the phenothiazine derivatives have been extensively investigated (Schmidt, 1957). Long courses of deep insulin coma have been largely abandoned, and replaced by E.C.T. and phenothiazines. There was also a more active approach to occupational therapy, with more attention to the individual and his needs *after* discharge. Factories were set up in hospitals and approaches were made to bring the family of the patient more into the therapeutic situation. The British Minister of Health verbalized all these views in his epoch-making address to the National Association for Mental Health (Powell, 1961) when he announced the intended abolition of the large mental hospitals. This particular speech was a great encouragement to our mental health work in Sarawak, and showed that we were on the right track.

The author took up his appointment in November 1958, and regarded it from the start as his personal challenge to prevent an enlargement of the existing mental hospital, and with his team to provide in due course some sort of a country-wide mental health service.

The Psychiatric Situation in Sarawak

The question is often asked, even by people who ought to know better, whether peoples who are less advanced in modern civilization have nervous breakdowns at all. It is not yet possible to answer this question exactly, however. Firstly, the methodology for incidence surveys is only in its beginnings and has not yet progressed much above the stage of "head counting", though better assessments have become possible today with the various available rating scales (Schmidt, 1957). Secondly, the "social tolerance" to mental abnormality varies from culture to culture, a subject commented on by many authors (Brooke, 1959; Soddy, 1961). A pilot survey carried out by the author in 1959 in the interior of the country showed a much lower frequency of psychiatric abnormality than one is used to in Western countries.

On the other hand, some cultures permit pre-psychotic, psychotic and neurotic (especially hysterical) personalities to find a role within their communities. At times, this may be a very harmful one. One has only to mention the strongly paranoid personalities of so many strong-men, political and otherwise. In Sarawak, for instance, there are people with visions who have found their niche as native healers, though by no means all native healers have such a psychopathology. We are inclined to the view that the incidence of psychiatric illness may be lower than elsewhere, and that differences are likely to exist between the various ethnic groups in Sarawak, which cannot be solely explained by accessibility to the psychiatric facilities (see Table 1).

TABLE 1.

Population of Sarawak Mental Hospital on 31.12.1959 grouped ethnically

Ethnic group	No. of people in each group (to the nearest thousand)	No. of patients from each group	Share of each ethnic group per 1000 people from it	Expected no. from each group according to the no. of persons in each group
Iban (or Sea-Dayak)	237,000	42	0·471	89
Chinese	229,000	170	1·707	86
Malay	129,000	36	0·739	49
Others	149,000	32	0·572	56
Total	744,000	280		280

Table 1 represents the ethnic distribution of patients at a certain date (31.12.1959). The differences between true numbers and expected numbers are significant at $P > 0·001$.

The question arises, especially as regards the Chinese, whether their high proportion represents a truly higher incidence in psychiatric illness, in comparison with the Iban or Malay.

Let us consider for a moment the proportions for schizophrenia (see Table 2).

TABLE 2.

Ethnic Grouping of Cases of Schizophrenia in Sarawak Mental Hospital, 1960–1

Ethnic group	Group size	True no. of cases in the hospital	Share of admissions for schizophrenia for 1000 of the group	Expected no. of cases
Native groups	336,000	78	0·448	175
Chinese	229,000	259	2·146	120
Malay-Melano	179,000	51	0·550	93
Total	744,000	388		388

The figures in Tables 1 and 2 were obtained as follows: the schizophrenic cases were extracted from the hospital population on 31 December 1960, and all cases with the above diagnosis who were admitted in 1961 were added to it.

Table 2 makes it clear that the ethnic distribution of the schizophrenic cases is similar to that for all psychiatric cases of Table 1. In other words, whilst over approximately 2 years, out of 4248 natives 1 person was admitted to hospital with the diagnosis of schizophrenia, with the Malay–Melano group, this occurred for 1 out of 1889, and for the Chinese, 1 out of 884. These figures unquestionably demand further investigation, and we are

TABLE 3.

Diagnostic and Ethnic Classification of First Admissions in 1964

Community	Chinese	Malay	Sea-Dayak	Land-Dayak	Others	Total	%
Diagnostic group							
Schizophrenias	81	14	25	7	14	141	43
Affective disorders	28	10	6	6	9	59	18
Organic psychoses	18	16	8	9	2	46	14
Epilepsies	4	2	1	1	1	9	3
Neurological disorders	2	—	—	1	—	3	1
Neuroses	17	2	11	6	10	46	14
Amentias	4	1	2	2	—	9	3
N.A.D.	7	1	3	2	1	14	4
Total	161	46	56	27	37	327	100
First-admission percentage by race	49	14	17	8	12	100	
Racial percentage by population	31	16	32	10	7	100	

probably in a unique position, in that these ethnic groups live closely together, but are at present still clearly delineated from each other. The Malay live in villages near the river estuaries, the Chinese in the larger settlements and ports, and the natives in longhouses further inland.

Table 3 shows that we still mainly deal with psychoses.

Special Conditions

Whilst the distribution of psychiatric conditions in Sarawak within the diagnostic spectrum is different from that of a Western culture, their forms are, on the whole, well encompassed within the usual psychiatric terminology. There are two exceptions to this. Firstly, *latah*. This, in this author's opinion, is a condition of increased suggestibility, usually on the basis of hysteria, but also occurring in organic conditions (encephalitis). It represents a dissociation, during which words or movements are repeated without inhibition, a kind of extreme echolalia and echopraxia.

Secondly, *amok*. This appears to represent a culture-bound behaviour pattern, within a certain group of cultures and within a certain geographical orbit. Aetiologically, the spectrum is so wide that almost all psychiatric conditions in the three main spheres (endogenous, organic, neurotic) may exhibit it, where the above conditions prevail. There is no doubt in the author's opinion that the longhouse community of the indigenous groups either offers a good protection against psychiatric illness, or that the tolerance especially for the psychoses is greater than in a Western society. A further phenomenon must be mentioned as regards the Malay. Whilst the diagnosis of schizophrenia is, of course, made for purposes of classification, in practice it would be more correct to describe most cases as schizo-affective psychosis, since it is rare to get a clear-cut schizophrenic amongst them. The clouding of the diagnosis is due to the hypomanic colouring of most of the endogenous psychoses occurring in Malays.

An Approach to the Problem

It is difficult to profit in this kind of work from the experiences of other workers who find themselves in a similar position as, for instance, Lambo (1964) in Nigeria, even if detailed studies of such experiences were possible; the setting and the problems are different. One major problem appears the same, however; the sparsity of medically qualified staff, so that the experience and co-operation of the senior nursing staff has to be taxed to the fullest. We felt that our particular problem was to provide the country with as comprehensive a mental health service as possible, within our modest staff-establishment and without enlargement of the Hospital.

Perhaps the main factor to date is the co-operation which the psychiatrist (who is also the only medical officer of the mental health section) got from his nursing staff, particularly the senior staff, who responded extremely well to the training, and to the encouragement to use their initiative freely.

Table 4 represents a summary of the case-load of the mental health section over the years.

TABLE 4.

Summary of Mental Health Work carried out

Year	Admissions to S. M. H.	Discharges from S. M. H.	Deaths in S. M. H.	New out-patients (total)	Total attendances at out-patient clinics
1954	112	90	27	—	—
1955	132	75	29	2	12
1956	154	110	24	13	40
1957	174	110	27	8	48
1958	195	120	34	19	88
1959	338	342	15	207	367
1960	429	405	24	209	1743
1961	581	567	21	600	3227
1962	544	542	16	424	3871
1963	577	581	11	455	4316
1964	630	586	17	262	4869

Table 4 shows that over the 6 years of active mental health service in Sarawak, the average number of admissions has been 500 per year. Of these, 53% (270) were new admissions. The average number of new registered out-patients has been 360 per year over the last 6 years. From the above figures, and the 4869 out-patient interviews carried out in 1964, it is quite obvious that the only medical officer could not possibly have carried out this work-load on his own. Though it is possible for the writer to maintain a therapeutic relationship with all the psychiatric patients in the country, now amounting to several thousand, this by necessity is often loose. However, all first admissions and all new out-patients are given an initial detailed diagnostic interview, when the treatment is outlined. The in-patients in three of the wards remain under the author's personal care from day to day, whilst he does a ward-round in each of the other five wards of the hospital once a week, changing from ward to ward daily. He is usually only able to conduct one-quarter of the out-patient interviews himself (i.e. in 1964, 1200 out of 4800), and for obvious reasons, these are the more time-consuming ones.

The rest of the work is done by senior nurses, who have been trained in this work over the years. To what extent this has been possible may be seen from the fact that they even give most of the modified E.C.T. within the hospital, though only if the writer is within earshot. In this way, time is found for dealing with the many other time-consuming duties of a medical super-intendent (especially as in our case, the catchment area is as large as the United Kingdom), with consultations from neighbouring countries, court work, training and supervision of staff, etc. It is thanks to the enthusiasm for work and study of some senior nurses that we are able to give something of a comprehensive mental health service to Sarawak, at least as far as the psychoses are concerned. Furthermore, the junior nursing staff, despite the enormous language difficulties with the eighteen different languages in the country, take an increasingly active part in psychotherapy, by seeking personal contact with the patients.

Once the therapeutic community was developed within the hospital, projection of psychiatric work into the country took place. Table 4 sum-marizes the evidence for this and also shows that more new patients are seen at out-patient clinics than on admission to the mental hospital. On the average over the 6 years, 360 new out-patients were treated, as opposed to 270 new in-patients, though 20% of new admissions to Sarawak Mental Hospital are in fact failures, for various reasons, of out-patient treatment.

It is therefore with some satisfaction that the psychiatric team at Sarawak Mental Hospital looks back on the way they have been able to provide a mental health service for the country with 350 psychiatric beds, of which, in fact, over the last 4 years, only 250 on the average have been occupied. This is with three-quarters of the beds being filled by chronic patients, for most of whom there is little hope of rehabilitation. Obviously, this is a very small number of beds indeed for the population and country of this size. If this policy had not been carried out, chaos would undoubtedly have reigned, and no personal relationship between the patients and the doctor would have been possible, in view of the larger numbers.

It also means that each of the acute-ward beds is used by more than 8 patients per year, which appears good usage (500 admissions annually). This is facilitated by the ease with which admissions can be obtained in-formally under the new Mental Health Ordinance, designed largely by the author.

In Table 3 a classification of diseases and their ethnic distribution is given for 1964. From Table 3 can be seen again the relative sparsity of neuroses treated. The proportions are very similar for out-patients, except that their share of neuroses is 20%.

A further factor which greatly helped us was the change in public attitude in Sarawak towards our unit. In this community, mental illness was something dreaded, brought about by "spirits" and "charms". A change of public attitude has been brought about by continual manipulation of public opinion, through lectures to various study courses and night classes, over the radio, in the press, and to the numerous groups who visit the hospital, such as senior pupils, students of the teachers' training colleges, groups of councillors and of chieftains, in-service training courses of the government service, and voluntary bodies such as women's organizations and boy scouts. In addition, the essentially curative nature of the mental health work in Sarawak is being explained continuously in every interview and informal person-to-person meeting, and, of course, our discharged patients and relatives have helped considerably. It can be seen from Table 5 that success has been forthcoming in winning the public's confidence.

TABLE 5.

Percentage of Non-law-committed Admissions
(i.e. Voluntary, Temporary and Non-statutory Patients)

Year	1958	1959	1960	1961	1962	1963	1964
Percentage	—	17	46	63	83	84	90

The aim is not to cut down further on the percentage of the legally committed cases, though this might be possible, since in some cases of patients from the interior of the country, the Mental Health Inquiry of a magistrate's court often constitutes the nearest to a case-history obtainable when the patient arrives without a relative. This is especially the case at the hill-rice planting and harvest times.

In order to cover at least the more severe forms of mental illness in the country, out-patient work was started in June 1959 with two sessions weekly at Kuching, the capital. Soon, work was proceeding independently in two separate rooms, the medical officer and a senior nurse interviewing patients and relatives, whilst physical forms of treatment were carried out by the rest of the team in another room of the maternity clinic, which was taken over for the purpose. At the mental hospital itself, out-patients are seen at any time if they live along the only major road in the country. This road, on which the hospital is situated, now extends for 120 miles.

With the object of reducing the flow of patients into the hospital further, an out-patient clinic has been held every 2 weeks since 1961 in the capital of the third province. This town, Sibu, is the main port on the country's largest river, and constitutes a good centre. It has relatively easy access by river from the surrounding catchment area, both up and down river. The need for this service can be seen from the fact that in the first 9 months of its establishment, 290 new out-patients were seen and 1006 out-patient interviews were carried out. That means that on the average, on each of these twenty occasions, with 3 half-days each, 15 new (mainly psychotic) patients were seen, and 50 psychiatric interviews were carried out.

Another out-patient clinic has been in operation fortnightly since 1963 in Sarikei, a river port on the way from Kuching to Sibu (per ship).

The question arises whether, in these circumstances, and with the staffing described, it is possible to do effective psychiatric work. One cannot, of course, be dogmatic about this, owing to the difficulties of measuring improvement or its maintenance, outside hospital (Schmidt, 1957). Neither has there been an opportunity to assess to what extent social functioning, especially work capacity, has been restored. Furthermore, the terms "work" and "earning capacity" are but peripheral aspects of a psychosis, however important to the patient's family. In our setting, consisting often of tribal work communities (hill-rice planting, hunting, fishing), these concepts are but poorly understood. There seems to be no doubt that a longhouse community finds a niche more readily for a member who is handicapped by a psychosis, if fairly well arrested, than in the case of a cash-economy community, where the employer–employee relationship is well defined. The impression is that our results on the whole do not differ materially from those of other units—that is, that the great majority of our patients return to their former employment, even if sometimes in a lower capacity.

An attempt is always made to bring the patient's family into the therapeutic situation, since most patients are being investigated and treated at the out-patient clinics. "Training of the family" is undertaken, both in "occupational therapy" and "psychotherapy". Table 6 gives an indication of the number of admissions which were prevented by out-patient management.

TABLE 6.

Year	No. of new out-patients	Subsequently admitted
1960	290	29 (10%)
1961	600	95 (15%)
1962	424	76 (18%)
1963	455	86 (19%)
1964	262	52 (20%)

These admissions became necessary not only for psychiatric reasons, but also for geographical ones, when the out-patient facilities are too far removed from the patient's domicile, especially in the interior of the country.

The saving in bed facilities is obvious from the above figures, even if it is not quite as extensive as might be assumed, since a proportion of the patients registered as new out-patients at the clinics are in fact follow-up cases, *after* direct admission to the hospital. However, a good proportion of the discharged patients is not followed up at the psychiatric out-patient clinics, but at the peripheral government dispensaries, static and travelling.

The hospital assistants who staff them, and to whom we refer the patients for follow-up, have all been trained in patient management, during training courses held over the last 2 years at Sarawak Mental Hospital.

In fact, a greater load is being put on the relatives if cases are treated as out-patients. This is unavoidable with the facilities at our disposal at present. The patient's relatives, are, however, assured during the initial discussion that should satisfactory improvement not occur quickly, or the condition deteriorate, admission is at their disposal.

As elsewhere, the considerations for out-patient therapy are:

1. Is it best for the patient?
2. Is it safe for the patient?
3. Is it safe for the community?
4. Is it fair to the family?

The chronicity rate has been assessed thus: of the patients admitted in the first 6 months of the year, 12% on the average were still in the hospital at the end of the year. At the end of the next year, their number had shrunk to 4%. This was so despite the relatively large number of cases of neurosyphilis in its late stages.

In Sarawak, it is only possible to undertake out-patient treatment if the patient either lives in or near the centres where psychiatric out-patient clinics are held, and if it takes no more than a day (by boat usually) to reach the clinic concerned, or if he has relatives there who are interested enough. The danger is that patients get lost to further treatment—that is, fail to attend because of rapid initial improvement. Without psychiatric social workers, it is very difficult indeed to keep a check on every case, and much reliance has to be placed on the patient's relatives. Also, Sarawak is by no means a fully literate society, as yet.

On the whole, families quickly get used to the idea of mental nursing, and in many cases do it very well. Since they are emotionally involved in the situation, it is relatively easy to teach them the importance of personal rapport with the patient, and of preventing or reversing the process of autistic withdrawal.

Treatment

The basic aim of therapy is to return the patient as a well-functioning personality into his social environment. As a practical approach, chemical and physical agents are employed to change the patient's mental state, so that he becomes accessible to psychotherapy and social therapy. At the same time, his social environment is manipulated to ease this process. As in all psychiatric units, the phenothiazine derivates, thymoleptic drugs and barbiturates are the main chemical agents, whilst the various forms of E.C.T. (including sub-convulsive applications) constitute the physical agents, in addition to modified insulin and abreactive agents.

This is coupled with trying continuously to impress upon the nursing staff "the conviction that the drug treatment of psychiatric illness can only ever be a palliative and symptomatic remedy for abnormality which grows, in every instance, out of a disturbed capacity for personal relationships and for direct or sublimated instructional qualifications" (Maddison, 1959). This goes together with the other conviction that a great part of the "real psychiatric revolution of our times has been not in the chemical or surgical spheres, but in a re-evaluation of the dignity and the capacities of psychiatric patients" (*ibid*).

As would be expected, the wards have been unlocked at Sarawak Mental Hospital since 1960, except for some security measures in one ward, which accommodates criminal patients. In our setting, psychotherapeutic functions have often to be carried out by nurses, or rather be carried on by them after initiation of the process by the psychiatrist. We think of it as neglect of the patient if the receptive void, created by the above therapies, is not filled with goal-directed activity and normal personal relationships, as soon as they become possible with improvement. This especially is the nurses' task.

In the case of out-patients, family members and employers are then encouraged to take over this function, even if not formally trained. Occupational therapy, play therapy, sport and social club are made use of widely. The Patients' Social Club has been successfully running now for almost 7 years. An out-patient club was also tried, but given up after 3 months' running; owing to the wide spectrum of diagnosis and culture among the patients who were able to attend, it was found that there were such difficulties that the therapeutic benefits seemed small in comparison. With the promised help of a temporary psychiatric social worker from Canada, another attempt is to be made at a fully functioning out-patient club.

These methods of treatment are therefore influenced by the following considerations:

1. To establish the best mental health service possible with our modest team, i.e. one full-time medical officer and 100 other staff, approximately half of them nurses of various grades. Of these, only two are fully qualified mental nurses—one of them a European. There is no clinical psychologist, no psychiatric social worker, no qualified occupational therapist, no matron and (most frustrating) no shorthand-typist.

2. To make the best use of the existing building of the new Sarawak Mental Hospital. However, this is co-ordinated with the policy of out-patient treatment and home visits by nurses and doctors, which has become possible with the advent of new drugs.

3. To provide as comprehensive a service as possible, i.e. to treat and supervise permanently all the severer forms of mental abnormality in

the country, in order to relieve the burden of the community. It is unavoidable in this poorly developed country that a gradient exists: the degree of abnormality which is brought for treatment increases with the distance from the urban centres. For example, a patient has to be much more mentally abnormal to obtain psychiatric treatment if he lives on the Kelabit Plateau, which before the arrival of army helicopters was remote by 2 or 3 weeks' travel, depending on the season.

It can be seen from Table 4 that a shift had occurred by 1961 to a situation when the major part of the psychiatric work-load was no longer carried out at the mental hospital, but in the out-patient clinics. In 1961, the number of admissions had increased to 581, but there were 600 new out-patients.

Problems of Communication

THE UNIQUENESS OF THE SETTING

Some idea has already been given, in the second section, of the complexity of the situation in Sarawak, both in respect of geographical problems and, more important, of interpersonal communication.

Communication between human beings and between groups of people, including nations, is a never-ending problem. In psychiatric illness, it is the development of the disease or its process which further interferes with normal relationships. In mental health work in Sarawak, the problem is again accentuated by language barriers (Harrisson, 1959). This applies not only to the expatriate worker in the field, but to Sarawakians also. The newcomer to such a unique setting is much impressed by it, although Sarawakians accept it as normal (Schmidt, 1961).

In addition to the eight different languages spoken by the Chinese communities, and to Malay, as spoken by that community, there are at least three different languages spoken by the various Land-Dyak groups (some would say that these are five). Then, there are the linguistically fairly uniform Sea-Dyak, the Murut-Kelabit, and in addition, at least the following ethnic groups, each with its own language: Melanau, Kayan, Kenyak, Punan and Kedayan, in addition to such small groups as Bisaya, Skapan, Kejaman. Also, there are non-natives such as Indians, Ceylonese, Sikhs, Javanese and Europeans.

The many languages constituting this Babelism have developed independently of each other, on each of the rivers or even tributaries, and thereby help to aggravate the problem of mental health care. The educated amongst the above eight groups of Chinese have, of course, the advantage that their script is a common means of communication, so that it is a not uncommon sight to see Chinese conversing with each other on scraps of paper in coffee shops, in the street or in the clinic room. As another example, a Land-Dyak, who is admitted from one river area may well find himself completely and utterly isolated from his fellow Land-Dyak patients or staff members reared in another river area, simply because the newcomer speaks an entirely different tongue. For this reason, the author considers that the transfer of a patient with contact disability from his own ethnic group to the wards of Sarawak Mental Hospital, containing a condensation of most ethnic groups and languages, is not desirable.

It is only to be expected that not all the languages spoken in Sarawak have representatives of their respective groups amongst the staff of the hospital, even though every endeavour is made to rectify this. In the whole length and breadth of the land, there is not one professional individual who masters even the greater part of the languages with a vocabulary sufficiently large to be of use in a psychiatric investigation. Many people speak some Malay, at least in the larger centres, but it is by no means uncommon, even in Kuching, to enter a house of a Chinese and find nobody who speaks either Malay or English. Whilst this is of course a difficult situation in any setting (Abercrombie, 1960), it is easy to see how its effect must deeply interfere both with diagnosis and treatment, in a field where interference with interpersonal communication is one, if not the most important, feature of the disease process.

Patients are therefore distributed within the hospital according to their language, as much as possible. The same applies to the nursing staff. Even so, this is not enough. It is therefore felt that only "failures" of out-patient treatment should be admitted to the hospital, apart from the numerous cases who for geographical reasons cannot be treated at home. In-patients must forgo the advantage which out-patients have, where members of the patient's family can take over the role of nurses and therapist to a large extent, in the patient's own language.

One also has to keep in mind that in most psychiatric illness there occurs some (often temporary) restriction of the field of effective intelligence. Most people in Sarawak speak at least one more language than their own, often several. But in a psychiatric disease process, it is precisely these "secondary-grafted" languages which first appear to be lost. It is astonishing to observe how a patient after psychiatric treatment may sometimes reveal knowledge of a language which he was not previously known to possess (see also Levy, 1943).

DIAGNOSIS

In the initial interview with the informant, every attempt is, of course, made to obtain as many facts as possible, and the admitting nurses have been trained to obtain this information if the medical officer is not available at the time of admission. There may also be some information forthcoming from the mental health inquiry, which will accompany the patient if he has been committed by law to enter hospital.

Patients about whom there is no information at hand often have to be interviewed at the Hospital, or at consultation in other hospitals. It often happens that there is nobody available who is able to speak the patient's language. Great importance is therefore laid, both in the training of nurses and in the day-to-day work, on detailed *behaviour* reports in writing by the nurses. Diagnosis has then often to be based largely on the following:

(a) Psychomotor activity.
(b) Appropriateness of such activity to the situation.
(c) Absence of or delay in any response.
(d) Gap between the affect displayed by the patient at interview and that appropriate to the situation.
(e) Facial expression.
(f) Bodily attitude.
(g) Amount of autistic mannerisms.
(h) State of nutrition and amount of dehydration if any.
(i) Dress and self-care.

Attitudes such as listening to voices or suspiciousness are carefully noted. Most of these factors have dimensions, to which scales can be applied, though some of them are overlapping (Schmidt, 1957).

All this, of course, is not new. However, the emphasis is of necessity changed. In any "normal" setting, these objective observational factors will more often have a confirming significance in diagnosis. In our setting, their significance is heightened and they are a diagnostic mainstay. Our diagnosis, therefore, often has to be based on examination alone, which in conventional practice leads to diagnosis in only a minority of cases. It is usually made from the patient's history and in a few from special investigations.

Features are taken into account such as Varaguth's fold, skin temperature of extremities, traces of oedema and trophic ulcers as evidence of long-standing immobility. The taking of the pulse rate and estimation of its volume provide an important avenue of rapport with the patient. The standard special investigations for patients entering Sarawak Mental Hospital are: Hb./ESR./WR. and K.T./Microfilaria and Malaria Test. M.S.S.U./F.E. Stools (Worms, amoebae)/Heaf-test and M.M.R.

Toilet habits are closely observed, even if they have to be matched against those normal to the community from which the patient stems. The native groups living in longhouses excrete under the floors from above (Schmidt, 1964) and pigs are kept there, acting as scavengers. Whilst the Chinese farmer makes direct use of excreta for fertilizing purposes, and the Malays excrete into rivers, most communities are being Westernized more and more. It hardly needs emphasizing how puzzled the majority of patients are by toilet facilities inside a hospital.

For the above reasons, the nurses' thrice-daily reports of patients' behaviour are of much greater importance in Sarawak than in a European setting. In principle, therefore, unless either the patient's mental or physical distress calls for quick action, the diagnostic interview is delayed for one to several days, in order to have a "package" of nurses' written reports on hand. These factors retain their importance, even in the many cases where direct communication between medical officer and patient is possible in the Malay medium without an interpreter. The Malay vocabulary of the population at large is so limited, as virtually to exclude detailed investigation by these means. For example, the Malay word for "fever" may mean almost any form of being unwell, and includes a wide range of psychopathological phenomena from hypomanic behaviour via catatonic excited stages to regressive actions, and, on the other hand, any form of withdrawal. Another example is that for "abdominal pain", which not only includes the whole gamut of physical symptoms of the abdominal and neighbouring cavities and structures, but also (and very often) psychotic or neurotic epigastric tension or epileptic phenomena. It must be remembered that detailed inquiries into mental states, both in phenomenological and dynamic psychiatry, have a comparatively recent history, dating back to about the turn of the century, and the same applies to the coining of many of the concepts with which we work.

In addition, it is notoriously difficult to obtain an exact sequence of events, since precise time scales are either absent or, as in the case of the Chinese calendar, differ widely from Western standards. As an example, an eminent native leader had no more accurate record of his age than that he was still a bachelor on the occasion that the spring flood reached the 7-foot mark on the wall of the fort in one of the district centres.

SPECIAL FEATURES OF TREATMENT

To start with, we always attempt to get into verbal contact with the patient. Whether or not verbal contact is successful, the patient is invited to sit down. It may, however, be necessary to coax the patient to come into the room, and in a great majority of cases, this is successful. Even so, there are cases where there is no choice but to conduct the interview in a place of the patient's choosing, which may be in the ward, near the fence of a garden, or in the entrance hall, apart from home visits, consultations in other hospitals or clinic attendances.

Fellow-patients are often called in to interpret at interviews—less often for diagnostic than for therapeutic reasons. Often, a staff member from another ward of either sex may have to be detailed to make contact with a patient from his ethnic group.

Nurses vary widely in their usefulness as interpreters; some lack vocabulary. More important, others are unable to achieve good rapport with the patients, through lack of ability or inclination. Therefore, it is not necessarily true that a poor interpreter is better than none at all. Sometimes, the interpreter has had to be sent out from the interview, because his attitude, unsympathetic manner of speech, or impatience has interfered with a relaxed and therapeutic situation. This is a point which has to be stressed time and time again during the training of nurses.

Once the patient and therapist have met, it appears that a handshake and some simple questions are often able to establish rapport, if offered in the right manner, by putting the patient at ease. The impact of even a few words spoken in the patient's own language, coming from a "foreigner", is usually considerably weightier than if it comes from a member of the patient's own community.

The questions need not be particularly meaningful, as long as they are put in the patient's language. A simple sentence such as "How are you?" can easily be learned, even in many languages, but the physical contact of the handshake appears often more important than spoken words. Physical contacts precede verbal ones in a person's life-history and functional hierarchy, and are therefore more likely to remain effective in states of pathological regression.

If, as is not uncommon with psychotic patients, the outstretched hand of the therapist is not met by that of the patient, it is necessary to get up from the chair, go round the table, and try again. If still unsuccessful, a hand placed gently on the patient's shoulder, or even stroking the hair, may help to break the ice. Obviously, this is never done without at least one staff member present. Often there are two—the presenting nurse and the interpreting one.

It is remarkable how little, on the whole, patients resent the presence of other persons at the interview. This fact is one example of the many differences between a Western and an Asian society. The requirements for privacy in the latter are much more easily met, and the differing European preferences are often thought of as peculiar by Sarawakians. The Asian, in the writer's view, is a much more sociable being than the average European.

A further approach is the regularly extended invitation to the patient to take a cup of coffee during the interview. This offer hardly requires verbal communication, or rather, the effect of the offer does not depend on the language in which it is made. These three simple therapeutic measures, the greeting and the invitation to sit down, the handshake or touch, and the offered cup of coffee, often create an initial rapport, which goes a long way to ease the patient out of the isolation imposed by his sickness.

Since human beings tend to push learned habits down the continuum from the conscious towards the unconscious, leaving the conscious free to deal with new phenomena and emergencies, it is important in the case of psychotic patients to engage the conscious self, and feed it with reality stimuli. They are made to compete as much as possible with the pathological ones, to prevent the establishment of pathological habits of thought and action. This point is a central one in the teaching of mental nursing to the staff of the hospital.

The writer explains the relationship between physical forms of treatment and psychotherapy to his nurses as follows. The patient in the grip of a psychosis is like a person thrown into the sea, who does not know how to swim and has sunk under the water. Physical methods of treatment will give him buoyancy, and his head will appear above water, so that he can be seen and reached. But it is for us, the doctors and nurses, to go out to him and pull him back to firm ground—back to the world we share. This is where psychotherapy and mental nursing come in, to ease the patient out of the isolation imposed by the sickness. The interview situation often provokes anxiety in the subject by its very unfamiliarity. This anxiety interferes with the therapeutic impact of the meeting. The therapist must therefore restructure the situation, by acting in ways with which the patient is familiar.

The psychotic patient may still not be able to differentiate clearly between a doctor, nurses and other professional workers, because there are none in his own community. He will, however, come out with—"You are the one who shook hands with me", or "You are the person who offered me coffee", even if there was no response, or only a negative one at the initial interview. The therapist, in other words, emerges increasingly from his non-existence for the patient. It is at this stage that reactive and social problems can be discussed, and adjusted as far as possible.

Early participation of patients in walks outside the hospital is insisted upon. Visitors are encouraged to take their sick relatives for outings, as are the members of the staff club on their excursions. There are many official, or unofficial visitors or bodies of visitors to the hospital, such as schools, women's associations, in-service training courses, delegations from district councils and so on. As they go round the hospital, they are made to enter the therapeutic situation in some way. So far, it has always been possible to find points of contact between the visitors and at least some patients. Either visitors come from the same area as the patients, who may otherwise have little contact with home, or they speak languages which enable verbal contact with patient, where otherwise there would be little.

In a similar way, every opportunity is given to members of the patient's family or to his friends to stay in the hospital as boarders, for as long as hospitalization is necessary. Thus, there is a familiar person present, who speaks the patient's language, and thereby aids treatment. This helps in rehabilitation, and assists in the follow-up medication and management, which can be explained to the relative. Occupational therapy, centred on local agriculture and handicraft (both for male and female patient), is of greater significance in this multiracial setting than in other therapeutic communities, since it does not depend on verbal communication. The social club has now been functioning weekly for almost 7 years, and works mainly on a non-verbal basis. There are two principal kinds of activities: firstly, native dances of the various ethnic groups, especially Malay and Iban (Sea-Dayak); secondly, nursery games, such as "musical chairs", the "donkey's tail", and various other contests and team games. The local drum, called *gendang*, has limitless uses in both. A token meal, in the form of orange juice and bananas, is taken in between. Nobody who has visited the hospital while the club is meeting has so far refused to take part. Visitors have either made contributions to the activities, or at least provided the stimulus of a new face. The visitor may be a chieftain from up-country, a bishop, or the Chief Justice.

While the described diagnostic and therapeutic procedures are by no means new, the necessary emphasis on non-verbal or para-verbal communication with the patient is an unusual feature. The extent to which it is practised at the Sarawak Mental Hospital is probably unique. There can be few communities in existence today with so many divergent complexities, especially as regards languages.

To make oneself felt as the main therapist, it is necessary to be continually with the patients in the wards. In the clinic room, the therapist should always have patients around him. Whoever enters the clinic room with administrative or other problems for the therapist stimulates the patients around him, thereby entering into the therapeutic situation. He, of course, shakes hands with the patient, after introduction. Often, patients are asked their views on whatever problem is discussed.

The author is fairly confident that a good proportion of our patients—40% as a rough estimate—receive at some stage treatment from folk medicine men of the communities to which they belong, or even from others, before we see them. The reason is that the native healer is often nearer at hand. This is undoubtedly changing, with the better penetration of all parts of the country by the government medical services, and with the increased capacity of such services to deal with mental illness.

It must be mentioned that there are no waiting lists, either for out-patient appointments or for admission of psychiatric patients, since all problems are dealt with at the time at which they arise, independent of duty hours. Any patient, with or without his relatives, can walk into our clinics or into the hospital and obtain examination and treatment, without appointment or referral. This, of course, is only in keeping with the tradition of the Brooke Rajahs and their officers—accessibility at all times and places.

Another question is whether the time which admitted patients spend in the hospital can be further reduced. It will be remembered that since each acute patient's bed is used by more than 8 patients a year, an average stay of something over 1 month is the rule. The author does not think that further shortening of stay can be achieved. One factor that rules against this is that co-operation has to be sought with other units as regards some of the special investigations, such as M.M.R. and its review by the chest clinic physician. The patients are transported to this clinic, which is situated in the capital, 7 miles away, by hospital transport. The same happens with consultations, dental care, spectacles or hearing aids, and it often takes a month to get through this ancillary programme. Furthermore, ships to take patients home may not be immediately available. This factor often delays discharge by weeks.

There are many shortcomings of this mental health service, such as in-sufficient care for the mentally subnormal, insufficient training of nurses, the absence as yet of a work hostel, and the staff shortage indicated earlier. Only limited use is made of the day and night hospital facilities provided, due to the distance of the hospital, not only from large parts of the country which constitutes the catchment area, but also from the capital itself. Also, the native healers have not yet been integrated on a large scale into the service, and there exists no Sarawak Mental Health Association as yet.

The main problem, however, "overwhelmed with a vast catchment area and a grotesque paucity of medical staff" (Smith, 1963), was to provide some sort of comprehensive mental health service on a country-wide basis. Step by step, we believe that this aim has been achieved, and the service described above is today considered by many as leading in South-East Asia. This has found its expression not only in the many interested visitors we get from overseas, and in the award of a Colombo-Plan Scholarship to a fellow-psychiatrist to study our methods of mental health management, but also in the interest from many parts of the world in research conducted in our unit.

The main plans for 1965 are the building of Early Psychiatric Treatment Centres in two provincial capitals, which are to allow for much wider use as day hospitals than is possible at the parent mental hospital. In March 1964, a psychiatric staff hospital assistant (an Iban male nurse) from Sarawak Mental Hospital was posted to the more distant of these two towns (Miri), to pioneer the more active mental health work, which will become possible with the building of one of these units (20 beds) there. Other plans for the immediate future are mainly directed towards more and better training of staff as nurse-therapists. Considerable experimenting takes place with group therapy, and a pattern is emerging from this which can be made fruitful, even if the discussion has continually to be switched from one language to several others.

Very recently, the experiences in the setting up of a mental health service in Sarawak have been made available to the neighbouring Malaysian State of

Sabah (previously British North Borneo) in a special communication (Schmidt, 1965). It must also be mentioned that the measures outlined in this account, whilst having been carried out in considerable geographical isolation, have been fashioned at least in part by association with such organizations as the World Federation for Mental Health and the Mental Health Section of the W.H.O.

Acknowledgements

My thanks are due to the Director of Medical Services, Sarawak, Dr. R. Dickie, for permission to publish this account, to M. Dickson, Esq., C.M.G., M.A. for editorial help, to Mrs. V. Porter for the considerable help in typing this account, to my staff at Sarawak Mental Hospital for their readiness to help and for their initiative, without which the task could not even have been attempted, and also to our patients and the people of Sarawak, who so readily co-operated and were prepared to shoulder the greater responsibilities of a non-custodial psychiatric service, and to experiment with us.

References

ABERCROMBIE, M. L. Y. (1960), *The Anatomy of Judgement*, London, Hutchinson.
BROOKE, E. M. (1959), *J. Ment. Sci.* **105**, 441.
HARRISSON, T. (ed.) (1959), *The Peoples of Sarawak*, Kuching, The Sarawak Museum.
LAMBO, T. A. (1964), In *Magic, Faith and Healing* (ed. Kiev, A.), Glencoe, Ill., Free Press.
LEVY, E. (1943), *Psychiatry*, **4**, 59.
MADDISON, D. C. (1959), Blueprint for a Model Psychiatric Hospital of the Future. Reprinted (1963) in *Trends in the Mental Health Services* (eds. Freeman, H. and Farndale, J.), Oxford, Pergamon Press.
NISSOM, M. P. and SCHMIDT, K. E. (1965), To appear in *Review of Transcultural Psychiatric Studies*, Montreal, McGill University Press.
POWELL, J. E. (1961), Annual Conference Report, London, National Association for Mental Health.
SCHMIDT, K. E. (1957), *J. Ment. Sci.* **103**, 430.
SCHMIDT, K. E. (1961), *J. Ment. Sci.* **107**, 446.
SCHMIDT, K. E. (1963), *Der Nervenarzt*, **34**, 9.
SCHMIDT, K. E. (1964), In *Magic, Faith and Healing* (ed. Kiev, A.), Glencoe, Ill., Free Press.
SCHMIDT, K E. (1965), *Int. J. Soc. Psychiat*. To be published.
SCHMIDT, K. E. (1965), *Psychiatry*.
SCHMIDT, K. E. (1965), *A Short Outline of a Mental Health Service for Sabah*. Available from the Director of Medical Services, Jesselton, Sabah.
SMITH, S. (1963), In *Trends in the Mental Health Service* (eds. Freeman, H. and Farndale, J.), Oxford, Pergamon Press.
SODDY, K. (1961), *Identity, Mental Health and Value Systems*, London, Tavistock.

13. The Family Doctor in a Programme of Comprehensive Psychiatric Care

COLIN M. SMITH

and

D. G. MCKERRACHER

Introduction

In the present paper a brief outline is given of a university-based Canadian programme of community psychiatric care. Its fundamental precepts are that all types of psychiatric patients should be treated locally; that the family doctor should play a major part in treatment; and that required hospital care should be provided by the general hospital. Following a description of the underlying philosophy, a more detailed account is given of an experiment in rural Saskatchewan, designed to increase the general practitioner's ability to recognize and treat a wide variety of psychiatric disorders.

It has been said that community psychiatry is more often denoted than defined. Its tenets are certainly more likely to be defended at the present time on the grounds of intrinsic reasonableness than of empirical verification. The testing of specific hypotheses arising out of these general theories forms an important part of present-day research. In Canada, there has been widespread assent to five principles of psychiatric care which were formulated in a report published by the Canadian Mental Health Association (Tyhurst *et al.*, 1963). These were as follows:

1. *Medical Integration.* Psychiatric services should be closely integrated with the physical and personnel resources of the rest of medicine.
2. *Regionalization.* Psychiatric treatment services should be established in centres of population on a regional basis, and a wide range of psychiatric services should be provided in the larger communities.
3. *Decentralization.* The management and administration of psychiatric facilities should be carried out locally.
4. *Continuity of Care.* The patient should not be passed around from one person to another, but as far as possible should be cared for by a small number of people who work closely together.
5. *Co-ordination.* Local psychiatric services in hospitals, clinics and other centres should be co-ordinated to promote maximum effectiveness.

In the University Hospital, Saskatoon, these principles have served as the guidelines for a series of studies. In particular, it has been felt that the general practitioner should play a key role in the treatment of all types of psychiatric patients before, during and after hospitalization. Where hospital treatment is required, the general hospital should be used and should continue to accept responsibility even for chronic patients. Naturally, it should provide adequate facilities for long-term patients. There is no good reason why the general hospital should be equated in the medical mind with a row of beds.

Background to the Present Project

Saskatoon is a university city with a population which rose from 62,500 in 1955 to 115,000 in 1965. The University Hospital was opened in 1955 and is the only facility providing in-patient psychiatric treatment in the city. The psychiatric ward is on the fifth floor of the hospital and is completely open. Since the nearest mental hospital is 100 miles away, most acutely disturbed patients come, at least initially, to the psychiatric ward. Despite this, recourse has never been made to barred windows, locked doors or mechanical restraint. All kinds of mentally ill patients are treated, although a proportion have to be transferred to the mental hospital (the 39 beds available are not sufficient to service both the city and the surrounding areas).

In 1961 an experimental project was designed, in which 6 beds were reserved for Saskatoon patients who had been committed on two medical certificates (Coburn, 1964; Smith and McKerracher, 1964; Smith, McKerracher and McIntyre, 1963), and who would normally have been sent to the mental hospital. The patients were completely unselected, for as soon as a bed was available, the next committed patient from Saskatoon was admitted to it and treated on the psychiatric ward. This programme was very successful in terms of patient management, but it was soon found that many of the patients needed a great deal of continuing support after they left hospital.

The need for a Home Care Programme (Smith, 1965; Smith and McKerracher, 1963) was now apparent and this was the next development. As a result, it was arranged to send nurses, social workers and psychiatrists into the community, as well as to provide home-maker services, drugs and certain other facilities, in order to help the general practitioner. This programme was more difficult to operate in Canada than would be the case in Britain, because in North America, general practitioners admit to hospitals and spend a considerable amount of time there. They are, therefore, less available to make home visits than their British counterparts. In addition to providing better after-care, an attempt was made to develop more adequate measures of change in patients, so that comparisons could ultimately be made between different groups of patients followed up in the community (Levey and Smith 1965; Smith and Levey, 1966).

As well as encouraging a movement of psychiatric personnel into the community, a reverse trend was established when two general practitioners were given admitting privileges to the psychiatric ward. These practitioners could admit and treat their own patients without being subject to direction and control, although, of course, consultation and advice were freely offered when requested. The experiment was highly successful and over a 3-year period, one of the practitioners admitted 64 patients, consisting of 37 psychotics, 23 neurotics, 2 alcoholics, and 2 character disorders. The large number of psychotics was due in part to referrals from other family doctors. The 37 psychotics consisted of 12 patients with organic brain syndromes (mostly senility or arteriosclerosis), 14 with affective disorders, and 11 with schizophrenia (McCorkell and McKerracher, 1962). The patients liked being treated by their own family doctor, and it was decided to extend the project by setting aside 4 beds which could be used by *any* general practitioner in the city who wished to admit and treat patients with psychiatric illnesses. The initial impressions are very encouraging, but because the project has only been operating for a short time, definitive conclusions are not yet warranted.

Another programme was commenced involving general practitioners, and this forms the main part of the present paper. It consisted of an attempt to have family doctors who were working in a remote country hospital treat all, or very nearly all, of their psychiatric patients, with the help of limited psychiatric consultations from Saskatoon. This was a good deal more ambitious than the previous undertaking, because the hospital, which is run entirely by the general practitioners, is 120 miles from Saskatoon, so that on-the-spot consultations and advice are less readily available.

The Rural Project

In a small town in Saskatchewan (600 population) there is a 25-bed hospital, attended solely by three family doctors. The nearest source of specialist help is about 60 miles away. The family doctors serve about 5000 persons, although it is difficult to be as precise about patient populations as in Britain, for the Canadian general practitioner does not have a list of registered patients. Two of the doctors had some previous psychiatric experience, from working for a short time in a mental hospital; all were actively interested in psychiatry. It was felt that they represented a well-informed type of family doctor, which it is hoped is likely to become increasingly common in the future. The three doctors were interested in attempting to treat all their own emotionally disturbed patients, helped by some psychiatric guidance. It was agreed that such help should be given, provided that research could be carried out on the undertaking. It was also agreed that throughout the project, a psychiatrist would travel down every second week and consult with the general practitioners on the more difficult cases. In addition, telephone advice was to be provided at any time and the University Hospital in Saskatoon agreed to admit cases which the general practitioners felt could not be handled in their hospital. During the visits by the consultants, seminars are held on different aspects of psychiatry. Members of the rural hospital staff have also come to Saskatoon for further experience. During the 7-month pilot phase, discussions were held with the general practitioners, in order to develop reasonable ways of collecting and analysing the data on the project.

Since the beginning of the research study, following completion of the pilot phase, all patients have registered when they came to the out-patient clinic or to the hospital. The registration form includes information on diagnosis, disposal and treatment, together with basic statistical data on age, marital status, date of birth, occupation, education and income. At each subsequent visit, diagnosis, disposal and treatment are recorded. This information is collected in order to give a good picture of the practice as a whole. In addition, careful records are kept of all psychiatric consultations and notes are recorded of all telephone calls relating to such patients. A special discharge form is used for admissions to the local hospital and includes information on emotional disturbance while in the hospital. The data is coded and punched on I.B.M. cards. The reliability of the psychiatric diagnosis is continually checked by having independent assessments made by the visiting psychiatrists, who see both in-patients and out-patients. Preliminary results show that a high degree of agreement has been obtained between general practitioners and psychiatrists.

Results

During the 7 months of the pilot phase, a considerable decrease was noted in the level of anxiety of the participants. Fewer telephone consultations were requested and good agreement was reached on the use of diagnostic labels. It was decided to retain the international statistical classification nomenclature, firstly, because the participants were familiar with it; secondly, because it is in widespread use across the country; and thirdly, because a set of written definitions was available for easy reference. Where a psychiatric condition co-existed with a physical one, both diagnoses were recorded.

A number of other papers have listed psychiatric diagnoses in general practice. In most cases, the general practitioners' diagnosis is used, or else the diagnosis is made by a psychiatrist who examined the records. The present study is distinctive because of the close degree of collaboration between the psychiatrists (who saw many of the patients) and the family doctor, both during the training period of the pilot phase and afterwards. Table 1 shows the diagnostic groupings for all 1394 patients seen during a

TABLE 1.

Diagnostic Groupings in all Patients seen by Three General Practitioners over a 12-week Period

Disease group and international statistical no.	Male	Female	Total	% of all patients seen
Infective and parasitic (001–138)	146	120	266	19·1
Neoplasm (140–239)	5	5	10	·7
Allergic, endocrine, metabolic and nutritional (240–289)	32	44	76	5·5
Diseases of blood (290–299)	7	21	28	2·0
Diseases of nervous system (330–398)	11	14	25	1·8
Circulatory diseases (400–468)	52	57	109	7·8
Respiratory diseases (470–527)	126	137	263	18·9
Digestive diseases (530–587)	52	50	102	7·3
Genito-urinary diseases (590–637)	29	73	102	7·3
Complications of pregnancy and puerperium (649–689)	0	57	57	4·1
Diseases of skin and cellular tissue (690–716)	34	36	70	5·0
Diseases of bones and organs of movement (720–749)	79	83	162	11·6
Congenital malformations (750–759)	0	0	0	0
Certain diseases of early infancy (760–776)	3	0	3	·2
Symptoms senility, etc. (780–795)	1	1	2	·1
Accidents, poisoning and violence (800–999)	81	46	127	9·1
Other and unspecified physical	49	39	88	6·3
All psychiatric categories	54	135	189	13·6
Total numbers of patients	645	749	1394	100

12-week period after the pilot phase had been completed. Psychiatric diagnoses (section 5 of the International Statistical Classification) are made in 13·6% of the patients seen. Considerable numbers of children are included in the patient population and when the analysis is confined to patients aged 15 or over, as in Kessel's (1965) study, the percentage of patients with a psychiatric diagnosis rises to 21. While this figure is considerably higher than the 8% of attenders found by Kessel, it can more legitimately be compared with his figure for conspicuous psychiatric morbidity (14% of attenders), since many of his cases with both psychiatric and physical symptoms were excluded from section 5 of the I.S.C. The sex ratio is very similar to Kessel's. More detailed analyses of the registration and follow-up data will be carried out at the end of the study and the present information is intended to give the reader a general overview of the practice.

Table 2 shows the major psychiatric groupings of the 189 patients with psychiatric diagnoses in Table 1. While neuroses account for the bulk of these patients (80%), there is a not inconsiderable residuum of other disorders. The notion that the general practitioner rarely sees a psychotic is mistaken, at least in this setting. If present-day policies of community care continue, the acquaintanceship will become greater in the future.

TABLE 2.

Psychiatric Diagnoses of Patients seen by Three General Practitioners over a 12-week Period

Diagnosis and international statistical no.	Male	Female	Total	% of all patients seen
Anxiety reaction (310)	24	70	94	6·7
Hysterical reaction (311)	0	6	6	·4
Obsessive compulsive reaction (313)	0	4	4	·3
Neurotic depression (314)	8	8	16	1·2
Somatization reaction (315–317)	1	12	13	·9
Other neurosis (312, 318)	6	12	18	1·3
Alcoholism (322, 307)	3	0	3	·2
Schizophrenia (300)	0	2	2	·1
Paranoid state (303)	0	1	1	·1
Manic depressive (301)	1	1	2	·1
Involutional melancholia (302)	1	8	9	·7
Senile, presenile and arteriosclerotic psychosis (304–306)	1	3	4	·3
Other organic psychoses (308)	1	0	1	·1
Disorders of character and behaviour (320, 321, 323, 324, 326)	2	2	4	·3
Mental deficiency (325)	1	5	6	·4
Other and unspecified psychiatric	5	1	6	·4
Totals	54	135	189	13·6

During the 12-week period, 37 of the patients with psychiatric diagnoses were admitted to the local hospital. They constituted 11% of all hospital admissions. The hospital group consisted of 12 neurotic depressions, 14 other neuroses, 1 toxic psychosis, 5 psychotic depressions, 1 schizophrenia, 1 drug addiction, 1 alcoholism and 2 senile psychoses. No patients were transferred to Saskatoon or to the mental hospital.

At the time of the present report, this experiment has been running for 16 months and final conclusions would be premature. So far, patients appear to have found it satisfactory, while the professional participants—psychiatrists, general practitioners and nurses—have benefited subjectively, at least. The family doctors have carried out a number of psychiatric treatments, both on their own and under supervision. These include brief psychotherapy, counselling, the use of psychoactive drugs, working with relatives, attempts to modify the environment and increased use of social agencies. The use of E.C.T., following consultation with a psychiatrist, is now planned.

Does all this mean the family doctor should replace the psychiatrist? Obviously not. It is reasonable to suppose, however, that the practitioner's increased psychiatric skills should be beneficial in a number of ways. Firstly, there should be an enhanced sensitivity to the emotional problems of patients in general, which certainly range in numbers far beyond the 14% labelled "psychiatric". Secondly, the many patients with psychiatric diagnoses who are *not* referred to a psychiatrist stand to gain. Thirdly, those psychotic patients who require to be maintained on drugs, but who frequently do not take them (Wing *et al.*, 1964), are more likely to do so if their family doctor actively participates in their treatment at all stages and is knowledgeable concerning it. Fourthly, the physician is better equipped to recognize emotional problems earlier, to refer more appropriately and to have a firmer grasp of his own knowledge and limitations as well as those of his patients. Finally, the practitioner is likely to feel more comfortable in handling these patients— a not unimportant matter, from both his viewpoint and that of the patients.

Clearly, none of these five propositions, however plausible, has been firmly established at this time, and an important purpose of the present project is to lay the groundwork for a series of ventures in which specific hypotheses in this area can be adequately tested.

Conclusion

There is no doubt from this and other studies that the general practitioner sees a very large number of emotionally disturbed patients. The literature on psychiatric illness seen by general practitioners is now very extensive and has already been reviewed by such investigators as Kessell and Shepherd (1960, 1962). Notable contributions have been made by some general practitioners like Watts (1952, 1964) and Primrose (1962). Nunnally (1961) carried out a survey of opinions and attitudes entertained by general practitioners towards mental illness in the U.S.A. He found that while their attitudes were "bad", as indicated by his scales, they would often treat many kinds of mental problems by themselves, even when psychiatric care was available. Smith, Badgley and McKerracher (1966) carried out a survey of opinions held by family doctors in Saskatchewan. It was encouraging to find that three-quarters of the group of doctors wanted a pattern of referral in which both the psychiatrist and the general practitioner played an active role in the treatment of emotionally disturbed patients.

Although there is general agreement that the general practitioner sees many such patients, particularly those with neurosis, there is less unanimity about what he should do with them. Kessel (1965) suggests that the large numbers of these patients preclude the general practitioner from devoting considerable time to each and every one of them. The same considerations, however, apply to the psychiatrist and it is important to determine how existing resources can be used most effectively and economically. This can only be done by studies in which shareable, reliable and multiple measures of change are applied to well-defined populations, under various treatment régimes. These studies have simply not been done at the present time and it is all too easy to attack or defend a variety of mutually contradictory propositions about neurosis by reference to impressionistic studies on ill-defined populations, which are scientifically worthless. Accurate recognition, careful descriptions and adequate follow-ups, using valid and appropriate criteria, are the cornerstones on which evaluations of different approaches can be made.

Studies such as the present one form an essential preliminary to comparisons of similar groups of patients treated under different conditions. Many family doctors feel anxious when they attempt to treat patients with emotional disorders. By helping the general physician to carry his psychiatric responsibilities more effectively and more comfortably, the basis is laid for collaborative studies between general practitioner and psychiatrist, in a group of patients for whom there seems to be no completely satisfactory treatment at the present time.

Summary

A brief outline is given of the University of Saskatchewan psychiatric service. Emphasis is laid on *local* treatment of all types of mental disorder, and *active participation by the general practitioner* is strongly encouraged. Following a description of the background and philosophy of the programme, an account is given of a rural Saskatchewan project, in which three general practitioners, advised by psychiatrists, are attempting to provide both in-patient and out-patient psychiatric treatment for all their emotionally disturbed patients—including those who would normally be referred to a psychiatrist for out-patient therapy or for in-patient treatment. An analysis is presented of the 1394 patients seen by the family doctors during a 12-week period, and it is shown that approximately 14% of them were diagnosed as having a psychiatric illness. Initial results of this project are encouraging and should lay the basis for future collaborative studies between psychiatrist and general practitioners.

Acknowledgement

Our thanks are due to the many persons who worked on this project; to Dr. Dallas W. Smythe who helped plan it; and in particular to Drs. G. W. Mainprize, L. W. Christ and E. K. Christ, who are chiefly responsible for its success.

References

COBURN, F. E. (1964), Psychiatry, the family doctor and public health, *Canad. J. Public Health*, **54**, 63–6.

KESSEL, N. (1960), Psychiatric morbidity in a London general practice, *Brit. J. Prevent. Soc. Med.* **14**, 16–22.

KESSEL, N. (1965), The neurotic in general practice, *Practitioner*, **194**, 636–41.

KESSEL, N. and SHEPHERD, M. (1962), Neurosis in hospital and general practice, *J. Ment. Sc.*, **108**, 159–66.

LEVEY, A. B. and SMITH, C. M. (1965), Follow-up and the measurement of change in psychiatric patients, *Acta. Psych. Scandinavia*, **41**, 236.

McCORKELL, W. J. and McKERRACHER, D. G. (1962), The family doctor and the psychiatric ward, *Mental Hospitals*, **11**, 300–2.

NUNNALLY, J. C. (1961), *Popular Conceptions of Mental Health*, New York, Holt, Rinehardt & Winston.

PRIMROSE, E. J. R. (1962), *Psychological Illness: A Community Study*, Springfield, Thomas.

SHEPHERD, M., COOPER, A. B., BROWN, A. C. and KALTON, G. W. (1964), Minor mental illness in London: some aspects of a general practice survey, *Brit. Med. J.* **ii**, 1359–63.

SMITH, C. M. (1965), Experiment in psychiatric home care, *Canada's Mental Health*, **13**, 8–13 (May–June).

SMITH, C. M. and LEVEY, A. B. (1966), The follow-up study in psychiatry, *Diseases of Nervous System*, **27**, 595.

SMITH, C. M. and McKERRACHER, D. G. (1963), Geriatric aspects of a psychiatric home care programme, *J. Amer. Geriatric Soc.* **11**, 399–346.

SMITH, C. M. and McKERRACHER, D. G. (1964), The comprehensive psychiatric unit in the general hospital, *Amer. J. Psychiat.* **121**, 52–7.

SMITH, C. M., BADGLEY, R. F. and McKERRACHER, D. G. (1966), Study of Mental Illness: II The General Practitioner. In *Trends in Psychiatric Care*, Royal Commission on Health Services, Ottawa.

SMITH, C. M., McKERRACHER, D. G. and McINTYRE, S. (1963), Care of the certified psychiatric patient in the general hospital: the Saskatoon project, *Canad. Med. Ass. J.* **88**, 360–4.

TYHURST, J. S. *et al.* (1963), *More for the Mind*, Canad. Mental Health Assoc., Toronto.

WATTS, C. A. H. and WATTS, B. M. (1952), *Psychiatry in General Practice*, London, Churchill.

WATTS, C. A. H., CAWTE, E. C. and KUENSSBERG, E. V. (1964), Survey of mental illness in general practice, *Brit. Med. J.* **ii**, 1351–9.

WING, J. K., MONCK, E., BROWN, G. W. and CARSTAIRS, G. M. (1964), Morbidity in the community of schizophrenic patients discharged from London hospitals in 1959, *Brit. J. Psychiat.* **110**, 10–21.

14. Development of a Day Hospital in Australia

W. J. HAMILTON

Introduction

In their preface to the first edition of *Trends in the Mental Health Services*, the editors noted that it was "a little paradoxical that three of our papers on the subject of day hospitals should be from overseas, since these facilities have so far been much more highly developed in Britain than in the U.S.A. or Canada". The present edition repeats the paradox. One out of two papers on day hospitals is from Australia.

In spite of the enthusiasm with which the Day Hospital movement has been espoused in many countries and the wealth of experience which must be accumulating, the indications for day hospital care are by no means clearly defined. Nor is there any unanimity of opinion that the day hospital venue has something to offer which cannot be provided by a well-designed and adequately staffed in-patient and out-patient service. Absence of many other papers in this volume may simply indicate that further evaluation is in progress, or it may imply a degree of disenchantment with the whole idea.

The goodwill shown by the Brisbane Hospital planners and administrators, together with the psychiatric consultant staff, in setting aside a whole floor of a new building for day hospital use makes it encumbent upon us to attempt to show usefulness and specific purpose. I doubt whether we can do both.

Useful the day hospital is; numbers are increasing, but there are still vacant places in spite of a considerable waiting list for in-patient beds.

While we have some clear indications and contra-indications for day hospital care in our particular setting, we agree with Moll (1963), Jones *et al.* (1963), and Peck (1963), that indications must be related to the overall psychiatric services at a particular time. Specific purpose must be a flexible concept. We believe we can show certain gains in patient management, but whether these would have been accomplished by the same enthusiasm and staff co-operation in another setting remains unknown.

History

In Brisbane, Australia, a city of some three-quarters of a million people, the public psychiatric services for adults prior to 1964 were centred around two large teaching hospitals, an out-patient department run by the State

Government Department of Psychiatric Services in the city proper, and a large mental hospital some 20 miles distant. One teaching hospital provided out-patient facilities only and the other out-patient, in-patient and (since 1958) a day hospital service.

The latter is the Royal Brisbane Hospital, the largest hospital in this city, containing approximately 1500 beds in its various departments. It is accommodated in a number of multistoried buildings on a single site, 2 miles from the centre of the city. It provides a large proportion of the clinical material for teaching in the Faculty of Medicine of the University of Queensland.

Prior to 1964, the Psychiatric Department was housed in two separate buildings, a single-storied one with refactory wards and a four-storied one with 66 beds for short-stay patients. The latter is Lowson House. In 1958, facilities for the care of day patients were first offered. These day patients were accommodated in and used the same facilities and ancillary services as the in-patients. An office was set aside for the visiting psychiatrist, who attended for five sessions per week. The part-time services of ancillary workers and two resident medical officers were available, and one assistant nurse spent all her time with the day patients.

I reviewed the first 6 months of its functioning, together with the relevant literature, in the *Medical Journal of Australia* in 1960, and commented that a case could be made out for the continuance of the day hospital experiment, both from a psychiatric and administrative point of view.

Premises

It had been realized that the psychiatric facilities of the hospital were quite inadequate to meet the demands upon it. The expansion planned was to include the provision of four redesigned wards in Lowson House, the building of a new three-storied block adjacent to it, and the provision of an intermediate-stay psychiatric hospital, some 3 miles away from the parent hospital. The ground floor of the new block was to accommodate the out-patient department, records and offices for the ancillary workers and secretarial staff. The second floor was to house the occupational therapy department and dining room, and the third floor to be occupied by the day hospital. These new additions were completed in June 1964.

During the planning stage, the literature on day hospital construction was reviewed and it was found that remodelling of old buildings, rather than the construction of new, had been general. At that time (1961), no description of a new construction could be found.

As it was proposed to use the facilities of the older building for physical treatments and those of the occupational therapy department, as well as the dining room on the first floor, the day hospital floor-plan was kept as open as possible. There are three consulting rooms, an office for the sister, a group therapy room and toilet facilities. The remaining large activities space is divided in two by folding doors. A further temporary subdivision of either of the resulting spaces is obtained by the use of hinged movable screens, approximately 6 feet high. While this floor is primarily set aside as a day hospital, space is available as a recreation area for in-patients in the evenings and at weekends. It is also used by professional groups of varying sizes for clinical meetings.

The Staff

The full-time day hospital staff comprises one psychiatric registrar, one nursing sister and one occupational therapist. The part-time services are available of a clinical psychologist, a social worker and the resident medical officers who carry out the physical treatments. The consultant psychiatrist attends for three sessions per week.

The average staffing of sixteen psychiatric day hospitals in the United Kingdom (Farndale, 1961) was as follows:

Registrar sessions per week per thirty places: 7
Nurses per thirty places: 2·1
Consultant sessions per week per thirty places: 4·9

Based on floor area and probable future needs, it is estimated that this day hospital will provide for fifty places. While we consider our registrar and consultant sessions adequate for the presently used thirty places, the deficit of nursing staff is apparent. This problem is shared by the other psychiatric services in this country.

The resonsibility for in-patient (120 beds) and out-patient services is divided amongst four units; one of these is the professional unit of the Department of Psychological Medicine of the University of Queensland. Each comprises a senior and junior consultant psychiatrist, two assistant psychiatrists, a psychiatric registrar and a resident medical officer.

The day-to-day management of day hospital patients has always been in the hands of the psychiatrist in charge of the day hospital, but prior to the move to the new building, consideration was given to whether each consultant psychiatrist should not refer and manage his own day patients. This idea was rejected for three main reasons:

1. Because of the lack of unanimity of opinion amongst the consultant psychiatrists as to the role of day hospital care.
2. Because of the number of consultants involved, it was a practical impossibility to provide a day-to-day opportunity to examine the living situation in the day hospital group. Without this, there was little possibility of any clear understanding of what was happening in the behavioural field, in both patient and staff worlds.

3. If the day hospital did not have control over its own admissions, it would never be possible by trial and error to reach some understanding of its limitations, or of the cases likely to benefit.

It is doubtful whether this arrangement is the best possible for the patients. As they come referred from the in-patient and out-patient departments, an inevitable change in psychiatrist occurs.

The alternative system is adopted by the Psychiatric Department of St. Vincent's, a large teaching hospital in Sydney, Australia. The in-patients and day patients share the same facilities during the day. At 5.00 p.m., the in-patients return to their wards and the day patients go home. This integration of all patients leads to the possibility of developing a therapeutic community atmosphere throughout the hospital (Woodforde, 1965).

At the Brisbane Hospital, it is very doubtful that this system would be practicable. The in-patient department also functions as a receiving house, and a programme suitable for acute admissions would not be of universal applicability.

The Patients

This day hospital must function as an integral part of the psychiatric services of the general hospital. If it is to preserve an acute treatment function and also to serve its administrative function of reducing the waiting list for in-patient beds, the criteria for selection of patients must be inclusive rather than exclusive. In addition, it should provide treatment for those patients for whom the contact frequency in the Out-patient Department is insufficient.

In common with Pitt and Markowe (1963), we have found that descriptive psychiatric diagnosis is not as important in patient selection as other factors. These are:

1. The degree of disturbance.
2. The real problem of the patient's transport to and from hospital.
3. The degree of supervision and support at home by family members in the evening.

Patients are referred to the day hospital from the out-patient and in-patient departments. They also are referred from the other teaching hospital and from certain psychiatrists in private practice. After work-up by the psychiatric registrar, which would include the factors mentioned above and may include a day or two's observation in the day hospital, a decision as to suitability or otherwise is made at the staff New Patient Conference.

Because there is less pressure to discharge patients from the day hospital, it can be seen that those conditions presenting to a general hospital which require prolonged care are likely to finish up in a day hospital; for example, patients with chronic neurotic conditions or personality disorders. The depressive illness which can be expected to respond promptly to physical methods of treatment, provided the suicidal risk is acceptable, is an admirable candidate for the day hospital.

The day hospital as part of an acute psychiatric treatment service is clearly not going to concern itself with the rehabilitation of chronic schizophrenics, deteriorating epileptics, nor with the industrial rehabilitation of patients recovered from other psychiatric disorders. On the other hand, many subacute and chronic schizophrenics are cared for in the community by well-motivated relatives. These relatives often present as acute psychiatric casualties themselves, their anxiety and depression being a reaction to the psychotic member of the family. We take the view that to admit the chronic schizophrenic to the day hospital for 2 or 3 weeks, to give some relief to the relatives and to provide some measure of resocialization, is a valid method of management of the relatives' acute reactive state.

In my earlier paper (Hamilton, 1960), I commented that it was our experience that the proportion of schizophrenics must be low and their degree of disturbance minimal. Further experience has shown that this is not the case, and, provided there is adequate communication between the various staff members, quite major degrees of disturbance can be managed. The out-patient who refuses but needs in-patient care can sometimes be motivated towards its acceptance by attendance at the day hospital.

There is little doubt that selection is biased by the interests and orientation of the psychiatrist in charge. I have always envisaged this day hospital as a therapeutic community, in which some help can be offered to patients with long-standing neurotic and personality disorders, who present so frequently both in the psychiatric and other departments of a general teaching hospital. Initially, we were unable to give a clearer idea to the referring psychiatrists of the patients whom we considered most suitable other than to specify as above, and to point out the value of the therapeutic community in the treatment of neuroses and personality disorders.

One hundred and fifteen patients were admitted to the day hospital in the last 14 months. There were 84 females and 31 males; the youngest was aged 15 years and oldest 79. The age distribution was as follows: 15–20 years: 14; 20–30 years: 27; 30–40 years: 27; 40–50 years: 26; 50–60 years: 14; older than 60: 7.

Diagnoses were as follows: schizophrenic disorders: 21 (acute 12, subacute 3, residual state 6); affective disorders: 22; neurotic depressive reaction: 30; personality disorders: 22 (immature, dependent, inadequate 14, aggressive 4, schizoid 1, with drug addiction 3); mixed neuroses: 8; obsessional phobic states: 9; juvenile behaviour disorders: 2; epilepsy: 1.

Compared with the distribution of diagnosis in 1959 (Hamilton, 1960), the proportion of schizophrenic disorders has increased, the proportion of depressive illnesses of all types has remained the same and the personality disorders, which now constitute one-fifth of the case-load, appear for the first time. This change is in accord with the predicted needs of the psychiatric department as a whole, and of the particular functions hypothesized for a therapeutic community existing in a day hospital setting.

Of these 115 patients, 14 stayed for less than 1 week. The severity of disturbance was underestimated in 6 cases and they were transferred to in-patient care; 8 lapsed because of poor selection. As we have become more adept at assessing motivation for help, and pay more attention to social circumstances in the home, this early lapsing has ceased. These 14 cases are excluded, leaving a sample of 101 cases.

Of these 101 cases, 27 are still attending day hospital, leaving 74 who have been treated. Of these, 25 were discharged in 1 month and 53 in less than 3 months. Of the 21 who attended for more than 3 months, 10 were discharged before 6 months, and 13 before 7 months. Five patients stayed for 12 months or longer (2 for 12 months, 1 for 14 months and 2 for 13 months). Thus, although the numbers are small, our patients are divisable into three groups; short-stay (less than 1 month), intermediate (about 3 months), and long-stay (12 months). The relatively simple anxiety and endogenous depressive ill-nesses are highly represented in the first group, while the schizophrenic disorders and abnormalities of personality stay longer. The average stay was $14 \cdot 5$ weeks and median $6 \cdot 5$ weeks.

Of the treated sample of 74 cases, results were recorded as: recovered or much improved in 21; improved in 25; ISQ in 20; and worse in 8. Those patients who were worse were transferred to the appropriate in-patient unit. Of the remainder, 52 were discharged to the out-patient department or their general practitioner for follow-up, and 14 lapsed.

Treatment

Therapeutic communities, whatever the ideology, share common aims. They see their function not only as caring for the sick, but as providing the opportunity for the sick to care for themselves and each other, believing this to be an important part of getting well. They try to avoid the authoritarian staff–patient relationship of the general hospital. They try to include in the framework, as realistically as the hospital permits, those interpersonal social activities, responsibilities, and hence anxieties, which the patient has found intolerable in the outside community from which he has retreated. This apparently simple idea means a profound change in the aims and organiza-tion of psychiatric hospital practice. The emphasis shifts from medication and symptomatic relief to understanding acquired through personal relation-ships (Heron, 1962).

A degree of "permissiveness" characterizes the relationship between patients and staff. "Permissiveness" does not mean lack of discipline, but rather it describes those attitudes and actions of the staff which enable the patient to determine the extent and limits of his own behaviour. It is to be considered as a useful technical device, not as an attitude classifiable as good or bad. It is of fundamental importance, and has been discussed in its general relationship to psychotherapy by Finesinger and Sheppard (1959).

It could be argued that the day hospital venue has no particular merit for the establishment of a therapeutic community, and that there is no reason why this atmosphere should not pervade the whole of the Psychiatric Department. If its usefulness can be demonstrated, it probably will.

There is no need for the therapeutic community idea to be oversold. In some hospitals, the observer is confronted with the harrowing spectacle of chronic psychotic patients valiantly trying to manage their own affairs in the teeth of angry non-intervention by the psychiatrists. Nor should the efforts of social theorists, repeating the errors of Faris and Durham (1939), be confused with the therapeutic atmosphere that we wish to establish. In the modern psychiatric hospital, many persons will be involved in the treatment programme of each particular patient. Each has something specific to offer from his or her particular field, but all have one thing in common, namely that they must meet with the patient in the discharge of their various duties. Apart from the specialized transactions at these meetings, the meetings themselves can be therapeutic or anti-therapeutic, depending on the attitude of the person involved.

It is important that an attitude to be used by all persons to a particular patient be clearly defined and adhered to. In this way, the patient is in the same emotional environment at all times, and the environment is specially selected to provide him or her with the greatest opportunity of getting well. We have found the system developed at the Menninger Clinic, with its five general attitudes of active friendliness, extra attention, passive friendliness, matter of factness, and firmness, together with special attitudes when making requests of a patient and when handling requests from patients, suitable to our own needs. But concepts of psychiatry provide a totally inadequate framework to describe the theoretical basis of a therapeutic community.

A full range of psychiatric treatments, both somatic and psychotherapeutic are available. Rather more attention is paid to the understanding of interpersonal relationships in naturally occurring groups than to the formation of artificial, closed, psychotherapeutic groups. Many of our patients are unreliable with regard to prescribed medication. To some extent, this problem is alleviated by the use of retard preparations of both phenothiazines and barbiturates, dispensed by the sister-in-charge once or twice a day.

Conferences

The presence of disturbed patients in a therapeutic community means periodic deviations from the general hospital's code of behaviour. The psychiatric staff's fear of disapproval can be considerable and instantly communicates itself to patients, with adverse effects. Psychiatric nursing staff are particularly vulnerable, as they may find themselves torn between a wish to please matron and her organization, of which they are a part, and the therapeutic community with its often contradictory aims. The handling by the psychiatrist of these staff anxieties is an essential part of the therapeutic programme.

For the first 12 months of its functioning in the new setting, the whole day hospital staff met with me each morning, 5 days a week, for 20 or 30 minutes, to discuss any difficulties that were arising with patients. As the communication and group cohesion between staff members has improved, the frequency of contact is quite satisfactory now at three times per week. Once a week, the whole staff and as many day hospital patients as can be persuaded to attend, meet for a "grumble group". This is followed by a staff meeting, which endeavours to understand the various interactions which have occurred.

The community has gone through the usual phases of authoritarianism and *laissez-faire* and is now reasonably democratic. The occupational therapist meets with the patients each morning for a discussion group, at which they are encouraged to plan at least some part of their day. All the usual facilities of an occupational therapy department are available. Where appropriate, use is also made of community recreational, educational and cultural facilities.

We are sensitive to the role diffusion between staff members mentioned by Cooper (1965). We tend to resist this, as it makes a mockery of an individual's professional skills. While the argument has force in an in-patient therapeutic community, its theoretical basis is perhaps too diffuse for acceptance in a general teaching hospital. Where role diffusion is of value is in the staff group meetings. An opinion on a social topic put forward by the occupational therapist would be received and discussed with as much care as the psychiatrist's tentative pronouncements about social factors in illness. The group atmosphere at the staff meetings ensures a free expression of opinion, both positive and negative, on any topic. When a problem is put up for discussion and the members try to associate to a theme of the patient and his problems, the atmosphere is informative, perceptive, challenging and at times, chaotic. Of course, we are beset by transference and countertransference contamination, but in the supportive atmosphere these are ventilated, and enrich rather than confuse understanding of the patient in this *milieu*.

Teaching

Final-year medical students, during their term in the Department of Psychological Medicine, attend the day hospital for two sessions. They see something of this venue of treatment, with its similarities to and differences from the in-patient and out-patient services. Some attention is paid to the dynamics of small and intermediate size groups, with illustrations drawn from patient and staff groups, and the idea of a therapeutic community is presented.

For post-graduate training, a psychiatric registrar is attached full-time to the day hospital and spends 6 months on the unit. During this period, in addition to his day-to-day clinical work with patients, he gains some insight into the psychodynamics of groups. He also receives training in individual psychotherapy with selected patients. Training is by way of recorded interviews and adequate supervision. Cases are selected to provide the trainee with experience in the various diagnostic categories, at a session frequency from one to four per week.

In a teaching hospital psychiatric department, where the average patient stays 3–4 weeks and out-patients are not seen more often than once per week, the day hospital provides a satisfactory venue for training in insight psychotherapy, which is not available with the short-stay in-patients nor with the infrequently seen out-patients. It is possible that more use will be made of this facility in the future.

Social work students are attached to the Department of Psychiatry. They work under the supervision of the senior worker and part of their case-load comes from day hospital patients. Each student is encouraged to attend patient–staff meetings and to be an active member of the therapeutic team.

A demonstration is given to second-year occupational therapy students of work in the day hospital. In their third year, there is a short period of active participation in the programme.

Conclusion

This day hospital seems to be serving specific functions, as part of the integrated psychiatric services of a teaching hospital. They are:

1. To provide treatment for those patients with neurotic and personality disorders, for whom in-patient care is not indicated and the frequency of contact in the out-patient department is insufficient.
2. To provide an alternative venue of treatment for some patients, who would otherwise require in-patient beds.
3. To provide a teaching situation in which the interaction between members of large and small groups may be studied and demonstrated.
4. To illustrate the principles of a therapeutic community.
5. To provide training at the post-graduate level in psychopathology and psychotherapy.

Acknowledgements

I am most grateful for the unfailing interest, co-operation and enthusiasm shown by the present and past members of the day hospital staff. My thanks are due to Dr. A. D. D. Pye, General Superintendent, and to the North Brisbane Hospitals Board for permission to publish this material.

References

BOAG, T. J. (1960), *Amer. J. Psychiat.* **116**, 801. Reprinted in *Trends in the Mental Health Services* (eds. Freeman and Farndale), Oxford, Pergamon Press, 1963.
BRODSKY, C. M. and FISCHER, A. (1964), *Am. J. Psychiat.* **120**, 793.
COOPER, D. (1965), Anti-hospital! An experiment in psychiatry, *New Society*, 11 March.
FARIS, R. E. L. and DURHAM, H. W. (1939), *Mental Disorders in Urban Areas*,
FARNDALE, J. (1961), *The Day Hospital Movement in Great Britain*, Oxford, Pergamon Press.
FARNDALE, J. (1963), In *Trends in the Mental Health Services*, (eds. Freeman and Farndale), Oxford, Pergamon Press.
FINESINGER, J. E. and SHEPPARD, G. K. (1959), *Amer. J. Psychiat.* **115**, 992.
HAMILTON, W. J. (1960), *Med. J. Aust.* **2**, 731.
HERON, M. J. (1962), *Brit. Med. J.* ii, 1529.
MENNINGER, K. (1952), *Manual for Psychiatric Case Study*, Menninger Clinic Monograph Series, No. 8, New York, Grune & Stratton.
JONES, A. L. *et al.* (1963), *Amer. J. Psychiat.* **119**, 973.
MOLL, A. E. (1963), *Trends in the Mental Health Services*, (eds. Freeman and Farndale), Oxford, Pergamon Press.
PECK, H. B. (1963), *Amer. J. Orthopsychiat.* **33**, 482.
PITT, B. and MARKOWE, M. (1963), *Brit. J. Psychiat.* **109**, 29.
WOODFORDE, J. M. (1965), Personal communication.

15. Psychiatric Aspects of Community Mental Health Center Planning in the United States

JOSEPH J. DOWNING

I. The Relationship of the Comprehensive Community Mental Health Center to Home, Job, Community and Beauty: a Plea for Therapeutic Aesthetics

A. PROLOGUE

Public psychiatric care in the United States is moving from the desocializing "out of sight, out of mind, so ship them off to the state hospital" past to the "let's solve this problem right here at home" present. By an evolutionary process, which will move faster than we now realize, home-town treatment in small comprehensive community mental health centers is replacing costly, inherently inefficient care in large, impersonal institutions.

Present community mental health centers are housed in makeshifts—in hospital wards, abandoned schools, homes, even in former institutional kitchens. We are planning facilities to be constructed specifically for this purpose. What existing institutions will they be like? Will they resemble schools, general hospitals, state hospitals, or office buildings? Undoubtedly there will be sufficient parking space, efficient first-aid rooms, ample linen-room space, efficient kitchens, reliable lavatories, drains and water closets. Will there be sensitive planning for the emotional and spiritual needs of the patient, whose overstressed mind and lacerated soul are the occasion for this structure?

What are those needs? What is the aesthetic of healing? The modern comprehensive mental health center will include a 24-hour emergency clinic, a part-time hospital equipped to give care on a day-, evening-, or night-time-only basis, a few attached 24-hour care facilities, a day-time out-patient clinic, and other doing-manipulative aimed facilities. Will it include a chapel, a quiet garden, soil and wood, an inviting library, the splash of water, fire-places—the amenities which add to construction costs and provoke frowns from public officials?

This is a plea to enlist the power of beauty to heal the soul, while the doctors heal the mind.

B. The Basic Mission of the Community Mental Health Center: Tangible Love and Security

The community mental health center of the future should be a social, not structural, institution joining a physical plant with a network of normal as well as special therapeutic social relationships. The psychiatric patient will be provided with calm, ever-present support, warm understanding, firm guidance, and tangible help in the form of medical care, food, shelter, occupation and friendship. Some will need help briefly, others for many years. The physical plant should be designed to protect, support, and further the all-important social relationships; its structure and form will either promote or hinder the main treatment objective: a secure relationship between the patient and the social and medical organization created to provide him with help.

C. A Sense of Security through Reliance on Institutional Security rather than Individual Therapist Dependency

1. *The majority of the patients coming to a community mental health center in the future will be the severe and long-term mentally handicapped and distressed,* i.e. primarily those who now go to state hospital care. A long-term supportive relationship will be needed for most of these people; this can be dependency on an institution made up of people and relationships in the local community, rather than a walled institution of locks and bars in an isolated state hospital. The unlocked community mental health center physical plant, in combination with the personal relationships, can give the essential sense of security and care which such sick and insecure patients must have, in order to live independently in the local community.

2. *The professional staff will come and go* but the physical plant remains, so the patients learn to rely on the permanence of the structure. Severely mentally ill people will frequently return to their place of treatment just to sit in the waiting room. They may drop in on the day center or clinic where they were treated, or otherwise "touch home base" in order to be reassured and gain a sense of protection and security that gives them the confidence to go ahead.

3. *For example, a proper, therapeutic waiting room should not be an architectual afterthought* or "front hall" located in the traffic pattern of every convenient draft, beset by clamor from the typing pool and hospital switchboard and casually furnished with discarded straight-backed chairs, too uncomfortable and disfigured to be used elsewhere. The children should not beset the waiting adults with clamor and high-spirited activity. It should be a place for quiet, soothing introspection, designed with intelligence and taste, to prepare the distraught patient or family member to talk with and receive the

maximum help of the highly expensive professional mental health worker. Commercial common sense tells us this; the supermarkets play music and serve free coffee; every bar uses comfort, quiet and pleasing surroundings to prepare the purchaser to separate from his money. How much more important similarly to prepare the patient to separate from his problems. (This is no sales pitch for piped-in music all day long.)

D. THE LONELY CROWD VERSUS THE FRIENDLY MENTAL HEALTH CENTER

1. *The treatment needs of the patient ought to precede the apparent needs of institutional efficiency.* Most public hospitals and similar institutions are designed with the cold and hard surface efficiency of a modern slaughter house. The endless efficient asphalt tile corridors weary and blunt the healthiest mind; better a converted dwelling with human turns and quirks to its plan, than endless halls marching to nowhere.

If patients were pigs, the aim to ship them out cold, quiet and sterile, the institutions would be of admirable efficiency. Fortunately, sterility is of little importance in a community mental health center, our patients are not to be quiet, they are to be normally self-contained and vocal, and we are not processing them through certain automated procedures on an assembly line fashion. Instead, we are aiming to treat each one like the individual human being that he is, and to make him a part of a therapeutic social *environment* that is as close to normal life process as we can possibly make it. And, let's face it, normal life is not "efficient", thank the Lord. Our test of efficiency is how quickly we help the patient back to health.

Our treatment aim is not automated, every-second-must-count routine. Isolation, impersonality and anonymity will further drive the disturbed person away from normal human contacts and into a withdrawal from society. The lonely crowd is a basic generator of illness in our society; we should not perpetuate it.

2. *Take, for example, the problem of dishwashing in the kitchen of our therapeutic community.* The patients serve the meals and do the dishes. We do not have a modern dishwasher, nor do we want one. Around the person-to-person aspects of dishwashing, who will do the dishes, why weren't they done, whose turn is it now, and so on, we are able to work out many more important personal problems. From the standpoint of therapeutic efficiency, hard work far outweighs the advantages of mechanical efficiency and higher sterility.

Another example: Stanton and Schwartz, in their pioneering book *The Mental Hospital*, cite one disturbed woman whose unintelligible, tense, highly speeded-up conversation was described in psychiatric slang as "a word salad", "confused", "excited and disoriented", and "manic and pressure of speech". This is a very common report on many severely ill hospitalized patients. However, the ward administrator took time to listen to her. One day, he caught the recurrence of the word "clothing" and asked the patient, "Are you mixed up about your clothes?" She nodded her head. With unusual but admirable tenacity, the administrator went ahead and discovered that for efficiency's sake, the patient's clothes were kept in an isolated clothing room locker. They showed the patient her clothing, and discovered that her excitement for a period of nearly 2 years had been based on misapprehension as to what had happened to her belongings. With demonstration and explanation, her incoherent talk cleared up almost immediately. Here is a striking example of how apparent efficiency in hospital operation, i.e. having a safe and secure clothing-room, resulted in prolonging one patient's illness. Understandably, you may say that this behavior was irrational, evidence of illness on the part of the patient. I agree; however, this is exactly the kind of person that we are dealing with.

E. THE THERAPEUTIC VALUE OF AESTHETICS

1. *For the long-term mentally ill patient, the community mental health center of the future may come to occupy somewhat the position of the Church in our pre-industrial America or in Europe in the Middle Ages.* Not that it will be a religious center for worship, but it will be a principal center of interest, concern, activity and help in the present, and security and hope for the future. The aesthetics will be extremely important, not as a secondary afterthought, to be glossed over in the interest of "architectual economy and efficiency" or placated with a two-bit terrazzo mural in the front lobby, but as a planned adjunct to therapy for the distraught mind.

2. *In an increasingly urban society, we will find that gardens and courtyards, running water and quiet pools, and the ability to sit refreshed under a shady tree will all be increasingly rare.* By the same token, they will be more necessary for that fraction of the population which is not able to adjust to urban tensions and demands, to living subway-style, buttock-to-buttock, eyeball-to-overly-familiar-eyeball. For such reasons, we should not waste the grounds and roofs around our institutions; rather, they should be planned with seats, benches, and parks that can be used for familiar occupations such as reading, shuffleboard, and quiet walks between the patient and his therapist.

3. *For similar tension reduction, the living space in the institution should admit of as much homely clutter and carelessness as possible.* In the proper mental health center, family rooms, game rooms and rooms for quiet reflection are all necessary. Many times, a wide hall with comfortable benches is a most excellent place for discussion and the gaining of understanding and insight, or a large kitchen with room to talk while serving a cup of coffee.

F. Healing through Gaiety and Light-heartedness

1. *I am recurrently impressed that the common-sense minded man of commerce, the businessmen who act as our arbiters of public institutional tastes, are very well sold on the commercial value of gaiety, beauty and aesthetics.* Modern shopping centers are coming close to my ideal of what I would like to see in a community mental health center, complete with open vistas, benches, flower boxes, fountains, statuaries, and occasional frivolous touches. I can do no better than to refer you to the Hillsdale shopping center development in San Mateo, California, or that charming, round, circus tent-like frivolous bank pavilion attached to the Crown-Zellerbach Building in San Francisco as illustration of this. Modern motels and factories are likewise intentionally pleasant and built to human needs. Why then is it that public care-giving institutions, with the exception of the spiritually-resonating Marin County, California, civic center, designed by Frank Lloyd Wright, must be built in the most constricted fashion of mail-order architecture? Money and costs? *I again repeat, the cheapest community mental health center is the one that gets people well and independent the fastest.*

G. Proximity, Accessibility and Size

1. *I have not mentioned the obvious items of hospital and shopping center proximity, accessibility to public transportation, and size.* In general, we should have a separate community mental health center for not more than 200,000 people. Standards of the National Institute of Mental Health define the necessary components of the community mental health center. The center will be a good neighbor; it will be no more disturbing than an elementary school to the neighborhood sense of propriety. In addition to close accessibility to public transport, it should take advantage of existing parks, public gardens, playing courts and fields.

2. *This is particularly worthwhile, since the community mental health center's peak hours will be during the working hours of the week,* when other citizens will not be using public recreational facilities. The community mental health centers will use such public facilities only slightly in the evenings and on weekends.

3. For the increasingly important day hospital program, there are patients who, for a brief initial period of treatment, have to be brought by their relatives or friends in the morning and then picked up in the evening. For this reason, the *facility should not be far from main traffic arteries.*

H. Medical Needs

The large majority of the community mental health center patients will not need physical medical care more frequently than the total population;

however, certain groups such as the alcoholic, aged, and the suicidal, will be in need of such specialized facilities. For this reason, working proximity to a general hospital, if not actual inclusion on the grounds and building, is advisable, although not essential.

I. Living Needs for Patients and Staff

Primarily a part-time facility, with a small fraction of 24-hour "hospitalized" patients, the community mental health center will operate around the clock with evening-only, night-only, and 24-hour emergency clinic services. Both staff and patients will need food service, bathing facilities, sleeping facilities, etc.

II. Alternate Approaches to Psychiatric Care in Community Mental Health Centers

A. Structure and Affiliation

1. *We are concerned with a total psychiatric care program.* The actual architecture is the expression of the means whereby the program objectives of a comprehensive CMHC can be achieved, rather than the end-product itself.

2. *The primary need is for a practical overall program directed primarily at the present known major public psychiatric load, i.e., those severely mentally ill or addicted persons who now have a high probability of being committed to a mental hospital.* This dictates design changes from the usual out-patient clinic or in-patient service in the direction of services close to home, services with a minimum of social and family disruption, services with a minimum of occupational disruption.

B. "Vertical", Decentralized, Geographically-based Organization

1. *The philosophy and treatment approach, I term "vertical" or "comprehensive service", team organization based on geographic decentralization* differs at certain points from conventional treatment methods and standards, such as those suggested by the American Psychiatric Association. The treatment approach given here, the entire philosophy of the therapeutic community as a treatment method, plus the highly specialized community mental health center as a community organization center is not based on theories of as yet untried effectiveness. The original experience of Dr. Maxwell Jones at Belmont (Henderson) Hospital, the later experience of Dr. Harry Wilmer at Oak Knoll Naval Hospital, Oakland, California, the San Mateo Community

Mental Health Services Program since 1957 in San Mateo, California, and the work of Dr. Maxwell Jones and Dr. Brooke at Salem State Hospital, Salem, Oregon, since 1960, and the Fort Logan State Hospital, Denver, Colorado, since 1960 under Dr. Allen Kraft, support this approach.

C. GENERAL HOSPITAL AFFILIATION

1. The program given herein envisions close and continuous co-operation through having the private practitioner, in psychiatric and other specialties and also in general practice, work co-operatively, in conjunction with specialized treatment teams in the CMHC.

2. *The specific dependence on the general hospital* for medical and surgical services, for the hospitalization of the acute-toxic states, for the intensive care of the suicidal overdose, and physically injured patients provides a treatment mode that could be transposed to almost any city. The pattern of close co-operation with community education, recreation, vocation and re-habilitation services could likewise be transposed, although it is recognized that in all general hospitals, there would not be the same variety of social and welfare services. It would be necessary perhaps for the CMHC to provide some ancillary services within its own facility. This could be provided for through space marked for "optional expansion" use. In locations in a higher income area in a large city, it is suggested that some of the optional space would be available for offices of private practitioners in psychiatry and the other specialties. It would be particularly valuable if the private practitioner in psychiatry found it worthwhile to locate all his professional operations in the intimate confines of the CMHC.

3. *Do the advantage of general hospital connection*, the medical advantages of accessibility to the wide spectrum of specialty for diagnosis and treatment, plus available skilled emergency care for toxic and injured psychiatric patients merit all community mental health centers being next to the general hospital? Certainly, it is impossible to have an effective 24-hour psychiatric service unless intensive care units for the care of drug overdosage, surgical treatment of injuries due to self-inflicted knife wounds or gunshot wounds, and care on medical wards of severe toxic states, due to prolonged alcohol ingestion, are available within a workable distance.

4. *Yet there are potential disadvantages to the medical location and orienta-tion which must also be recognized.* Social welfare and public health needs must be met, particularly among those patients who have a high probability of mental hospital commitment. The individual private practitioner usually deals with a sick individual in an intact family. In public psychiatric services, there are nearly always severe familial, vocational, social and economic problems, frequently of long-standing and stubborn nature. These multiple problems require multiple professional skills—psychiatric social work,

psychology, and many others. Such patients are often in need of a psychiatric treatment plan, which envisions lifelong responsibility for a relapsing illness of chronic and remittent nature. Financial and social work assistance for essential life maintenance frequently must be gained from local social welfare departments through the mechanism of aid to the chronically disabled, because psychiatric treatment facilities cannot provide it. Necessary contact and follow-up supervision must be provided through the Visiting Nurse Association and public health nurse departments.

5. *Since vocational programs for the psychiatric patient are particularly important* in the maintenance of self-esteem through a degree of independence, close working-level co-operation with employment and vocational rehabilitation agencies is essential. For these reasons, an exclusively medical approach, directed entirely to the symptomatic alleviation of immediately presenting psychiatric symptoms, oftentimes with the aim of shunting the patient off to another responsible service as quickly as possible, only ends in complicating an already complex and tangled situation. Thus *the general hospital location must not overshadow the fact that the complex problems of the psychiatric patient are medical, social, and economic*, requiring long-term work with patient, family, and community, as well as through specific psychiatric and other medical intervention.

6. The local general hospital is traditionally the point for *emergency medical care of all types.* For this reason, emergency psychiatric care is well located within the admitting room of the general hospital. This means that there has to be special planning, however, for the integration of 24-hour care in a CMHC and in a general hospital. In certain locations, it may be preferable to locate the emergency care entirely in the general hospital. As psychiatric emergencies are grouped largely from 3 p.m. to midnight, it is also possible for the physician providing this coverage to provide necessary coverage in the CMHC, and in the general hospital psychiatric service during the night.

7. *The key to successful management of the acutely disturbed patient* on an open ward is initial control by heavy tranquilizing medication while still in the emergency room. Before making the decision to admit, observation in secure holding rooms for up to 8 hours is necessary. A large percentage of emergency room patients (over 50% in San Mateo experience) can be referred out next day for follow-up services, thus lessening the hospital load to an extremely important degree.

D. Plans for Continuous Care

1. *A variety of functions does not inevitably dictate a variety of separate services.* The classical psychiatric operational plan has been modeled on general medical care, which has separated out the "in-patient" or 24-hour

residential hospital patient who is provided sleeping service and "round-the-clock" attention, from the out-patient, ambulatory, i.e., "walking" patient seen by pre-arranged appointment, and able to utilize specific intermittent direction with a minimum of overseeing. Extending this either total-super-vision or not-at-all pattern to psychiatric care has resulted in needless and indeed socially and individually harmful removal of large numbers of individuals from their usual functioning and placing them in an enforced total dependency situation. Other patients, who for their own and society's benefit need more than intermittent attention, fail to benefit because total hospitalization is also not the answer. Further, brief 1–7-day total (24-hour) care can precede part-time care with safety, if the same minimally pro-fessional team can treat in the same situation the same patients. There are individuals in disturbing life situations which are best handled by temporary brief removal from the situation for a few days by total hospital care. Others need longer-term care for a matter of months. The functional need is for ease of rapid and flexible movement of the patient back and forth from one type of treatment situation to another.

2. *"Professional judgment" of behavior* is far less important in medicine and surgery than in psychiatry; indeed, it is traditionally ignored, in favor of specific laboratory data plus recording of signs and symptoms. Extending the classic medical in-and-out pattern to the psychiatric patient has en-countered a major problem in the necessity of communication from one treatment situation to the next of a large amount of what can be best called "professional judgment" regarding future behavior, based on close and continued observation of the patient in the living situation of the treatment service. Such communication of "judgment" has been a major barrier to efficient, rapid co-ordination of clinical care by the traditionally structured services based on specialization of function, such as in-patient (24-hour care), out-patient, day center (part-time), appointment only, and so forth. The psychiatrist, in contrast to medical-surgical practice, is concerned with primarily the patient's *behavior*. Traditionally, medicine and surgery are concerned with the presence or absence of constellations of observed or reported manifestations of bodily function or dysfunction, *not* social function or dysfunction. A competent physician or surgeon can read an adequately recorded case file and usually provide a reliable prediction of future course before ever seeing the patient. With the addition of the interpersonal and social levels of functioning, evaluation of present behavior and extrapolation from the evaluation, in order to predict future behavior, are expected from the psychiatric physician. Experience to date suggests such prediction cannot be reliably based on the usual type of clinical case notes, no matter how meticulously maintained. (It should be parenthetically added that, often, psychiatric case records are notoriously idiosyncratic and inadequate, even for routine administrative purposes.)

3. *A continuous relationship between doctor and patient* is much more efficient in terms of conserving the valuable relationship and information gathered by observation. A great deal of understanding of the patient is based on a continued doctor–patient relationship, and on the subliminal perception of subtle behavior, which is difficult, if not impossible, to communicate by written records. For this reason, private practice of psychiatry is able to maintain much sicker patients with less hospitalization because of a continuous relationship between therapist and patient, family and environment. The therapist sees the patient, whether in or out of the hospital, and directs his treatment. Unfortunately, economic realities dictate such care be confined to those well-to-do persons able to pay for large amounts of expensive professional time. In contrast, the present *discontinuous* system of public psychiatric care, based on specialization of function, transfers the patient to a new group of professionals each time his needs change. This forces each new responsible professional to repeat with the patient and the family the entire time-consuming process of "evaluation".

A frequent complaint in any public psychiatric service is the fact that other services refused to accept the recommendations and evaluations of the previous referring service. This is so common that it cannot be held to be generated by a superciliousness or professional "one-upmanship". Rather we must recognize that the present keystone of psychiatric care today continues to be guided by an interpersonal relationship between therapist and patient, supplemented by a wide gambit of physical, social and other therapies. Each time the patient gains a new therapist, the new relationship must be slowly and expensively formed, before the new therapist has a sound opinion.

4. *Common to almost every psychiatric patient is a deficiency in his ability to form and maintain meaningful, useful, co-operative, trusting interpersonal relationships.* An alienation, estrangement or extreme shyness oftentimes is at the root of the interpersonal difficulties which constitute his illness, and in the acute form, such as a suicide attempt, lead him to enforced psychiatric care. The traditional system of discrete, discontinuous and separate services, based on intensity of care, is almost perfectly calculated to magnify and aggravate this underlying major source of the patient's disorientation, his difficulty in relating to and trusting other people.

5. *Based on this reasoning, the mental health center operational plan given here has been radically changed to maintain continuity of relationships* with the community, and with all treatment, and help-providing persons in the CMHC. Essentially, the patient remains with the same treatment team throughout the period that he receives care in the center, regardless of his "out-patient", "day-hospital" or "in-patient" status. Even during the "after-care", he sees the same team with whom he began. That this is of value in public psychiatry as well as in private practice has been well shown by the

work of those public institutions which have set up this program, specifically Fort Logan Colorado State Hospital. One team functions flexibly to provide all necessary functions, as in private practice.

E. Assessing Existing Local Resources

Our cities present in heightened fashion all the problems of mental illness: the metropolitan core problems of social stratification, isolating poverty, increased non-white population, increased numbers of desocialized or "skid row" individuals, broken homes, a greater proportion of aged and single person households.

1. *All over the U.S. co-ordination of multiple services at the individual case level is minimal.* Nowhere in the extensive facilities for public psychiatric care is there one service facility which takes responsibility for the total range of conditions, for reaching out to meet needs unmet by other agencies. The CMHC can and must take this dual co-ordinating and supplementing responsibility for the mentally ill.

Since the CMHC is not seen as a diagnosis and referral service only, but rather as a definitive treatment service, it is expected that a certain proportion of the existing load in any community would soon be carried by the center. In particular, the affiliated general hospital psychiatric service would soon refer all psychiatric applications from study area residents to the adjacent CMHC, unless they were urgently in need of immediate medical or surgical care.

2. *Looking beyond the psychiatric treatment and medical services to the equally essential vocational, educational, social and health services,* a major problem exists in the matter of designating the agency which will accept continuous follow-up responsibility for the psychiatric patient to whatever service he may be currently receiving. The psychiatric patient is in need of the same complex range of services as any other citizen, and in conformity with the principle that these services should be provided by existing agencies solely for the subgroup designated as "psychiatric patients", an elaborate system for insuring the existence of available services and the effective movement of the patient among them is needed. This suggests the existence of a central psychiatric case file in the CMHC which takes on the essential characteristics of a case register combined with a follow-up "tickler" system. Notoriously, psychiatric patients "get lost" between agencies, through failure of the patient or the family to follow-up on referral, or due to inaccessibility of needed service at the time of application. Major effort and continued attention to this transfer and follow-up problem is absolutely essential if the community is to provide services readily, at the time needed and in an effective manner.

F. Estimating Use Rates

1. *Existing data extrapolated from clinics and hospital are misleading,* particularly of the need for 24-hour care. It has been established in a number of centers that immediate treatment, beginning at the point of initial contact in the admissions room, can singly reduce the in- or out-patient bed days required. The San Mateo, California, services through use of spectrum-co-ordinated services have reduced their state hospital commitment rate to one-half the expected, while at the same time maintaining a hospital day rate of 280 per 100,000 a year in the county general hospital.

2. *Typical projection of need for CMHC.* We can expect rates of use to go up as there is more immediately available service. Patients will come in for help earlier in their illness, and with the expectation of working out their problems while still in their normal life situation, rather than of being removed from that life situation and sent to a state hospital. We can also expect that a greater proportion of women would become patients than at the present time because of their general greater suitability for part-time care, due to their passivity, docility, and due to the fact that fewer women work during the day than men, who are therefore not available for treatment.

3. *In the children's services we can expect a high proportion of anti-social acting-out and the necessity for close working with juvenile probation and with the police.* In a middle-class or an upper-class area a greater proportion of school learning problems and neurotic illness would dominate. A necessity for specialized programs for culturally undeveloped children from minority groups will be evident. It may also be necessary to consider the establishment of a crèche for the care of the infants or very young children of day center patients, within the CMHC.

4. *Social agency referrals will become a high proportion of the patients seen.* Undoubtedly, the courts would continue to be a principal source of referrals, as at the present time, to the general hospital (four out of ten). With the emphasis on consultation as a means of dealing with symptomatic behavior, the patient being retained as the primary responsibility of another care-giving agency, we can expect that the socially dependent (welfare) population and the social population (police, courts and probation) would be more highly represented.

5. *In the CMHC, part-time care would replace about 50% of the existing general hospital 24-hour care.* Emergency room interviews with a follow-up limited to five times or less would take care of perhaps 20% of those persons now admitted to the general hospitals. We would find that 24-hour care of the type now given on the treatment ward of the general hospital would be at a higher rate than now given locally, but would reduce to perhaps 60% of the existing level of state hospital care from this area.

6. *Gaps in data.* The previous estimates, based on the work of Leighton *et al.* (1963), are in close correspondence with those issued by the National Institute of Mental Health, Washington. On this basis, we can reasonably calculate the patient load for the entire CMHC at $1\cdot75\%$ annually of the adult population. In view of the fact that various populations will have differential rates of use, an important feature of any plan presented here is its modifiability and expansibility. It should be emphasized that the outline here is based on minimal estimates and it is felt that only by experience extending over a period of 3–5 years will it be possible to know how much treatment space each team will need, in order to meet the total eligible load from its own catchment area.

7. *Areas in which existing data might be misleading in terms of CMHC program.* Since existing data is based on "committable" patients, who are only a minority of the total persons in need of CMHC care and eligible for such, and because the pattern of care in state hospitals up to now has been long-term 24-hour care, usually separated from the community, existing figures on use are undoubtedly erroneous in three directions:

(1) In terms of underestimating the potential case-load;
(2) In terms of overestimating the proportion of persons who will need to be removed from their homes of residence and receive 24-hour care; and
(3) In terms of underestimating the numbers of persons who will need attention by social work, in terms of referral and co-ordination of activities of other community agencies. For this reason, social work activities will be more intensive and will require more workers than in the conventional clinic or state hospital.

III. Establishing a Treatment Program

A. ALTERNATIVE MODELS

1. *The traditional psychiatric care model has been usually a locked ward, in conjunction with the public charitable general hospital.* In most instances, an in-patient, 24-hour, receiving, diagnosing and disposition service is maintained. Because of a lack of alternative services, particularly 24-hour emergency definitive treatment at the point of application, nearly all applicants are admitted. The serious understaffing of public general hospital services has resulted in a very small minority of patients receiving definitive service at the point of admission. The consequence of this is to postpone definitive treatment until the person enters the mental hospital, at which time essential sources of information regarding the social genesis of dysfunction such as the

family, the arresting policeman, the employer and so forth are distant and not available. The final result is that patients pile up in the mental hospital because of the difficulty of gaining reliable information regarding the patient's status and working out arrangements for their discharge.

2. *The single, centralized, general hospital-based service comes to be viewed in isolation,* as a dumping ground for the problems that other community agencies lack the time, inclination or resources to deal with. It has been the experience in the San Mateo Health Program that through dealing with the problems at the point of application, providing immediate specific psychiatric treatment for every patient, providing social case-work, and working closely with available resources, the majority of applicants for hospitalization can be cared for without hospitalization at all. Of those who are admitted, the large majority (80%) can be returned to the community within a 2-week period. Screening and detention without treatment, awaiting mental hospital transfer, average nearly the same length and the same cost per patient admitted, as an intensive, effective treatment service.

B. CENTRALIZED TREATMENT PROGRAM

1. *Within the area served, all public psychiatric cases needing emergency attention or possible state hospital commitment* are taken to a psychiatric ward or building connected with the general hospital. In such areas, there is usually an admissions ward for screening and disposition, the majority of whose occupants are then sent on to the mental hospital for definitive diagnosis and treatment. A small minority, who are considered "most treatable" or who are considered "legally eligible for service", go to much less crowded treatment wards. As given in the statistics for San Francisco, which may be considered typical for most American cities, only 10% of admissions received any form of treatment. Transfer to the treatment ward was recommended for only 4% of the patients. The effect of this is to lose the extremely valuable attributes of immediate treatment at the point of maximum receptivity, greatly to increase the work of the committing courts, to lose the benefits of treatment planning and execution in co-operation with the family, employers, and local social service agencies, and to act inhumanely, as though ill persons were criminals to be incarcerated, sorted and disposed of. One wonders if such a cold, impersonal disregard of need for medical care is also tolerated in the medical and surgical wards of the same hospitals. Is the cardiac or appendicitis sufferer also held for days, pending eligibility for care?

2. A low local cost per patient admitted is one of the seeming advantages to the centralized ward at a local general hospital, with a maximum amount of treatment cost being transferred to the state hospital. However, in San

Mateo it has been found that actual treatment costs little more than detention and disposition elsewhere. In view of the inherent inefficiencies of prolongation of treatment and planning, the total public cost of delayed treatment is much increased.

3. *A disadvantage of existing patterns* of administrative service structure on the horizontal model is that it requires large numbers of supervisory personnel, in terms of the service-giving professionals. The result of this is that the numbers of persons engaged in supervision increase geometrically, while the number of professionals giving service increases only arithmetically. Through the decentralized, geographically-based, multiple-purpose team approach, co-ordination of services within a given secondary area is the responsibility within the team and it is of considerably lesser concern to the supervisory personnel. As a result, the number of supervisory administrative personnel is lessened.

4. *Another perplexing integration obstacle* is the hierarchy of professional prestige connected with the various facilities, the top of the hierarchy being occupied by the out-patient staff, who engage in high prestige psychotherapy, and at the bottom of the status-seeking order, the state hospital personnel who receive patients who are legally restrained against their will and must take care of the long-term problems which the other facilities either are not interested in or have failed with.

5. *The main advantage of the "horizontal" type* of organization for care is that it fits into the conventional pattern, overwhelmingly predominant across the country. Further, it is the pattern to which the majority of professionals in the mental health field have been trained and with which they are familiar and in which their social roles, attitudes and gratifications are clearly established. Also, it provides for a high degree of specialization and ready sorting by status and type of care, so that a young social worker may become a highly skilled psychotherapist, a psychiatric graduate of a university center becomes a well-paid private practitioner, a foreign-born state hospital psychiatrist skilled in administering electric shock, and a psychologist may be particularly skilled in providing psychological diagnostic tests of certain types of mental illness.

6. *The main disadvantages are the serious discontinuity of patient care*, a tendency to mold the patient to the Procrustean bed of the service available, rather than adapting the service to the changing needs of the patient's condition, a pattern of intensive use of large numbers of highly skilled psychiatric professionals to provide psychotherapy for a relatively small number of out-patients, most of whom are of less social concern than a greater number of severely ill and maladjusted psychotic patients. These latter receive scanty attention from the few overworked, low-status hospital professionals.

C. Decentralized Treatment Programs

1. *Characteristics of the new program proposed here are that* the services given are intended to be definitive, short-term treatment services, maintaining the individual in the normal home environment, in contact with the important small social groups of family and work, with but a minority of patients receiving 24-hour care. The decentralized service teams are linked directly to small geographical and social area subgroups, so that the mental health professionals providing help can know through personal contact the important formal and informal social group leaders in the area in which the patient resides.

2. *Observation in existing mental health centers has shown* that many psychiatric patients are brought to hospitals not because of a change in their intrapsychic condition (their inherent mental illness) but because of a breakdown or change in the social situation in which they have resided. In these cases, it is seldom necessary to provide definitive medical psychiatric treatment, but rather to provide effective social service and social planning for the patient.

3. *Another advantage of the decentralized service in a CMHC* is that it tends to be identified by the community as a friendly, concerned place with a hopeful prognosis, rather than a way station to court and then to a mental hospital. For this reason, there is less resistance encountered by the persons who are persuading the disturbed individual to seek voluntary care, rather than forcing police and court action.

4. *A major disadvantage in the present climate of social opinion* is that decentralized care is most effectively based on specific geographical catchment areas. In nearly any large city, this means that certain residential areas will be entirely or predominately Negro and that the patients served will be all Negro. Protests may arise over this kind of seeming segregation. It would seem advisable, wherever at all possible, to draw geographical boundaries so as to include some persons of both white and colored races in a given catchment area in order to avoid charges of intentional segregation. However, in large areas such as New York's Harlem, the population receiving service is so large and the numbers of persons needing service is so large that it would be impossible to have a mixture of white and non-white. This fact, together with the great advantages of geographically-based services, should be faced in advance with leaders of the service area.

5. *A further advantage of the decentralized service* is that it is located closer to the person served so that, thereby, they identify this service as being an element of their own neighborhood. We can both decentralize the CMHC to a primary area of approximately 200,000 people, and further decentralize it by subdividing the region served into three secondary subdistricts, which relate to one of the three general-purpose service teams.

Each service team is planned to have its own two or three evenings a week clinic, in conjunction with an existing secondary subdistrict neighborhood center. This center might be either a library, a public health center, a church, a neighborhood house, or a private physician's office. In any case, the existing patterns of community service within a smaller district of approximately 55,000 persons are already established. The decentralized team would thus be even more in touch with the community resources of the areas served.

6. *A disadvantage of the decentralized scheme* is that the persons served are on a geographical basis, i.e. that of residence. Due to the heightened mobility of our population, particularly in the West, fully 1/3 of the inhabitants can be expected to move to a new place of residence within 5 years. This means that if a patient goes from one home to another, he will have to enter into another team's treatment area, thereby breaking the continuity of service. As it is not possible to have both geographical continuity and service continuity from the point of entry into the treatment program, it is felt that the advantage of the teams being fully equated with the area served, resources, the population characteristics and needs outweigh that of continuity of service based on assignment at times of entry into the treatment program.

D. Use of existing Facilities and Agencies

1. *The CMHC is not solely the problem and province of those public psychiatric services which are available in the area served.* The CMHC must concern itself with the totality of care, both public and private, in the area for which it has responsibility. Treatment responsibility is only one facet of its total over-all program. Additional responsibilities are for surveying needs of the area, in conjunction with existing service and planning agencies, such as community councils, in providing non-critical services of a specialized type such as agency consultation, and in initiating and carrying out a systematic mental health education program directed at the particular needs of the area served. Other important responsibilities are co-ordination with agencies outside the geographical area which provide service, such as the mental hospital and veterans' hospitals. In order to carry out effectively these multiple responsibilities, many of which are not at the present time being met by anyone, the CMHC must work closely with all types of private and public medical facilities, private practitioners of medicine, with welfare, public health, rehabilitation and educational agencies. In order to do this, there should be formed an advisory board or council, having within it representatives of these and other publicly concerned agencies within the area. Local private medicine should be heavily represented on such an advisory board. In addition, local private practice professionals and any private psychiatric service may form a regular professional advisory committee to the director of the CMH service.

2. *It is particularly valuable* if the boundaries of the CMHC primary service area and of the secondary team service areas can be largely continuous with the boundaries of public health nursing and social welfare worker service areas.

3. *To the extent that religious organizations* and private religious schools can be interested in mutually working on existing neighborhood problems, an extremely valuable resource is gained.

4. *Through the educational program*, many activities of direct treatment benefit to the patients in a CMHC, and in the important educational aspects of the CMH program can be gained. Vocational resources should be sought; particularly, rehabilitation services connected with local schools should be utilized. As in many places there is still suspicion and lack of understanding, coupled with fear of those persons labeled "mentally ill", there must be a systematic attempt in the program of the CMHC to bring the citizens of the area into programs at the center. It is worthwhile, for example, to offer the use of the meeting rooms in the center on an "as available" basis to all neighborhood organizations needing such facilities.

E. Relationship to Mental Hospitals

1. *The traditional pattern of local facilities has been to shift* what was considered a long-term chronic care burden to the State as soon as possible, rather than to attempt treatment on a short-term intensive basis within the local facility. The reasons for this are the now outmoded experience that the care of the mentally ill was a long-term custodial cost, beyond the ability of local facilities to meet, as well as a general governmental tendency to shift tax costs to other jurisdictions wherever possible. Modern psychiatric care has shown it is much more expeditious, effective and humane, and but little more expensive, to treat most patients locally at the point of application, rather than to shuffle them off to the mental hospital, to the delays and lack of effective intensive care inherent in caring for large populations at a distance from the area served. *However, some persons requiring medium and long-term 24-hour care are better served in treatment-orientated hospitals, than in the community mental health center.*

2. *Some types of patients, most particularly the aged patient*, are admitted to the general hospital in a state of mental confusion based on brain diseases, which is not usually considered "psychosis". Such persons are better cared for through consultation by the psychiatrists of the local mental health center with nursing homes and homes for the aged in the area served. In this fashion, many individuals who are admitted and transferred to state hospitals as "senile psychotic" can be cared for more effectively, more cheaply and with greater humanity in non-psychiatric facilities near their own family.

3. *The state mental hospital suffers from the inherent disadvantage of distance, isolation, overload and lack of sufficiently skilled professionals.* It is much to the advantage of both the state hospital and the CMHC if a close, personal and working relationship is established, through regular scheduled exchange of visits and through personal acquaintance, and through the fullest exchange of actual case records between the local mental health facility and the mental hospital. The CMHC should take the responsibility for providing whatever information is needed by the mental hospital when a patient is transferred to state care, and for receiving any and all referrals for after-care from the mental hospital at the point of discharge. In this fashion, the mental hospital is able to accelerate the process of admission, diagnosis, evaluation, and definitive treatment and discharge planning, to the extent that its total patient load is reduced. As a result of the reduced patient load, the mental hospital staff is able to do a more intensive, satisfactory job on the patients who are admitted.

4. *Of particular advantage and worthy of emulation* is the special designation of subunits or buildings of the existing mental hospital, to work with designated geographic catchment areas or regions. The so-called "Kansas Plan", which has been particularly effective at Osawattomie State Hospital, and the Salem Oregon State Hospital "regionalization" have shown the advantages of such a plan. In effect, certain units or buildings within the existing mental hospital plan are limited in their patient reception and treatment to designated cities or counties. The reception, treatment and discharge of both acute and long-term patients has been shown to be materially speeded up by this plan.

5. *The new change in national social welfare regulations*, making the mentally ill eligible for aid to the disabled, has opened major new resources for the support of the indigent mentally ill, who require public maintenance but do not require close custodial care. Through co-operation between the CMH services, the mental hospital and the local welfare department, those persons discharged from the mental hospital to welfare support can be known and evaluated by the CMH facility. Many of these individuals will require maintenance medication or occasional supportive follow-up. It is to be strongly recommended that at the point of mental hospital discharge, they be interviewed in the CMH services, so as to be known to them as well as to welfare.

6. *The state vocational rehabilitation agency* should also be aware for planning for local mental health services. More and more, it becomes apparent that one of the basic supportive services to the discharged mental hospital patient is employment. In many instances, this feeling of self-esteem and worthwhile endeavor is essential to maintaining a psychic balance without regression into mental illness.

IV. Professional Staffing and Utilization

A. STAFF AVAILABILITY AND TRAINING

1. *Despite the huge cost of the present, less than adequate public psychiatric care*, the governmental bodies and civil service refuse to set payment for public psychiatric care at an equivalent level for private psychiatric care. In effect, the public psychiatric services must content themselves with a much lower rate of doctor–patient ratio, with the marginal, not psychiatrically trained physician who is frequently foreign born, and with the younger man just out of training, who is frankly using the public service as a stepping stone to a more lucrative and less demanding private practice.

2. *The CMHC staffing given here* is based on the firm reality that far less than adequate psychiatric and medical coverage will be available, that the majority of preventive care must be given by non-medical staff and non-psychiatrists, and that the treatment program must be based heavily on the social organization of the treatment service—the so-called "therapeutic community approach". Since the pattern given here is only effective if immediate emergency care is available, which dictates the attention of the physician at least on the diagnostic basis, then routine administrative duties must be carried out by other than the psychiatrist on the team. Availability of non-psychiatric physicians is higher than of psychiatrists, and of non-physicians higher than of physicians.

3. *Although trained social workers are in short supply*, there is a general preference for working in psychiatric centers over working in welfare or other agencies, so it can be expected that adequately trained social workers can be found.

4. In regard to nursing, it has generally been found preferable not to have nurses trained in the traditional psychiatric hospital, because of their emphasis on jail-like, locked and searching techniques, their indoctrination in a rigid separation of roles between patients and staff, and their insistence on the traditional medical model for conduct in the ward. It has been found generally preferable to receive young registered nurses and practical nurses without other than the minimal psychiatric training and to allow them to learn through on-the-job training. Availability of trained vocational rehabilitation, recreational therapy, and occupational therapy personnel can be considered moderately difficult, but not impossible.

5. *Training, both in-service and through attendance at short courses* sponsored by other institutions and by the university training centers, is essential for effective staff morale. A study by Passamanick *et al.* in Ohio showed that intellectual stimulation ranks well above any other aspect of professional work, as far as professional staff morale is concerned. A separate specific professional concerned primarily with staff training is essential. (We should

provide an office in administration.) Preferably, this person should be a
psychiatrist, but this is not absolutely necessary. Continuous on-the-job
training including supervised experience, seminars, and lectures is necessary,
due to the fact that a continuous staff turnover can be expected even in a
high-morale institution.

   6. *Of particular importance are those persons generally considered as
"psychiatric aides"*. These individuals have the most continuous contact
with the patients and are frequently the "carriers of culture". By this, is
meant that the aides have the most frequent and intimate contact with
patients, and being usually of the patients' own class, are looked to as guides
and mentors in how to act within the hospital community. For this reason,
attendants and aides should be fully involved at all points in staff conferences
and activities.

B. ORGANIZATION OF THE TREATMENT PROGRAM
IN THE COMMUNITY

   1. The program presented here is aimed at three important characteristics:

   (a) Provisions of immediate care at the point of entry into the treatment
        facility or immediate and effective care by another community
        social agency;
   (b) Minimizing of social and psychological regressions;
   (c) Maintenance of normal, existing social relationships and strengths.

As discussed previously, the existing patterns of delayed psychiatric care for
the socially maladjusted and severely mentally ill postpone the point at
which the individual is given definitive help with his problem. The result of
this is that many times, the already bad situation is aggravated by the manner
in which the so-called diagnosis and treatment is provided. Through providing
24-hour care at the point of admission, social stress can be minimized or
aggravation avoided. If a skilled physician sees patients at the point at which
they are brought to the emergency room of the hospital, in the majority of
cases, he may provide preventive treatment at that point, without admission.

   2. *Maintenance of doctor–patient relationship* from the time the individual
enters into the treatment program until he is no longer receiving follow-up
after-care is the pattern which has always existed in private medicine and is
of even greater importance with the socially disorganized and extremely
mentally ill persons seen in a CMH set-up. This is provided through having
one team, in which the patient is able to receive whatever type of service is
needed, without changing the individual's professional persons giving the
service. The manner in which the team is able to provide such service is as
follows:

(a) Each team has within its service patients who are receiving inter-mittent after-care, perhaps even through a public nurse home visit rather than through direct contact with team members.

(b) By having a pre- and post-mental health care center in the satellite clinics, located in the actual neighborhood served.

(c) By having scheduled social group and vocation activities, such as patient social groups and sheltered workshops, in which the individual is not formally in a treatment program but has regular weekly contact on a group basis with mental health professionals.

(d) Through scheduled after-care visits on an office basis.

(e) Through "open house" activities in the team area on a certain after-noon or evening each week, in which the former patient knows he can go without schedule and participate in group activities and see a professional regarding a problem, if necessary.

(f) Through scheduled part-time or full-time hospital or evening activities.

(g) Through a 24-hour sleep-in facility, which is located in the team area and can be used flexibly, so that a day patient may stay overnight if there is some particular disturbing home situation or exacerbation of illness.

(h) Through consultation to neighborhood residential centers, such as half-way houses, nursing homes or children's foster homes.

(i) Through periodic consultation with the regionalized mental hospital building serving the particular CMHC.

(j) Through regular consultation with other community professionals and agencies, so that the information available to any one care-giving group can be available to all, as needed.

It is entirely feasible for all these treatment programs to go on in the same area and be provided by the same professionals.

3. *Experience has shown* that when a patient is referred from one facility to another, say from an in-patient hospital facility to an out-patient clinic, that only 1 out of 10 patients actually makes the follow-up contact. Even with the most vigorous, close and willing goodwill between the two services, this pattern of care violates the fundamental precept of psychiatric treatment care, i.e. continuity of therapist–patient relationship. Basic to psychiatric illness is the fact that the individual has a disturbance in the ability to form interpersonal relationships. As our goal in the community service is to provide care to these patients which is effective and gains their co-operation, we must have a pattern of service which avoids the breaks in treatment continuity, inherent in the present fragmented system.

4. Services are generally provided by a great variety of agencies, having different policies, different attitudes, and oftentimes rivalries between each

other. In many cases, such agencies will not even exchange records, as they do not trust each other sufficiently to be "professionally responsible". Geographical separation, often of many miles, further aggravates the problem, even with the best goodwill between agencies. The serious result of this is that the agencies are able to avoid facing really widespread social problems and seeking for solutions. This inappropriate evasion can be avoided in the CMHC by giving responsibility in one area to one team, who must give assistance to all applicants, regardless of their commitments otherwise.

C. ORGANIZATION OF THE TREATMENT PROGRAM IN THE CMHC

1. *Based on the Fort Logan Colorado State Hospital model.* Rather than having a number of separate psychiatric services or agencies, each performing a specific specialized function, such as out-patient care, hospital care, etc., a general-purpose team consisting of a number of mental health specialists provides all types of care within its own service area, without subdifferentiating into specialized groups.

(a) The physical setting within which the team function is designed to provide for total activities and group facilities needed for either a day hospital, an out-patient or a 24-hour hospital treatment service. For example, professional offices can be used either for group sessions or individual care; day rooms become sleeping facilities, as these are needed for 24-hour care.

(b) The team receives patients regardless of their type of illness, and within a widely flexible program provides care for them, regardless of their residential status, intensity of treatment, or type of mental illness, age or sex, or any other characteristic. In this fashion, it is very similar to private practice, particularly that based on a private hospital.

(c) Thus, the private practice of medicine provides for continuity of care, the private practitioner in the smaller center tends to take care of all types of problems in children, adolescents, adults or the aged, follows the patient into hospital care if indicated, and treats him afterwards on discharge. The vertical pattern is much more similar to the private practice of psychiatry than to the traditional public medical practice.

(d) In the variant given here, the team would receive patients in whatever degree of disturbance, as long as they were not in need of bedside medical nursing care. As the CMHC under study is attached to a general hospital, we assume that the general hospital would take care of persons needing medical or surgical care within its own facility. It has been found, particularly for the suicidal patient, both the self-injured and the overdose of medication patient, that these are best cared for in the intensive care unit of the hospital, with daily visits from the psychiatrist. At the point that the patient improves and is ambulatory, he is then transferred to the psychiatric unit.

2. *The San Mateo County General Hospital experience* shows that the alcoholic patient needing bed care can be cared for very well on the general medical wards of the hospital, regardless of the intensity of the alcoholic stupor or the presence of brain symptoms such as delirium tremens. This, of course, presupposes that the medical staff of the hospital is acquainted with modern methods of medication and with the methods of minimizing delirium. Thus the patient, from the point of application at the emergency room, enters into treatment with the team which will provide care from that point on.

3. *In order for the team to take care of the acutely disturbed individual*, close co-operation with local police authorities is absolutely essential. Experience of the San Mateo County Unit has shown that by the use of heavy doses of intramuscular tranquilizers in the admission room, all but $0·3\%$ of admissions can be cared for in an open ward setting. The police bringing the disturbed patient in can give the necessary restraint, while the admitting physician gives a large dose of a tranquilizer to the acutely disturbed individual. If the police officers will wait 30 minutes, a second dose can be given, if needed. Once tranquil, the patient is taken to his bed in the team area and further medication given as needed.

4. *Once the patient is introduced to this treatment mode, the type and intensity of service depends on current needs of the patient*. He can go flexibly from a residential status or 24-hour care to either evening care, at which he can return to his job during the day, to night care only (if his family relationships are disturbed) and if he is unable to hold employment, but can reside at home, he can come in during the day. As he improves and is undertaking specialized rehabilitation services such as vocational training or sheltered workshop, then the patient can come in one morning or afternoon a week, an evening a week for social club meeting, etc.

5. *A major advantage is that this service can be carried out with the minimum* of psychiatric attention. The psychiatrist acts in the traditional medical diagnosis and treatment prescription role, but the majority of care can be carried out either by non-psychiatric physicians, by the nursing team in the group program, by social work, or whatever is indicated. This, however, has a negative side, in that few psychiatrists are trained today to work with a team in such fashion. They tend to be threatened by the dilution of their contact with the patient, and they often feel that their status and traditional physician's role is jeopardized by this kind of interaction.

6. The team is not allowed to pass the buck for local care, except for long-term patients sent to mental hospitals, for patients who can be cared for by non-psychiatric services locally, and for patients able to afford private psychiatric care. Even if a patient is referred to one of these other agencies, he remains the responsibility of the individual team, until such a time as he is accepted by the other facility and is actually in care with them. This puts considerable strain on the team, and in addition, as cases are treated and go into less intensive care on a maintenance basis, the load piles up. It is impossible at this time to estimate the extent of this continuous and maintenance load, but it may approximate somewhere around $2\frac{1}{2}\%$ of the adult population. This means that the team has to work for maintenance of such patients by other community agencies, through consultation with the team, and must have adequate group activities which lessen the individual load.

7. *It does not seem likely that a comprehensive children's program* could be ensured within the general purpose team. Children's activities are specialized and experiences show that they are not well carried out within an adult program. There is no harm in having children in the same area as the adults, but children's and adolescents' needs are different from those of the adult. It has been found, however, that aged patients can work quite effectively in any adult group. A separate children's–adolescents' team would share certain eating and activity facilities with the other parts of the center but have its own area, staff and program.

8. *General experience has shown that the alcoholic* does not fit in easily to a general program for the mentally ill patient and that the alcoholic in general refuses to come to a program for mentally ill persons, who they feel are different from themselves. Further, the needs of the alcoholic are different from those of the mentally ill patient. For all these reasons, and for the practical reason that, generally speaking, if you have a combined program for the mentally ill, the neurotic and the alcoholic, the alcoholic tends to be shoved out or to withdraw and not get treatment at all, it is recommended that there should be a separate alcoholic treatment team and program. This does not mean that all individuals who have alcohol as a symptom of their disability would be referred to the alcoholism team. The General Purpose Teams would be expected to keep as many as possible within their program but those who do not fit into the general teams program would be referred to the alcoholic program.

9. The team members, as outlined, care for 12 in-patients, for 20 day hospital patients, and for 30–40 out-patients at a time. This is considerably more than can be cared for by any other type of facility. The reason for this is that the greater efficiency of this flexible arrangement means that less time is spent in unnecessary overhead transfer, evaluation of new patients, etc. There are very definite efficiencies and gains in professional time, which can be used for more effective and extensive patient care.

D. Closed (Locked) Compared to Open (Unlocked) Wards

1. *A characteristic of closed wards is that the patients* are viewed as de-socialized, unable to meet social expectations, as potentially dangerous to themselves and to others, and as a social obligation for protection, through coercion and restraint. In this, the characteristics of such services are a distrust in the patient, the use of overt restraint and authoritarianism and covert force and punitive measures.

The closed program is an extension of the traditional medical attitude that the patient should be the passive recipient of medical direction. If the patient is not the passive recipient, but on the contrary expresses his own views of his problems and what should be done about them, the physician tends to label the patient as "unco-operative" or "untreatable". He (the physician) then feels justified, indeed obligated, to use coercive measures. Extending this to a psychiatric area, unless the patient docilely accepts the psychiatrist's direction or (much more frequently) the direction of the designated representative—the attendant or nurse—he is labeled as "psychotic", "dangerous", or "untreatable".

With the person receiving care pushed into the traditional "patient" role, the gulf in role between the person intended to provide care and treatment (the "staff") and the person receiving them (the "patient") is very similar and, in fact, often identical with the situation in a prison. Attempts to assist the person with his problems, however gentle or well meaning, are effectively blocked by the gulf in communication between the two cultures, that of the staff and that of the patient. The staff, being uncertain as to the patient's thoughts, feelings and motives and basically viewing the patient as being unpredictable and unstable, nearly always emphasizes "security" measures, which lead to an authoritative, punitive, suspicious atmosphere. Since the characteristic of the psychiatric patient is his inability to form normal relationships and his fear and insecure distrust of others, this poisonous atmosphere further accentuates and severely aggravates the underlying personality problem.

2. *Among the few advantages of this authoritarianism* "security-based" is that it fits into the traditional social role that is assigned to persons who are labeled "mentally ill". The community rarely questions the care or the administration of a psychiatric ward which is locked, regardless of proven instances of brutality, of despair-driven suicide or homicidal attempts on the part of the patient, or of needless prolongation of illness due to aggravation of the patient's mental pathology by the detention situation.

3. *Another advantage of the closed ward* is that it makes it possible, in fact inevitable, for the staff to disregard the patient's pleas for help. If the patient becomes bothersomely demanding or persistent in his seeking for help, it is

easy to lock the importunate fellow in an isolated room, where he cannot bother the staff.

A locked ward makes it possible to disregard the condition of the patients and to keep them under a minimum of attention, by providing only the minimal level of food, clothing, shelter, and medical care. From this standpoint, it makes it possible to maintain a seemingly low patient/day cost. The basic fallacy in this, of course, is that it prolongs the period that the patient is in the hospital and makes the total cost-per-patient stay much higher. Also, low-quality untrained personnel can be used to act in the position of jailers and supervisors.

4. It is claimed that locks and "security precautions" reduce the number of homicides and suicides among the mentally ill. This is not borne out by the facts; in those services which have not been locked but are true treatment-orientated open wards, the number of suicides and homicidal attacks has been reduced to the vanishing point.

5. The jail-like atmosphere creates a feeling of fear in the surrounding community, and the conviction that individuals within the jail-like psychiatric ward must be dangerous and therefore fearful. This potentiates the fear of psychiatric illness and the suspicion which is already rampant.

6. *The characteristics of the open ward* are not that there is unlimited freedom, but that the principal entrance and exit of the ward is unlocked. The other doors are usually locked, so that in order for a patient to leave, it is necessary for him to pass in front of some degree of control station, such as the secretary's desk and out through a public corridor toward the front of the hospital. It is found in the majority of cases that under these circumstances, the patient who leaves can be found and persuaded to return, without ever actually entering outside of the mental health center. Through the use of a patient system, whereby a "door watch" is maintained by the patients, together with a sign-out and pass system, it is found that it is a rare occasion for a patient to actually leave the ward and then to proceed out of the hospital undetected. Since there is no locked door and the patients know that they come and go at will, it is found that the explosive, oppressive prison-like atmosphere of the usual locked psychiatric ward, together with the feeling of apathy and helplessness, is not created. A further advantage is that through the easy coming and going, a healthy normal atmosphere can be created on the ward. The open ward, of necessity, lends itself to total lack of the usual security measures, so that the searching fear, suspicion, and other prison atmosphere is not created.

Reference

LEIGHTON, D. C. *et al.* (1963), *The Character of Danger*, New York, Basic Books.

16. Community Psychiatry in Israel *

Louis Miller

COMMUNITY psychiatry in Israel, as in any country, is a close reflection of the attitudes prevailing generally in this discipline. One may speak of the psychiatry of a country in several senses. Today, it may be concerned to include in its purview the following phenomena, in order to influence them for individual or general mental health:

(a) Socio-cultural forces at work in the formation of personality. Such are social relations, values and prohibitions, institutions and educational methods and economic sources, promotive or destructive of personal satisfaction and support.
(b) The personality patterns which tend to be produced by and in the society by these strivings and social techniques.
(c) The patterns of personality deviation, in thought, behaviour and emotional reaction, produced by relative failure in personality formation through social or biological accident.
(d) The intrinsic or expressed attitudes to deviation deriving from the social or cultural situation, and hence the type and quality of treatment or service made available to or sought by the deviants, or employed to prevent deviation.

Hospital psychiatry has little contact with most of these forces and can hardly influence them. Psychiatry in the community has, in the main, accepted its role as the agent for influencing such social and personal forces. Community psychiatry has special opportunities for fulfilling the goals of psychiatry, such as prevention, mitigation, early diagnosis, early treatment and rehabilitation which are not available to hospital psychiatry, however much hospital psychiatry moves towards the community and those functions. With these opportunities, community psychiatry and its services tend to develop techniques specially suited to the goals towards which they strive.

The establishment of psychiatric clinics in hospitals—or in the community—is not necessarily a form of practice which is suited to preventive or promotive mental health work, or to the mitigation of the many forms of human suffering and deviation. The shift of psychiatric clinics into the community, however, has several advantages over hospital care for many

* This chapter is based on a paper which appeared in *The Israel Annals of Psychiatry and Related Disciplines*, 2, No. 4, April 1964.

patients. Psychiatric services set in the community may help reduce harmful attitudes in the community and family *vis-à-vis* a particular patient or to psychiatric disorder as a whole. Contact with community enables the psychiatrist to mobilize material as well as emotional forces for the support of the patient. General community services may thus be involved in the rehabilitation of patients. Communities may be spurred to develop new and more extensive psychiatric services. These activities are often termed "community psychiatry". Perhaps it would be advisable to see them as the employment of community psychiatric principles in clinical psychiatry. In all events, the shift towards the community in clinical psychiatry has added to it many important dimensions for early diagnosis, treatment and rehabilitation, which when judiciously and selectively employed, have resulted in greater capacity for the alleviation of individual stress.

Community psychiatry perhaps is best seen as action designed to promote, in the particular socio-cultural *milieu*, the best possible social relations for the development of the personality of the growing child (or for that matter the functioning of the adult or disengagement of the aged), and the reduction of the intensity of deviation. It is concerned as well, to foster constructive and human attitudes to the deviant and distressed, and to promote in the society suitable and positive methods of care for them.

These extensive and deep-running trends in community psychiatry demand of the people working in it a particular view of life, and a preparation and kind of activity quite different from that of the clinical psychiatrist, who is ever concerned with a particular patient and the exploitation of social and other resources for the individual patient's restitution.

Nonetheless, the community psychiatrist is a clinical practitioner working for the individual patient. But the patients he will be best able to handle will be those whose problems bear a direct and immediate relation to the environment and emotional *milieu* in which they are growing up or living. Such are children in disturbed and broken families, children whose cultural situation leads to problems of learning and behaviour at school and younger and older delinquents. The psychiatrist in the community will encounter adults in family or social conflict, who have difficulties at work and problems of physical health, behaviour or addiction. Older people facing problems of ageing and retirement or physical incapacity become an increasingly important part of his practice.

These difficulties appear especially in the developing and changing society of the Western city. They may be classed professionally as problems of behaviour, psychopathy, addiction, criminality, apathy, neurosis, early psychosis or simply as the unregenerate nature of the won't-works, the poor or the pampered. Community psychiatry is concerned with these personal problems, which are directly, if not solely, related to social situations and the reflections of them in the family or groups.

Practice with individuals who are the products of general social stress, disadvantage or malaise fits the community psychiatrist at least to attempt to participate in their alleviation. He acquires through a particular individual practice an awareness, and possibly an understanding, of the relation between a particular situation, say poverty, and the personal problem, such as learning and social difficulties, which the child has at school and the conflicts it may have with its parents or people. Generally, the community psychiatrist should become expert in the effect of the social order on the nature of the personality, its attitudes and on the type of emotional or behaviour deviation it tends to develop.

Of course, the community psychiatrist, practising with such individual cases of personal malfunction on the basis of social difficulties, cannot himself develop any sort of machinery capable of making an impress on social pathology, dysfunction or disadvantage. Without such machinery for social action, his efforts with the individual are doomed and his work in the community frustrated. (It may be quite as depressing to struggle with individuals from a middle-class environment as from a slum.)

A prime interest of the community psychiatrist is to support the development of an apparatus in the community, capable of incisive action for change in the social situation. Experience to date has been that the most potent social technique available has been community organization. This method demands of a specially trained worker, who is not a member of the psychiatric team, skills in stimulating the community to action, to meet its own needs and to attack its own problems. It is a technique which, while more embracing, has something in common with group methods of adult education and even with family case-work and psychotherapy. It has, however, little of their hedged-in nature in the treatment of the client, or their isolation from the crucial social realities around the client.

Community organization is not directive. It should be more concerned with the individual's growth, through his participation in the tackling of mutual problems, than with material goals. Psychologically, it is concerned with healthy ego-growth and social attitudes, co-operation and identification with the general needs. However, it best attains this through the fostering of social tactics in the group, so that it and the people in it may attain what they wish with legitimate means and resources, that are theirs by democratic right. In helping people to employ their resources to the best of their ability, to develop a social *savoir faire* in finding these resources, and to decide jointly how to use them, community organization is a political method for mental health.

The community psychiatrist attempts as well to promote and exploit other resources in the community for mental health. Chief among these are the personnel in services who participate in child care, the services at school and in education generally, and the agencies in the community. All may be front-line workers in mental and social health. They may often be ready to infuse new social and psychological principles into their service to people. At times, their organization and self-image makes of them bureaucrats and even actual sources for the creation of dependence and resentment in their clients. The community psychiatrist should attempt to free these community resources from such limitations and guide them towards mental health action in their professional fields.

Problems of mental ill-health are not infrequently the result of social policy and economic organization. This may be true even in affluent societies. Community psychiatry may be powerless to effect improvements in the spheres of personal mental health if it does not also find methods of influencing social policy. This influence, which is certainly attainable in the open and humanitarian atmosphere of the modern democracies, should not be exploited only for the development of psychiatric services, but also for the mitigation of social problems. Mental health problems relate directly to the socio-economic struggle of the modern city with its housing difficulties, the burdens on the working mother and the problems of ageing. The stresses on the isolated city family result often in deep injury to the emotional integrity and identity of its children.

The community psychiatric team should be composed of psychiatric as well as social specialists. There is certainly a place in it for the sociologist or the community worker specialized in mental health. All members of the team should be at home in the problems of the group and society, and aware of their effects on the personality, since human function and deviation take root in human relations as well as in biological impulses. The understanding of the variety of interpersonal and social determinants of personal deviation and a contribution to an attack on them demands flexibility of the team, and at times, unusual tactical changes in leadership.

Social psychiatry should become the discipline concerned with the diagnosis of group and community forces, making for general behaviour patterns or deviation and ill-health. In making its diagnoses, it should use such methods as field studies in mental ill-health, epidemiology and the techniques of sociology and anthropology. Social psychiatry studies the effects on the individual of social and cultural changes in the group, and the impress on him of social and economic class differences and pressures. It measures his attitudes to himself and others to leadership and to services. Social psychiatry has a special task to perform in the assessment of the needs and priorities for psychiatric and mental health programmes, and the evaluation of the results of social and mental health action. It is a mass diagnostic and evaluative technique, vital to clinical and community psychiatric operations.

Clinical psychiatry will be dependent on the work of the community psychiatrist for early diagnosis, for the fostering of the acceptance of treatment and for the proper employment of psychiatric services. Community psychiatry, however, should not place too great an emphasis on its contribution to clinical psychiatry. Its goals should be essentially the general social and mental health of the community and should be determined mainly by them.

Although it may be said that the State of Israel and its present social structure go back for only a century, it has already a largely formed socio-cultural being. The recent processes of actual state formation and the fore-gathering of Jews in the State have wrought changes in the nation and have modified it, enriching its cultural contents.

For all its varied ethnic and cultural roots, Israel is the product of a millennial urge of Jews to return to national life. This urge is the strongest substratum of the nation. Infused and bound into this element in Israel now are the principles and goals of Western egalitarian society, modulated by the values and themes of group responsibility and mutuality, toward which the West is still evolving. This is something of the atmosphere and its background in which the Israeli personality pattern is being formed, stands or falls and must be promoted or supported.

The pattern of Israeli society was already in evidence before the establishment of the State. For all its special group formations, such as the rural collective, the urban co-operative and youth movements, its structure and problems were of course predominantly those of the West. Little research was done, but it was evident that group living had fostered character formation of a special variety, suited to the intensely co-operative life, which also coloured the type and quality of deviation.

Relatively large migrations to the national home in pre-State Palestine had occurred before the establishment of the State in 1948. Statehood was accompanied not only by military attacks from the surrounding countries, but also by massive immigrations from a variety of countries and cultures. At first, the immigration came from the remnants of the concentration camps of Hitler's Europe and was composed of people who had suffered physically and psychologically as grave a hurt as the human spirit can suffer. To this day, many of Israel's people are scarred emotionally and socially from that experience and families rebuilt here carry the heritage of that history.

Flight to Israel had been accompanied by marked anxieties in the refugees. Escape from countries that resemble police states brought individuals stamped with fearful suspiciousness, which subsided only at length and by dint of constant social reassurance. Generally, all the emotional and social problems concomitant on migration were renewed with each migration. However, since Israel is in its nature uniquely a society and a State planned to receive and integrate immigrants, problems of migration were largely dealt with as they appeared, with sympathetic identification and through great material sacrifice. Among these problems of migration one may mention the strain for the aged and the incapacity of the immigrant family to cope with its handicapped members or the emotional difficulties among its own

members. Many, especially Oriental, immigrants, confused by the strange
ways of the new society, reacted with aggressive behaviour difficulties and
somatic and hysterical neuroses. This was especially evident in the Oriental
people from the rural areas of the countries of Islam.

These states, reactive to immigration, were also seen in the European
immigrant, if perhaps in more sophisticated forms, although abnormal
personality and behaviour reactions were also unusually frequent. Even the
hosts to the immigration were not without their reactions to it.

With the economic settlement of the immigrants, a great deal of these
acute reactions seem to have disappeared. Today, therefore, the urgent mental
health problems in Israel's new communities are less reactions to migration
and more the problems encountered through cultural change in non-Western
peoples, which have set in after the settlement of the mass immigration.
Relatively large numbers of people from non-Western ethnic groups strive
to adjust to Israel's Western patterns of living. They frequently exhibit
problems associated with rapid cultural change to Western standards, which
are complicated also by the problems of urban living. The powerful social
forces making for homogeneity in the country are underlaid by marked
differences in the groups. This is hallmarked by the fundamental differences
in family structure and content of Western and Eastern ethnic groups. The
situation of the Western family and its problems are fairly well known in
psychiatry. Those of the large Eastern family are less understood. The
understanding of the vicissitudes of the large Eastern family in its struggle
to adjust its size, structure and activity to urban, industrial and Western
demands is still in its infancy.

Because of its rapidity, the cultural change among Easterners occurring
in the country is accompanied by appreciable personal difficulties. Problems
extensive enough to be thought of as general social problems arise as a
result of the stresses of change. Among the more obvious ones is the educational lag, accompanied by behaviour difficulties in children of school age.
Learning difficulties result from a diversity of causes, such as the attitudes
to education in the Eastern family and differences in the intellectual processes
between the educators from the Western groups, who determine educational
standards, and Eastern culture groups who receive the education. Economic
failure of the large Eastern family and parent–child conflicts in the changing
family certainly play a part.

The Oriental family is generally at a disadvantage. Immigrant parents
were often illiterate, untrained for any occupation and at a loss in the competitive culture of Israel's growing cities. The family was not organized in its
relations and roles for material survival in the new and alien culture. Its
educational influence on its children was dissipated.

Social failure, then, threatens in the city by virtue of the formation of
conglomerations of poor Eastern families. These neighbourhoods tend to

show the first signs of social and economic failure in higher rates of delinquency and a drift to fringe occupations. Such neighbourhoods, if they do crystallize out as such, will also tend to draw towards themselves social failures or deviants. For some large families in the city, the struggle is weathered with the establishment of a smaller second-generation immigrant family. In villages of rural areas, the process of cultural change is much less rapid and generally more solid.

Specific personality problems revealing themselves during this type of social and cultural change include resentful and aggressive behaviour or apathy, difficulties at work and emotionally reinforced reactions to minor injury. Confused reactive states to social and family difficulties are frequent among the ageing, who least tolerate the social upheaval. Frank magical beliefs and thinking often colour the personal difficulty. Alcoholism is relatively rare still, and compulsion, depression and suicide are of lower frequency in the Oriental groups. With advancing social change, they may increase. A curious concomitant of rapid social and cultural change in Israel was the excess of work and road accidents.

The focus of community psychiatry in Israel is the *mental health centre*.

The mental health centres take various forms. In the major cities, there are still separate child guidance clinics, loosely related to adult mental health centres. Both of these urban types of centre are staffed by interdisciplinary teams of psychiatrists, psychiatric social workers, clinical psychologists and therapists. The adult mental health centre of the Mental Health Services of the Ministry of Health is the seat of the regional community organizer for mental health, whose function it is to foster a closer relationship between it and community organizers and agencies. The centre may be the seat of the regional psychiatrist, who co-ordinates psychiatric services.

In the small regional towns, progress has been made with the establishment of combined community and family mental health centres. The teams in these centres, if on a smaller scale, serve mental health and psychiatric functions for all ages. This allows of a type of family and community approach to mental health promotion which is difficult to attain in the classical child-guidance setting, or in the adult mental health centre in the city.

The modes of action of present-day Israeli psychiatry in the community may be summarized as follows.

(a) *Consultation with and counselling to agencies* in the social, health and education fields as to the mental health requirements of their clients. Such direction is given to all public agencies. This service is employed especially by social welfare, the public health service, schools, youth probation services and the courts. These consultations are designed to enrich the service to the client by the professional agency, but may result in all gradations of concerted treatment programmes of the community psychiatric service and the agency, in the attack on the case and family.

Case counselling of this sort extends not only the efficacy of the psychiatric service, but is the first step towards the establishment of mental health and preventive practice through the recruitment to these activities of agencies and services deeply involved with families and groups in the community. The national public health services (mainly pediatricians and nurses), for example, are today profoundly conscious of their mental health, early diagnostic and care functions. The teacher is less so, but noteworthy changes are already in evidence at school, with efforts to reorganize the educational-psychological services and to integrate them with the mental health services in the community.

Community psychiatry in Israel is adjusting itself. With less facility to the support of the community organizers at work in the new communities of cities and new towns, there is increasing awareness at the centres that the community organizational effort is a prime mental health instrument. Community organizers see as their goal the mobilization of community agencies and leadership for mental health programmes, such as for youth, the aged or for refractory or handicapped groups. Inevitably, therefore, the organizer and the community mental health team are moving towards a common line of action.

(b) *Early diagnosis and community care of psychiatric patients*. The mental health centres, because of their connection with community agencies, are in the most favourable position for early case-identification and early psychiatric treatment of the patient in the community. They are also well placed for the mustering of social resources for the support of the patient and the family, by virtue of their intimate working relation to all agencies, especially those in the welfare and public health fields.

(c) *Preparation of cases for hospital care; case-work with families of hospitalized cases; after care*. The increasing activity of psychiatric treatment in mental hospitals and the shortening of patients' stay there make increasing demands on community psychiatry. Relatively more patients are being prepared to enter hospital and must be cared for on returning to the community. The shortened stay in hospital limits the amount of work that can be done with the patient and his family while he is there. This tends to shift the burden of continuing psychiatric care and rehabilitation work onto the community services, especially at mental health centres in the smaller and rural towns. These functions of the mental health centre are absolutely vital for the success of the modern psychiatric hospital. Without it, the out-patient stituation at hospital, because of the increasing number of patients under care, tends to become chaotic and empirical.

The mental health centre shares the increased burden on the patient's family that results from the shortened hospital stay. Without this support, the family and community alike tend to revolt against the resulting burdens. A most important contribution of the mental health centre is its effort to increase community tolerance of the psychiatric patient and the assessment of the limits of that tolerance.

There is still a variety of mental health centres in the communities of Israel. Some still tend to duplicate the work of traditional out-patient departments, relying heavily on drug therapy and techniques of social manipulation for the patient's benefit. Others, being analytically orientated, tend to be highly patient-centred and intensive in their pursuit of intra-psychic forces. Most centres, however, attempt to retain through their teams a balance in their attention to the intrapersonal, family and group influences in the patient's life.

While the mental health centres remain essentially orientated on the individual patient, they are beginning to see as their main and specialized function the care of the individual, whose development or functioning is being impaired by virtue of the impact of pressures or deficiencies in his family and social group. This approach has become inescapable, in the light of the fact that the community centres are in the midst of communities undergoing rapid cultural and social change in Israel.

Recently, in addition to the community organizer for mental health, a new member has been added to the mental health centres of the Ministry of Health—the public health nurse. The nurses are still few in number and their work is still rather tentative. These nurses are either psychiatric nurses who have been trained in public health or public health nurses who have under-gone training in mental health. At the mental health centre, they have become a link with the public health nursing service. The Israel public health nursing service is profoundly involved generally with family and community problems and, freed from tasks in physical preventive health, they have become active in the family and community mental health programmes. The public health mental health nurse brings the mental health centre to their aid in the same way as the clinical psychologist, the social worker and community organizer link the centre to the school psychological and welfare services and the community programme. It is intended that the nurse should link the mental health centre to curative programmes for the chronic sick, the handicapped and the aged. The tendency for curative medical services to work in professional isolation may make this extension of mental health function in the community a much more difficult proposition than the integration with preventive services and community programmes.

Hospital Psychiatry

At the inception of statehood in 1948, psychiatric hospitals in Israel, with the exception of one or two small units, were of low standard and very inadequate in number. There were about 1000 beds for a population of 800,000.

Several small, open neurotic and psychotic hospitals were developed as part of the programme of military psychiatry and at the cessation of hostilities in 1949, these units were transferred with their personnel to the Ministry of Health. They became the core for the programme of State psychiatry.

Immediately on statehood, the flood of immigration brought many neglected chronic psychotics, remnants of the holocaust and patients from situations of neglect in the Middle East and North Africa.

The programme of hospital psychiatry which was implemented immediately, in spite of lack or absence of staff and buildings, adhered to definite principles. These principles called for small, active psychiatric units of several types, according to patient needs. The whole range of these services, if economically feasible, was to be made available for each region in the country. A limit was placed on size of the hospitals—a maximum of 400 beds, so that community and group therapy could be employed.

It was established that even for longer-stay patients, the whole spectrum of psychiatric personnel should be employed and that the staff concentration for them should approach that of the active psychiatric hospital. This approach to the long-term rehabilitation of the chronic patient led to the crystallization of the "work village", of which there are now four. The work village is an active community of chronic psychotics and staff, in which the patient is progressively involved in community life and productive occupation.

The range of services today in the four psychiatric regions of Israel is as follows.

1. *Psychiatric night hostel.* There are only two of these now. They cater in the main for younger patients who are at work. In one hostel, the majority of the patients who are psychotic have not been to hospital. Day sections are being added to the hostels.

2. *Psychiatric service in general hospitals.* There are three hospital wards in general hospitals. Out-patient care is a growing feature of these units, as is consultation in the general wards. With the activation of psychiatric care, it seems that the accent will shift from in-patient care to out-patient and day treatment. In-patient care for children and geriatric cases is being planned to replace in-patient practice with adult early psychotics and severe neurotics, who will be cared for extramurally.

3. *The city psychiatric hospital.* This hospital, of up to about 400 beds, has been the mainstay of Israeli clinical psychiatry to date. There are six in the country now. They are multi-purpose but length of stay now rarely exceeds 3–4 months. Out-patient services, which are most active, have been added and day sections are now being developed. It is planned that these hospitals shall not exceed 250 beds and about 50 day cases, and should each serve a population of about 250,000.

4. *Work village.* The work villages are undergoing a revision. They have been provided with facilities for the direct admission from the community

of longer-stay patients and for their intensive treatment in a reception section, before going on, if necessary, to a resocialization and rehabilitation section (the work village itself).

5. *Custodial care.* While some of the government hospitals carry custodial sections, this function has been allocated temporarily to small private homes. This is an unsatisfactory arrangement, as the private hospitals are generally of low standard. The custodial facilities, especially those for patients requiring nursing and physical care, will have to be rebuilt by the State, either as separate units or as annexes to the longer-stay settings.

6. *Children.* Although facilities for severely disturbed children have grown in number and improved in quality over the last few years, they are still in short supply. In two regions now there are in-patient facilities for children and youth. The first day-hospital for children was opened recently. Plans provide for the extension of children's in-patient and day centres to the remaining regions. Facilities for children, especially those with brain damage, will be developed at general hospitals.

7. *The aged.* A geriatric service was established at first as a single national project. It comprised geriatric physical and psychiatric in-patient care, with out-patient and day sections. Consultation was provided to homes for the aged and, by means of a mobile team, a rehabilitation programme was promoted, with the co-operation of local authority welfare and other services. This geriatric service is now being extended to a further region. The dearth of general hospital provision in Israel for the chronic sick and geriatric organic cases may prove a stumbling block.

8. *Special services.* There are particular functions for which one facility is still able to supply the needs of the small nation. Such are the prison psychiatric ward and consultation service, a small unit for tuberculous disturbed patients and a unit for adult high-grade defectives.

The interlocking range of facilities on the regional level makes for homogeneity of the patient community and intensification of individual care. It has also contributed greatly to the depth of relation between the psychiatric hospital, the patient in the community, and the community and its services. This development has allowed the mental health centre more time to cater for the type of personal and social dysfunction with which the psychiatric hospital is not really qualified to deal. The mental health centre, consequently, is increasingly fitted to support and exploit action for mental health in the community.

17. Soviet and American Approaches to Mental Illness: a Comparative Perspective*

MARK G. FIELD

Introduction

It is practically an article of faith among Soviet writers on the subject that the nature of the Soviet social order is such that mental illness is bound to decline from year to year, that it is indeed declining, and that it is bound to disappear altogether once full Communism has been achieved. By the same token, it is also apparently a matter of conviction among the same writers that mental illness is bound to increase, and is indeed increasing, under the conditions of "decadent" Western capitalism. Kerbikov, for example, commenting on the steady decline since 1940 of first visits by schizophrenics to the Moscow psychoneurological clinics, attributes it to the "constant rise of the material standard of living and of the cultural level of Soviet citizens, which leads to a general strengthening of their health", [1] and Adlai Stevenson, who visited the Soviet Union a few years ago, was told by Dr. Grashchenkov, a professor of neurology in Moscow, that the unity of the Russian people in building up their country accounted for the lower rate of mental illness in the Soviet Union when compared, for example, with the United States. The professor went on to say that at one time the American people had also been imbued with the goal of developing and building their country, particularly at the time of the Civil War and the opening of the West. "In those days," he observed, "the incidence of mental illness in the United States was very low because [the American] people were imbued with common, simple, big aims— victory, social justice, national development."[2] The implication, of course, was not only that American society had lost the pioneering spirit and the *élan* that characterized it as a young nation, but that its population, mercilessly exploited by capitalism, threatened by economic crises, depression, unemployment and misery, and thus prey to anxiety and fear about the morrow, was afflicted by ever-increasing rates of mental illness.

---

* Reprinted from *Review of Soviet Medical Sciences* (1964), **i**, 1. Some slight changes were made in the preparation of this article for reprinting here; in particular, statistical materials were brought up to date.

[1] O. V. Kerbikov, *Lektsii po psikhiatrii* (Lectures on Psychiatry), Moscow, 1955, p. 232.

[2] Address by Adlai E. Stevenson to the National Association for Mental Health, Kansas City, Missouri, November 20, 1958.

Valid comparisons in this field are notoriously difficult and often impossible. Lack of common terms and definitions, the absence of standardized terms, differences in diagnostic procedures and therapeutic orientations may indicate differences (or uniformities) that do not exist in reality. Furthermore, it seems to be fairly well established that the so-called "increase" in mental illness (particularly psychosis) that has allegedly accompanied the process of industrialization and urbanization over the last 100 years or so may be due primarily to better case-finding, greater diagnostic sophistication and an improved reporting system.[3] By the same token, it is at least conceivable that the "decrease" in mental illness claimed by the Soviets is (to some degree) the result of an artifact, this time working in the opposite direction to prove a point.[4]

What seems to be clear, on the other hand, from an examination of the scanty evidence available to us is that at the present time mental illness is not a salient medical problem in the Soviet Union, or at least it is not considered so by the health authorities or the regime; certainly, on a comparative basis, the interest and concern with this problem nowhere approach that displayed in most Western countries, the United States in particular. The reasons for this are many, and far more complicated than the simplistic and almost naïve theory of a direct correlation between social structure and mental illness.[5]

In this paper I shall attempt the task of unraveling some of these reasons and providing some comparative insight into the Soviet approach to mental illness by looking at the Soviet psychiatric system in particular. By psychiatric system I mean the totality of formal efforts a society invests in the handling, treatment and rehabilitation of individuals with diseases or impairments of the psyche. I shall leave aside, for examination at a later time, such areas as research in psychiatry or the training of future psychiatrists, and I shall not venture too far onto the treacherous shoals of comparative statements. This is one area, then, in which circumspection is mandatory, and this paper can only be an incomplete and necessarily unsatisfactory statement of a difficult question.

[3] Herbert Goldhammer and Andrew Marshall, *Psychosis and Civilization*, Glencoe, Illinois, 1953.

[4] In a personal conversation, a Soviet authority suggested that the decline, for example, of first visits by mental patients to the Moscow psychoneurological clinics from 1940 to 1956 (see Table 6) may have been due primarily to the fact that these clinics had been established toward the end of the thirties. As such, there had been a "bunching up" of patients around 1940 needing treatment and/or an official certification of mental illness. Once this backlog (itself a result of a previous lack of facilities) had been taken care of, the rate (or incidence) of "fresh" cases began to decline.

[5] For a good study on this, see Joseph Eaton and Robert Weil, *Culture and Mental Disorder*, Glencoe, Illinois, 1955.

Nature and Size of the Problem

GENERAL MORBIDITY

Since Stalin died in 1953, the Soviet regime has been more generous with statistics on many aspects of its social and economic life. Unfortunately this generosity has not extended, so far, to information on national morbidity: for instance, two statistical handbooks on medicine and public health, one published in 1957,[6] the other in 1960,[7] do not contain any data on causes of death or on the incidence and prevalence of disease. Fragmentary information applying to certain regions, cities, industrial or agricultural enterprises may sometimes be found in professional journals. Attention tends to be focused on those medical and public health problems that cause loss of work capacity, and on the measures that should be taken to reduce these causes. Conditions such as upper respiratory infections, influenza, diseases of the gastrointestinal tract, cancer, heart disease and industrial injuries occupy the limelight of Soviet medical concern, as might well be expected in a country undergoing rapid industrialization, urbanization and mechanization. Mental illness, by contrast, receives much less attention. Nonetheless, according to Kline, a most competent observer, Soviet authorities told him they believe that the prevalence of psychoses in the Soviet Union does not differ materially from that in other countries and ranges between 3 and 7 per 1000 of the population.[8]

More accurate Soviet data are available for one of the cities of the Belorussian SSR (unspecified, but presumably Minsk) for 1955.[9] According to a survey, the reported prevalence of all illnesses (except those of the mouth and teeth) was 1106.1 per 1000, or slightly over one illness per person. Psychiatric illnesses are included in these rates and are given as follows.

	Prevalence of illness per 1000 of population		
	Men	Women	All
Psychic disturbances	5.7	3.1	4.2
Diseases of the nervous system	57.9	59.7	58.9
All illnesses	1198.2	1036.7	1106.1

[6] *Zdravookhranenie v SSSR* (Health Services in the USSR), Moscow, 1957.

[7] *Zdravookhranenie v SSSR* (Health Services in the USSR), Moscow, 1960.

[8] Nathan S. Kline, The organization of psychiatric care and psychiatric research in the Union of Soviet Socialist Republics. *Annals of the New York Academy of Sciences*, New York, **84**, 1960, Art. 4.

[9] *Bolshaya Meditsinskaya Entsiklopediya* (Large Medical Encyclopedia), 2nd ed., **10**, Moscow, 1959, col. 520.

The first figure apparently refers to the psychoses, and is thus within the limits of the estimates reported to Kline; the second figure presumably refers to the neuroses and other mental disturbances and is probably a less accurate one for comparative purposes because of the greater importance of cultural factors in recognizing, defining and diagnosing neuroses and mental disturbances. It is significant to note, however, that if one totals the Soviet figures for psychiatric illnesses (using the Soviet rubrics of "psychic disturbances" and "diseases of the nervous system"), the results are strikingly similar to those of some of the American intensive prevalence studies on the subject.[10] If we consider only the psychotics this would mean that the Soviet Union, with a population conservatively estimated at 220 million in mid-1962[11] would have (very roughly) between 650,000 and 1½ million psychotics. Using such estimates, the sheer *magnitude* of the Soviet problem would not seem to be too different from the one faced by the United States, with its population of over 186 million in mid-1962.[12] It is interesting to note, however, that Rapoport, reviewing Kline's paper and without giving any statistical evidence, disputes the figure reported by Kline and insists on the relatively low rate of mental illness in the Soviet Union when compared to foreign countries.[13] Some of his reasoning is as follows:

> . . . the index of 3 to 7 per 1000 does not mean anything: for, if the index of 3 is basically correct then it means a morbidity significantly lower in the USSR, and if the index is 7 then it only approaches the lowest levels [given in] foreign statistics . . . and besides, one must consider that many [out-patient] clinics take a broad view of the term mental illness, including in it alcoholism, epilepsy, drug addiction, reactive states, arteriosclerosis and many other groups without psychosis as such. Further, American statistics essentially are based on data on the number of mental patients who are hospitalized, only partly supplemented by data from physicians in private practice and are therefore far from complete. Soviet statistics are based not only on information from the hospitals, but also on the card files of [out-patient] clinics, where all the mental patients of a given city or district (including also patients with "borderline" states—neuroses, psychopathies, alcoholism) are accounted and treated.

While Rapoport (who still does not give any numerical data) may or may not be correct in that Soviet statistics have a broader definition of the term "mental illness", he does not recognize that the prevalence studies done in United States communities are attempts to find the total morbidity existing in the population at large, without restricting it to those who are under

[10] See, for example, Paul Lemkau, Mental hygiene problems in an urban district, *Mental Hygiene*, Concord, New Hampshire, **24**, 1941, pp. 624–46; **26**, 1942, pp. 100–19, also W. P. Roth and F. H. Luton. The mental health program in Tennessee, *American Journal of Psychiatry*, Hanover, New Hampshire, **99**, 1943, p. 662.

[11] Estimate based on a population on January 1, 1961 of about 216 million and a rate of natural increase of about 1·7% (*Narodnoe khozyaistvo SSSR v 1960 godu* [The National Economy of the USSR in 1960], Moscow, 1961, p. 7).

[12] Figure issued by the Bureau of the Census on July 19, 1962, giving a population as of June 1, 1962 of 186,367,000, including Armed Forces overseas. (Boston Regional Office of the Census Bureau, personal communication.)

[13] A. M. Rapoport, In *Zhurnal nevropatologii i psikhiatrii imeni S. S. Korsakova*, **62**, 1962, No. 3, pp. 453–60, quotes N. S. Kline (see footnote 8).

treatment, whereas obviously Soviet morbidity figures are based only on those patients presently or formerly under either hospital or clinic treatment.

Furthermore, Rapoport, citing the Lemkau (1936) and the Roth (1938) surveys, indicates that they do not include the mentally retarded and epileptics, who are apparently included in the statistics of Soviet clinics. This is not quite correct: the Lemkau survey, otherwise known as the Eastern Health District Study, included psychosis, psychoneurosis, psychopathic personality, personality disorder (adults), behavior disorder (children), minor or possible disorder, epilepsy, mental deficiency, school progress problem and adult delinquency. It also included social problems such as school maladjustment, delinquent behavior, work adjustment difficulties, marital difficulties, difficulties over relations with social agencies, sex problems, alcoholism, drug addiction, suicide and institutionalization.[14] The Roth survey of mental illness in Tennessee, covering the entire population of three rural districts, used 87 diagnostic categories to classify three broad forms of mental illness: (1) mental disorders, personality and behavior problems; (2) mental deficiency; (3) organic and miscellaneous cases.[15]

At any rate, given the information at our disposal and granting the many difficulties in this area, it is not likely that this controversy will soon be settled. What emerges, however, is that the Soviet claim of a lower rate of mental illness often appears to be in the nature of an *a priori* assumption, based more on ideological premises than facts: indeed, in theory (from the Soviet viewpoint, of course) there *should* be less mental illness in a socialist society of the Soviet type than under American "capitalism". By the same token there *should* be less alcoholism, crime and juvenile delinquency. Again, the absence of statistics makes it difficult to verify the claim. However, from what can be inferred from the qualitative evidence in the Soviet press this may not necessarily be the case.[16] Thus, in the absence of contrary evidence and using Kline's estimate (which does not seem unreasonable), the magnitude of the Soviet mental illness problem seems quite similar to that of the American. This similarity would then (if true) tend to highlight a major *dissimilarity* in the disposition of psychotic patients, particularly with respect to their hospitalization, which does reflect, as we shall see later, rather favorably on the Soviet psychiatric system.

TREATED MORBIDITY

For comparative purposes it is also unfortunate that the Soviet Union does not issue statistical reports of *hospitalized* mental patients similar to

[14] Richard J. Plunkett and John E. Gordon, *Epidemiology and Mental Illness*, New York, 1960, pp. 71–2.

[15] *Ibid.*, p. 72.

[16] Mark G. Field, Alcoholism, crime and delinquency in Soviet society, *Social Problems*, **3**, No. 2, New York, 1955, pp. 100–9. Attempts to obtain such figures during a visit to the Soviet Union early in 1963 were unsuccessful.

those of the US Public Health Service.[17] The only data of a somewhat comparable nature were given by Snezhnevskiy in 1959 in an article presenting what purports to be the percentage distribution of hospitalized mental patients in the Soviet Union according to diagnosis for the years 1950–4.[18] An attempt to compare these figures with American data is not only an exercise in frustration but also presents several methodological problems to which no categorical answer can be given until we know much more about the Soviet psychiatric system. For one, the Soviets (in general, and in the cited table in particular) use a smaller number of diagnostic categories than the American reporting system. The problem is further compounded by the fact that the American reports sometimes tend to be inconsistent and to change from year to year. Thus, the difference in the sheer number of categories means that the more than 30 entries in the American sources must be collapsed into the 16 used in the Soviet table given by Snezhnevskiy. I made an attempt, with the assistance of two American psychiatrists (Drs. Jason Aronson and Nathan S. Kline), to reduce the American categories to the Soviet ones, and the result of this effort was given in my original paper on this subject.[19] My colleagues and I were fortunate, subsequently, in having the opportunity to check this reduction with Professors Snezhnevskiy and Kerbikov in the course of one of their visits to the United States, and the results of that discussion were published in the *American Journal of Psychiatry*.[20]

It appeared that we had been essentially correct except for the following points: we had placed the American "Birth Trauma" category under the Soviet category of "Traumatic Psychoses". It would fit better under the Soviet category of "Oligophrenia", and the revised table presented here (Table 1) incorporates this change. Another place where we went wrong concerns the group we know as paranoid states or paranoia. Since no such category was given in the Soviet table, we had assumed it would fit under "Schizophrenia". According to our informants, patients with fixed but limited paranoid delusions who are free from hallucinations and show no "primary changes" belong under the classification of reactive disorders, since this is where, in the Soviet Union, transient paranoid episodes and paranoia are listed. There must be other changes in personality beside the paranoid delusion in order to establish the diagnosis of schizophrenia. This

[17] US Department of Health, Education and Welfare, Public Health Service, *Patients in Mental Institutions*, Washington, D.C. (yearly reports).

[18] Prof. A. V. Snezhnevskiy, Dispensary method of registering psychiatric morbidity and the Soviet system of psychiatric service, *Living Conditions and Health*, World Medical Council, Vienna, **1**, 1959, No. 4, pp. 236–41.

[19] Mark G. Field, Approaches to mental illness in Soviet society: some comparisons and conjectures, *Social Problems*, **7**, No. 4, 1960, pp. 277–97.

[20] Nathan S. Kline, Mark G. Field and Jason Aronson, Soviet psychiatric nomenclature, *American Journal of Psychiatry*, Hanover, New Hampshire, **118**, August 1961, pp. 178–80.

correction has also been incorporated in the table. Another difficulty is that the Soviet data give no indication of the numbers, age and sex of the patients these percentages represent, the numbers and types of hospitals reporting, or the geographic areas surveyed. On the American side, the problem was to decide which kinds of hospitals reporting to the federal government should be included in the comparison. American data are given for four categories of mental hospitals: (1) public institutions for mental defectives and epileptics; (2) public hospitals for the mentally ill; (3) private hospitals for the mentally ill and general hospitals with psychiatric facilities; and (4) private institutions for mental defectives and epileptics. Since the Soviet Union does not have, to my knowledge, any private medical institutions it would seem appropriate to include, in the American figures, private as well as public hospitals on the assumption that a patient hospitalized in a private hospital in the United States would have to go to a public one in the Soviet Union.[21] The same considerations would apply to epileptics, so that epileptics in private institutions were included in the American figures. The placing of the mental defectives was done as follows: we know there are special institutions for the mental defectives or oligophrenics in the Soviet Union (under either the Ministry of Education or that of Social Welfare), so that it might be reasonable to exclude from the American figures patients in public and private institutions for the mental defectives (but retaining, as is probably the case in the Soviet Union, mental defectives in mental hospitals).

It must be recognized, however, that in the light of differences in cultures, psychiatric organizations and of gaps in knowledge strict comparability is problematical and the decisions taken must, in the nature of the case, remain somewhat arbitrary. It is in the light of the above questions, limitations and qualifications that one may look at Table 1. One similarity is immediately apparent: according to the data, hospitalized patients who suffer from schizophrenia constitute the largest single group in the two societies, accounting for slightly over one-third of all patients, and that proportion increased slightly from year to year in the two societies. It may be noted, furthermore, that in 1954 schizophrenics accounted for only 28.8 percent of admissions to Soviet mental hospitals, but represented 58.6 percent of all patients occupying beds in these hospitals at the beginning of that year, and 54.9 percent at the end of the year, as against 37.6 percent and 37.1 percent respectively in American hospitals. While the increase in the percentage of patients diagnosed as schizophrenics from 1950 to 1954[22] cannot, of course, be taken as evidence of an increase in the incidence (i.e. "fresh cases") of schizophrenia in the

[21] In the table presented in the original paper I had excluded patients in the United States who were not in public mental hospitals. Further work on the Soviet psychiatric system led me to believe that this might not be justifiable.

[22] A. M. Rapoport, On the composition and movement of patients in the psychiatric institutions of the USSR, *Zhurnal nevropatologii i psikhiatrii imeni S. S. Korsakova*, **57**, 1957, No. 1, pp. 95–103.

TABLE 1.

Distribution of Diagnoses per 100 Patients in Soviet Mental Hospitals and in American Public and Private Mental Institutions (1950–4)

Diagnosis	Soviet Union			United States		
	1950	1952	1954	1950	1952	1954
Schizophrenia[a]	32.3	34.7	37.4	33.80	35.71	37.10
Epilepsy[b]	10.5	10.7	9.7	7.04	6.73	5.52
Manic Depressive Psychosis[c]	2.2	1.9	1.7	6.82	6.93	5.77
Cerebral Arteriosclerosis and Other Circulatory Disorders[d]	4.0	3.8	4.4	6.03	5.87	6.68
Senile Psychosis[e]	3.1	2.8	3.1	5.26	5.70	5.16
Lues Cerebri (Cerebral Syphilis)[f]	1.1	1.1	1.0	0.68	0.61	0.53
Progressive Paralysis[g]	1.0	0.9	1.1	3.61	3.53	3.22
Infectious Psychoses[h]	2.8	2.1	2.1	0.37	0.40	0.26
Intoxication Psychoses[i]	1.0	0.8	0.4	0.32	0.33	0.08
Alcoholic Psychosis and Chronic Alcoholism[j]	7.1	9.0	10.4	9.72	8.69	7.73
Narcomania (Drug Addiction)[k]	0.9	0.5	0.4	0.37	0.42	0.47
Traumatic Psychoses[l]	5.6	5.8	4.8	0.38	0.42	0.40
Psychopathies[m]	4.6	3.8	3.8	6.54	7.21	6.57
Oligophrenia[n]	3.9	3.5	3.4	1.90	0.84	0.88
Neuroses and Reactive Disorders[o]	7.3	7.0	6.8	7.78	8.91	10.28
Other Neuro-psychiatric Diseases and Examination Cases[p]	12.6	11.6	9.5	9.38	7.71	9.34

[a] Includes the American diagnosis of "Schizophrenia (dementia praecox)".

[b] Includes "psychoses with convulsive disorders".

[c] Includes "manic depressive psychosis".

[d] Includes "psychosis with cerebral arteriosclerosis" and "psychosis with other disturbances of the circulation".

[e] Includes "psychoses—senile".

[f] Includes "psychoses—with other forms of syphilis of the central nervous system".

[g] Includes "chronic brain syndromes associated with meningoencephalitic syphilis", sometimes given as "psychoses—with general paresis".

[h] Includes "chronic brain syndromes associated with epidemic encephalitis" and "other intracranial infections".

[i] Includes "acute brain syndromes associated with drug or poison intoxication", and "chronic brain syndromes associated with drug or poison intoxication".

[j] Includes "acute brain syndromes associated with alcoholic intoxication", "chronic brain syndromes associated with alcoholic intoxication", and "personality disorders: alcoholism addiction".

[k] Includes "personality disorders: drug addiction".

[l] Includes "psychoses—traumatic".

[m] Includes "personality disorders: anti-social reaction, dyssocial reaction", sometimes given as "psychopathic personality".

[n] Includes "chronic brain syndromes associated with disease and conditions due to prenatal influence", "birth trauma", and "mental deficiency".

[o] Includes "psychotic disorders: paranoid reactions", "psychophysiologic autonomic and visceral disorders", "psychoneurotic reactions", "personality disorders: personality pattern disturbance, personality trait disturbance, sexual deviation, special symptom reaction", and "transient situational personality disturbance".

[p] Includes "acute brain syndromes associated with all other conditions", "chronic brain syndromes associated with diseases of unknown cause", "chronic brain syndromes of unknown cause", "psychotic disorders: other mental disorder", "intracranial neoplasm", and "undiagnosed".

SOURCES: *Living Conditions and Health*, World Medical Council, Vienna, 1959, No. 4, p. 240; *Patients in Mental Institutions 1950 and 1951, Patients in Mental Institutions 1952, Patients in Mental Institutions 1954*, US Department of Health, Education and Welfare, Washington, D.C.

society at large, since the increase may be due simply to a decrease in the number of patients suffering from other disorders, it nevertheless seems to indicate that in the two societies the condition known as schizophrenia is still a major (and unresolved) psychiatric problem, as most Soviet psychiatrists and their American colleagues would agree. An attempt to explain the major differences in the other conditions (outside of the weaknesses inherent in any such type of reporting) must make use of the factors listed below, either singly or in combination. These factors, which are not necessarily exhaustive, and most of which will be examined in greater detail subsequently, are suggestive of the multiplicity of causes behind the make-up of the resident population of mental hospitals in any society. Furthermore, these factors should not be restricted only to a comparison of tables of hospitalized patients; they also suggest some of the basic elements at work in the two (and other) societies that might account for similarities and dissimilarities in mental illness. Their relevance, it is suggested, is thus broader than this specific comparison.

1. Nature of the Problem

(a) It is quite possible that the two social structures produce different types and rates of some mental illnesses. (b) The differences in the age[23] and the sex ratio of the population may account for such differences as are visible in the figures for the senile psychoses (which include involutional psychotic reactions), cerebral arteriosclerosis and other circulatory disorders, progressive paralysis, and perhaps manic-depressive psychoses.[24] (c) The differences in the traumatic psychoses might be accounted for, as Soviet specialists often suggest, by the many head injuries suffered by the civilian and military population as a result of the Second World War.[25] Additional explanation may lie in the nature of an expanding economy with an inexperienced work force drawn from the rural population and the rudimentary safety precautions that often accompany the early stages of industrialism. This may then lead to a relatively high level of industrial

---

[23] For example, 13 percent of the population in the United States in 1960 was 60 years old and older, as against 9.4 percent of the Soviet population in 1959 (*Statistical Abstract of the United States*, Bureau of the Census, Washington, D.C., 1961, p. 28, and *Narodnoe khozyaistvo SSSR v 1960 godu*, p. 11).

[24] On January 1, 1961, it can be estimated that there were about 20 million more women than men in a total Soviet population of 216 million. This surplus of women was not distributed evenly among all age groups but was located primarily in the age group over 32, i.e., those members of the population affected by the Second World War. Thus, while for the entire Soviet population the sex ratio was 45 percent male and 55 percent female, in the older age categories this ratio was much more unbalanced in the direction of more females than males. In the United States the sex ratio was 49 percent males and 51 percent females (*Vestnik statistiki*, 1962, No. 3, p. 91, and *Statistical Abstract of the United States*, 1961, p. 28).

[25] Rapoport, *op. cit.*, p. 455.

traumatism, including head injuries. (See also 4 (a) below for another suggested explanation.)

2. Nature of Social Organization

(a) Differences in social organization may, for example, permit the Soviets to maintain a relatively greater proportion of mental patients within a family surrounding because of the greater proportion of rural households (about half) than would be the case in a more urbanized society such as the United States. This would apply particularly to the so-called senior citizens who are sometimes admitted to American public mental hospitals because they have nowhere else to go. (b) The nature of the Soviet system of social welfare benefits, pensions and other aids makes it possible (and sometimes financially advantageous) for a family to keep a mental patient at home, particularly if the mental hospital or psychoneurological clinic provides an additional stipend to the family explicitly for that purpose, as it sometimes does.

3. Nature of the Psychiatric Resources Available

(a) Relative differences in the availability of psychiatric institutions and in the number of psychiatric beds may limit the hospitalization of certain categories of psychiatric patients, schizophrenics and oligophrenics, for example. (b) The existence of *alternatives to hospitalization* (out-patient care, day hospitals, family or foster-family care and sheltered workshops) may affect the composition of the hospitalized population.

4. Nature of the Therapeutic Orientation and Practices

(a) A greater Soviet emphasis on, for example, an organic, physiological or sociological interpretation (in Marxist terms, a "materialistic" approach) of the etiology of mental illness may mean a greater propensity on the part of Soviet psychiatrists to diagnose patients in organic (rather than dynamic) terms. This might apply, for example, to the traumatic psychoses (in addition to other factors mentioned under 1 (c) above). (b) Although the figures of Table 1 do not reflect this, Soviet psychiatrists apparently (and for many reasons, some of which will be examined below) try not to hospitalize psychotics if they can at all be maintained in the community, but will be more ready to hospitalize neurotics than their American colleagues, on the assumption that neuroses are the result of environmental factors and that the hospital provides a different and more therapeutic *milieu* in which the patient's "tired" nervous system may rest. It is interesting to note, just in passing, that if one were to remove from the American figures those neurotics hospitalized in private hospitals for the mentally ill and general hospitals with psychiatric facilities, the percentage of neurotics in American public hospitals would fall to a figure significantly lower than that of the USSR. Indeed, according to the computations made in the original article, as well as those made by Kline (both of which excluded American private mental hospitals and psychiatric sections of general hospitals), the percentage of hospitalized neurotics in the Soviet Union would be about six times larger than that in the United States. Commenting on these figures as they appeared in the Kline paper, Rapoport wrote:

> ... this can be explained by the efforts of Soviet physicians to remove the patient with a neurosis from a traumatizing milieu (as Kline suggests) and by the preventive work of psychiatric clinics which strive to provide hospital care also for patients with "border-line" conditions . . . neurotics are almost never admitted to mental hospitals in the USA. . . .[26]

What seems to happen in the United States is that patients admitted to public mental hospitals and who come from lower socio-economic backgrounds tend to be diagnosed in most instances as psychotics rather than neurotics, while the reverse phenomenon obtains for middle and upper socio-economic class patients admitted to private mental institutions, as Redlich and Hollingshead have pointed out in their study of social class and mental illness.[27] (c) Differences in general medical organization and philosophy may also mean differences in the paths and barriers (financial, for example) to psychiatric care (socialized medicine as against private practice), which may then be reflected in the composition of the hospitalized population.

This is about as far as one might want to pursue this comparative examination. Generally speaking, the impression emerges that the problem posed by mental illness in the two societies is not strikingly dissimilar. At the same time it should be clear that the statistics of the resident population in mental hospitals (or of admissions to these hospitals, or first visits to clinics) cannot be interpreted as accurately reflecting the true incidence and prevalence of psychiatric morbidity in the community and this for the reason that many conditions never come to the attention of psychiatric personnel and institutions. As one study of the Joint Commission on Mental Illness and Health has pointed out: "Hospital data have been of limited value . . . because they exclude the great majority of the mentally ill who escape institutionalization by virtue of the relative mildness of their symptoms."[28]

26 Rapoport, op. cit., p. 455.

27 August B. Hollingshead and Frederick C. Redlich, Social Class and Mental Illness, New York, 1958, pp. 220–50. An additional problem is that this category includes not only the neuroses but also reactive disorders (including paranoid reactions).

28 Plunkett and Gordon, op. cit., p. xi.

Personnel and Facilities

We are on statistically firmer ground when we turn our attention to psychiatric personnel and facilities.

PERSONNEL

There does not seem to be a sharp differentiation between neurologist (or neuropathologist) and psychiatrist in the Soviet Union. The neurologist often acts as a psychiatrist and the psychiatrist as a neurologist. As Zilboorg pointed out, the tradition of Russian and Soviet psychiatry is more French than German, and the orientation as a whole that of the neuropsychiatrists of whom Henri Claude is the typical representative.[29]

At the end of 1962, there were 20,100 psychiatrists and neuropathologists in the Soviet Union, about 40 percent belonging to the first category. I shall refer to both categories as "psychiatrists", although a relatively small number of neuropathologists handle primarily neurological rather than psychiatric cases.[30] As a rule, however, the *neuro*pathologist is more likely to treat *neuroses*, or what the Soviets call "nervous diseases", and the *psychiatrists* the psychoses, or what the Soviets call "psychic diseases" or "disturbances". But psychiatrists who work in out-patient clinics also treat neurotic patients, referring them, when indicated, to hospitals for treatment.[31]

At the gross national level, the proportion of psychiatrists (as defined above) to the population appears to be higher in the Soviet Union than in the United States (as is also, incidentally, the proportion of physicians to the population). As can be gathered from Table 2, there were in the United States an average of 7–8 psychiatrists per 100,000 of population as against 9 in the Soviet Union (1962). These figures, of course, cannot reflect regional variations. Such variations can be observed when one examines the number of psychiatrists per constant units of population in the Soviet constituent republics and in the different American states. We find, for example, in 1959 that Latvia and Estonia had about 50 percent more psychiatrists per population than the national average; while Georgia, Armenia, the RSFSR and the Ukraine were slightly above the national average; and such Central Asian republics as Tadzhikistan and Uzbekistan had from about one-third to one-half less than the national average. In the United States, in 1956, the Northeast had a number of psychiatrists per population that was 70 percent higher than the national average, the West about 15 percent higher, the North Central states about 25 percent below that average and the South

[29] Gregory Zilboorg, Some aspects of psychiatry in the USSR, *American Review of Soviet Medicine*, New York, August 1944, p. 563.
[30] Kline, *op. cit.*, p. 150.
[31] Rapoport, *op. cit.*, p. 453.

(less the District of Columbia) 43 percent below the average for the nation. Among the factors that account for these variations, the degree of urbanization (resulting from industrialization) is undoubtedly the major one for the two countries. Ranking the Soviet republics according to urbanization and the supply of psychiatrists results in a rank order correlation of .76; the same ranking done for the ten most and ten least industrialized American states yields a correlation of .84 (.87 if all the states are included), indicating in both the Soviet and American cases a substantial relationship. Further, in the United States the ten most urbanized states of the union (including the District of Columbia) had 65.8 percent of all psychiatrists in 1957, while the ten least urbanized ones had only 4.6 percent. In the ten most urbanized states there were about three times as many psychiatrists per population than in the ten least urbanized states.[32]

Similar trends may be observed in the Soviet Union using the statistics for the fifteen constituent republics. Thus, as Table 3 shows, the five republics with the most highly urbanized population have about three-fourths of all

TABLE 2.

Estimate of Population and Psychiatric Professional Personnel,
Soviet Union and United States (1962)

	Soviet Union[a]	United States[b]
Total population	223,100,000	186,656,000
Psychiatrists	20,100[c]	13,000[d]–15,000[e]
Population per psychiatrist	11,099	14,358–12,443
Psychiatrist per 100,000	9	7–8

[a] Figure for December 31, 1962 from *Narodnoe khozyaistvo SSSR v 1962 godu* (The National Economy of the USSR in 1962), Moscow, 1963, pp. 8 and 617.

[b] Figure for July 1, 1962 from US Bureau of the Census, *Statistical Abstract of the United States, 1964*, Washington, D.C., 1964, p. 5.

[c] Includes 7928 psychiatrists and 12,172 neuropathologists.

[d] Estimate based on American Psychiatric Association, *Biographical Directory of Fellows and Members of the APA*, as of May 8, 1962 (R. R. Bowker, New York, 1963).

[e] A higher estimate for the number of psychiatrists in the United States may be derived from those who list themselves as psychiatrists with the American Medical Association, and includes physicians who are working in a situation of a psychiatric nature. For example, a foreign physician working in a state hospital may list himself as a psychiatrist; in addition, there are a number of residents in psychiatric training who have not yet become eligible for APA membership or who have not applied for membership. (Information from a letter from Walter E. Barton, M.D., Medical Director, American Psychiatric Association, January 6, 1965.) The number of psychiatrists in active practice rose from 5800 in 1950 to about 13,000 in 1960, and the projected estimate for 1965 is 17,800, so that an estimated 15,000 psychiatrists for 1962 is within these limits. (Blue Cross Reports, *New Directions Toward Community Mental Health*, **2**, No. 3, July–Sept. 1964, p. 10.)

[32] George W. Albee, *Mental Health Manpower Trends*, New York, 1959, Appendix I, Table 30, p. 302.

TABLE 3.

Urbanization and the Number of Psychiatrists to Population, by Soviet Constituent Republics (1959) and by America's Ten Most and Ten Least Urbanized States (1957)

SOVIET UNION

Urbanization rank	Population	Number of psychiatrists per 100,000	Rank: psychiatrists to population
1 Latvia	2,093,000	11.56	1
2 Estonia	1,197,000	10.02	2
3 RSFSR	117,534,000	8.22	5
4 Armenia	1,763,000	8.62	4
5 Azerbaidzhan	3,698,000	6.73	8
6 Ukraine	41,869,000	8.05	6
7 Turkmenistan	1,516,000	7.19	7
8 Kazakhstan	9,310,000	4.40	14
9 Georgia	4,044,000	9.62	3
10 Lithuania	2,711,000	5.49	11
11 Uzbekistan	8,106,000	3.95	15
12 Kirghizia	2,066,000	5.62	10
13 Tadzhikistan	1,980,000	5.00	12
14 Belorussia	8,055,000	5.96	9
15 Moldavia	2,885,000	4.93	13

SOURCE: *Zdravookhranenie v SSSR* (Health Services in the USSR), Moscow, 1960, pp. 16, 19, 86–100.

UNITED STATES

Urbanization rank	Population	Number of psychiatrists per 100,000	Rank: psychiatrists to population
1 District of Columbia	866,000	24.1	1
2 New Jersey	5,403,000	4.8	14
3 New York	16,195,000	13.2	2
4 Massachusetts	4,812,000	10.5	4
5 Rhode Island	828,000	5.0	11
6 California	13,433,000	7.9	6
7 Connecticut	2,232,000	11.3	3
8 Illinois	9,432,000	4.9	12
9 Michigan	7,516,000	4.6	16
10 Pennsylvania	10,964,000	5.4	9
40 Idaho	625,000	1.8	41
41 Kentucky	3,017,000	2.9	29
42 South Carolina	2,353,000	1.5	45
43 Vermont	370,000	4.9	13
44 West Virginia	1,983,000	1.5	46
45 North Carolina	4,423,000	2.7	32
46 South Dakota	696,000	1.6	44
47 Arkansas	1,815,000	3.3	25
48 Mississippi	2,124,000	1.5	48
49 North Dakota	657,000	1.4	49

SOURCE: George W. Albee, *Mental Health Manpower Trends*, New York, 1959, Appendix I, Table 31, pp. 302–3.

Soviet psychiatrists; the five republics with the least urbanized population only about 7 percent. Or, interpreted as the number of psychiatrists per population, the five most highly urbanized republics have a proportion of psychiatrists to population that is 7 percent higher than the national average, the five least urbanized a proportion that is lower by 35 percent than the national average. While the American states cannot strictly be compared with the fifteen Soviet republics, it may be interesting to note that with the exception of the District of Columbia (which is atypical in any case) the trends are somewhat similar, but that the least urbanized American states have considerably fewer psychiatrists per population (with the exception of Vermont) than the least urbanized Soviet republics. Indeed, the Soviet republic with the lowest number of psychiatrists (Uzbekistan) has more psychiatrists than the ten least urbanized American states (again except Vermont). Actually, if we examine all American states, 32 have fewer psychiatrists than Uzbekistan.

At the same time, not only is the number of psychiatrists (at the national level) more favorable in the USSR than in the United States, but the rate at which the Soviets are training physicians should permit them, if they so choose, to increase substantially the number of psychiatrists in the near future.

TABLE 4.

Physicians and Psychiatrists, Soviet Union and United States, 1950–62

SOVIET UNION (Figures for End of Year)

	1950	1955	1958	1959	1960	1961	1962
Physicians	247,346	310,175	361,544	379,501	401,612	425,745	445,116
Psychiatrists[a]	8,237	12,353	15,000	15,996	16,932	18,485	20,100

SOURCES: *Zdravookhranenie v SSSR* (Health Services in the USSR), Moscow, 1960; *Narodnoe khozyaistvo SSSR v 1961 godu* (The National Economy of the USSR in 1961), Moscow, 1962, pp. 744–6; *Narodnoe khozyaistvo SSSR v 1962 godu*, Moscow, 1963, p. 617.

UNITED STATES (Figures for Mid-year)

	1950	1955	1958	1959	1960	1961	1962
Physicians	204,100[b]	218,061	231,700[c]	236,818	241,617	245,796	257,035
Psychiatrists	5,856	8,354	9,801	10,420	11,037	11,637	13,000

a Figures include both psychiatrists and neuropathologists. The psychiatrists make up between 33 percent and 40 percent of the total.

b This figure is an estimate based on the given figures of 201,277 for 1949 and 218,061 for 1955.

c This figure is an estimate based on the given figures of 226,625 for 1957 and 236,818 for 1959.

SOURCES: *Statistical Abstract of the United States: 1961*, US Bureau of the Census, Washington, D.C., 1961, p. 69; *Statistical Abstract of the United States: 1962*, US Bureau of the Census, Washington, D.C., 1962, p. 74; *Statistical Abstract of the United States: 1963*, US Bureau of the Census, Washington, D.C., 1963, p. 74; *Statistical Abstract of the United States: 1964*, US Bureau of the Census, Washington, D.C., 1964, p. 70; American Psychiatric Association, *List of Members*.

Thus, for example, between 1955 and 1962 the Soviet medical profession increased from 310,175 to 445,116, or had an average *net* annual increment of about 19,000 as against an average net annual increment of about 5,600 for the United States.[33] Table 4 shows the increase in total medical and psychiatric personnel in the Soviet Union and the United States from 1950 to 1962.

HOSPITAL FACILITIES

While at the gross national level the proportion of professional psychiatric personnel to the population appears more favorable in the Soviet Union than in the United States, the difference between the psychiatric systems of the two societies is nowhere more marked than in the number of mental hospital beds, or rather in the proportion of psychiatric beds both to the population and to non-psychiatric hospital beds. Using the latest available figures (for 1962), it can be seen that in the United States, as the title of a popular book

TABLE 5.

Population, Psychiatric and Non-psychiatric Hospital Beds
Soviet Union and United States, 1962

	Soviet Union[a]	United States[b]
Total population	223,100,000	186,656,000
Non-psychiatric beds	1,718,900	906,272
Psychiatric beds	222,600	783,142[c]
Total number of beds	1,941,500	1,689,414
Percentage, psychiatric beds of all beds	11.46	46.35
Proportion, psychiatric to non-psychiatric beds	1: 7.72	1: 1.16
Psychiatric beds per 1000 of population	.99	4.19
Number of persons per one psychiatric bed	1002	238

[a] For December 31, 1962.

[b] For July 1, 1962, includes Armed Forces Overseas.

[c] Estimate based on proportion of Federal Psychiatric Beds to All Federal Beds for 1957 and projected to 1962 (66,142) plus 717,000 Non-Federal Psychiatric Beds.

SOURCES: *Narodnoe khozyaistvo SSSR v 1962* (The National Economy of the USSR in 1962), Moscow, 1963, pp. 8 and 617; *Statistical Abstract of the United States*, 1962, p. 5; 1963, pp. 79–84; and 1964, pp. 5 and 70.

[33] It should be noted that Soviet statistics of physicians include stomatologists, i.e. dental doctors (who account for about 4 percent of the total). In addition, a much greater proportion of Soviet professional medical personnel are engaged in the administration of health services than is true in the United States. Recent statistics of American medical professionals have included, in some instances, doctors of ostheopathy. Thus the *Statistical Abstract* indicates a grand total of 271,700 physicians for the United States in 1962; this figure includes 257,035 M.D.s (the figure used in Table 4) and 14,665 D.O.s.

on the subject once suggested, *Every Other Bed*[34] is a mental hospital bed.
By contrast, in the Soviet Union only about *every eighth bed* is used for psychiatric purposes. If, furthermore, we consider the fact that the *total* number
of hospital beds for the two societies is of about the same magnitude we
conclude there is a vastly different pattern of hospital bed utilization. As the
figures in Table 5 show, for every psychiatric bed in the USSR there are
7.72 non-psychiatric ones; in the United States for every psychiatric bed there
are only 1.16 non-psychiatric beds. This means, of course, a significant
difference in the supply of psychiatric beds to the population: in the Soviet
Union there is about one such bed per 1000 of the population as against over
four (4.19) in the United States. Expressed in terms of persons per one
psychiatric bed, there were in the Soviet Union 1002 such persons per bed as
against only 238 in the United States. While these figures are valid for 1962,
it is unlikely that they would have changed significantly in the past few years.
Again, several not mutually exclusive explanations (apart from therapeutic
considerations to be examined later) suggest themselves:

1. The possibility, as the Soviet sources suggest, that Soviet psychiatric
morbidity is so much lower than the American that only a much smaller
proportion of beds need be earmarked for mental illness;

2. The further possibility that the nature of psychiatric morbidity is such
that only a small proportion of mental patients need hospitalization;

3. The impact upon the health of the population of high speed, massive
industrialization, with its concomitant transfer from rural areas to the
crowded, unsanitary, and environmentally different living conditions in
urban areas and factory towns. These conditions initially provide fertile
ground for the spread of infectious diseases, including tuberculosis (which is
still a major Soviet health problem), as they did in Europe in the nineteenth
century following the Industrial Revolution. Under those circumstances it
makes sense to devote as much bed capacity as possible to these diseases
rather than to mental illness;

4. The need on the part of the regime for the maximum utilization of manpower in industrialization, particularly in the light of grievous population
losses and birth deficits following both world wars and associated social and
political traumas. Under those circumstances it would appear logical to
encourage any treatment or handling of the mentally ill that could be carried
out without hospitals and their expensive "hotel" functions, and would simultaneously utilize their residual work capacity in industry and agriculture;

5. The general scarcity of roofed facilities in the Soviet Union, accentuated
by massive programs of industrialization and urbanization carried out since
the beginning of the Five-Year Plans at the end of the twenties and aggravated by the massive destruction of housing capital during the Second
World War. With topmost priority going to industry, with the concomitant

[34] Mike Gorman, *Every Other Bed*, New York, 1956.

scarcity of capital and other resources medical buildings (as well as housing) have had to assume, perforce, a secondary if not a residual priority. In the Soviet Union hospitals, and particularly mental hospitals, are likely to be housed either in facilities built before the Revolution or in buildings that originally had been erected for non-medical purposes and were then converted;

6. In spite of rapid industrialization and urbanization still about half of the Soviet population[35] lives in rural surroundings where the mentally ill are less disturbing and better accepted and cared for in the community than in the over-crowded urban conditions. The village idiot does not have an equally accepted city counterpart. As Dubos has remarked, the problem of our times may be less an actual increase of the mentally ill than a decrease in the tolerance of our (urban) society of them;[36]

7. The existence of collateral channels for the disposition of patients outside of the hospitals reduces the need for these facilities; further, a more *intensive* utilization of hospital facilities (as appears to be the case) may permit the psychiatric system to operate with a smaller number of beds than would be feasible otherwise.

Nevertheless (and in spite of a heavy commitment to non-hospital treatment of mental patients, as we shall see below) Soviet authorities are aware of a shortage of psychiatric beds and admit that "if more beds were available they would certainly be used by mentally ill people who are now in the community".[37] It should be noted, for example, that the absolute number of psychiatric beds in the USSR has more than doubled in the past decade and the number of mental hospitals has increased by more than 60 percent, while the population increased by only 16 percent. In addition, the rate of increase of psychiatric beds has been considerably more rapid than the rate of increase of general hospital beds over the same period. Rapoport states:

> Actually, many of our psychiatric hospitals are overcrowded, and although we do not need as many psychiatric beds as the USA, England and other countries (4 and more per 1000), the problem of an increase in the number of psychiatric beds is included in the plans of health protection for the next few years.[38]

Apparently the goal is in the vicinity of 1.3 to 1.5 (and perhaps slightly more) per 1000 population. The Moscow region, for example, which presently has a higher proportion of psychiatric beds to population than the national average, proposed to raise the number of these beds from 9675 (January 1, 1959) to 11,500 by the end of the Seven-Year Plan (January 1, 1966), an increase of over 18 percent that probably will be greater than the natural

[35] *Narodnoe khozyaistvo SSSR v 1961 godu* (The National Economy of the USSR in 1961), Moscow, 1962.
[36] René Dubos, *Mirage of Health*, New York, 1959, p. 173.
[37] Robert H. Klein, A visit to Kashchenko Mental Hospital, Moscow, *Mental Hospitals*, Washington, D.C., December 1958, p. 25.
[38] Rapoport, *op. cit.*, p. 455.

increase of the population, particularly since the relatively high rate of natural population increase maintained over the last few years (about 1.7 to 1.8 percent) is bound to decline as a result of serious birth deficits of the Second World War, and as a smaller number of persons will be having children in the mid-sixties and early seventies.[39] If the plans for the Moscow region are carried out this would mean about two psychiatric beds per 1000 by 1966.[40]

It may be interesting to note, in the comparative perspective, that while Soviet plans are to about double the rate of psychiatric beds per capita, the so-called Kennedy Program on Mental Illness and Retardation envisions, as one of the goals of the United States for the next decade, a reduction in the number of hospitalized mental patients by about one half. It thus appears that the two societies are converging toward approximately the same ratio of psychiatric beds to the population (about 2 beds per 1000 of population).

One of the consequences of this smaller proportion of beds to population (particularly when compared to the United States) is, thus, their more intensive use to accommodate the needs of mental patients, i.e., short periods of hospitalization and a relatively high turnover of patients. The policy is thus one of active treatment, the aim being to return the patient to the community as quickly as possible, even at the price of subsequent re-admissions. These readmissions are apparently no cause for undue concern on the part of Soviet psychiatrists, but simply an indication that the patient needs, at a certain point, the specific services available only in a hospital. For instance, at the Kashchenko Hospital (in Moscow), of the 9000 yearly admissions, 8500 are really readmissions and 500 are first admissions, while the hospital has a capacity of 2400 beds.[41]

The ratio of three admissions yearly per bed was also reported by Kline, who visited psychiatric institutions in the Leningrad area.[42] This is confirmed by Rapoport, who reports a yearly turnover of beds in 1954 of 2.8 with an average length of stay of 129 days for the USSR, RSFSR and Belorussian Republic; for the Ukraine, the turnover was slightly less, 2.5, and it was slightly higher in the Azerbaidzhan Republic (3.9), Uzbek (3.6), Estonian and Lithuanian Republics (3.1–3.2). In 1955, in the RSFSR the turnover was 2.7 and the average length of stay 130.7 days.[43] This must be contrasted with the use of hospital beds in the United States. In American public prolonged-care hospitals for mental diseases, with about 550,000 beds in 1956, there were 122,585 first admissions, 58,892

---

[39] Harry Schwartz, Birth rate shows decline in Soviet, *The New York Times*, September 9, 1962.

[40] Lapchenko, N. S., "Perspectives of the development of the public health network of Moscow for 1959–65", *Sovetskoe zdravookhranenie*, Moscow, 1959, No. 4, p. 10.

[41] Klein, *op. cit.*, p. 19.

[42] *Ibid.*, p. 158.

[43] "On the Composition and Movement. . . .", p. 95.

readmissions and 12,098 transfers,[44] or a ratio of about one admission to three beds. Contrasting these figures, it could be said that psychiatric beds are utilized nine times more intensively in the Soviet Union than in the United States.[45]

With more psychiatric personnel available than in the United States and fewer beds a greater staff to patient ratio can be maintained in Soviet hospitals. Most visitors emphasize that this certainly was the case in the facilities they visited,[46] and official Soviet norms confirm these impressions. This patient-to-staff ratio is in the vicinity of 1 to 1. In the United States the average is about 4 patients per full-time employee in public mental hospitals.[47] In the Soviet hospitals, for example, published figures indicate that a physician normally has 27.4 patients under his care,[48] whereas in American public mental hospitals this number is 183.9, or about seven times as many patients per physician.[49] The Soviet figure for physicians in mental hospitals is thus even better than the one recommended by the American Psychiatric Association of one physician per 30 patients in admission and intensive treatment hospitals.[50]

Observers have reported that mental patients (or for that matter any hospitalized patients) are treated with a great deal of gentleness and genuine "tender loving care".[51] According to the Alts: "The quality of competence, adequacy and warmth displayed by the staff toward the [mentally ill] children could only evoke our admiration and respect."[52] It should be pointed out that the medical profession in the Soviet Union is primarily a *female* profession with 75 percent of all doctors women, who may find it easier than male psychiatrists to give emotional support to patients.

The Soviet Union thus seems to have avoided the American pattern of

[44] US Department of Health, Education and Welfare, Public Health Service, *Patients in Mental Institutions*, Washington, D.C. (Yearly reports).

[45] This pattern of utilization, it must be noted, applies only to American public hospitals. In private psychiatric hospitals there were about five times as many admissions as beds, and in psychiatric facilities in general hospitals 25 times as many admissions as beds (figures for 1956 in US Department of Health, Education and Welfare, Public Health Service, *Patients in Mental Institutions*, Publication No. 632, Part III, Tables 1 and 2). It is also probably true that this pattern of intensive utilization reported by Western visitors must apply primarily to urban and research facilities. Rapoport points out in his review of Kline's report that alongside patients with acute forms of mental illness Soviet psychiatric hospitals (particularly large suburban ones) also hold a significant percentage of patients with chronic diseases (Rapoport, *op. cit.*, p. 454). The turnover of these patients must thus be correspondingly smaller.

[46] Herschel Alt and Edith Alt, *Russia's Children*, New York, 1959, p. 222; Klein, *op. cit.*, p. 20; Albert Maysles, Russian mental hospitals, *Boston University Graduate Journal*, January 1956, p. 71; personal observations.

[47] Albee, *op. cit.*, p. 284.

[48] Snezhnevskiy, *op. cit.*, p. 240.

[49] Albee, *op. cit.*, p. 294.

[50] *Ibid.*, p. 287.

[51] Klein, *op. cit.*, p. 23.

[52] Alt and Alt, *op. cit.*, p. 222.

huge public mental hospitals with their thousands of patients, their institutionalized atmosphere, their depersonalization, their isolation from the
community, and their dubious therapeutic efficiency.[53] Most Soviet hospitals
visited by Western observers were of modest size, one of the largest being the
Kashchenko Hospital in Moscow, already mentioned, which has 2220 beds
(including 240 pediatric beds) plus a 180-bed branch hospital outside the
city limits.[54] In 1963, according to data gathered by the American Hospital
Association, while American psychiatric hospitals constituted only a small
proportion (7.6 percent) of hospitals listed in the Directory of the Association
for that year they accounted, as we have seen, for about 46 percent of the
beds, so that their size was considerably greater than the average size of
non-psychiatric hospitals (1440 beds per psychiatric hospital as against 139
per non-psychiatric hospital). Some American state mental hospitals have,
of course, many more beds than the average figure given here.[55]

The mental hospital does not, therefore, occupy a central position in the
Soviet approach to mental illness. Rather it is considered as one (and only
one) of the facilities in the psychiatric arsenal, to be used for treatment
whenever indicated and whenever treatment cannot be given outside,[56] and
thus not merely as a dumping ground for society's rejects. This, of course,
could be interpreted as only a rationalization for an existing shortage of beds
and, as pointed out earlier, plans provided for a modest increase in such beds
during the recently completed Seven-Year Plan. And yet, it is also conceivable
that this shortage may well be a blessing in disguise since it compels psychiatric
authorities to devise methods of maintaining a certain number of the mentally
ill in the community rather than removing them to the potentially desocializing atmosphere of the mental hospital, where many receive (in the US, at
least) little active treatment and where their chances of release and useful
participation in the community's life diminish with each year of hospitalization. As the American Psychiatric Association has pointed out, it is suspected
that the very existence of hospital beds has created a tradition that militates

[53] One might also add the degradation, mortification and loss of personal autonomy that
often accompanies the commitment of the individual to what Irving Goffman calls a "total
institution" (*Asylums*, Garden City, 1961).

[54] Klein, *op. cit.*, p. 19. Observers usually agree that mental hospital buildings, while not
new (indeed, most of them appear to have been built before the revolution) nor of good
construction (as judged by American standards), are kept in excellent cleanliness and in
good repair, inside and out. Governor Meyner, however, reports after having visited
Kashchenko Hospital in Moscow that "in New Jersey the entire building would be condemned by one of our fire marshals because of poor construction, wood floors, windows
and doors and inaccessible exits" (Meyner praises Soviet hospital, *New York Times*,
August 3, 1959). Grounds surrounding the hospitals are said to be attractively landscaped
with flower beds, benches and statues of famous psychiatrists or political figures, particularly Lenin and (formerly) Stalin. Priority to housing is given as an explanation for the
lack of new hospital construction.

[55] Hospitals, *Journal of the American Hospital Association*, 38: No. 15, Part Two (August
1, 1964), *Guide Issue*, pp. 467–552.

[56] O. V. Kerbikov et. al., *Uchebnik psikhiatrii* (Textbook of Psychiatry), Moscow, 1958

against the use of simpler methods of dealing with mental illness and that countries that do not have elaborate hospital systems may find better ways of treating and managing the mentally ill.[57]

It may also be remembered that it was precisely a shortage of psychiatric beds that launched one of the more promising approaches to mental illness in the West. This is the system of emergency psychiatry or psychiatric first-aid pioneered by Dr. A. Querido in Amsterdam, Holland. One of the basic tenets of Dr. Querido's philosophy is not only to bring psychiatric aid *to* the patient wherever and whenever he needs it (without red tape and other administrative barriers) but, insofar as possible, to maintain him in the community, with help given to his family. Querido believes that:

> . . . in the last analysis, the cure or the adaptation of the mentally disturbed can be accomplished only in society and a successful stay in society is the only real test of any therapeutic endeavor. The removal of the mentally disturbed from his background implies the sidestepping of the nucleus of the problem.[58]

The Soviet viewpoint expressed by Rapoport is that the reduced need for hospital beds is due to four factors:

> 1. A system of widespread free out-patient psychiatric care sharply diminishes the need for hospitalization by providing preventive services and the early uncovering of psychic diseases;
> 2. A more active treatment of patients in the hospitals, giving the possibility of early release with the continuation of treatment at the out-patient clinic (which is made possible by the large number of personnel, particularly physicians);
> 3. The extensive possibility of the vocational placement of quiet mental patients in medical-vocational workshops and the many cooperatives of invalid collaboration as well as the placement (of recovered patients) in ordinary production (insofar as there has been for many years no unemployment in the country);
> 4. The relatively low nervous and psychic morbidity as the result of many social conditions—availability of employment, medical care, right to rest, education (including higher education), pensions, confidence in the morrow, absence of war hysteria and of pornography, prostitution, poverty, vagrancy, etc.[59]

While some of these points (particularly Number 4) may or may not be valid, it is quite evident that because of necessity or therapeutic conviction, or more probably because of both, Soviet psychiatry has developed a sophisticated approach to the treatment of the mentally ill *on an out-patient basis*. The reader should be cautioned that what is to follow is more a description of the Soviet blue-print or model of psychiatric treatment rather than of actual institutions available all over the Soviet territory. And yet, even as a programmatic statement, this blue-print deserves careful attention on the part of Western psychiatrists and administrators.

[57] American Psychiatric Association, *Mental Health Needs and Resources of Costa Rica,* Washington, D.C., 1956.
[58] A. Querido, Early diagnosis and treatment service, *Elements of a Community Mental Health Program,* New York, 1956, pp. 138–69.
[59] Rapoport, *op. cit.,* p. 454.

OUT-PATIENT FACILITIES

In the United States the focus of out-patient psychiatry is the psychiatric or mental health clinic and the private practice of psychiatry. In the Soviet Union out-patient psychiatry is centered in the so-called psycho-neurological clinic (*psikhonevrologichesky dispanser*), although there is a small but statistically insignificant private practice by some psychiatrists who see patients on a part-time basis. In order to better understand the nature and functions of that clinic it will be necessary to examine briefly certain aspects of Soviet medical organization.

Medical care in the Soviet Union is available either on a territorial (area) or an occupational basis. While the larger industrial organizations maintain medical facilities for their workers (occupational basis), the greater part of the population is assigned for its primary medical care to an out-patient clinic serving a specific district (*raion*). The district clinic thus constitutes the individual's first point of entry or contact with the medical system. Usually the territory of the district is subdivided into smaller medical sub-districts or sections (*uchastok*) of about 4000 people each. A district may have as many as ten or more medical sections. Each section is the responsibility of two full-time physicians (therapists); specialists, on the other hand, serve more than one section. Soviet tables of organization provide for 6.85 medical positions for each section (including the two therapists). One-quarter of one position is budgeted for the psychiatrist (or neuropathologist), indicating that, working full time, the psychiatrist serves a population of about 16,000.[60] The psychiatrist is based either at the district clinic (being assigned to its psycho-neurological office) or at an independent psycho-neurological clinic also serving the district population or the population of several districts. The independent clinic is thus a specialized medical facility in the community (as is, of course, the psycho-neurological office in smaller communities)[61] and is considered by Soviet psychiatric authorities as the kernel of the psychiatric network in the community, and is by its nature part and parcel of the general system of medical facilities and public health; the clinic psychiatrist is called "the pillar of that system".[62] Conditions are established for close cooperation between the therapist and the psychiatrist, each one helping the other in his own field of competence, and in providing care

[60] K. V. Maistrakh, *Organizatsiya zdravookhraneniya* (Organization of Health Services), Moscow, 1955.

[61] In 1956 there were 2327 psycho-neurological clinics, 119 of which were independent ones (not part of a district clinic) (*Zdravookhranenie v SSSR*, Moscow, 1957). In 1959–60, the number of psycho-neurological clinics (presumably independent) was reported as 146 (WHO Expert Committee on Mental Health, 1960). The figures for 1960 and 1961 were 157 and 167 respectively (*Bolshaya Meditsinskaya Entsiklopediya*, 2nd ed., **30**, Moscow, 1963, cols. 1111–12, Table 71).

[62] Snezhnevskiy, *op. cit.*, p. 238.

either at the clinic or at the patient's home.[63] The fact that both the psychiatrist and therapist (as well as other specialists) work in the same medical organization permits (in theory, at least) continuity and consistency in the treatment of the mentally ill and emotionally disturbed. Moreover, medical care provided without direct charge under socialized medicine permits the elimination of the financial considerations, eligibility criteria and other administrative and financial barriers that so often interpose themselves between patient and treatment in a system of mixed public and private care as we know it in the United States. With the provision of a partial continuation of income for salaried employees or workers while the individual is ill, the only barriers to treatment that might remain are the motivational ones, i.e., the patient's (or his relatives') unwillingness to recognize that he needs psychiatric care and his readiness to undergo treatment.

The psycho-neurological clinic, as it appears in Soviet psychiatric thinking, is, however, much more than a series of offices for psychiatrists to hang their hats in and see patients. The clinic is truly conceived as a comprehensive medical health center *in the community*, equipped to ensure the whole gamut of psychiatric treatment except for long-term hospitalization. Its main contribution is that it is geared to provide continuity of care through the changing phases of psychiatric illness and to keep, insofar as possible, the patient outside of the mental hospital, socially useful and whenever possible gainfully employed.[64] As such the clinic is conceived as giving all or most of the following services:

1. MEDICAL-DIAGNOSTIC SERVICE

This is the major clinical service of the clinic. It is usually divided into the following phases.

(a) *Out-patient service*

Treatment is offered by the section psychiatrist to adults and children (in a special pediatric division) in the form of psychotherapy, narcotherapy, pharmacotherapy, speech therapy, and such adjunct procedures as physiotherapy, injections and laboratory tests. The psychiatrist (whether formally psychiatrist or neuropathologist) is responsible for the mental health of the

---

[63] *Sorok let sovetskogo zdravookhraneniya* (Forty Years of Soviet Health Services), Moscow, 1957, p. 177.

[64] It should be noted that to some extent out-patient clinics in the United States perform the same functions. As Blain put it: "The techniques of treating patients in out-patient clinics have so advanced that it is probably safe to say that as many as one-third of the patients who are now treated successfully in the clinics would, several years ago, have been regarded as suitable only for hospital treatment." (Statement by Daniel Blain, M.D., Medical Director, American Psychiatric Association, during House Interstate and Foreign Commerce Hearings, October 8, 1953, Washington, D.C.)

population of his section, arranges for treatment when needed either at the clinic or at home if necessary, refers the patient to a mental hospital if that is indicated, and provides after-care at the time he is released from the hospital.[65]

When referring the patient to a mental hospital the psychiatrist is expected to send the hospital a summary of the patient's medical and psychiatric history (diagnosis, course of illness, treatment given), and when the patient is released, the hospital is similarly expected to notify the referring psychiatrist (and the clinic) and to supply pertinent information about treatment received while in the hospital and further recommendations. Should the patient fail to report to the psycho-neurological clinic, the initiative then passes to the psychiatrist, who sends for the patient or visits him at home. The constant supervision of the area population by the same psychiatrist (apparently Soviet psychiatrists have more job stability than their American colleagues)[66] permits him to know the mentally ill under his supervision (just as the resident physician of a hospital is expected to know the patients in his ward)[67] and the families of his patients; with the resources of other medical specialists at his disposal he should be in a good position to detect, prevent, mitigate, diagnose and treat mental illness. By becoming familiar with the occupational resources of his area he is also in a favorable position to recommend transfers to different, more suitable work for his patients. Finally, the ability to give attention and treatment at the time it is needed (there are apparently no waiting lists) and if necessary where it is needed (i.e., where the psychiatric crisis has occurred) creates optimal conditions for treatment. Experience has shown that such help often prevents the need for hospitalization, and again Querido has stressed the importance of psychiatric help at the time of an acute crisis (suicidal attempt, psychotic episode) and of seeing and studying the problem *in situ*:

> . . . we have the advantage of observing the conflict as a complex occurrence in which, of course, the personality of the patient and symptoms of his illness play an important part, but in which we have at the same time an opportunity to note the interplay of all that is related to the conflict. We note the quality of the surroundings; we feel the influence of the wife and the children; we see how the patient is feared, loved or respected; we note the burden of material care that rests on the family; we see the tensions originating from bad family conditions; we note the reactions of the neighborhood and attitudes of the patient toward authority; we see signs of hobbies and cultural activities.

And, Querido adds, "one psychiatrist in this service is more effective than the whole personnel of a 60-bed ward".[68]

In the larger cities emergency psychiatric care is also a function (presumably when the psycho-neurological clinic is closed) of emergency

[65] Snezhnevskiy, *op. cit.*, p. 239.

[66] Transfers must receive administrative approval, salaries and conditions of work are fairly uniform throughout the country, and private care does not create a strong pull.

[67] Kerbikov *et al.*, *op. cit.*, pp. 330–1.

[68] Querido, *op. cit.*

psychiatric teams composed of psychiatrists and junior medical personnel (*feldshers*),[69] ready to move by ambulance to the scene of an emergency. Snezhnevskiy says that such services are available in all major cities;[70] and Kline reports that in Leningrad there are eight such emergency psychiatric teams strategically located so as to be able to reach any part of the city.[71]

(b) *In-patient service*

Historically, out-patient care has developed as an extension of services provided by the mental hospital. The Soviet psycho-neurological clinic reverses the procedure by providing psychiatric beds as a community extension of its out-patient functions. These beds, it should be noted, are *not* intended to replace the mental hospital. Rather, they permit the psychiatrist to carry out certain procedures he could not otherwise do. They permit, for example, short-term hospitalization without having to remove the patient from the community to a distant mental hospital. The general functions performed by these beds are then the following: (i) they serve as a receiving center for psychiatric patients, particularly when the mental hospital is distant and there are transportation difficulties. This also permits the immediate hospitalization within a medical setting of violent patients who otherwise might be, as they sometimes are in the United States, tossed into the local jail or lock-up; (ii) they permit diagnostic workups; (iii) they provide clinical services, particularly the ones that require brief periods of hospitalization;[72] (iv) they serve as a temporary haven for psychiatric patients who require separation from a disturbed home environment.[73] As such, these beds play, perhaps, a similar function to that of our psychiatric beds in general hospitals. Naturally, in isolated settlements, or in the face of great distances and transportation difficulties (in the winter and early spring) these beds will tend to assume, temporarily at least, some of the functions of the mental hospital. The number of such beds varies from 15 to 100, the variation depending on local conditions and the availability of an easily accessible mental hospital.

(c) *Work-shops*

Work therapy, as distinct from occupational therapy, plays an important role in the Soviet psychiatric system and permits the gainful employment of psychiatric patients under conditions that are carefully controlled and under

---

[69] A *feldsher* is a physician's assistant, a sort of high-grade nurse.

[70] Snezhnevskiy, *op. cit.*, p. 239.

[71] Kline, *op. cit.*, p. 154.

[72] N. A. Vinogradov, *Organizatsiya zdravookhraneniya v SSSR* (The Organization of Health Services in the USSR), Moscow, 1958, Vol. II, p. 255.

[73] Stanley Lesse, Current clinical and research trends in Soviet psychiatry, *American Journal of Psychiatry*, Hanover, New Hampshire, **114**, 1958, p. 1018.

the supervision of medical and psychiatric specialists. The system of work-shops attached to psycho-neurological clinics had its beginnings as early as 1932 at the Bekhterev Neuropsychiatric Institute in Leningrad; these shops are said to be available in Moscow, Leningrad and a few of the other large cities[74] and provide different types of activity for psychiatric patients, graded to their capacities and abilities, but more nearly resembling work under normal conditions than "occupational therapy", which keeps the patient busy in more "artistic" but economically sterile activities such as painting, drawing, wood-burning and basket-weaving. Patients employed in these work-shops receive payment on a scale comparable to that of regular industry. It should be noted that the primary function of these work-shops is understood to be the preparation of the individual for work either under normal conditions or in so-called "invalid co-operatives".[75] Thus, the aim of the work-shops is also to imbue the patient (or former patient) with the values and attitudes necessary for industrial work (discipline, punctuality, accuracy, diligence). Experience has shown in the Soviet Union that 95 percent of psychiatric patients need such training or re-training after their illness.[76]

(d) *Day hospital*

The idea of providing certain patients with the treatment procedures available in a hospital but without keeping the patient overnight also has a long history in the Soviet Union; the first day hospital was opened (because of a shortage of beds) in Moscow in 1933.[77] The day hospital may also be used for patients who have been released from a hospital and who still need treatment and supervision, or who cannot yet assume their full work and other responsibilities in the community. It thus often assumes the position of a half-way station between hospital and community. Most patients in the day hospital receive treatment and work in the work-shops.

2. SOCIAL AND VOCATIONAL SERVICE

Medical treatment alone is not conceived as sufficient to restore the individual to a position of usefulness in society. The psycho-neurological clinic therefore maintains an office or offices whose function it is to provide assistance to the patient in the following spheres:

[74] G. B. Abramovich *et al.*, *Voprosy organizatsii vnebolnichnoi trudovoi terapii* (Problems of Organizing Out-patient Work Therapy), Moscow, 1956.
[75] Work groups made up of disabled individuals, producing primarily consumer goods. The income from the sale of these goods is divided among the members of the cooperative.
[76] Abramovich *et al.*, *op. cit.*
[77] M. A. Dzhagarov, Experience in organizing a day hospital for mental patients, *Nevropatologiya i psikhiatriya*, Moscow, **6**, 1937, No. 8, pp. 137–47.

(a) *Improvement of the living conditions or arrangements of the patient*

While about half of the Soviet population still lives in the countryside, where mental patients are much less of a disturbance than in the towns, the other half lives under incredibly crowded conditions in the urban areas. Indeed, the housing shortage caused by the extremely rapid increase of the urban population, and the inability of the housing program to keep pace with this increase are salient features of the round of daily living in the Soviet city.[78] The typical arrangement is that of a family living in each room of an apartment and sharing cooking, washing and toilet facilities. These conditions, bad as they are for the average individual, are even worse for a mental patient and his family, particularly if the patient is psychotic. Recognition of this problem led, as early as thirty years ago, to measures aimed at providing a single room for mental patients living in the community.[79] One of the clinic's tasks is that of providing a certificate of mental illness that will help a patient to secure such a room and of initiating further steps to the same end. In addition, the clinic may provide the patient (or his family or any family that takes care of him) with a modicum of financial and other assistance to improve his living conditions. Since the patient may also be entitled either to a temporary disability compensation or a pension for a permanent condition, this will ease his (or the family's) financial burden.

(b) *Social and welfare assistance*

This includes such assistance as may be needed in solving family conflicts and quarrels occasioned by the patient's condition and the cramped living accommodation, in applying for social welfare benefits to which the patient (or his family) may be entitled, in placing children into crêches or kindergartens, and in referring the patient, when indicated, to other medical institutions. The role performed by the clinic staff in this respect is thus similar in its essential aspects to that of the social worker in the United States; this role is undertaken, in most instances, by a nurse (*sestra*) and more particularly by the visiting nurse (*patronazhnaya sestra*).

---

[78] See, for example, Timothy Sosnovy, *The Housing Problem in the USSR*, New York, 1954.

[79] Decision of the Party Central Executive Committee and the Council of Peoples' Commissars, February 28, 1930.

(c) *Vocational assistance*

This consists in efforts at placing the patient in a job, or in a job better fitted to his condition, or in changing his type of work (for example, a transfer from the night to the day shift). This is done, primarily, with the help of the trade union organizations of local factories and plants. Thus whenever possible an attempt is made to maintain the patient at work in the community, even if he has only partial or residual work capacity. The emphasis on work as a rehabilitative factor is further reinforced by the Marxist view of labor as the primary activity of man. Soviet experience has also shown that this approach facilitates the preservation of a certain "tone of life" for many years, tends to prevent chronic states of illness and the deterioration that almost inevitably accompanies long-term hospitalization. Vocational placement is also facilitated by the manpower shortage the Soviet Union is experiencing as a result of losses and birth deficits suffered in the Second World War.

(d) *Legal assistance*

There may be many instances in which a patient requires legal assistance, either directly by having someone on the staff with legal experience help the patient, or by referring him to what is called a legal consultation.

(e) *Certification*

The clinic also has as its function the certification of the degree of disability and residual capacity of the patients as well as the provision of expert testimony in cases that come before the courts.

(f) *Home visiting*

Home care is an important element of the work of the clinic. While the psychiatrist has as his primary function the giving of treatment to the patient, a great many of the ancillary services in home care are given by the visiting nurse, who plays, in this instance, the role of doctor's assistant and social worker: she gives injections and other prescribed treatment, and gathers the necessary information that the psychiatrist will want to have. The visiting nurse thus establishes a direct and personal link between the patient and his family in the community and the clinic, and stands ready to assist him in most non-clinical aspects of his life situation.

3. PREVENTION, MENTAL HYGIENE, INTRA- AND EXTRA-MURAL EDUCATION

The theory of Soviet medicine puts a great deal of emphasis on the prevention of disease, and indicates that preventive medicine is the medicine of the future. There is good reason to believe that prevention is as important in psychiatry as in other areas of medicine. In some mental illnesses, for example, early detection and prompt treatment may well prevent the illness from becoming chronic and irreversible. By its position in the community the psycho-neurological clinic is well placed to engage in activities of a preventive nature. The child psychiatrist, for instance, is expected to work in close contact with the educational and economic institutions of the area under his supervision (i.e., schools and the factories that employ adolescents). The child psychiatrist is expected to remain in touch with teachers, parents, and supervisors in order either to detect and to prevent illness or to give early treatment to those children and adolescents who might need it. The psychiatrist must also be consulted on measures that might affect the mental health of the population, particularly the construction of new industries. Furthermore, the Soviet psychiatrist, like all other physicians, must devote some time each month (a minimum of 4 hours)[80] to educational talks or other activities of the same general nature, either to personnel (usually junior) at the clinic or to groups of the population. Intra-mural education takes the form of in-service education (talks, lectures, courses, seminars); extra-mural education may take the form of lectures, evenings of questions and answers, consultations, showing of slides or educational movies, or meetings with special groups (pregnant mothers, young workers).

4. Accounting of Morbidity

As the institution responsible for the state of the mental health of the population of its area, the psycho-neurological clinic must maintain a dynamic accounting of morbidity. The statistical department maintains a card file of the persons who have come or who are under the care of the clinic. A further function is the uncovering (presumably through surveys, communications or referrals) of patients who need psychiatric treatment or ancillary care. The Soviet literature also emphasizes that this picture of the state of psychiatric morbidity must be a dynamic one, i.e., it must reflect the changing nature of morbidity. This is done, primarily, through keeping the card file "active", i.e., each card must be kept up to date and must record every type of treatment or intervention, whether received at the clinic, at home, or at the mental hospital (or any other medical institution) as well as changes in condition. As indicated earlier, this card (or an extract) accompanies the patient when he is hospitalized and presumably returns to the clinic when the patient is discharged. These files permit a statistical accounting of morbidity and permit better staffing and planning. Soviet psychiatrists seem to be aware, however, that morbidity registration (even if really dynamic) is not enough to provide

80 Vinogradov, *op. cit.*, **2**, p. 572

an accurate picture of the incidence and prevalence of mental illness in the community since many of the persons who suffer from mental illness are not identified as such (at least not for a long time) or do not identify themselves. In a well-organized clinic, Kerbikov, for example, contends,[81] practically all those who are mentally ill should be on the clinic books. Whether this is done or even possible is a moot point, of course, in view of the difficulties posed by such a survey.

This description of the psycho-neurological clinic, however brief and incomplete, should be enough to suggest that it is a model for the comprehensive treatment of mental patients in the community and as such is either in line with, or even ahead of, the most advanced psychiatric thinking in the West, and this regardless of whether these clinics are widespread in the Soviet Union or exist only as models or demonstration institutions in a few of the larger cities.

Treatment Methods

GENERAL CONSIDERATIONS

One of the striking aspects of Soviet psychiatric theory (at least until very recently) has been its heavy reliance on Pavlov, and its violent rejection of Freud, his theories and the treatment methods derived from them. The attack on "Freudism" is couched in ideological and political as well as scientific terms. The psycho-analytical method is branded as "one of the most reactionary and pseudo-scientific manifestations of bourgeois ideology," and is identified with all that is unscientific, reactionary and "imperialistic." According to Professor D. Fedotov, Director of the Institute of Psychiatry of the USSR Ministry of Health, Freudism

> . . . is basically false and speculative, ignores the role of etiology, the physiological mechanism of disease, and denies the deterministic significance of the external milieu. . . . Precisely because of the assertion of the primacy of instincts over conscious action and the limiting of the role of social factors in determining human conduct, Freudism constitutes a weapon of bourgeois reaction. The center of contemporary Freudism is the USA, which, as is well known, is also the center of world imperialism.[82]

Freud's theories thus not only fail to fit the concepts of dialectical materialism and are thus "idealistic," i.e., unscientific,[83] but they wrongly exaggerate the role of instincts. Man's life, according to Soviet contemporary psychiatric theory, his desires and aspirations, his acts and actions, his behavior in

[81] Kerbikov et al., op. cit., p. 331.

[82] D. Fedotov, Freudism—a reactionary manifestation of bourgeois ideology, Meditsinsky rabotnik, Moscow, November 25, 1958. (I am indebted to Ina Schlesinger for an English translation of this article.)

[83] S. V. Bassin, Freudism in the light of contemporary scientific discussions, Soviet Survey, London, January–March 1959, pp. 82 ff.; P. P. Bondarenko and M. Kh. Rabinovich, Problems of ideological struggle with modern Freudism, ibid., July–September 1959, pp. 29–38.

general, are the product of the society's social and economic conditions and not of blind, instinctive forces. As a product of his environment, man's instincts are repressed by social forces and the primary method of treatment in mental and emotional illness should be a combination of re-education plus physiological, or pharmacological and sociological treatment. Most Soviet psychiatrists like to emphasize the profound difference between Pavlov and Freud and officially tend to see red when anyone tries to reconcile their theories. Pavlov, for example, is quoted approvingly as having compared himself and Freud to

> ... two parties of miners who began to drive a tunnel at the foot of a big mountain in order to come to light—the understanding of the human mind. But Freud started digging downward and has dug himself into the labyrinth of the unconscious, whereas we shall some time come out into the open ... and shall finish building the tunnel ... we are on the right track. .... We have learned to reproduce the neuroses and have joined the clinic to physiology while Freud is only trying to guess the inner states of man.[84]

"Psychoanalysis interests itself in the depths," recently said a Soviet specialist (who himself had earlier been interested in psychoanalysis) to an American visitor. "*We* are interested in the *heights* (points finger heavenward) ... in the nervous system of the highest type and its regulatory mechanism."[85] And yet one may wonder whether the violence of the attack on psychoanalysis does not reflect some ambivalence on the subject. For instance, Rentchnik, on his visit to the Soviet Union a few years ago, felt he detected, in private conversations with psychiatrists, a bit of nostalgia about this method.[86] This would be particularly true in view of the existence, in the late twenties and early thirties, of interest in psychoanalysis, and even of a Society of Psychoanalysts. It may perhaps be surmised that some of the premises of psychoanalysis still lurk in the minds or sympathies of certain psychiatrists and that these psychiatrists use these concepts *sub rosa* in the treatment of patients.[87] At least, as Kalinowsky reports, while psychoanalytical psychiatry does not exist, its principles are well known.[88] Be that as it may, the main treatment methods reported are the following.

SOMATIC OR PHYSIOLOGICAL THERAPIES

These include insulin coma therapy, following the Sakel method with coma periods of 30 to 90 minutes, prolonged sleep treatment induced by a weak

[84] L. Rokhlin, *Soviet Medicine in the Fight Against Mental Illness*, Moscow, 1958, p. 125.
[85] Zigmund M. Lebensohn, Impressions of Soviet psychiatry, *AMA Archives of Neurology and Psychiatry*, Chicago, **80**, December 1958, pp. 735–51.
[86] Dr. Pierre Rentchnik, *Esculape au Pays des Soviets*, Geneva, 1955.
[87] The term "psychoanalysis", incidentally, is used in the Soviet Union but refers to "rational", i.e., non-Freudian, analysis. The patient undergoes autobiographical analysis to determine what environmental factors gave rise to the illness. (Kline, *op. cit.*, p. 165.)
[88] Lothar B. Kalinowsky, Practice of psychiatry in the Communist countries of Eastern Europe, *American Journal of Psychotherapy*, New York, **16**, 1962, pp. 301–13.

current, narcotherapy, electric shock (its use is said to be declining), and pharmacotherapy, which at the present time is the treatment of choice with such agents as chlorpromazine (called *aminasin*), reserpine and other tranquilizers. Radical surgical interventions such as lobotomies and leucotomies have been forbidden by a decree of the Health Ministry of December 9, 1950.

THE PSYCHOLOGICAL THERAPIES

These include what we would call psychotherapy, but primarily directive psychotherapy. Narcotherapy and hypnosis are used as adjuncts to "rational" or "autobiographical" psychotherapy in an effort to re-educate the patient through changing his attitudes to his environment (or through changing the environment by periods of brief hospitalization). Relatively little attention is paid to infancy and sexual problems.[89] It should be noted that until about 1950 psychotherapy as such was looked upon with disfavor because of its obviously "idealistic" character.[90] In that year a joint session of the Academy of Sciences and Academy of Medical Sciences devoted its efforts to putting Soviet medicine on a truly Pavlovian basis. This session, oddly enough, helped to re-establish psychotherapy as an ideologically and scientifically acceptable form of treatment. This was done simply by pointing out that Pavlov's theory of the second signal system in man, in which verbal stimuli replace physical stimuli in the conditioned-reflex arc, had been neglected by Soviet psychiatrists and theorists. Since psychotherapy uses words, a psychotherapist would be a good Pavlovian.[91]

Indicative of this interest in psychotherapy was the All-Union Conference of Psychotherapy, held in 1956 in Moscow. The basic materials of the conference have recently been published in book form,[92] and consist of more than 50 papers on the use of psychotherapy in a variety of conditions, both somatic and psychological, either as the main method of treatment or as adjunct therapy. Among the conditions for which psychotherapy was indicated were not only neuroses but also psychoses, psychogenic impotence, stuttering in children, the treatment of alcoholism and tobacco smoking; it was also recommended, with other therapies, for use in such conditions as bronchial asthma and hypertensive diseases, in obstetrics and gynecology, eye operations and dermatology. While one paper refers to "Group Psy-

[89] George Serban, The psychotherapeutic approach to neurosis in the Pavlovian school, *Journal of the American Medical Association*, Chicago, **170**, August 1, 1959, pp. 1651–7.

[90] Ivan D. London, Therapy in Soviet psychiatric hospitals, *American Psychologist*, Baltimore, Maryland, **8**, 1953, pp. 79–82; Toward a realistic appraisal of Soviet science, *Bulletin of the Atomic Scientists*, Chicago, Illinois, **13**, 1957, pp. 169–73 and 176.

[91] Ivan D. London, Toward a realistic appraisal of Soviet science, *Bulletin of the Atomic Scientists*, Chicago, Illinois, **13**, 1957, pp. 169–73 and 176.

[92] M. S. Lebedinsky (ed.), *Voprosy psikhoterapii* (Problems of Psychotherapy), Moscow, 1958.

chotherapy and Cinema", in general the attention is focused on individual, rather than group, psychotherapy.

THE SOCIOLOGICAL THERAPIES

These are based on the Soviet theoretical conception of the importance of the milieu for mental health and mental illness, and the assumption that the care of the mentally ill is the responsibility not only of the psychiatrists, but also of others.[93] As Rentchnik suggests, the Soviet theory is that health, and particularly mental health, is much too important to be left exclusively to physicians.[94] The idea is very strong that in many instances the patient may be treated more effectively through the environment: transferring him to a different and more congenial job, encouraging treatment at home or in the community, i.e., in familiar surroundings and with people who care for the patient (in the sense of both treatment and affection), by having the psychiatrist or a visiting nurse see the patient on his home ground if necessary, by sending him to a resort or sanatorium to give him a change of pace and rest in pleasant surroundings, and even, as Berman has suggested, using the laws and legal institutions as instruments of mental health.[95] We have already touched on the importance which attaches to work therapy; this type of treatment finds additional ideological reinforcement in dialectical materialism, which holds that the consciousness of the individual is a reflection of the objective world, is formed by the process of social labor, and appears early during human activity.[96] Thus work "has an extraordinary effect on the psyche of the individual. It follows that this effect must be used to normalize psychic activity when it has been disturbed."[97] While it can be suggested that the use of the labor of mental patients in a society that is short of manpower may be motivated by other than strictly therapeutic concern, it can also be suggested that the needs of the society and those of the patient may well coincide, so long as therapeutic considerations are not neglected in favor of the needs of production alone.

The Outlook

The Soviet approach to mental illness raises, particularly in the comparative and cross-cultural context, certain interesting and as yet unresolved questions. We shall touch here, in conclusion, briefly and speculatively on some of them.

[93] Harold J. Berman, "Law as an instrument of mental health in the United States and Soviet Russia." Address given at the Second Institute on Preventive Psychiatry, State University of Iowa, April 11, 1959.

[94] Rentchnik, *op. cit.*

[95] Berman, *op. cit.*

[96] Serban, *op. cit.*, p. 1653.

[97] Abramovich *et al.*, *op. cit.*, p. 5.

1. CULTURE AND MENTAL ILLNESS

As seen earlier, the Soviets claim, time and again, that their type of society, which has a clear-cut, well-defined goal and a collectivistic orientation in its culture, leads to a lesser degree of mental illness than a capitalistic society with its antagonistic classes, its violent competition, its irresponsible individualism and its multiplicity of goals.

While we may be permitted some skepticism about the inverse relationship between common goals and schizophrenia, it is still possible that both the psychoses and the neuroses are affected by the nature of the social system. In the Soviet Union this relationship would be as follows.

Psychoses

Improvement in the standard of living of the population, improvement in medical care and public health, and particularly in maternal and infant care permit an attack, at least upon the infectious and organic psychoses. As to the other psychoses, the work of Hollingshead and Redlich at Yale suggests that the individuals of the lower socio-economic groups are "populations at risk" to a significantly greater degree than those of the upper socio-economic groups of the society. They show, for example, that the rate of schizophrenic psychoses is eight times larger in the lowest socio-economic groups of the population than in the highest.[98] While there are a variety of suggested reasons for this, it is possible that a rise in the standard of living and greater accessibility of psychiatric care will decrease the impact of the psychoses on the population through earlier detection, diagnosis and treatment. And indeed, the number of first visits of mental patients to the psycho-neurological clinics of Moscow would generally seem to bear out this contention (see Table 6), though, as we have indicated above, some of these changes may have been an artifact of special conditions.

Kerbikov, who feels that the halving of "fresh" cases of schizophrenia is ample demonstration of the importance of the external environment in the etiology of mental illness, and particularly of this "so-called 'endogenous' nosological form", probably rejects, as most Soviet psychiatrists would, the more "pessimistic" theory of the hereditary nature of schizophrenia and other psychoses, and of man's helplessness in dealing with them.[99]

Neuroses

If there is an inverse relationship between common goals or culture and mental illness, it is perhaps in the area of neuroses where it will be most

98 Hollingshead and Redlich, *op. cit.*, p. 232.
99 Kerbikov, *op. cit.*, p. 232.

TABLE 6.

First Visits of Mental Patients to Psychoneurological Dispensaries, City of Moscow, 1940–56 (per 10,000 of Population)

Diagnosis	1940	1945	1946	1947	1948	1950	1953	1954	1955	1956
Schizophrenia (all forms incl. neurotic and latent)	5.5	5.5	4.7	3.9	3.8	3.0	2.5	2.4	2.9	2.4
Epilepsy	3.5	5.5	4.7	3.5	3.0	2.3	1.5	1.5	1.8	1.4
Manic-depressive psychosis	0.7	0.4	0.5	0.3	0.2	0.2	0.13	0.07	0.14	0.11
Psychoses with brain circulation disturbances	2.6	5.2	4.2	3.8	4.3	3.0	2.7	2.7	3.2	2.7
Pre-senile psychoses	0.7	0.6	0.5	0.6	1.8	0.4	0.44	0.46	0.42	0.4
Senile psychoses	0.5	0.5	0.3	0.4	0.3	0.5	0.49	0.48	0.4	0.5
Lues cerebri	0.6	0.5	0.4	0.3	0.4	0.2	0.14	0.1	0.3	0.1
Creeping paralysis	0.3	0.1	0.05	0.67	0.1	0.05	0.08	0.02	0.02	0.02
Psychoses with infectious and virus diseases	0.5	1.1	0.8	0.8	0.8	0.49	0.12	0.33	0.4	0.3
Intoxication psychoses	0.1	0.1	0.01	0.08	0.08	0.08	0.04	0.04	0.05	0.02
Alcoholic psychoses and chronic alcoholism	8.1	2.0	3.1	3.0	2.0	5.5	5.9	5.6	6.0	5.0
Narcomania	0.09	0.04	0.02	0.06	0.04	0.03	0.06	0.03	0.08	0.07
Mental disorders with diseases of internal organs	1.6	1.7	1.1	0.7	0.7	0.7	0.3	0.6	0.9	0.6
Mental disorders (incl. neurotic) with brain trauma	1.3	9.1	8.5	7.4	7.2	4.5	4.2	3.9	3.7	2.8
Psychoses with organic trauma of the central nervous system	2.6	3.7	2.8	2.6	2.6	2.2	2.2	2.6	2.6	1.7
Oligophrenia	1.1	1.1	1.1	0.8	0.8	0.7	0.8	0.6	1.3	1.0
Psychopathy	3.3	2.7	4.3	3.3	2.8	2.4	1.7	1.8	2.0	1.9
Neuroses, psychoneuroses and reactive disorders	16.4	17.4	11.7	10.5	12.8	9.6	7.5	6.9	8.4	6.0
Others (neuro-psychic and undetermined diseases)	5.2	4.5	2.9	2.5	2.2	1.7	2.9	2.4	3.0	2.8

SOURCE: Living Conditions and Health, World Medical Council, Vienna, 1959, No. 4, p. 236.

evident. Western and particularly American culture, for example, is one that puts a great deal of insistence on individualism, on individual happiness, on individual rights; it is a society that often romanticizes life, human relations, love and marriage; the contrast between these conceptions of the individual's place in society and the realities of everyday living may well be an important wedge for the neurotic pattern. In Soviet society, the *Weltanschauung* (*mirovozzrenie*) encourages the resolution of personal ambivalence by presenting the individual with a series of goals and decisions made for him, thereby relieving him of these decisions and often of the anxieties of choice.[100] Personal mental adjustment is to be found in the submerging of one's wishes and desires to the needs of the group or society, in the assumption that society has rights against the individual and not *vice versa*, and in the lack of romanticization about human relationships. It is stressed to the patient that he must "give to others and not be concerned with himself", that he must not isolate himself from others. Even if his family rejects him, his fellow citizens are ready to welcome him "with open arms." He is told: "There is an obligation of the individual to society in return for the love which society has for the individual."[101] Some twenty-five years ago, Frankwood Williams argued that the type of social order existing in the Soviet Union was conducive to mental health, and recent advances in the field of social psychiatry should make it possible to examine this proposition more critically.

2. INDUSTRIALIZATION, THE PSYCHOSES AND THE NEUROSES

Still on the subject of the neuroses, it is probable that the Soviets have not paid much attention to neuroses, at least until a few years ago, since more concern was given to the psychoses because of their disruptive impact on the individual as a productive unit, i.e., as a "hand".

And yet, as the nature of Soviet society gradually changes under the impact of the industrialization drive set into motion by the regime, the decrease in the importance of physical work (replaced by mechanical power and machinery) is matched by an increase in the importance of mental work and in the proportion of those engaged in this type of work. In this kind of society, intellectual capacity, at most levels of production, becomes much

---

[100] Kent Geiger reports a conversation he had in 1958 with the director of a "tourist base" which bears on this. The director was asked why people come to a tourist base or a camp, rather than being on their own. He answered: "First, because it is more secure; they are guaranteed a place at which to stay before they leave home. Second, it is more organized; they can get food, hiking equipment, etc. Third, it is a collective organization and people are used to it. People's stamina is greater in a collective. . . . We transport them from one town to another, give them food, showers and equipment. Just like children, they have no problem. We receive them, wash them, feed them, and send them off to bed." (Kent Geiger, personal communication, author's file.)

[101] Kline, *op. cit.*, p. 166.

more strategic than muscular power and good physical health. As such, mental stability, personality integration and organization will become just as important as, and even more important than, physical health. Moreover, the kinds of pressure that are put on individuals in this type of society, particularly in the occupational sphere and in decision-making, will make it imperative to devote more attention to the neuroses and other emotional disturbances. The growing interest in, and use of, psychotherapy may be a portent. The present approach to the neuroses is that they are the results of bad social conditions or traumatic events (such as war or unemployment) and that with an increase in the welfare and the security of the population they are bound to disappear. It is perhaps this approach to the neuroses that makes it so difficult for Soviet medical and lay authorities to understand certain social problems that plague Soviet society. Juvenile delinquency, crime and alcoholism are examples of such problems. Stealing among children, for instance, is interpreted as due to weak parental education or school training, or to the need of objects stolen by "poor" children.[102] What is particularly baffling to Soviet authorities is that juvenile delinquency often appears among children of the élite and privileged classes, i.e., precisely those whose lives are free from want and who do not need to steal, *objectively speaking*. "Nowhere", the Alts remark with amazement, "did we find any recognition that stealing might be a symptom of the child's emotional conflict."[103] Nor is it easy for Soviet psychiatrists to understand why, in the United States, there are so many neurotics in the upper socio-economic groups of the population. Such recognition and understanding may well be forthcoming in the future.

3. Industrialization, Urbanization and the Changing Morbidity

It is also possible that, as the industrialization drive and the mass transfers of population from the countryside to the urban areas reach a plateau and level off, the health problems of the population will change in the direction of the decreased importance of the infectious diseases (tuberculosis, for example), to be replaced by the illnesses that are major problems in heavily industrialized societies, such as cancer, heart disease and mental illness. The first two of these already are important in the Soviet Union, and it may be expected that mental disease will sometime in the future follow suit. In this respect, the Soviet Union has the initial advantage of not being saddled with a tradition of hospitalization of mental patients, and may then be able to escape Parkinson's Second Law (Psychiatric Section), to the effect that the number of mentally ill rises to meet the number of psychiatric beds and then proceeds to surpass it.[104]

[102] Mark G. Field, Alcoholism, crime and delinquency in Soviet society, *Social Problems*, New York, 3, October 1955, pp. 100–9.
[103] Alt and Alt, *op. cit.*, p. 202.
[104] I am indebted to Dr. Aronson for this analogy.

4. MENTAL ILLNESS AND THE MEDICAL MODEL

Finally, a comparison of the Soviet and American psychiatric systems makes one wonder whether, in the last analysis, the medical and public health approach (so often advocated in the United States) is a suitable one or an exclusive one for this illness and even whether the concept of "illness" is an appropriate one for this range of phenomena. The classical medical model is still tied down to the search for the "offending agent", its isolation and neutralization. In mental illness and emotional disturbances there is probably (except in some clear-cut instances) no single "offending agent", but a multiplicity of etiological factors, some in the individual but many in the society and the culture and in the specific constellation of such factors that impinge upon the individual.[105] The concept of "cure" may also be inadequate and may have to give way to another one such as adaptation or adjustment. The problem of providing the kind of setting in which those who are mentally ill or emotionally disturbed can still function to the best of their abilities, without the stigma that traditionally attaches to the word "mad", is an important challenge to the contemporary industrial society of the Soviet or American type. Again, Kerbikov expressed the idea of broadening concepts of care by advocating "not only treatment in the direct and narrow sense of the word, but all-round active help to the patient, with the aim of preserving him as a useful member of society".[106] By paying more attention to the social (or socio-cultural) aspect of mental illness, by a judicious arrangement of the individual's social environment (including the home and the work situation) it may be hoped that these broadened concepts may be reached.[107] In many respects, the Soviet approach to the mentally ill (particularly the psychotics) and Soviet social structure, in theory at least, are well adapted for the implementation of these goals. The main contribution the Soviets have made lies probably in their principle of not condemning the psychotic patient to the idle, demoralizing, de-socializing, untherapeutic and wasteful life of the chronic patient in the large mental hospital, where with the passage of time the chances for a return to the community constantly decrease. Concomitant with this approach is the bringing of psychiatric care into the community, even into the patient's home if necessary, and the linking of this treatment with the general network of medical facilities maintained under a system of socialized medicine as well as those of the organs of social welfare. By contrast, it may be that their contribution to the treatment of the neuroses is hampered both by the collectivistic nature of their social order and philosophy and by the dogmatic intolerance of schools that do

---

[105] Dubos, *op. cit.*

[106] Kerbikov, *op. cit.*, p. 231.

[107] Morris S. Schwartz and Charlotte Green Schwartz *et al.*, *Social Approaches to Mental Patient Care*, New York, 1964.

not fit their theoretical and ideological commitments. Mao Tse-tung's gentle reminder of letting "a hundred flowers bloom, a hundred schools contend" applies with equal force to psychiatry, whether the school is that of Pavlov's, Freud's or any other "miner's".[108]

[108] It may be a straw in the wind that Academician P. L. Kapitza recently gave Freud equal billing with Pavlov, naming both as founders of the science of higher nervous activity; he also specifically mentioned the "influence of the subconscious on the activity of the individual" (P. L. Kapitza, The future of science, *Nauka i zhizn*, Moscow, 3, 1962, pp. 18–23, 96–7).

18. The Double Life of American Psychiatry

HENRY A. DAVIDSON

IN AMERICA, private practitioners of psychiatry are, for the most part, readily classifiable into one of two categories: the essentially psychotherapeutic and the eclectic. The latter utilizes medication, electroconvulsive therapy, counselling, learning theory, advice-giving and, to a lesser degree, the traditional psychotherapy, usually at a superficial level. The other type of practitioner relies on psychotherapy as the prime or exclusive method of treatment. More prestige attaches to psychotherapy, while the higher incomes generally go to the more flexible therapist.

The Structure of Private Practice

Most psychiatrists in private practice assert that they are not bound to any one method and will give whatever treatment is indicated. However, the one kind of doctor finds that, to handle anxiety, psychotherapy is indicated; the other practitioner will see anxiety as an indication for tranquilizers. (He may seek the prestige of the psychotherapist by asserting that the purpose of the tranquilizers is to make the patient more receptive to psychotherapy.)

In all, there are about 14,000 psychiatrists in the U.S.A. Of these, some 8000 are largely in private practice, though many supplement their incomes by part-time work in clinics, teaching institutions or (more rarely) hospitals. And about 6000 American psychiatrists are on salary and devote most of their professional time to working in hospitals and clinics (Davidson, 1965), though many of these have part-time private practice, too.

To the average American, the word "psychiatrist" conjures up a picture of a private practitioner, sitting in his chair while the patient is on a couch. The doctor is listening to a report of his dreams and childhood memories. This is so compelling an image (Davidson, 1964b), that more than half of the cartoons about psychiatrists show a couch as an essential part of the office furniture. In American folklore, the psychiatrist is rarely thought of as a doctor who uses a stethoscope or prescribes medication. Actually, more than half of the psychiatrists in the U.S.A. *do* prescribe, but the popular image remains that of the psychotherapist.

The psychodynamically orientated psychiatrist practises in this way. He sees each patient two or three times a week. He allocates 50–60 minutes for each visit. He does not write prescriptions, fearing that if medication is used, the patient may assume that his condition is of physiological or biochemical origin. This would interfere with dynamic therapy—which requires faith in the psychogenic nature of the illness. The psychotherapist will usually not sign certificates committing his patient to a psychiatric hospital, lest this be seen as a hostile gesture—which in a way it is. He will not do physical examinations, even of the most cursory sort, because he worries that the patient may construe the hand-to-body contact as a kind of seduction. He will not undertake to treat the brain-damaged, the homicidal, the senile, the seriously suicidal, the severely psychotic, the grossly disorientated or the poorly motivated patient. He recognizes that these are poor subjects for psychotherapy. Because the psychotherapist gives the patient an hour of expensive professional time (thus shutting the doctor off from other patients during the same time periods), he charges fees which, in the more urban areas of the U.S.A., average 20–25 dollars (about 7–8 guineas) a contact (Davidson, 1956). Since this therapeutic transaction is a highly verbal one, the relatively inarticulate, unintelligent or non-intellectual patient is excluded.

The more eclectic psychiatrist writes prescriptions—usually for tranquilizers, occasionally for mood-stimulators, less often for the older hypnotic and sedative drugs. He may do electroconvulsive therapy in his office, in which case he is likely to have a nurse, resuscitation equipment, cots or beds, and stimulating medication available. More often, he has an arrangement with a private nursing home, sending his patients there for electrical therapies. He is available to testify in court on behalf of his patients, usually in litigation concerning claims of neurotic reaction or brain damage to personal injury. When indicated and when requested by the family, he is willing to sign medical certificates on commitment papers. He may make wide use of physical medicine (as well as psychiatric) equipment, either to "tone up" muscles, to produce relaxation through heat, or because of the psychological or suggestive effect of electricity, massage, baking and similar modalities. Since this practitioner can see several patients an hour, he is likely to charge lower fees than his more "purely psychotherapeutic" colleague. In the aggregate, he is going to earn more money than the psychoanalyst. The more eclectic doctor will average about 15 dollars per patient-contact; and if he sees three to five an hour, he will be earning from 45–75 dollars an hour (15–25 guineas), compared with the 25 dollar-an-hour standard income of the psychoanalyst.

The former's income is somewhat reduced by the expectation of his rendering unpaid service to "clinics" or community agencies. In the U.S.A., the word "clinic" refers to the out-patient department of a hospital, where patients may be treated gratis or at nominal fees. The psychoanalyst is almost certain to do no free or nominal-fee work. For this, there are two reasons. One is a matter of doctrine; a theory that the patient who is getting his service gratis does not value it. The other reason is that the psycho-therapist has an appointment book filled with private patients. And when that happens, any abrupt departure from the office for unpaid attendance elsewhere would be seen both as an unethical abandonment of a patient and a quixotic gesture, like throwing money away.

The Salaried Psychiatrist

About 40% of the psychiatrists in the U.S.A. draw their income essentially from salaried appointments. One recent survey (Davidson, 1965) divides the specialty as follows:

58% are primarily in private practice,
14% are in psychiatric or child guidance clinics,
13% are in public mental hospitals,
 6% hold salaried positions in general or university hospitals,
 4% hold salaried positions in private institutions.
_____
95%.

The remaining 5% are in industry, correctional institutions, military service, social agencies, schools for the retarded, in research or in educational institutions.

The psychiatrist in a clinic or child guidance center usually has a 35-hour week and does a good deal of work for community installations—schools, courts, and the like. Certain aspects of this work are reviewed below at the end of the section on The Financing of Psychiatric Care.

Psychiatric clinics usually pay their staffs somewhat less than could be earned in private practice, but more than public mental hospitals offer. Most of these clinics are child-guidance installations, though some mental health clinics for adults are available in the larger metropolitan centers.

The many small private hospitals in the U.S.A. vary in their staffing patterns. In some, there is only a rudimentary house-staff, most of the psychiatric and medical service being supplied by the private practitioners who send patients in. Others, however, have well-trained psychiatric staffs who supply direct care to the patients. Salaries in private hospitals are usually higher than those paid in the tax-supported or rate-supported public mental hospitals, where the range is from 9000 to 18,000 dollars (3000–6000 guineas) a year—sometimes with free or low-cost maintenance.

The Financing of Psychiatric Care

One of the unsolved problems in the U.S.A. is how the average American can afford to pay for private psychiatric care. Attention was called to this in an editorial (Davidson, 1963) in the official organ of the American Psychiatric Association. This leader reads in part:

> Most American psychiatrists in private practice have so good an income, that they are unable to devote time to unpaid, or modestly paid community services in clinics, public hospitals, guidance centers and the like. Most psychiatrists received part or all of their graduate education with an assist from the community in the form of in-service training in public or community-financed facilities. There is, one would think, something owed to the community in return for this.
>
> Almost every public hospital, community clinic, or similar installation is desperately understaffed. Most of them cannot afford fees that compete with private practice. Not enough private practitioners recognize the moral obligation to serve the community that has been so good to them. If they work for 10 dollars an hour in a community clinic or public hospital, they are—in effect—donating 15 dollars of their valuable time for each such hour, since they can earn that much more in private practice.
>
> But where does the average (90 dollars a week) American get psychiatric care? He can hardly pay 50 dollars a week for private psychiatric attention. In other branches of medicine, Blue Shield or another insurance might pay the bills; or he can go to a public clinic. But Blue Shield does not, as a rule, pay standard psychiatric fees; and the community clinic is no solution if the better-trained psychiatrists turn up their noses at serving in them.
>
> And what happens to the doctor–patient relationship if the private psychiatrist commits his patient to a public hospital? Will the private psychiatrist visit the institution, see the patient, attend staff meetings about him, make therapeutic suggestions, and show any interest in his previously paying patient? No—he cannot afford the time.
>
> The private practitioner will not serve Americans in public hospitals or community clinics; but he will fight vigorously against other therapists who *are* willing to render this service; psychologists, clergymen, psychiatric social workers, and so on.
>
> Only a small proportion of psychiatrists are now in community clinics and public hospitals. Those who cannot afford private care are piled on to the shoulders of the few doctors willing to work in such installations—and their loads are increasing to the point where they cannot give first-grade service; or where they too, no matter what their ideals, are being driven out from the less remunerative clinic and hospital service into the far more prosperous arena of private practice—thus making the problem even more desperate.
>
> The solution of this lies in the hands of our organized profession. We cannot forever accept a two-class society in terms of psychiatric care. Having private practitioners contribute some of their time to community enterprises is one possible way out. And surely the soaring mind of man is capable of thinking of other solutions.

The difficulty with providing private psychiatric out-patient care has been that psychotherapy, when the preferred method, takes up an enormous amount of the practitioner's time. If a doctor spends 50 or 60 minutes with a patient, he expects to be compensated adequately—and the stipend varies between 15 dollars (5 guineas) an hour in southern or rural areas, and 25 or even 30 dollars (10 guineas) a visit in the West and in urban centers throughout the country.

It does not take many patients to fill an appointment book, when the doctor can interview only eight or nine a day, and wants to see each patient two or three times a week.

As a result of his crowded schedule, the private psychotherapist has no way of knowing how many people need his help, but cannot afford it.

To meet this need, a system of clinics has been developed. Known variously as mental hygiene (or mental health) centers or clinics, as "development" or guidance centers or clinics or services, some facilities of this type exist in every state. To permit the therapist (who may be a psychiatric social worker, a psychologist or a lay analyst) to devote the necessary time to each patient, it has been found necessary to operate on an appointment basis. A one-visit-a-week pattern is generally considered too infrequent for effective psychotherapy; but even on that basis, the clinic cannot actually have on its books more than 25–35 patients per therapist.

(Some clinic time is diverted to meetings, research, teaching, administration and conferences.) Since the demand is much greater than can be met at this ratio, nearly all clinics have had to set up waiting lists. In many centers, a patient may not get his first therapeutic contact until he has been on the waiting list for several months.

Some clinics are sponsored by general or mental hospitals; some are sponsored by educational agencies. Government, at city, county or state level, is also a frequent supporter of out-patient mental health centers. Throughout the U.S.A. are many local mental health associations which operate or support mental hygiene clinics.

Most clinics are plagued by staff shortages. The difficulty with staffing is that the centers can not compete with private practice incomes. Typically, a clinic might offer its psychiatrist a salary of 35–50 dollars (12–17 guineas) for a half-day. The young doctor, just completing his residency, is happy to accept an appointment for perhaps three or four mornings a week, since this income will more than cover his rent and office expenses. However, as his private practice grows, he learns that he can earn 75–100 dollars (25–35 guineas) a morning in his private office. He is reluctant to keep working in the clinic at half that. After a short time, the doctor—at least the more successful one—is likely to leave the clinic. This causes further difficulties. Either the clinic recruits a new young doctor—or it reduces its case-load of patients—or it turns treatment over to psychologists or psychiatric social workers. While there are some noteworthy exceptions, in general, the level of out-patient care for the indigent or low-income patient is impaired by these problems.

In private psychiatric hospitals in the U.S.A. there are usually as many employees as patients. Typically, an 80-bed private mental hospital will have 80 patients. Each patient must, in effect, then pay the salary of one employee, plus all the costs for food, equipment and overhead expenses. Charges of 150 dollars (50 guineas) a week are at the lower end of the price scales. Costs in many private institutions come closer to 250 dollars (83 guineas) a week. Health and hospital insurance may cover much of this, but usually this insurance is limited in the amount of the indemnity and the number of weeks it will cover. A common pattern is for the patient to remain in a private institution until this insurance coverage is exhausted. By then, if he has not recovered, he is transferred to a public mental hospital. In the public institutions, indigent and low-income patients usually do not pay for their care. The actual cost to the State will be between 6 dollars (2 guineas) and 12 dollars (4 guineas) a day. Patients who can afford this (or their responsible relatives) are expected to meet these costs. The average length of stay in public mental hospitals usually outruns the insurance coverage.

The Widening Acceptance of Psychotherapy

Over the past half-century, the doctrines of psychotherapy in general, and psychoanalysis in particular, have become the prestigious modality of psychiatric treatment in the United States. This represents an extraordinary reversal of older American concepts in this field.

Certainly, the earlier American soil was unfavorable for psychotherapy. At the turn of the twentieth century, American psychiatry was colored by physiological rather than psychological thinking. For example, the Wier Mitchell "rest cure" was one of the popular panaceas of those days. It was based on theory that fatigue and anxiety were due to a "wearing out" of the nerves, and that rest was needed to recharge the batteries. Then, in the first decade of the century, the hope was that the endocrines had the magic key that would unlock the mind. Again, in the period after World War I, a surge of interest developed in focal infection as the cause of mental symptoms. One public hospital in the U.S.A. was so convinced that colon bacilli were the culprits, that removal of half the colon became a standard therapeutic procedure. And with all that medical, surgical and nursing care, colectomized patients did, indeed, seem to improve. The whimsy of the 1920's was that psychiatrists were persuading the surgeons to convert the colons into semi-colons.

The only non-medical thesis that won acceptance then was the concept that mental illness was the fruit of social and cultural pressures. But this ran a poor second to the biological explanations of emotional sickness. And all this seemed to provide little welcome for any psychodynamic thesis.

Somehow, the stone that the builder rejected became the capstone. The Freudian hypothesis, prior to perhaps 1940, was the subject of ridicule. It was the butt of a thousand jokes, cartoons, and contumacious references. Physicians who should have known better said that Freud ascribed all emotional illness to sex or that he blamed everything on incest wishes. This distortion resembled the misunderstandings of the late nineteenth century, when the anti-evolutionists insisted that Darwin had said that men were descended from monkeys.

In 1940, very few medical schools had placed analytically orientated psychiatrists on their faculties. The analysts then had to form their own institutes to train, examine and certify their aspirants. Neither the regular psychiatric organizations, nor the schools, nor the mental hospitals, would offer policy-making positions to psychoanalysts.

By 1960, the situation had been reversed. Nearly all medical schools had analysts in leading positions on psychiatric faculties. The typical private mental hospital boasted of the "dynamic" orientation of its staff. Even huge state hospitals, traditionally the stronghold of conservative leadership, began to accept some analysts. In metropolitan areas, psychiatric societies rapidly passed under the leadership of the more dynamically orientated specialists.

No one has satisfactorily explained this metamorphosis. Sargent (1963), viewing the phenomenon from Britain, hinted that the reason for the change was that during World War II, the proper psychiatrists of America entered the Army. The resulting vacuum he suggested, was then filled by aliens from Mittel Europa who seized control of the psychiatric machinery while its caretakers were in their country's service. Few Americans have accepted this colorful explanation. The analysts have a simpler thesis. It was a case of truth, crushed to earth, rising on its own merits. The very popularity of psychodynamics was seen as proof of its validity.

A number of more plausible, if less interesting, possibilities have been advanced. One was that the milder emotional illnesses—the psychoneuroses largely—were treated by private practitioners in urban offices, while the severer ones retreated into the overcrowded, understaffed human warehouses, identified as state hospitals. These institutions then had an essentially static view of mental illness, since their patients were, in essence, the rejects of society: the treatment failures abandoned by the private practitioners. Private practitioners were treating only the milder cases. By screening out the sicker ones—and sending them to state hospitals—the doctors in private offices automatically accumulated a reservoir of more treatable patients. Thus, their results were better. This implied that their methods were more effective and their theories more valid.

The Enchantment with Psychotherapy

The psychodynamic explanation of mental illness soon acquired prestige. Psychoanalysis as a treatment method was available only to those patients who were well enough to stay out of hospitals, articulate enough to talk freely, prosperous enough to pay substantial fees, sophisticated enough to talk comfortably about matters previously dismissed as unmentionable, and intelligent enough to co-operate in a complex program. Thus, analysis became identified with the smart, the articulate, the mildly ill, the wealthy, and the sophisticated. So, it acquired the glamor which it has never lost.

Physicians who want to become psychiatrists now stand at the branching of two roads: one leads to the public hospital, one to the greener backed pastures of private practice. In American public mental hospitals, the 600,000 patients have 3000 doctors, an average ratio of 200 patients per psychiatrist. The other road, as the aspirant sees it, would place him in an office, listening to articulate (and prosperous) young patients (old ones are not wanted). The doctor could practice in this way, content in the knowledge that a "difficult" patient could always be abandoned as poorly motivated; a violent or seriously psychotic one could be dismissed as too sick for out-patient care. He could, at a gentlemanly pace, see only a small number of patients, work intensively with their problems, never leaving his office to make house calls, testify in court, handle hospital emergencies or otherwise become involved in the labor and drudgery that is the lot of other physicians.

Faced with these alternatives, most American physicians (if free to do so) will elect the second image. Thus, the prestigious training programs in the U.S.A. are now the analytically orientated ones. The physicians who do not have the standing to win acceptance at the better known (analytically orientated) training institutes, must accept the hospitals which use non-analytic approaches. And, following the law of nature that the rich get richer and the poor poorer, it has come to pass that dynamic programs in America attract the better doctors. This is now cited to prove the first assumption: that the psychotherapeutic approach must be better because it enrolls the better doctors. Q.E.D.

Most American medical schools, especially in the more populous northern half of the country, have psychiatric departments under the leadership of dynamically orientated chairmen. Medical students are thus offered the psychotherapist as the very model of the modern psychiatrist, and are taught that all psychiatric treatment (other than psychotherapeutic) is "palliative" because it does not root out the trouble. The effect is to down-grade any non-analytical type of treatment. This is even more pronounced in the graduate training programs.

The psychiatrist who leans on psychotherapy must have a small case-load. If he works a 45-hour week, and wants to see his neurotic patients for three interviews a week, he can handle only 15 patients. On an average of a 2-year treatment course, he can manage only 7 or 8 new patients a year. Thus, he can accept only an infinitesimal proportion of the patients who need psychiatric care. But something like 90% of all of the more prestigious psychiatric training is geared to this kind of program. So, 90% of training time is spent in teaching its happy beneficiaries to handle only 5% of the patients. The remaining 10% of the trainees have to treat the remaining 95% of the patients.

There has developed in this area a self-fulfilling prophecy. The better-trained psychiatrists limit their practice to the patients most likely to be helped by psychotherapy, and thus exclude the sicker ones. They then achieve better results by psychotherapy than the less restrictive doctors do by eclectic treatment methods. This is taken to demonstrate that the psycho-dynamic approach is better. It reinforces the determination of the rising generation of new psychiatrists to limit themselves to psychotherapy, and the cycle continues.

Challenges to the Validity of Psychotherapy

Efforts to question the validity of the psychotherapeutic approach meet a strange resistance (Fisch, 1965). Even raising the question exposes the challenger to the feeling that he himself must be sick. For example, one psychoanalytical spokesman ascribed the challenge to psychotherapy to "pathologic narcissism and the persistence of the challenger's transference neurosis". This, it was further suggested, meant that the teachers of psychiatry had not been authoritarian enough; in Gittel's words (1962):

> Our failure to be uncompromising in the application of our insight into our authoritarian roles as teachers and educators may have something to do with the fact that at least some of our colleagues and students find solace for narcissistic injury in alliance as dissident coteries.

In all other branches of medicine, results are used to measure the validity of the therapeutic theory. A surgical doctrine that led to bad operative results would soon be abandoned. In American psychiatry, however, good results are dismissed as being merely palliative, if they seem to violate the doctrine. Fisch (*ibid.*) puts it this way:

> New forms of therapy are often discounted on the basis that the results achieved are only transference cures or flights into health. Thus, what in all other fields is the criterion is relegated to a secondary position, in favour of consistency with a prevailing theory. I have heard therapists claim that, should symptom relief without insight prove to last the lifetime of the patient, they would still regard it as a transference cure and something less than desirable. The concept is an unfortunate and devastating one. One wonders how often patients who have achieved marked relief and ego enhancement in early stages of treatment are subsequently convinced of the illusory nature of their improvement and seduced into lengthy, if not interminable treatment, with loss of confidence in their ability to gauge improvement because symptom change was labeled as flight into health. Telling patients that we are not interested in results may be a useful stratagem of treatment, but to disregard results in evaluating any form of therapy is dangerous.

This attitude has become self-perpetuating. A psychiatric apprentice who is paying 5 guineas a session for his didactic training analysis, knows that he will not be set free from his "learning" until he can accept the doctrines of his analyst. When he approaches the end of his training period, he finds it hard to keep saying "no", when it means more and more training sessions. If it costs 5 guineas every time he says "no", he soon learns to say "yes".

Some observers see other methods of persuasion which mold the aspiring psychiatrist. Fisch (*ibid.*) tells us that:

> In more subtle forms, supervisors in residency training programs may discourage innovation by asking that supervisees explore their own motivation for deviation

from conventional treatment. Residents who hope to practice in the area in which they are taking their training are particularly vulnerable to this kind of discouragement, since they will have to depend on senior clinicians and their hospital for recognition and sources of referral. The same applies to young psychiatrists in the community who also depend on the senior members of the profession to introduce them into the professional community and provide referrals. A reputation for being far out may seriously jeopardize the newcomer's practice.

The Community Mental Health Center

The newest development on the American psychiatric scene has been the promotion of "community mental health centers". This is intended to fill the gap between the private psychiatrist's office (or public clinic) and the mental hospital. In most of the U.S.A., a patient too sick to be handled, even briefly, in an office, has to be sent to a distantly located, badly over-crowded and seriously understaffed state hospital. Only a minority of American general hospitals will knowingly admit patients with primary psychiatric diagnoses. Furthermore, many of the private health insurance corporations either refuse to cover emotional illness, or place tight restrictions on such coverage and impose limitations on the indemnities they do offer. Typically, for example, a policy may pay benefits for 120 days in any year for a non-psychiatric illness or other disability; but for mental illness or emotional disability, the indemnity might be limited to 21 days in a life-time. The insurance plan developed by the hospitals (known in the U.S.A. as "Blue Cross") also generally puts limits on their coverage of mental illness, although this varies from state to state. Thus, even the meagre general hospital facilities that *are* available are often unused, since most Americans cannot afford private room care in general hospitals, which now runs to some 27–51 dollars (9–17 guineas) a day, if insurance is not available to cushion that financial blow.

To fill this gap, the U.S. Government is providing funds to states that will construct community mental health centers. These, it is expected, will be combined in-patient and out-patient facilities, to be set up at the ratio of one center per every 200,000 population. The model center will have 120 in-patient beds and be open 24 hours a day. Here, it is expected, acutely psychotic patients will be received—the depressed person on the verge of suicide, the man in a sudden catatonic excitement, the severe anxiety reaction, the overactive manic, and the suddenly disabling conversion reaction. A large proportion of these patients, it is hoped, would never need to be sent to the distant state hospitals, since they should recover promptly in the intensive treatment facility of the community mental health center.

So far, only a handful of these centers has been constructed. One dilemma has been the fear that these installations would rapidly silt up with untreatable cases. If that happens, the center would, in effect, be out of business because, with all its beds occupied, it could no longer accept the acute patients most responsive to treatment. The other horn of the dilemma, however, is that with a rigid admissions policy, the centers would be used only for the milder cases, for the patients least in need of treatment. Already, the few community mental health centers now in operation have listed such exclusions as: no seniles, no narcotic addicts, no brain damaged patients, no assaultive ones, no deteriorated patients, no defendants in the hands of civilian authorities, no alcoholics, no mentally retarded children, and so on. One unanticipated by-product of this exclusiveness has been that better doctors, nurses, psychologists and social workers, are moving out of the state hospitals (where eventually, only chronic and untreatable cases would be sent) into the more interesting and stimulating community centers. Thus the state hospitals, which so recently have lifted themselves above their status as custodial storage bins for the rejected, will find themselves forced back into that bleak position. This would happen if the more acute, more hopeful, and more treatable patients would get only as far as the community centers. One answer to this has been suggested: that is, to construct some community centers on the grounds of existing state hospitals.

The future of American psychiatry may lie in the success of community mental health centers, with 1966 and 1967 promised as the years when this program will move into high gear.

References

DAVIDSON, H. A. (1956), *Amer. J. Psychiat.* **113**, 41.
DAVIDSON, H. A. (1963), *Amer. J. Psychiat.* **119**, 796.
DAVIDSON, H. A. (1964a), *Amer. J. Psychiat.* **121**, 279.
DAVIDSON, H. A. (1964b), *Amer. J. Psychiat.* **121**, 329.
DAVIDSON, H. A. (1965), *Opportunities in a Psychiatric Career*, New York, Universal Publishing and Distributing Corporation.
FISCH, R. (1965), *Arch. Gen. Psychiat.* **13**, 359.
GITTEL, M. (1962), *J. Int. Psychoanalytical Assoc.* **43**, 375.
SARGENT, W. W. (1963), *Atlantic Quarterly*, July.

19. Links and Barriers between Hospital and Community *

BERNARD M. KRAMER

How is the mental hospital linked to or barred from the outside world? What forces are at work to foster or hinder the outflow of patients into the community, or the inflow of community elements into the hospital? How does the hospital reconcile contending pressures to keep the patient under protective wraps on the one hand, and to ease the patient into the community on the other?

Moving the patient into the community depends partly on how strong the attachments of the hospital are to the community. If the connection is weak, the likelihood of successful return is correspondingly weak. If it is strong, the conditions are more conducive to successful return.

I assume *a priori* that strong hospital–community linkages are associated with successful rehabilitation. What, then, are the link-barrier characteristics of the mental hospital? More specifically, what are the implications for hospital–community ties of such elements as physical characteristics, policy characteristics and day care?

Physical Characteristics of Hospitals

A mental hospital's location bears significantly on its relation to the community. Its distance from the center of population reveals something about its posture toward its service area. When a hospital is located in a distant, inaccessible place, the community's lack of contact with the hospital tends to foster avoidance which, in turn, tends further to reduce contact. In the present era of high-speed transportation, of course, distance is not so crucial as an isolating factor. Still, physical isolation, acting as a psychological barrier between hospital and community, is a potential deterrent to success in rehabilitation.

Size may also contribute to the bond between hospital and community. This is amply demonstrated by the experience of early nineteenth-century psychiatry. That period, known as the "moral treatment era", revealed the therapeutic value of a small mental hospital (Bockoven, 1956). A large hospital serving thousands of patients yields a bureaucratic atmosphere

* Reprinted from *The Community Mental Health Journal*, **1**, 69.

impeding therapeutic change, and weakening ties between the hospital and its service area. A hospital or community mental health center of not more than a few hundred patient-places is more human in scale, and would seem to be more inviting to hospital–community interaction.

Hospital architecture may likewise foster or hamper community participation. Imposing walls and fences tend to evoke a taboo against fraternization. On the other hand, inclusion of community facilities such as stores, theatres, gyms and art galleries would evoke encouragement of interaction.

Policy Characteristics

Hospital–community relations may also be affected by policy decisions. A classic example is the policy decision around the turn of the century to transfer responsibility for the care of the mentally ill from local government to state government (Hunt, 1959). Although the reasons for the shift were various—some good, some bad—the consequences were enormous. A major consequence was the almost fatal weakening of the bonds between the institutions and the local communities. The structure needed to administer the state-wide network became too ponderous to serve as a bridge between hospitals and localities.

Gradually, but inexorably, localities became less and less involved in the care of the mentally ill. It was no surprise, therefore, that the hospitals declined gradually from the grand stature of the moral treatment era to the miserable custodial atmosphere we have come to know so well (Bockoven, 1956). Some of the decline can be attributed to legislative and administrative policies that removed responsibility from the local to the state level. Happily, we now witness many significant efforts to strengthen local involvement through such mechanisms as the comprehensive community mental health center.

Another example of policy influences on community–hospital linkage lies in the realm of hospital trustees. Some administrators take the view that hospital affairs are of a professional order and that the influence of trustees should be minimal. They encourage weak appointments to boards of trustees, meet infrequently with them, and hold them at a distance. As a consequence, channels of communication to the outside world tend to be restricted, and opportunities for profitable dialogue are limited. Some hospitals, on the other hand, formulate a conscious policy of encouraging structural linkages. They appoint strong trustees with substantial civic roots. Likewise, they seek representation of all segments of the population, including labor and minority groups, as a way of tying the hospital to the entire locality. This alone, of course, does not effect a full bond between the hospital and the people it serves—but it does illustrate the thought that conscious hospital policy may influence hospital–community relations.

Other policies with potential relevance for hospital–community ties include those concerning admission and discharge, length of stay, relative weights in the service–research–teaching triad, reception of patients, visiting hours and patient classification. All these may exercise influence on how open or closed the hospital is to the community at large or to patient-related individuals.

Day Hospitals

Perhaps the most important factor shaping the hospital's openness to the community is its pattern of rehabilitation facilities. Today the "therapeutic *milieu*" tends to make the very hospital itself a rehabilitation facility. Orientating itself to returning the patient to the community, it becomes a facility not only for care but also for rehabilitation. This philosophy enhances the hospital's intercourse with the community as it seeks to improve its rehabilitation potential. Let me focus on the community implications of one current approach—the day hospital.

It is intriguing to watch the extraordinary rise in popularity of day care in the past several years (Epps and Hanes, 1964; Farndale, 1961; Kramer, 1962; National Clearinghouse, 1964). This growth is reflected in the federal regulations concerning the Community Mental Health Centers Act of 1963. They specifically refer to partial hospitalization as a key element of service in comprehensive community mental health centers (U.S. Department of Health, Education and Welfare, 1964). There is now hardly a state in the union that does not have some sort of day care facility for its mentally ill.

More important than the geographic spread, however, is the diversity in character of the various units which, by now, must number in the several hundreds. Some units operate as wards within large state hospitals, some as separate, quasi-autonomous services; some are related to, but located at a distance from, the hospital; some units are small, others large; some are administered by a local community mental health center, some by a mental health association, and a few are altogether independent. Some focus on the chronically ill, while others focus on rehabilitation of acutely ill patients. Some emphasize the transition from full hospital-status to community living, and others focus on day care as a means of preventing initial hospitalization.

To my knowledge, no studies have definitely shown whether any of these approaches is superior to any other. Nor, in fact, have studies shown whether day care is more or less effective than traditional care, from a therapeutic or rehabilitative standpoint. A reasonable statement, nonetheless, would seem to be that day care is not grossly less effective than full-time care. Yet it has, at the same time, the advantage of preserving the patient's communal ties. Likewise, it would seem fair to say that the various approaches to day care are equally valid if adequate provision is made for efficient transfer of patients to other facilities when day care appears not to be in their best interest.

In the long run, the most distinctive and enduring feature of the day hospital is its intrinsic character as a link between the hospital world and that of the community. This linkage takes shape in several ways. First, and probably most telling, is the fact that day patients return home nightly to their families and neighborhoods. Patients are reminded each day of their continuity with their own setting. Local sights and sounds retain their familiarity. Expected behavior and activity hold their customary force. Social skills in moving back and forth between hospital and community do not become atrophied through disuse. The daily trips to and fro declare concretely that, despite illness, they are not irreparably cut off from their homes. To be sure, some patients would prefer to do just this, and withdraw into the narrower and perhaps less trying world of the hospital. On the whole, though, preservation of neighborhood ties is probably the most important single value of day care.

A second involvement of day care in the community is through patients' families. When a patient is admitted on a full-time basis, the hospital takes responsibility for his care and the family recedes into the background as an interested, but psychologically distant, party. Under day care, by contrast, the family is always in the foreground, in that it shares responsibility with the hospital.

Although the patient is away at the hospital during the day, the family has to help the patient muster ego-strength to execute the often taxing job of just getting to the hospital. The family must also often assist the patient to make it back home. Although coming and going is for many patients quite simple and smooth, the family is never really quite sure how well the process will work, and therefore tends to remain in a poised position, ready to step in when needed. Likewise, caring for the patient at home, evenings and weekends, carries with it special problems and difficulties which call for a relationship of mutuality between family and hospital. Episodes of turmoil will arise which call for special family reflexes and the day-care unit must be ready to assist when needed. In brief, the hospital cannot execute a day program without the co-operation of the family, and the family cannot carry out its end without the assistance of the hospital. This interdependence between hospital and family operates as a continuing link between the institution and an important segment of the community.

A third nexus between day hospital and the community is represented by neighbors and other individuals in the patient's orbit. If the patient's activities proceed fairly smoothly, neighbors and significant others, seeing his daily movement between home and hospital, may undergo significant changes in attitudes toward the mentally ill. Indirectly this may heighten community receptivity for psychiatric rehabilitation. If, on the other hand, these individuals experience recurrent episodes of violent or other disturbing behavior by the patient, a boomerang effect may occur. People in the locality might call for greater strictness in the control of patients or for abolishing partial hospitalization. Under such a circumstance, a strong relationship with the community stands the hospital in good stead. Expression of negative community attitudes provides an opportunity for the hospital to encounter directly the feelings of the community and, through the process of confrontation, assist the community to develop workable attitudes toward mental illness.

Finally, serving to bind the community and the day hospital are the unit's workers. They are directly involved in the whole process of keeping the patient in the community. They work with the family, interpret to the local population, deal with health and welfare agencies, arrange placements in sheltered workshops, maintain ties with employment resources, seek out recreational and educational opportunities, and stay alert to community developments that bear on the welfare of their patients. If they carry out these activities effectively, they serve as indispensable bonds between hospital and community. Without a well-trained and effective staff in sufficient numbers, all the hospital's efforts at community relations would fail, and the chances for success in rehabilitation would be diminished.

In summary, links between hospital and community may be affected by such physical characteristics as size, location and architecture; by policy characteristics, such as State versus local initiative and policy concerning trustees; and by the nature of hospital-based rehabilitation facilities, such as day care. Since rehabilitation has the objective of maintaining the patient in the community, and since this requires a fertile soil of community acceptance, it is important to identify and strengthen those forces which tend to link together the community and the hospital. We may hope that as this process gathers momentum, those afflicted with mental illness will be led along toward higher levels of rehabilitation.

References

BOCKOVEN, J. S. (1956), Moral treatment in American psychiatry, *The Journal of Nervous and Mental Disease*, **124**, 167–320.

EPPS, R. L. and HANES, L. D. (1964), *Day Care of Psychiatric Patients*, Springfield, Ill., Charles C. Thomas.

FARNDALE, J. (1961), *The Day Hospital Movement in Great Britain*, London, Pergamon Press.

HUNT, R. C. (1959), Rehabilitation Potential of the Mentally Ill, In *Rehabilitation of the Mentally Ill* (eds. M. Greenblatt and B. Simon), Washington, D.C., 1959, pp. 25–36.

KRAMER, B. M. (1962), *Day Hospital*, New York, Grune & Stratton.

NATIONAL CLEARINGHOUSE FOR MENTAL HEALTH INFORMATION (1964), Selected Bibliography on Psychiatric Day–Night Services. Brochure distributed by National Institute of Mental Health, Bethesda, Maryland, January 1964.

U.S. DEPARTMENT OF HEALTH, EDUCATION AND WELFARE (1964), Community Mental Health Centers Act of 1963, Title II, Public Law 88–164, Regulations. *Federal Register*, May 6, 1964.

20. A Five-year Survey of a Psychiatric Service in a Geographically Delimited Rural Population

JOHANNES NIELSEN and ERIK STRÖMGREN

THE purpose of the present study is to give a survey of how many and what type of patients were referred to the psychiatric service in a delimited, relatively small rural area, given very easy access to this service which was set up in the community in close co-operation with the physicians and the general hospital in the community, a service which was extended from the Århus State Hospital in 1957 as part of a psychiatric-demographic research project comprising a project in Århus County and the Samsø-Project.

The Samsø-Project as a whole can hardly be compared with any other community psychiatric project, but it is in some of its aspects similar to the community psychiatric projects described by Carse *et. al.* (1958), Sainsbury and Grad (1962), Grad and Sainsbury (1963), and Macmillan (1958, 1962, 1963).

The Samsø-Project

One of the purposes of the Samsø-Project is to investigate to what extent a geographically delimited population will make use of a psychiatric service, when given easy access to such service through the general practitioners in the island and the physicians at the general hospital serving the area. It also has the purpose of collecting psychiatric incidence and prevalence data in this population, and to determine to what extent there is a need for psychiatric treatment in the population concerned, and to study the effects of such treatment in those who are in need of it.

Samsø was chosen for this project because it offers opportunities of studying a geographically delimited and relatively stable population within the receiving area of the Århus State Hospital where the project was started. It was not chosen because the population was considered especially in need of psychiatric treatment, nor because the population was found to be representative of the population in Denmark, except perhaps of the population in other rural districts. The purpose of the Samsø-Project is not to compare the population with the rest of the Danish population, but rather to compare it with

* Reprinted from *Comprehensive Psychiatry*, **6**, No. 3 (June), 1965.

itself; follow it for many years through the service of the psychiatric out-patient clinic on the island, and include prevalence and incidence studies. It is hoped that it will be possible to arrive at some quantitative results with regard to possible changes in the mental health status of the population when it is given maximum opportunities for psychiatric treatment. It is also anticipated that some hints will be obtained as to how, where, and by whom psychiatric treatment is best and most practically given to patients in the different diagnostic and age groups.

THE PSYCHIATRIC CLINIC

The psychiatric clinic in Samsø was started in 1957 in co-operation with the general practitioners and the chief of the hospital in the island. There are two general practitioners and a general hospital with 36 beds. The psychiatric clinic is for out-patients only; it is located in the same building as the general practitioners' consulting rooms, and in the general hospital there is a room available for E.C.T.-treatment of patients who either stay in the hospital during the treatment or are treated as out-patients. The hospital has in this and several other ways played an important role for the psychiatric service. Only the general practitioners and the physicians at the hospital refer patients to the psychiatric clinic—patients who are considered by these physicians as psychiatric cases in need of treatment and patients who are willing to see a psychiatrist. There are no fees for consultations in the clinic. The physicians in the island have been urged to refer all psychiatric cases to the clinic. Practically no cases have been referred to psychiatrists outside the island.

The conditions that distinguish the Samsø psychiatric clinic from other psychiatric out-patient clinics in Denmark are the great number of patients seen in their homes and the close co-operation between the psychiatrists and the physicians in the island.

Before a referred patient is seen, he is usually discussed briefly with the referring physician, and the case record which is kept by the general practitioner is studied and quoted in the psychiatric case record.

The patients might be seen first either in the clinic or in their homes. Elderly people are nearly always seen in their homes all through the treatment period. Psychotic patients who do not wish to go to the clinic, but who are willing to accept visits by the psychiatrist are also visited in their homes when referred. Later during treatment, most patients are visited in their homes as described under Results.

When a new patient has been seen for the first time, the referring physician is usually contacted again, and a preliminary opinion of the patient is given by the psychiatrist. As soon as the case record is written up, a summary of it with the preliminary diagnosis, opinion about the patient, and treatment plan is sent to the general practitioner. Patients in treatment in the clinic are discussed with the general practitioners at monthly or more frequent intervals. Follow-up notes giving information about the patient's condition, the anticipated length of treatment, etc., are sent to the general practitioner approximately once a month.

Before the Samsø-Project and the psychiatric clinic in the island were started, practically the only psychiatric service in the island was provided by admission of patients to the Århus State Hospital, but a few patients were admitted to psychiatric institutions in Zealand. There was practically no opportunity for referring patients to a psychiatrist or to a psychiatric out-patient clinic, as has also been the case in many other rural districts in Denmark.

During the 5 years the clinic has existed, there has been a psychiatrist on the island at least once a week and there has been assistance by psychologists who have tested patients when needed. The clinic has been run by young psychiatrists supervised by senior psychiatrists. Treatment has comprised supportive psychotherapy, drug therapy, and E.C.T., but not psychoanalytic therapy. The psychiatrists working in the clinic have spent approximately 2 days per week in the clinic, working in other research projects the rest of the time. During the 5-year period the clinic has existed, 600 patients have been referred, those under 15 years, constituting 8%, have been described by Lange (1960). Patients above 15 years constitute 10% of the adult population in the middle of the 5-year period (Nielsen et al., 1962). During the same period, 73 patients aged 65+, constituting 8% of the population 65+, have been referred to the clinic (Nielsen, 1962a).

The Island

Samsø is situated in the Kattegat between Jutland and Zealand, 2 hours by ferry boat from Århus in Jutland and Kalundborg in Zealand. The island is not very isolated because of daily ferry connections with Jutland and Zealand and a tourist invasion in the summer. Samsø belongs to the county of Holbaek in Zealand and until recently it was divided in five parishes which by now are united in one parish administrated from Tranebjerg, which is the largest village in the island with approximately 800 inhabitants.

Samsø consists of 28,151 acres of which 22,396 are farming land and 1961 forests and plantations. More than half of the farms have less than 50 acres, most of the bigger farms have about 75–100 acres, and only very few have more than 150 acres, but there is one big estate that has 5930 acres of which 1900 are forests and plantations.

The Population

The population in Samsø has increased from 4049 in 1801 to a peak of 7500 in 1911. From 1911 to 1961, the population has decreased from 7500 to

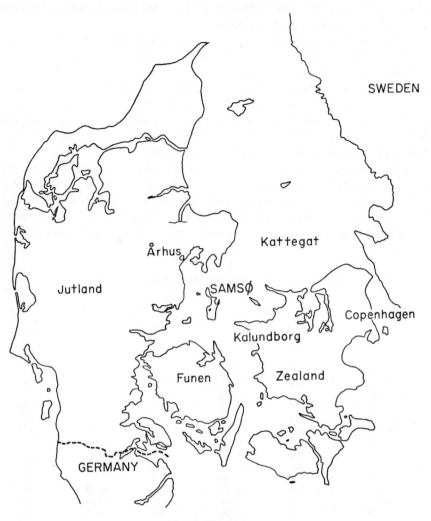

Fig. 1. Denmark.

6189. In other rural districts in Denmark there has also been a considerable decrease in the population resulting from the moving of younger people to the cities. The rate with which young people have been moving away from Samsø has, however, been higher than in other rural districts during the last decade and, consequently, the percentage of people in the age group 20–24 is approximately half and in the age group 25–29 three-quarters of the percentage found in those age groups in other rural districts in Denmark. The population in the age groups 15–20 and 30+ is, however, distributed as elsewhere in rural districts in Denmark. The population is relatively stable with only 33% born outside the island.

Of the 1634 married couples on Samsø on 1 January 1960, 11 were first-cousin marriages; this gives a consanguinity rate of 0·7%, which corresponds with what is found in other rural districts in Denmark. Economically, the population can best be characterized as a relatively wealthy rural population with farming as the main source of income. Of the male population above 15 years, 54% are occupied with farming, 19% with commerce, trade, and industry, 3% with fishing, and only 2% with unskilled labour. Only very few of the married women work outside their homes.

As background population for the present 5-year survey of patients aged 15+ referred to the psychiatric clinic in Samsø by the general practitioners and the physicians in the hospital, we have chosen the population aged 15+ in the middle of the 5-year period (4860). The distribution of this population according to sex, age and marital status is seen in Table 1, Fig. 2, and Fig. 3.

TABLE 1.

The Population aged 15+ on 1 January 1959. Distribution by Age and Sex

	Male		Female		
Age	Total	%	Total	%	M + F Total
15–19	240	9·72	206	8·62	446
20–24	171	6·93	138	5·77	309
25–29	139	5·63	163	6·82	302
30–34	175	7·09	155	6·48	330
35–39	213	8·63	204	8·53	417
40–44	189	7·65	182	7·61	371
45–49	228	9·23	236	9·87	464
50–54	258	10·45	238	9·95	496
55–59	202	8·18	197	8·24	399
60–64	200	8·10	212	8·87	412
65–69	171	6·93	161	6·73	332
70–74	123	4·98	140	5·86	263
75–79	96	3·89	80	3·35	176
80–84	42	1·70	51	2·13	93
85–89	16	0·65	22	0·92	38
90–94	4	0·16	6	0·25	10
95–99	2	0·08	0	0·00	2
Totals	2469	100%	2391	100%	4860

THE CENTRAL FILE OF SAMSØ

Information about the population gained within the frames of the Samsø-Project are recorded in the central file which comprises punch-cards and

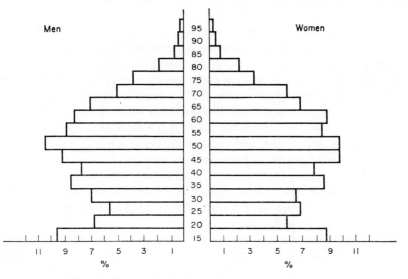

FIG. 2. The population aged 15+ on 1 January 1959.

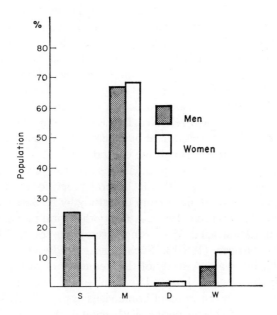

FIG. 3. The population aged 15+ on 1 January 1959;
distribution by marital status.

corresponding file cards for the whole population in Samsø, made in collaboration with the Statistical Office and Punch Card Office of the City of Århus, set up on 1 January 1959, and since then checked every 6 months, adding cards for new-borns and newcomers in the island and removing the cards on those who died or moved away from the island. It should be mentioned that in Denmark registration in the parish or city where one lives is compulsory and the registration files are nearly 100% complete. When moving to a new parish or city, registration has to be completed within 5 days after arrival.

On each card in the central file, there is information of age, sex, marital status, address, occupation, and birthplace. It is thus possible to get information about the stability of the population every 6 months, and the distribution according to sex, age, marital status, occupation, birthplace and address on the island. The central file is set up alphabetically for the whole island with a card for each person, and also with all persons in a family recorded on the card of the head of the family.

Whenever a person is referred to the psychiatric clinic in Samsø, information is obtained about all relatives, especially those living in the island. The name of the patient referred is then recorded on the central file card of all relatives together with the case record number and the type of family relation.

Within the framework of the Samsø-Project, a psychiatric-psychological study of 122 10-year-old children and their parents has been made by Lange et al. (1960), and a study is being made by a psychologist and a social worker, aiming at a psychological and social study of 59 children, their homes, and parents when the children are 6, 10, and 14 years old. Preliminary data from this study have been presented by Haslund (1962). An evaluation of the Binet–Simon system evaluated from an unselected sample of children in Samsø has been made by Mogensen et al. (1960). The information obtained in these special studies is also recorded in the central file cards of the persons examined and their near relatives. In these different ways, psychological, psychiatric and social information about the whole population is expected to be collected and available through the central file.

A census study of the whole population aged 15+ has been made by a psychiatrist in co-operation with the general practitioners in Samsø. Preliminary reports have been given from this study by A. Sørensen and Strömgren (1961) and A. Sørensen (1962). A 6-month-period prevalence investigation of the population aged 65+ using several sources of information has been made by Nielsen (1962b). Such census studies are planned to be made at regular intervals. A study of the frequency of mental illness among the patients in the general hospital in Samsø has been made by Nielsen (1962c). Reports about the value of home visits by psychiatrists and treatment in the community of elderly people with mental illness has been given by Nielsen (1963, 1965), and a study of mental disorders in married couples has been made by Nielsen (1964).

DIAGNOSES

The diagnoses are with a few modifications in accordance with the diagnostic list established by the Danish Psychiatric Association.

The concept of *schizophrenia* is used in a narrower sense and the concept of *manic-depressive psychosis* in a considerably wider sense in Denmark than in most countries (Arentsen and Strömgren, 1959). Most of the manic-depressive psychoses are cases that do not have the typical oscillations between mania and depression. One-fourth of the manic-depressive cases are mild depressions as described from the Samsø-Project by Florian Sørensen (1961), patients who manifest signs of mild depression, reduced zest of life, feelings of insufficiency and self-reproach—but with such somatic complaints as tiredness and hypochondria as the prevailing symptoms—cases that respond well to antidepressive treatment.

Psychogenic psychoses are psychoses which arise in immediate connection with mental stress, and the symptomatology and course of such psychoses are in most cases determined by mental trauma (Faergeman, 1963). In Anglo-Saxon psychiatry, a number of these cases are usually labelled schizophrenia or neuroses.

Paranoid psychoses are those dominated by delusions that are not accessory psychiatric disturbances in schizophrenia, manic-depressive psychosis, mental deficiency, or organic dementia.

Senile and arteriosclerotic psychoses follow the usual diagnostic lines in Anglo-Saxon psychiatry.

Other organic psychoses comprise patients with psychiatric symptoms in connection with cerebrovascular attacks or *sequelae* from such attacks, patients with previous encephalitis, patients with delirious reactions or severe depression in relation to somatic disease.

Epilepsy, Neuroses, Character-disorder, and *Alcoholism* are in diagnostic accordance with Anglo-Saxon psychiatric classification.

Mental deficiency also comprises patients with I.Q. between 70 and 90.

Legal abortion comprises patients referred to the psychiatric clinic for evaluation of a possible indication for legal abortion because of mental disease.

Unspecified mental disorder comprises patients with neurological disorders and mild psychiatric symptoms, patients with hypochondria, and patients with fluctuating mild anxiety or nervousness.

Of the patients with *no mental disorder*, 80% are neurologic cases.

Results

During the first 5 years, 472 patients age 15+ were referred for the first time to the psychiatric service in Samsø.

The distribution of the 472 patients according to sex and age in relation to the population is shown in Fig. 4. In the population, the percentage of men is 50·8, and among the patients it is 39·6.

The percentage of women in the population is 49·2 and among the patients 60·4. Figure 4 shows that the excess of female patients falls in the age group 20–34, rising to 18% in the age group 20–29 and having another peak at the age group 50–54 years. The total percentage referred of the female population is 11·9, and that of the male population is 7·9. It is seen in Fig. 4 that the referral rate of men is exceptionally low in the age group 35–39.

Figure 5 shows that there are only small differences in the distribution of the population and the patients according to marital status. The only statistically significant find is in divorced women with 1·4% found in the population and 3·7% in the patients referred ($p < 0·05$).

The percentage of patients born outside Samsø is higher than the percentage of the total population born outside the island, but the difference is statistically significant only for women with 36·7% in the population and 44·2% among the patients ($p < 0·01$). For men the figures are 31·1% of the population and 33·7% of the patients born outside Samsø.

The distribution by age and sex of the 283 patients born in Samsø and the 189 born outside the island is shown in Fig. 6. It is seen that the difference in sex of patients referred is caused by the higher referral rate of women born outside Samsø, and it further shows that the highest percentage of patients born outside the island is primarily found in the age groups 20–39 for women and 40–49 for men.

Table 2 shows that there are only slight differences in diagnostic distribution of the patients born outside Samsø and the total number of patients, the only statistically significant deviations found in character disorder with 7·8% among the total number of patients compared to 11·6% in the group of patients born outside the island ($p < 0·02$), and in legal abortion comprising 4·9% of the total number of patients compared to 7·9% of the patients born outside Samsø ($p < 0·02$).

Figure 7 and Table 3 show that the number of patients referred per year has varied only from 70 to 102 giving a referral rate per 1000 per year of 20·6, 21·0, 20·4, 14·4, and 20·9 in the 5 years respectively.

The number of patients referred more than once has been rising from 3 in 1957 to 32 in 1961, an increase in referral rate from 0·6 in 1957 to 7·6 per 1000 per year in 1961. The total referral rate per year has thus actually gone up from 21·0 per 1000 in 1957 to 28·5 in 1961 with the lowest total referral rate of 19·0 per 1000 in 1960.

Table 3 further shows that there are some changes in the percentage of patients referred within the different diagnostic groups from year to year. The percentage of patients with psychoses has been rising from 30·0% in 1957 to 46·5% in 1961. The percentage of neuroses has been falling from

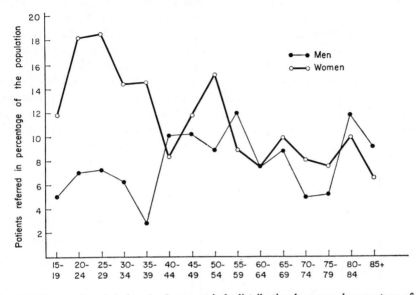

FIG. 4. Patients referred during the 5-year period; distribution by sex and percentage of the population in the corresponding age groups.

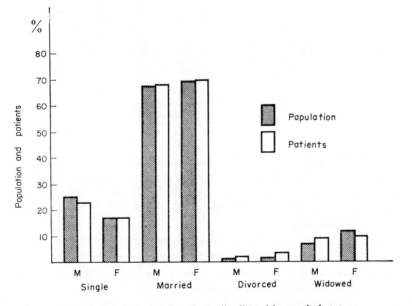

FIG. 5. Population and patients distributed by marital status.

37·0% to 24·8% and character disorders from 12·0% to 4·9%. In the other diagnostic groups, the changes are small and insignificant.

The distribution of patients according to diagnosis, age, and sex is seen in Tables 4 and 5. The percentage of patients and the rate of patients for the 5-year period calculated in relation to the population aged 15+ in the middle of the 5-year period are given for the different diagnoses and age groups. For psychoses there are only slight differences in the rates for men and women, 34·4 and 36·2, whereas the rate for neuroses is 42·2 for women and 10·9 for men. The rate of patients referred is highest in the age group 20–29

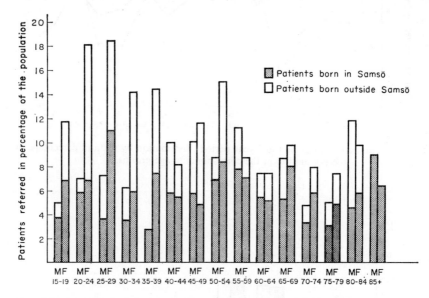

Fig. 6. Patients referred during the 5-year period; distribution by sex, age, place of birth and percentage of population in the different age groups.

for women as seen from Fig. 4 and Table 5, and the rate for men highest in the age groups 40–60. The total rate for mental illness is higher for women than for men, 119·2 compared to 75·6 per 1000. The rate for men and women taken together is 97·0 per 1000. Of the patients referred, 37% had psychoses and 27% had neuroses.

In Table 6 it is seen that 51% of the patients had at least one home visit paid by a psychiatrist. A total of 1451 home visits were paid to these 241 patients making up 45% of the total number of 3228 consultations. Nearly all the manic-depressive patients and schizophrenic patients have been seen in their homes and 68% of all the psychotic patients have been visited at home.

TABLE 2.

Distribution of Patients according to Place of Birth—in Samsø or Somewhere else in Denmark

	Patients totals		Patients born outside Samsø	
	Total	%	Total	%
Schizophrenia	5	1·1	1	0·5
Manic-depressive psychoses	65	13·8	24	12·7
Psychogenic psychoses	36	7·6	14	7·4
Paranoid psychoses	6	1·3	2	1·0
Senile and arterioscl. psychoses	35	7·4	13	7·0
Other organic psychoses	26	5·5	12	6·3
Psychoses total	173	36·7	66	34·9
Epilepsy	12	2·5	2	1·1
Neuroses	128	27·1	45	23·8
Character disorders	37	7·8	22	11·6 $X = 6·24$ $(p < 0·02)$
Alcoholism	6	1·3	2	1·1
Mental deficiency	19	4·0	6	3·2
Legal abortion, obs.	23	4·9	15	7·9 $X = 6·35$ $(p < 0·02)$
Unspecified mental disorders	52	11·0	20	10·6
No mental disorders	22	4·7	11	5·8
Totals	472	100·0	189	100·0

Ninety-one patients have been paid more than 10 consultations (Table 7). It is seen that it is mainly the patients with manic-depressive psychoses, schizophrenia and paranoid psychoses who have been treated for longer periods, whereas none of the patients with senile and arteriosclerotic psychoses have been seen more than 10 times.

In Table 8 it is seen that 75 of the 472 patients have been referred more than once, the highest percentage of patients referred again is found among the schizophrenic and manic-depressive patients. There are, however, no great differences between the percentages of patients with psychoses total, neuroses and character disorders who have been referred. Of the 75 patients referred, 12 were referred twice, the number of re-referrals being thus 88 during the 5-year period.

In Table 9 is shown the diagnostic distribution of the 46 patients admitted to psychiatric hospital. The highest admission percentage of the referred patients was 40% of the schizophrenic and 50% of the patients with paranoid psychoses. The percentage of patients with psychoses who were admitted was 17% and that of neuroses and character disorders 7 and 8%. No patients with neuroses and character disorders have been admitted during the last 2 years of the 5-year period.

In Table 10 it is seen that there was no great difference in the diagnostic distribution of the patients referred by the four general practitioners A, B, C and D. The percentage of psychoses was slightly higher among the patients referred by D and there was a slightly lower percentage of patients with neuroses, and a higher percentage of patients with unspecified mental disorders among the patients referred by C and D. E represents the physicians at the general hospital. It is seen that the percentage of psychoses referred by the physicians at the hospital was relatively high.

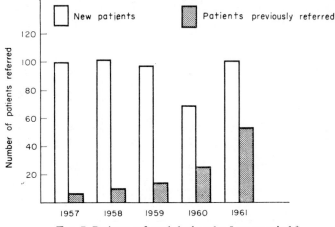

FIG. 7. Patients referred during the 5-year period.*

The total number of patients has been divided into three groups according to where and by whom they were considered to be treated best and most practically (Table 11). This judgement has been made by psychiatrists working in the Samsø psychiatric clinic and is based on the special circumstances in this clinic, comprising close contact and good co-operation with the general practitioners and the physicians in the general hospital, home visits, free and long-term treatment possibilities.

It is seen in Table 11 that 43% of the patients referred might be treated by the general practitioners after examination by the psychiatrist and advice to the general practitioner concerning treatment. Forty-six per cent of the patients referred could be treated on an ambulatory basis, and 11% were judged as being in need of treatment in a psychiatric hospital. The difference between the 10% admitted and the 11% who were thought to be in need of hospitalization stems from patients who did not want to be admitted.

* 1957 was not a complete year, as the psychiatric clinic was not opened till May.

The time spent in the clinic by the five young psychiatrists has not been recorded, but they each worked approximately 2 days per week in the clinic counting also the travelling time to and from the island. All five together spent 138 months in the Samsø-Project. On the average there were two psychiatrists working simultaneously at all times during the 5 years. Calculating from these approximate figures one psychiatrist working 4 days per week could have taken care of the ambulatory psychiatric treatment in this population with 4860 people aged 15+ where the referral rate of new cases was 19·4 per 1000 per year and the admission rate 1·7 per 1000 per year.

In Table 12 is shown treatment results in the 270 patients who were actually treated by the psychiatrists; 202 patients were examined by the psychiatrists, and then treated by the physicians in the island if needed.

Treatment of the 270 patients comprised mainly supportive interview therapy in 139 cases, mainly antidepressive drug therapy in 48 cases, E.C.T. in 9 cases, mainly phenothiazine derivatives in 42 cases, and drugs of different kinds such as chlorprothixene, chlordiazepoxide, phenobarbitone, meprobamate, migraine drugs, anti-epileptic drugs, and antiparkinsonism drugs in 32 cases.

Treatment results are seen in Table 12, 73 patients were unchanged, 36 of whom were neurotics. One hundred and thirty-six improved, and 61 were cured. Forty-five per cent of the patients with psychoses improved, and 41% were cured compared with 52% improved in the group of patients with neuroses and only 10% cured in this group.

Discussion

During the 5-year period 1957–61, a total of 472 patients aged 15+ have been referred as new patients to the psychiatric clinic on Samsø by the general practitioners and by the physicians in the general hospital in the island. That gives a rate of 19·4 per 1000 per year when calculated in relation to the population aged 15+ in the middle of the 5-year period. The rate for patients re-referred rose from 0·6 per 1000 in 1957 to 7·6 in 1961. The rate for admission to mental hospitals in Denmark outside Copenhagen in 1959 was 2·32 per 1000 for men and 3·23 for women (*Medical Report for the Kingdom of Denmark, 1961*). In Samsø, the admission rate during 1957–61 was 1·7 per 1000 per year a rate about half the rate for the whole country, but corresponding to the average admission rate from Samsø during the 5-year period previous to 1957.

In Chichester where all patients referred to psychiatric service are seen either at home or in the ambulatory clinic before admission is decided upon, the referral rate in 1960–61 was 6·3 per 1000 but only 27% were admitted to psychiatric hospital, the rest was treated as out-patients. This gives an admission rate of 1·7 per 1000 or the same as the average admission rate in Samsø during the 5-year period.

TABLE 3.

Patients referred First Time distributed by Year, Diagnosis and Rate/1000 and Patients referred More than Once distributed by Year and Rate/1000

	1957 Total	1957 %	1958 Total	1958 %	1959 Total	1959 %	1960 Total	1960 %	1961 Total	1961 %
Schizophrenia	1	1·0	1	1·0	2	2·0	0	0·0	1	0·9
Manic-depressive psychoses	16	16·0	10	9·8	16	16·2	10	14·2	13	12·9
Psychogenic psychoses	4	4·0	6	5·9	9	9·1	7	10·0	10	9·9
Paranoid psychoses	1	1·0	0	0·0	3	3·0	1	1·4	1	0·9
Senile and arteriosclerotic psychoses	7	7·0	7	6·7	6	6·0	7	10·0	8	7·9
Other organic psychoses	1	1·0	4	3·9	5	5·1	2	2·9	14	13·9
Psychoses total	30	30·0	28	27·5	41	41·4	27	38·6	47	46·5
Epilepsy	3	3·0	6	5·9	1	1·0	1	1·4	1	0·9
Neuroses	37	37·0	34	33·3	13	13·1	19	27·1	25	24·8
Character disorders	12	12·0	7	6·9	10	10·1	3	4·3	5	4·9
Alcoholism	1	1·0	1	1·0	1	1·0	1	1·4	2	2·0
Mental deficiency	3	3·0	3	2·9	5	5·1	3	4·3	5	5·0
Legal abortion, obs.	2	2·0	3	2·9	11	11·1	3	4·3	4	3·9
Unspecified mental disorders	8	8·0	15	14·7	14	14·1	7	10·0	8	7·9
No mental disorders	4	4·0	5	4·9	3	3·0	6	8·6	4	3·9
Patients referred first time										
Total	100	100·0	102	99·8	99	99·9	70	99·9	101	99·7
Rate/1000	20·6		21·0		20·4		14·4		20·9	
Patients referred more than once										
Total	3		5		7		23		37	
Rate/1000	0·6		1·0		1·4		4·7		7·6	

TABLE 4.

Patients referred First Time to the Psychiatric Clinic during the 5-year Period 1957–1962. Distribution According to Sex, Diagnoses and Rate/1000 of the Population aged 15+ on 1 January 1959

| | Patients | | | | Patients/population rate/1000 | | Total | % | Patients/population rate/1000 |
| | Total | | % | | | | | | |
Population aged 15+	M 2469	F 2391	M	F	M 2469	F 2391	M + F	M + F	M + F 4860
Schizophrenia	2	3	1·1	1·1	0·8	1·3	5	1·1	1·0
Manic-depressive psychoses	29	36	15·5	12·6	11·7	15·1	65	13·8	13·4
Psychogenic psychoses	12	24	6·4	8·4	4·9	10·0	36	7·6	7·4
Paranoid psychoses	1	5	0·5	1·8	0·4	2·1	6	1·3	1·2
Senile and arterioscl. psychoses	21	14	11·2	4·9	8·5	5·9	35	7·4	7·2
Other organic psychoses	20	6	10·7	2·1	8·1	2·5	26	5·5	5·4
Psychoses total	85	88	45·4	30·9	34·4	36·9	173	36·7	35·6
Epilepsy	2	10	1·1	3·5	0·8	4·2	12	2·5	2·5
Neuroses	27	101	14·4	35·4	10·9	42·2	128	27·1	26·3
Character disorders	20	17	10·7	6·0	8·1	7·1	37	7·8	7·6
Alcoholism	6	0	3·2	0·0	2·4	0·0	6	1·3	1·2
Mental deficiency	16	3	8·6	1·1	6·5	1·3	19	4·0	3·9
Legal abortion, obs.	0	23	0·0	8·1	0·0	9·6	23	4·9	4·7
Unspecified mental disorders	24	28	12·8	9·8	9·7	11·7	52	11·0	10·7
No mental disorders	7	15	3·7	5·3	2·8	6·3	22	4·7	4·5
Patients aged 15+	187	285	99·9	100·1	75·6	119·3	472	100·0	97·0

In Salisbury, the area without community psychiatric service used by Grad and Sainsbury (1963) for comparison with the Chichester area, the referral rate was 5·2 per 1000 in 1960–61, and 57% were admitted to psychiatric hospitals. This gives an admission rate of 3·0 per 1000, about the double of the admission rate in Chichester and Samsø, and about the same as the admission rate in Denmark in 1959 with 2·32 per 1000 for men and 3·23 per 1000 for women. The population in Samsø is, however, too selected, comprising only a rural district, and too small to make any reliable comparisons with Denmark total, Chichester, and Salisbury.

In comparisons between referral rates in different areas, distance from the hospital should also be taken into consideration. Bille (1963) found a highly significant difference in admission rates to Århus State Hospital from a city 90 kilometres away from Århus. Admission rates per 1000 population were 3·38 for men and 4·07 for women from the city 90 kilometres from the hospital, while they were 6·88 for men and 7·52 for women from the city where the hospital is situated.

Macmillan (1963) found a rise in admission rate when a well-integrated community psychiatric system was introduced in the Nottingham area with a population of 400,000. This has to be seen on the background of a previous relatively low admission rate compared with that of the Worthing area, for instance, where there was a 50% fall in admission rate (Carse et al., 1958) when community psychiatry was introduced. In Nottingham there was a considerable rise in referral rate and in the percentage of patients treated as out-patients after the introduction of a community psychiatric system, and Macmillan emphasizes, that in spite of the rise in admission rate, there has been a fall in the number of beds needed on account of a fall in the average length of stay in the hospital, and a more efficient use of the beds available because of the screening of patients before admission, and the integration of all psychiatric services in the area.

The unchanged admission rate during the first 5 years in Samsø after introduction of the community orientated psychiatric service is most probably due to the low admission rate of approximately 2 per 1000 before introduction of this service and to the tremendous rise in referral rate from around 2 per 1000 to 19·4 per 1000, three times the referral rate in Chichester of 6·3 per 1000.

It is most probably a fact that the admission rate to psychiatric hospitals cannot be brought very much below 2 per 1000 even in a well-integrated community psychiatric service.

The type of patients admitted has, however, to some extent changed and since 1957 only patients really in need of hospitalization have been admitted, primarily schizophrenics, severe depressions with suicidal risk, and patients with severe senile and arteriosclerotic psychoses, as seen in Table 9. No patients with neuroses or character disorders have been admitted during the last 2 years of the 5-year period.

TABLE 5.

Distribution of Patients according to Age, Sex, and Diagnoses in Relation to the Population aged 15+ on 1 January 1959

	15-19		20-24		25-29		30-34		35-39		40-44		45-49		50-54		55-59		60-64		65-69		70-74		75-79		80-84		85-89		M + F
	M	F	M	F	M	F	M	F	M	F	M	F	M	F	M	F	M	F	M	F	M	F	M	F	M	F	M	F	M	F	
Schizophrenia	0	0	1	0	0	0	0	0	0	1	1	1	0	0	0	0	1	0	0	0	0	0	0	0	0	0	0	0	0	0	5
Manic-depressive psychoses	0	0	0	2	0	0	0	3	1	2	4	3	7	5	2	9	4	9	4	2	4	3	1	2	0	1	0	1	0	0	65
Psychogenic psychoses	0	2	2	1	2	3	1	2	0	4	2	3	2	0	1	7	1	0	2	3	0	1	0	3	1	0	0	0	0	0	36
Paranoid psychoses	0	0	0	0	0	1	0	0	0	0	1	0	0	2	0	0	0	0	0	2	0	1	0	1	0	1	0	0	0	0	6
Senile and arterioscl. psychoses	0	0	0	1	0	0	0	0	0	0	0	1	2	0	0	2	0	0	2	1	2	2	3	3	3	2	2	4	2	2	35
Other organic psychoses	0	1	1	1	1	0	0	0	1	0	0	1	2	0	7	2	2	2	1	1	2	0	1	1	1	1	0	0	0	0	26
Psychoses total	1	3	2	4	3	1	2	4	2	7	9	5	13	6	10	18	11	4	9	9	8	7	5	9	5	4	3	5	2	2	173
Epilepsy	0	2	0	3	1	1	0	1	0	2	0	3	0	1	1	1	1	0	0	2	1	0	0	0	0	0	0	0	0	0	12
Neuroses	1	4	3	5	2	13	2	12	0	13	3	6	4	15	3	12	3	9	2	8	2	4	1	0	0	1	0	0	0	0	128
Character disorders	2	2	3	0	2	3	3	0	1	1	3	2	3	0	1	0	1	2	2	0	0	2	0	0	1	0	0	0	0	0	37
Alcoholism	0	0	0	0	0	0	0	0	1	0	1	0	1	0	2	0	0	0	0	0	1	0	0	0	0	0	0	0	0	0	6
Mental deficiency	5	8	0	6	2	0	0	3	0	0	0	2	0	1	0	1	0	3	1	0	0	0	0	0	0	0	0	0	0	0	19
Legal abortion, obs.	0	1	1	6	1	8	0	3	0	3	0	2	0	2	0	5	0	0	0	0	0	2	0	0	0	1	0	0	0	0	23
Unspecified mental disorders	5	0	2	2	0	3	3	2	1	0	2	2	2	1	5	0	0	3	1	0	0	0	0	0	0	1	0	1	0	0	52
No mental disorders	0	0	2	4	1	3	0	0	1	0	0	0	0	1	0	2	4	1	0	0	2	1	0	2	0	0	0	0	0	0	22
Total M + F	36		37		40		33		36		34		51		59		42		32		30		17		12		9		4		472
Population	446		309		302		330		417		371		464		496		399		412		332		263		176		93		50		4860
Rate/1000 of population	80·7		119·7		132·5		100·0		86·3		91·6		109·9		119·4		105·2		77·7		90·4		64·6		68·2		96·8		80·0		97·1

Sixteen patients with psychoses who previously had been admitted to a mental hospital have for long periods been treated as out-patients in the Samsø clinic, 12 patients with psychoses would definitely have been admitted to a mental hospital if no out-patient clinic had been available.

The rate of patients with psychoses treated as out-patients in the psychiatric clinic per year has been as high as the rate of patients admitted before and during the period 1957–61.

At the moment, less than 5 per 1000 of the Danish population aged 15+ are examined or treated by psychiatrists per year. This rate is, of course, known not to cover the incidence of mental illness, and the results from the psychiatric clinic in Samsø show that neither does it cover the incidence of patients with mental illness in need of treatment. The 19·4 per 1000 population referred to the psychiatric clinic per year do not give a complete account of the incidence of mental illness in the population. The number of patients referred to such a clinic depends on several factors, such as the number of people in the population with mental illness, and the number of those feeling in need of psychiatric treatment and wanting to see a psychiatrist; the latter again depends on the population's attitude towards psychiatric examination and treatment. Admission to a mental hospital is still regarded as a shame for the patient and his family by most people in Denmark. Consulting a psychiatrist was also considered in this way by many people in Samsø when the clinic was started in 1957, but this has changed considerably by now. The number of patients referred also depends to a great extent on the referring physicians—do they find all cases with mental illness; how many of them do they treat themselves; to what extent will they try to convince the patient with mental illness that it might be worthwhile to see a psychiatrist in the clinic on the island or at the patient's home if this is considered more convenient?

Referral rate in Samsø of patients with psychoses aged 65+ was 16·4 per 1000 while the total rate of psychoses in this age group was 67·5 per 1000 as found by Nielsen (1962c) in a 6-month period prevalence study. The total referral rate in this age group was 77·7 per 1000 while the rate of mental illness was 378·3 per 1000. Such comparisons will be made between referral rates and rates of persons with mental illness in the total population, comparing a prevalence investigation made by A. Sørensen (1962) (not yet published) and the present study.

Kessel and Shepherd (1962) and Kessel (1963) found that young adults are more likely to be referred than older people. Pressure from the patient or his relatives exerts considerable influence, and also the physician's own attitude is important. Non-clinical considerations are among the most weighty ones in the choice of patients, Kessel concludes (1963), and he suggests that this is because few general practitioners know what psychiatrists do.

Rawnsley and Loudon (1962) found that the difference of referral rate of six general practitioners from 1·5 per 1000 to 3·7 per 1000 for men

TABLE 6.

Patients visited in their Homes at Least Once. Distribution according to Diagnoses in Relation to the Total Number of Patients

	Total number of patients	Patients visited in their home at least once	Percentage of patients visited in their home
Schizophrenia	5	4	80
Manic-depressive psychoses	65	55	85
Psychogenic psychoses	36	20	56
Paranoid psychoses	6	4	67
Senile and arterioscl. psychoses	35	21	60
Other organic psychoses	26	14	54
Psychoses total	173	118	68
Epilepsy	12	5	42
Neuroses	128	59	46
Character disorders	37	18	49
Alcoholism	6	4	67
Mental deficiency	19	5	26
Legal abortion, obs.	23	6	26
Unspecified mental disorders	52	19	37
No mental disorders	22	7	32
Totals	472	241	51%
Home visits total	1451		
Consultations total	1571		
Consultations in the general hospital	206		
Totals	3228		

and from from 1·1 per 1000 to 3·9 per 1000 for women could not be accounted for by social and demographic variations in the population at risk, nor by selective recruitment of psychiatric patients to the list of certain practices. The difference in referral rates did not seem to be related to variations in the clinical severity either, nor to major diagnostic category, age, civil state or occupation of the patients referred. Interviews with the six general practitioners suggested that they were influenced to a varying degree by social and attitudinal factors in deciding whom to refer for psychiatric service.

In Samsø there was practically no difference in the number of patients referred by the two general practitioners who were in the southern part of the island when the psychiatric clinic was opened in 1957. As seen in Table 10, there are no great differences in the diagnostic composition of the patients referred by the 4 general practitioners. Our experiences concerning the small

TABLE 7.

Patients paid More than 10 Consultations in the Clinic and in their Homes.
Distribution according to Diagnoses in Relation to the Total Number
of Patients referred

	Patients paid more than 10 consultations		Patients total
	Total	%	
Schizophrenia	3	60	5
Manic-depressive psychoses	28	43	65
Psychogenic psychoses	5	16	36
Paranoid psychoses	4	40	6
Senile and arterioscl. psychoses	0	0	35
Other organic psychoses	1	4	26
Psychoses total	41	24	173
Epilepsy	2	17	12
Neuroses	37	29	128
Character disorders	11	30	37
Alcoholism	0	0	6
Mental deficiency	0	0	19
Legal abortion, obs.	0	0	23
Unspecified mental disorders	0	0	52
No mental disorders	0	0	22
Totals	91	19%	472

differences in referral rate among the 4 general practitioners go along with the above mentioned findings by Rawnsley and Loudon (1962).

The importance and influence on the referral rate of close co-operation between the psychiatrists and the referring physicians is also emphasized by the fact that there was a rise in the number of patients referred to the psychiatric service from the general hospital in Samsø from 0–8 during the first 4 years 1957–60, to 35 patients in 1961, when weekly visits were paid in the hospital by a psychiatrist who treated patients referred, discussed problems concerning patients with mental illness, with both physicians in the hospital, and made ward rounds with them off and on. The reason for the rise in referral rate was also due to the change of chief of the hospital.

The higher percentage of female patients in the age group 20–40 (Fig. 5) may to some extent be explained by the 23 women referred for legal abortion, who are all in this age group with the peak in the age group 20–29. But the finding of a relatively high referral rate in the younger age groups corresponds with the findings of Kessel and Shepherd (1962) and Kessel (1963) that general practitioners are more prone to refer younger neurotic patients than older ones. Kessel gives two reasons for this: (1) the general practitioner

TABLE 8.

Patients referred to the Psychiatric Clinic More than Once. Distribution according to Diagnoses in Relation to the Total Number of Patients referred

	Patients referred more than once		Patients total
	Total	%	
Schizophrenia	4	80	5
Manic-depressive psychoses	23	35	65
Psychogenic psychoses	3	8	36
Paranoid psychoses	0	0	6
Senile and arterioscl. psychoses	7	20	35
Other organic psychoses	4	16	26
Psychoses total	41	24	173
Epilepsy	2	17	12
Neuroses	27	21	128
Character disorders	1	17	37
Alcoholism	0	0	6
Mental deficiency	0	0	19
Legal abortion, obs.	1	4	23
Unspecified mental disorders	3	6	52
No mental disorders	0	0	22
Totals	75	16%	472

TABLE 9.

Patients admitted to Psychiatric Institutions during the 5-year Period. Distribution according to Diagnoses in Relation to the Total Number of Patients

	Patients admitted to a psychiatric institution		Patients total
	Total	%	
Schizophrenia	2	40	5
Manic-depressive psychoses	13	20	65
Psychogenic psychoses	4	11	36
Paranoid psychoses	3	50	6
Senile and arterioscl. psychoses	5	14	35
Other organic psychoses	3	11	26
Psychoses total	30	17	173
Epilepsy	2	17	12
Neuroses	9	7	128
Character disorders	3	8	37
Alcoholism	2	33	6
Mental deficiency	0	0	19
Legal abortion, obs.	0	0	23
Unspecified mental disorders	0	0	52
No mental disorders	0	0	22
Totals	46	10%	472

TABLE 10.

Patients referred during the 5-year Period. Distribution according to referring Physician.
A, B, C, D are General Practitioners, and E the Hospital Physicians

Referring physician	A		B		C		D		E	
Patients referred	Total	%	Total	%	Total	%	Total	%	Total	%
Psychoses	41	34	59	37	19	37	38	44	25	51
Neuroses	36	30	54	34	10	19	17	19	13	27
Character disorders and alcoholism	14	12	16	10	1	2	7	8	3	6
Legal abortion, obs.	6	5	7	4	5	10	4	5	1	2
Mental deficiency	5	4	3	2	5	10	4	5	2	4
Unspecified mental disorders	12	10	15	10	8	15	13	15	—	—
No mental disorders	5	5	4	3	4	8	4	5	5	10
Totals	119	100	158	100	52	101	87	101	49	100

(Seven patients came to the clinic without being referred by the physicians, three of them suffered from psychoses, two from neuroses and two from character disorders.)

TABLE 11.

Distribution of Patients according to Judgement by the Psychiatrists, Where and by Whom the Patients Might Be Treated Best and Most Practically

	To be admitted to mental hosp.	To be treated by psychiatrists as out-patients	To be treated by the general practitioner	Total number of patients
Schizophrenia	5	0	0	5
Manic-depressive psychoses	17	42	6	65
Psychogenic psychoses	2	22	12	36
Paranoid psychoses	6	0	0	6
Senile and arterioscl. psychoses	2	8	25	35
Other organic psychoses	3	7	16	26
Psychoses total	35	79	59	173
Epilepsy	3	2	7	12
Neuroses	4	78	46	128
Character disorders	5	25	7	37
Alcoholism	1	4	1	6
Mental deficiency	0	2	17	19
Legal abortion, obs.	1	22	0	23
Unspecified mental disorders	3	5	44	52
No mental disorders	0	0	22	22
Totals	52	217	203	472
Percentage of the total number of patients	11	46	43	

may have higher hopes for successful treatment of the neurosis in young adults; (2) there is more pressure on him to take action, because neuroses at this age are more eruptive and difficult for the family to tolerate.

The percentage of neuroses in the present survey is, however, about the same in the six female age groups from 25 to 49 and 55 to 64, varying only from 43 to 55% whereas in the age group 15–19 neuroses only comprise 17% and in the age group 20–24 only 20%. That the percentage of female patients born outside the island is significantly higher than the percentage of the female population born outside the island ($p < 0.01$) may be due to several facts. Those born outside the island may consult the general practitioner more often as they might come from cities or areas where it is more common to consult a physician or a psychiatrist. Coming to live in a relatively small island may be a special stress for women in their twenties and thirties, and again during the menopausal years (Fig. 6), and cause a higher incidence of manifest mental illness than among those born on the island and used to living there, and having more of the members of their family around them.

TABLE 12.

Distribution of Patients according to Treatment Results and Diagnoses

	Un-changed	Im-proved	Cured	Total treated	Ex-amined not treated	Total number of patients
Schizophrenia	2	2	0	4	1	5
Manic-depressive psychoses	4	24	30	58	7	65
Psychogenic psychoses	3	12	13	28	8	36
Paranoid psychoses	3	1	0	4	2	6
Senile and arterioscl. psychoses	4	7	0	11	24	35
Other organic psychoses	1	8	6	15	11	26
Psychoses total	17	54	49	120	53	173
Epilepsy	4	1	0	5	7	12
Neuroses	36	49	9	94	34	128
Character disorders	8	14	0	22	15	37
Alcoholism	1	2	2	5	1	6
Mental deficiency	2	0	0	2	17	19
Legal abortion, obs.	1	1	0	2	21	23
Unspecified mental disorders	4	15	1	20	32	52
No mental disorders	0	0	0	0	22	22
Totals	73	136	61	270	202	472

If this was the reason we might, however, expect to find another diagnostic distribution of the patients born outside the island. But in Table 2 it is seen that the only statistically significant difference is found in character disorder ($p < 0.02$) and in legal abortion ($p < 0.02$), with a higher percentage among the patients born outside the island. The percentage of psychoses among the total number of patients and the patients born outside Samsø is nearly the same, 36.7% and 34.9%. The percentage of neuroses is slightly lower among those born outside Samsø. The percentage of patients with unspecified mental disorder and no mental disorder correlates well (Table 2).

When the clinic was started in Samsø in 1957, nobody could know what the referral rate would be nor if it was going to rise or fall during the following years. One of the most interesting facts found in this 5-year survey is the stable first-time referral rate per 1000 of 20.6, 20.9, 20.4, 14.4, and 20.9 during the 5 years 1957–61, calculated with the population aged 15+ in the middle of the period as background population (Table 3). An explanation for the relatively low rate in 1960 is given in the discussion of the individual referral rates of the general practitioners.

There was a 55% rise in the percentage made up of patients with psychoses from 1957 to 1961, a figure which suggests that the close contact and good co-operation between psychiatrists and the general practitioners taught the latter to select the psychiatric patients who really need psychiatric treatment, and who respond better to treatment than neurotic patients.

During the same 5-year period there was a 41% fall in the percentage of patients with neuroses from 37 in 1957 to 24·8 in 1961. A fall that most probably might be explained in connection with what has been said about the rise in the percentage of psychotic patients. The general practitioners realized that at least chronic neurotic patients have poor prognoses, even when treated by psychiatrists, from the fact that 41% of the psychotic patients treated and only 10% of the neurotic patients were much improved. Only 14% of the psychotic patients were unchanged, whereas 38% of the neurotic patients did not improve. There was a 59% fall of patients with character disorders from 1957 to 1961, a fall which most probably is due to the same factors as mentioned for neuroses. There is no reason to expect the changes in diagnostic composition to be caused by a different diagnostic classification, nor by a change in the incidence of psychoses, neuroses and character disorders in the island.

In Table 7 it is seen that long-term treatment was given to psychotic as well as neurotic patients and to patients with character disorders. Of the 472 patients referred to the clinic during the first 5-year period, 26 were still in treatment at the end of the 5-year period, 7 had been followed for 3–5 years, 6 for 2–3 years, 2 for 1–2 years, and 11 from 1–11 months; 13 of these patients suffered from manic-depressive psychoses.

The patients with manic-depressive psychoses are especially suitable cases for treatment in the community. Florian Sørensen (1961) emphasized this concerning the mild endogenous depressions, but it also holds true for more severe cases of endogenous depressions which can be kept on a low dosage of antidepressive drugs during long periods, and visited with monthly intervals if needed. Keeping in close contact with such patients by monthly home visits, or even by a telephone call once a month, may often be of great value by offering a chance of early intervention whenever a depression starts. During depressions, weekly home visits together with antidepressive drug treatment is an ideal way of treating most cases of endogenous depressions. In some instances it might be necessary to give E.C.T. treatment, but during the last 2 years of the 5-year period, only one patient with manic-depressive psychosis was treated with E.C.T. She was admitted several times to the general hospital and given E.C.T. treatment, as antidepressive drugs had no effect on her agitated severe depressions. Case histories of this and other cases of manic-depressive psychoses are given by Nielsen (1963, 1965). The treatment as seen in Table 8 comprised most of the usual therapy forms in ambulatory psychiatry. Most important factors were, however, the possibility of home visits and the close co-operation with the physicians in the island. A total of 3228 consultations were given, 45% of which were home visits. The 1451 home visits were paid to 51% of the 472 patients as seen in Table 6. The highest percentage of home visits were paid to patients with psychoses and especially to patients with manic-depressive and schizophrenic psychoses. There was a variation in the extent the 5 different psychiatrists used home visits, from 20 to 60% of their total number of consultations paid.

It is our experience from the Samsø-Project that one or more home visits to nearly all psychiatric patients are of great importance for diagnostic and for therapeutic purposes. A home visit gives the opportunity of dealing with the acute situation by investigation of the family dynamics and the relatives' attitudes towards the patient, and towards mental illness in a way which is not otherwise possible.

Domiciliary visits are always of diagnostic as well as therapeutic importance to psychotic patients with the exception of paranoid psychoses, to whom it is usually not advisable to pay home visits. Elderly people with all kinds of mental disorders are preferably treated at home, or at least in an institution in their own community as emphasized by, among others, Macmillan (1960, 1963), Kemp (1962), and Nielsen (1962a, 1962b, 1965).

It has been the opinion of most of the psychiatrists working in the Samsø-Project that neurotic paients ought not to be treated in their homes, and that wife and husband should never be treated by the same psychiatrist. It is, however, very doubtful if any generalization can be made along these lines. There are by now several patients with neuroses as well as married couples with neuroses treated in their homes as well as in the clinic by the same psychiatrist, as pointed out by Nielsen (1964).

It is our experience that the possibilities for diagnosing and treating a "sick family situation" or using healthy family members in the therapy of the patients are greater by making home visits than by only seeing the patients and their family separately in the clinic or the hospital. We are aware of the danger that home visits used uncritically or schematically might lead to increased secondary gain for neurotic patients or to family difficulties not helpful for the patients. We feel, however, that through home visits and close contact with the patient's physician, there is a possibility of breaking down the too rigid boundaries between home and hospital, and general practitioner and hospital, although we are aware of the contra-indications and indications for home visits and treatment of patients in their homes as for any other psychiatric treatment.

Of the 472 patients, 57% were judged by the psychiatrists to be in need of psychiatric treatment to be given by psychiatrists, 46% could be treated as out-patients in the set-up of the Samsø psychiatric clinic with close co-operation among the psychiatrists and the general practitioners, and the physicians at the general hospital, and with the possibilities of giving consultations in the patients' homes. The 57% in need of treatment give a rate of 9·3 per 1000 per year calculated in relation to the population aged 15+

at the midpoint of the 5-year period. The 11% of the patients that needed admission to a psychiatric hospital give a rate of 2·1 per 1000 per year, and the 43% of the patients referred in need of psychiatric examination by a psychiatrist give a rate of 8·7 per 1000 per year (Table 11).

During the 5 years' experience in the Samsø psychiatric clinic, it has been established that when easy and free access to psychiatric service is given to a geographically delimited rural population, with the general practitioners and the physicians in the general hospital in the area as referral sources, the incidence of mental illness, previously recorded through referral of patients to psychiatric institutions, increases approximately 10 times. The 19·4 per 1000 of the population aged 15+ referred to the psychiatric clinic per year is not the real incidence rate for mental illness. The latter is probably much higher, but it is an important incidence rate from a community psychiatric point of view. It is a rate which might be very useful when planning a well-integrated community psychiatric service for a rural district. It is also a rate that ought to modify the many very high and misleading incidence rates of mental illness quoted in the literature. If such very high rates for mental illness are published in an uncritical way, they may do more harm than good to the development of a reasonable psychiatric service, by giving the impression that the number of people in need of psychiatric treatment is rising and rising, and is by now so high that it is rather hopeless even to think of offering psychiatric treatment to those in need.

In the Samsø-Project it has been shown that there is a great need for community psychiatric service in close co-operation with the physicians in the community, but it has also been shown that 90% of the patients referred to this service can be treated without being hospitalized—leaving the hospital admission rate as low as 2·0 per 1000 per year, even with maximum opportunity for psychiatric treatment offered to the population concerned.

In the Samsø psychiatric clinic, a psychiatrist has spent approximately 2 days per week taking care of 20 first-time referred patients per 1000 population per year in a grown-up population of 4860. He has had no assistance of social workers or nurses and only occasional assistance of a psychologist.

If community psychiatric clinics like the Samsø clinic were established all over Denmark, at least one psychiatrist, one social worker, one nurse, and a half-time psychologist would be needed per 20,000 inhabitants aged 15+ to run these clinics if 20 per 1000 population are referred as in Samsø. This would mean a total of 170 psychiatrists. At the moment there are approximately 300 psychiatrists working in the psychiatric institutions in Denmark, 112 of whom are not yet specialists in psychiatry (Udsen, 1964).

From the experience in the small rural area of Samsø, it is impossible to say anything definite about the possibility of a fall in the number of admissions when such a community psychiatric service is introduced. But from the experience in Chichester, as reported by Carse and Sainsbury, a slight fall might be expected.

It will be necessary to make a community psychiatric project in a much bigger area comprising a city of at least 100,000 inhabitants, together with its surroundings, in order to study the practical as well as the economical aspects of such service.

A community psychiatric service gives the population of the community where it is situated a much better service than the present hospital-orientated system. Such service has to develop slowly, mainly because of lack of trained personnel.

Summary

This is a 5-year survey of the work in the psychiatric clinic in Samsø which is situated in the Kattegat between Jutland and Zealand, 2 hours by ferry boat from Århus in Jutland and Kalundborg in Zealand. The island consists of 28,151 acres of which 22,396 acres are farming land. The population of 6189 is a rather wealthy farming population.

During the first 5 years, 472 patients aged 15+ were referred to the clinic, counting only patients referred for the first time. These patients made up $9 \cdot 7\%$ of the population of 4860 aged 15+ in the middle of the 5-year period, giving an average referral rate of $19 \cdot 4$ per 1000 per year. Of this population, $50 \cdot 8\%$ were men and $49 \cdot 2\%$ women, compared to $37 \cdot 9\%$ men and $60 \cdot 4\%$ women among the patients referred to the clinic. The percentage of women referred is especially high in the age group 20–34 with a peak of 18% in the age group 20–29. The percentage of men referred is exceptionally low in the age group 35–39. The average referral rate is $7 \cdot 9$ for men and $11 \cdot 9$ for women.

The only statistically significant difference in the distribution by marital status (both among the population and the patients) is found in the group of divorced women with $1 \cdot 4\%$ among the population and $3 \cdot 7\%$ among the patients ($p < 0 \cdot 01$).

The percentage of female patients born outside the island is higher than the percentage of the female population born in the island; $44 \cdot 2\%$ compared to $36 \cdot 7\%$ ($p < 0 \cdot 02$).

The percentage of patients with psychoses has increased from 30% in 1957 to $46 \cdot 5\%$ in 1961, the percentage of character disorders has decreased from 12 to $4 \cdot 9\%$, and the percentage of neuroses has decreased from $37 \cdot 0$ to $24 \cdot 8\%$ during the same period. The total number of patients referred is about the same per year during the 5-year period the clinic has existed.

For the 5-year period, the rate per 1000 for psychoses is $34 \cdot 4$ for women and $36 \cdot 8$ for men, whereas for neuroses, the rate is $42 \cdot 2$ for women and $10 \cdot 9$ for men. The total rate for mental illness is higher for women than for men:

119·2 per 1000 for women and 75·7 for men. When women and men are taken together, the rate is 97·0 per 1000 for the total 5-year period.

The number of consultations to the 472 patients has been 3228 with 1571 consultations in the clinic and 1451 in the patients' homes; 241 patients have been visited at least once in their homes and many of those have been visited many times in their homes.

Of the 472 patients referred, 270 were treated by the psychiatrists, 61 of those were much improved, 136 were improved and 73 were unchanged. The total number of patients was divided into three groups according to where and by whom they were considered to be treated best and most practically; 43% might be treated by the general practitioners after examination of the patients by the psychiatrist and advice to the general practitioner concerning treatment; 46% might be treated as out-patients in the psychiatric clinic in the island, and 11% were in need of treatment in a psychiatric hospital. Of the 472 patients referred, 242 had a clearly-defined subjective need of treatment.

In the Samsø-Project it has been shown that there is a great need for community psychiatric service in close co-operation with the physicians in the community, but it has also been shown that 90% of the patients referred to this service can be treated without being hospitalized—leaving admission rate to psychiatric hospital as low as 2 per 1000 per year, even with maximum opportunities for psychiatric treatment offered.

Acknowledgement

The work was supported by a grant from the Ford Foundation to the University of Århus.

References

ARENTSEN, K. and STRÖMGREN, E., Patients in Danish psychiatric hospitals, *Universitetsforlaget, Århus and Munksgård*, Copenhagen, 1959.

BILLE, M., The influence of distance on admission to mental hospitals, *Acta psychiat. Scand.* Suppl. 169, **39**, 226–33, 1963.

CARSE, J., PANTON, N. E. and WATT, A., A district mental health service, *Lancet*, **i**, 39–41, 1958.

FAERGEMAN, P. M., *Psychogenic Psychoses*, Butterworths, London, 1963.

GRAD, J. and SAINSBURY, P., Mental illness and the family, *Lancet*, **i**, 544–7, 1963.

HASLUND, L., Planning and Beginning of a Longitudinal Study of Fifty-nine Unselected Schoolbeginners. Paper read at the Vth International Congress of Child Psychiatry, Scheveningen, September 24–30, 1962.

KEMP, R., Old age is not a disease, *Lancet*, **i**, 94–6, 1962.

KESSEL, N., Who ought to see a psychiatrist, *Lancet*, **i**, 1092–4, 1963.

KESSEL, N. and SHEPHERD, M., Neurosis in hospital and general practice, *J. ment. Sci.* **108**, 159–66, 1962.

LANGE, B., Børnepsykiatriske patienter, *Ugeskr. Laeg*, **122**, 1335–7, 1960.

LANGE, B., MOGENSEN, A. and FENGER, G., Nogle resultater ved intelligensundersøgelser af uudvalgte 10-års børn i en landbefolkning, *Nord. psykiat. T.* **4**, 286–93, 1960.

MACMILLAN, D., Mental health services of Nottingham, *J. soc. Psychiat.* **4**, 5–9, 1958.
MACMILLAN, D., The Need for Integration of Mental Health Services. Proceedings of the Third World Congress of Psychiatry, Montreal, 1962.
MACMILLAN, D., Recent developments in community mental health, *Lancet*, **i**, 567–71, 1963.
MEYRICK, R. LL., A geriatric survey in a general practice, *Lancet*, **ii**, 393–5, 1962.
MOGENSEN, A., LANGE, B. and FENGER, G., Binet-Simon systemet vurderet ved prøveresultaterne fra et uudvalgt børnemateriale, *Nordisk Psykologi*, **12**, 302–15, 1960.
NIELSEN, J., Geriatrisk-psykiatriske problemer i en afgraenset befolkningsgruppe, *Ugeskr. Laeg.* **124**, 1652–6, 1962a.
NIELSEN, J., Geronto-psychiatric period prevalence investigation in a geographically delimited population, *Acta psychiat. Scand.* **38**, 307–30, 1962b.
NIELSEN, J., Psykiatriske lidelser på et blandet sygehus, *Ugeskr. Laeg.* **124**, 1108–12, 1962c.
NIELSEN, J., Home visits by psychiatrists, *Compr. Psychiat.* **4**, 442–60, 1963.
NIELSEN, J., Mental disorders in married couples, *Brit. J. psychiat.* **110**, 683–97, 1964.
NIELSEN, J., Geronto-psychiatric treatment in a rural community, *J. Clin. Geront.* **2**, 148, 1965.
NIELSEN, J., JUEL-NIELSEN, N. and STRÖMGREN, E., Psykiatriske lidelser i almen laegepraksis, *Ugeskr. Laeg.* **124**, 1103–8, 1962.
RAWNSLEY, K. and LOUDON, J. B., Factors influencing the referral of patients to psychiatrists by general practitioners, *Brit. J. prev. soc. Med.* **16**, 174–81, 1962.
SAINSBURY, P. and GRAD, J., *Evaluation of Treatment and Services. The Burden on the Community. The Epidemiology of Mental Illness*, Oxford University Press, 1962.
SØRENSEN, A., Praevalensen af neuroser i en dansk landbefolkning. Paper read at the XIII Nordiske Psykiaterkongres, Helsinki, June 13–16, 1962.
SØRENSEN, A. and STRÖMGREN, E., Prevalence. The Samsø Investigation, *Acta psychiat. Scand.* Suppl. 162, **37**, 62–8, 1961.
SØRENSEN, B. F., The ambulant treatment of endogenous depression (with special reference to the role of the general practitioner), *Acta psychiat. Scand.* Suppl. 162, **37**, 105–111, 1961.
The National Health Service of Denmark. Medical report for the Kingdom of Denmark, 1961.
UDSEN, P., Dansk psykiatri gennem 50 ar 1934–1984, *Yngre Laeger*, **11**, 81–91, 1964.

21. Human Relations Training as a Response to a Need for Effective and Economical Psychiatric Treatment

Dale L. Johnson, Philip G. Hanson and Paul Rothaus

The Human Relations Training Laboratory, or Patients' Training Laboratory, at the Veterans' Administration Hospital in Houston, was established to meet a need for an effective and economical form of treatment for the psychiatric patient. Individual and group psychotherapy in psychiatric hospitals are costly. The results have been less than spectacular. One problem regarding effectiveness is that patients often appear to be relatively symptom-free upon discharge from hospital treatment, but on returning to their home environments find that their symptoms reappear, as they encounter problems they have been living with for years. Longer periods of treatment are not feasible, because many patients are from lower socioeconomic levels and cannot afford the expense or time required for extensive psychotherapy. Furthermore, even when psychotherapy was available, many found its emphasis on talking too remote from pressing problems which demanded action.

It occurred to Robert Morton (1965), the first director of the Patients' Training Laboratory, that a new approach to this persistent problem was necessary. He drew on the literature of social psychology for its theories and research on attitude change, group processes, and communication procedures. In 1961, he established the Patients' Training Laboratory (PTL) as a continuing treatment program in a hospital setting. The original form of the program was closely adapted from the Southwestern Training Laboratories for industrial supervisors and managers, developed by Blake and Mouton (1962).

The primary goal of the PTL is to help the psychiatric patient become an agent of change; to be sufficiently sensitive to his own behavior with others and to know enough about the processes of personal change to be able to diagnose interpersonal problems accurately and to cope with them effectively. A second goal is that this should be accomplished in a reasonably short period of time and at moderate expense.

To achieve these goals, a program was developed which, in the period of one month, would (1) help the patient see himself as an active participant in the change process, (2) facilitate a high degree of personal involvement,

(3) provide the patient with opportunities to receive information on his behavior (feedback) from significant others, and (4) offer opportunities to learn new concepts and to practice them in simulated vocational and family settings.

Patient Selection

Participants for the PTL are selected from all wards of a large general medical and surgical Veterans' Administration Hospital, upon referral from a ward physician, and by direct admission from the receiving clinic. Most are referred from psychiatric wards, and the PTL program is administratively a part of the Psychiatric Service of the hospital. The criteria for selection are (1) literacy at a level expected of persons having four or more years of formal schooling, (2) ability to see some interpersonal relevance of symptoms, (3) freedom from gross psychosis, and (4) ability to stay in the program for 1 month.

Since 1961 approximately 800 men have completed the program. They have ranged in age from 20 to 70, with a mean age of 39, and 10.6 years of education. Seventy percent of them are married. The population is drawn primarily from the skilled and semi-skilled labor ranks, and most are from the lower middle-class to lower-class socioeconomic levels. Approximately 70% have received diagnoses of anxiety or depressive reactions, 12% schizophrenic, and 8% personality disorder. The remainder are from other psychiatric and nonpsychiatric classifications. About half of the participants have been hospitalized previously for a psychiatric condition, and some have had many previous hospitalizations.

Basic Design of the Training Laboratory

Each new training group works together for a period of 4 weeks. The activities of the 4 weeks are carefully scheduled, but no attempt is made to adhere strictly to any pre-planned format. Exercises, lectures, ward meetings, and other elements of the laboratory are shifted to make the most of current problems, or used when opportunities for learning seem maximal. See Table 1 for a schedule of a typical day's activities.

The basic idea in regard to scheduling is that each week's activities are designed to provide learning experiences that can be amplified in the next week. Thus, the first week introduces procedures of the laboratory and emphasizes the learning approach to problems and basic means of learning in and through groups. In the second week, focus is placed on relationships within the self-directed groups; that is, on such issues as styles of group participation and the consequences of different kinds of group action. The third week brings in problems of intergroup competition and of improvement of social skills. The final training week is designed to allow integration of

TABLE 1.

*Basic Schedule of Human Relations Training Activities
for One Day*

8:30–10:30	Human Relations Exercise
10:30–12:00	Development Group Meeting
12:00–1:00	Lunch
1:00–3:00	Lecture and Training Exercise
3:00–4:30	Recreation or Medical Consultations
4:30	Free Time

Wednesday Evening: Husbands and Wives Meeting

new concepts and older ways of thinking, and exercises are introduced which present problems of the home environment.

Of the various elements in the program, the development groups, or D-groups, are very likely the most important part. The entire participant body is divided into three or four D-groups, ranging from six to ten men, who meet together for $1\frac{1}{2}$ hours each day. In a typical training session, there are about twenty D-group meetings. During these meetings no member of the staff is present as a therapist or trainer, and no agenda is set for the group. An additional $3\frac{1}{2}$ hours a day are spent in structured general sessions where participants may be involved as intact D-groups or as individuals in one large group. The focus of attention is primarily on the events occurring in the *here and now* and on the processes of behavior in groups, rather than on the content of the discussions. The D-group is designed to help its members make constructive changes in their social selves by analyzing their experiences with each other in their on-going, developing relationships. The implicit goal of the D-group members is to obtain an understanding of their own interactions as a group. Initially, there are no stated rules or procedures, topics or agendas, and groups members find that they have to draw from their own resources to organize and function as an effective working group. When problems arise and are handled solely by the group, the members gain new confidence in dealing with other problems in their social relations. Most groups discover they can use their own resources to function effectively and need not become entangled in a web of dependency on staff leaders. Problems of authority and dependency relations do arise and are issues for group work, but the organization of the program does not foster reliance on authority. On the contrary, a high level of productivity of the D-group sessions is promoted by instruction in group dynamics during general session lectures and exercises. Furthermore, the D-group sessions are "instrumented"; that is, members rate group behavior after each session and post the results for their group on charts in the general session room. These ratings focus the group's attention on such important characteristics of groups as participation, trust, interest, content versus process, and emotional climate.

The exercises are introduced as experiments in important areas of inter-personal relations, and are complex enough to perform more than one service in training. For example, an exercise on power relationships is useful in developing insight into the effects various power styles have on interpersonal relations. The same exercise also helps develop role-playing skills and offers a relatively secure kind of interaction for the socially awkward participant. Whenever possible, the exercises are run with outsiders—student nurses, dietetic interns, state employment counselors—interacting in some of the roles. Exercises are in a continual state of development. Many begin as spontaneous role-playing sessions but develop into exercises, in order to illustrate the issues involved more clearly. Others have been adapted from the research literature in social psychology. For example, two-person games using the Prisoner's Dilemma Problem (Luce and Raiffa, 1957) are currently being used to stimulate thinking about competition and cooperation. The key feature of the exercises is that each is instrumented; participants complete rating scales on the pertinent issues involved, e.g. "satisfaction felt" and "styles of leadership". This information is summarized and returned to the participants in discussion sessions.

When lectures are presented, they usually run from 20 to 30 minutes and are used to raise questions or to point up certain group problems. We have interviewed participants as to the usefulness of these lectures and have found that their value lies in providing terms and ideas with which to con-ceptualize the learning experiences. In another sense, the lectures help to reinforce the idea that the laboratory is a setting for learning, and different from ordinary treatment approaches. Many participants have entered the laboratory with the expectation of undertaking a nonthreatening, intellectual course, but soon find themselves deeply involved and having to draw on personal inventiveness and imagination.

Role-playing sessions are introduced to provide more spontaneous, less structured experiences in several important areas. Role-playing has been especially useful in dealing with the problems of obtaining employment, with attitudes toward those who have been hospitalized, and with family problems. Wives or other family members are urged to participate in group meetings held once a week in the evening, to explore family problems through role-playing and discussion. Again, in these sessions, the emphasis is placed on discovering more effective ways of reacting to problems by choosing intel-ligently from an array of available alternatives.

Role-playing has been especially helpful in presenting concepts in meaning-ful ways. For example, we have found that lectures on ways of giving and receiving feedback on interpersonal behavior tend to be abstract, and beyond the level of understanding of many of the participants. When these lectures are supplemented with role-playing, however, the concepts take on a great deal of meaning.

Distinctive Features of the Training Laboratory

Four characteristics distinguish the training laboratory from traditional group therapy and are basic to the training laboratory approach. These characteristics are (1) the use of autonomous groups, (2) pre-set time limits, (3) here-and-now orientation, and (4) a problem-centered rather than a mental-illness approach.

Autonomous Groups

There is currently a rising wave of interest in the use of autonomous groups with psychiatric patients. Fairweather (1964) has reported on a highly imaginative treatment program for chronic schizophrenic patients that is based on autonomous groups. Berzon, Farson, Solomon, Gibb, and others at the Western Behavioral Sciences Institute have met with success in exploring the feasibility of using autonomous groups with outpatient neurotics (Berzon, 1964). In these investigations and in our work in Houston, there has been much interest in this form of group for the economic advantages that it offers (i.e. fewer staff members are necessary to work with a given number of patients). There are, however, even more important benefits. The autonomous or self-directed group appears to be especially valuable in leading the patient to see that *he* is capable of instigating change in himself and in his environment. In a group led by a therapist, group members expect him to determine the course of the group's development and will wait for him to raise questions or protect vulnerable members. If it is possible to involve patients in a long series of group therapy sessions, they can be trained by the therapist to assume greater responsibility for the group's development. But when, as is so often the case, patients can participate only in a relatively small number of group meetings, changes in group structure are necessary to accelerate this process of personal involvement. In the self-directed group, the patient interacts with his peers; other members are no more or less "expert" in human relations than he is, and he need not be dependent upon another with greater skill or deferent to a person of greater authority.

The use of autonomous groups has been criticized on the grounds that the absence of a therapist deprives the patient of an opportunity to work through authority and dependency problems with the therapist. This is a valid point, for some patients especially, and it does appear to be true that the authority-dependency issue is one that occupies much of the time of conventional group therapy. But our argument is that this issue is not necessarily the problem with which most men have most difficulty. Our contention is that the main problems in living involve peers: friends, relatives, work associates, and wife. In any event, while autonomous groups do focus attention on peer relations, problems of authority-dependency are not absent, and when they do arise, they are worked out by the group members themselves (Gibb, 1964).

We have just completed a study of six self-directed and six trainer-led groups (all other aspects of the training laboratory activities remain the same). An analysis of sociometric and participation data (Rothaus, Johnson, Hanson, Lyle, and Moyer, in 1966) have revealed that trainer-led groups have more evenly moderated patterns of participation, while self-directed groups tend to form a more rigidly structured hierarchy or participation, with the brighter men assuming leadership roles. Analysis of drop-out data shows that the more active members drop out of trainer-led groups, while in autonomous groups, those members whose participation is low tend to leave the group. Men in the self-directed groups showed significantly greater improvement as measured by the MMPI, given before and after participation in the program. A 9-month follow-up of post-hospital adjustment, however, failed to show any difference between the two group approaches.

TIME LIMITS

When patients are interviewed for the PTL program they are told that the sessions will last 1 month; but if they are not ready to leave the hospital at the end of that period, special provisions are made for a longer stay. While most of the participants do stay for 1 month and return home, a smaller number stay on in the hospital for vocational training or further therapy.

The decision to set a time limit for the program was due partially to the desire to preserve the educational flavor of the venture; i.e. school sessions are limited to specific time periods as are industrial management development workshops. The primary rationale, however, was that a prearranged time limit provides a structure for the learning process which facilitates the patient's involvement. The patient is less prone to postpone getting into serious matters because he knows that he has only so much time available. A specified period of time also provides patients with a target date which appears to motivate them to remain in the program until completion. Drop-outs have never been a serious problem in the laboratory.

A major reason for closed groups is that they create a social content that is the same for each group member. There are no "new men" or "old pros." All begin and end group sessions together.

PRESENT ORIENTATION

Participants in the PTL are trained to become participant-observers and to be aware of group processes. In focusing attention on process instead of content, and on here-and-now events rather than past experiences, the PTL is more akin to the human relations training laboratories utilized in industry and adult education than group therapy (Frank, 1964).

The emphasis is one of degree only; if a participant wants to discuss past experiences or events occurring apart from the D-group, he is, of course, able to do so. In an exploratory investigation of the content of group meetings, using tape recordings, we found that most of the discussions were indeed of there-and-then matters. It is evident that this is the realm of group discussion that is most natural and easiest for group members. Learning to observe and describe such group processes as struggles for leadership position, attention-getting maneuvers, and the like, is more difficult. Nevertheless, an important part of our rationale is that personal change occurs when the person who wants to change is involved in the social process and receives immediate, relevant feedback on his on-going interpersonal behavior. During this critical time, while the behavioral incident is sharply in focus by the person and by his fellow group members, he can review the implications of the incident and relate it to other aspects of his life. As an example of this, one participant, a 30-year-old photographer, who received a diagnosis of socio-pathic personality on his entry to the hospital, adroitly assumed a leadership role in his group during one of the laboratory problem-solving exercises. He persuaded, cajoled, and coerced the group members to adopt his point of view, only to find that he had led them to failure. The group delighted in reviewing his behavior and the patient reported the incident as a major event in his life. Because of the clarity of the happenings in this here-and-now event and the cooperation of his group members, he was able to examine his exploitive attitudes toward others and was helped to adopt other ways of behaving.

PROBLEM-CENTERED VS. MENTAL-ILLNESS APPROACHES

The mental-illness concept has recently been soundly criticized by Szasz (1961) and others. While many professionals have responded sympathetically, there is relatively little evidence that treatment programs have changed accordingly. The PTL represents one attempt to base a psychiatric change program on concepts other than those of mental illness (Rothaus and Hanson, 1965; Rothaus and Morton, 1962).

In the PTL the participant is seen as a person who experiences problems in living rather than a person suffering from an illness. The mental-illness approach was useful historically in dispelling the widespread notion that psychiatric symptoms were the products of witchcraft or demon possession, but it now fosters attitudes in the patient and his family that have undesirable consequences. A mental-illness orientation classifies the patient as a victim of his heredity or environment and engenders attitudes of hopelessness and helplessness not conducive to change. In treatment he is also perceived as having a passive role. He is the receiver of treatment rather than an active agent in his own improvement.

Our approach to the problem of initiating a change from a mental-illness to a problem-centered point of view requires a series of steps. First, a lecture is given on the two concepts, followed by small group discussions of the ideas presented. Finally, men are encouraged to try out the merits of each point of view for his own problems by role-playing the two self-description styles with other laboratory participants.

Perhaps the most significant effect comes from the staff attitude. The staff psychiatrist, nurse, and psychologists wear ordinary civilian clothing instead of hospital whites. Official titles are rarely used. Furthermore, the men are referred to as "participants", not "patients", and they conceive of the program as educational rather than curative. The participants are also expected to take a responsible role in the operation of the program. Such questions as whether or not a man may have a pass for the weekend is decided by the members of his group. Infractions of hospital and laboratory rules are dealt with by participants (Rothaus, Hanson, Johnson, Lyle, and Moyer, in press). This concern with involving patients in the solution of problems that arise in the hospital milieu derives to a large extent from the work of Maxwell Jones and his associates (Jones, 1952).

The problem-centered approach may have its greatest significance in the vocational area. If a man believes he is mentally ill, he depreciates himself and is inclined to believe that others will also depreciate him and will be unwilling to hire him. Research on this question, involving counselors of the Texas Employment Commission in roles of prospective employers, suggests that employers are more favorably impressed with men describing their difficulties in problem-centered terms than with men using mental-illness terms (Hanson *et al.*, 1964; Rothaus, Hanson, Cleveland, and Johnson, 1963). Recently, Blank (1965) found that participants shift their orientation from a mental-illness to a problem-centered approach to problems after going through the training laboratory.

Effectiveness of the Program

When the PTL was begun in 1961, the critical question was whether it would be at all possible to place psychiatric patients in groups that lacked professional leadership and expect them to function at all constructively. After 4 years we are very clear on the answer to that question; it is indeed possible. The first groups worked out well despite predictions from many psychiatrists and psychologists that the group meetings at best would be "bull sessions" and at worst provoke uncontrolled aggression. Research on the outcome of the first groups to complete the program—showed a decrease in complaints made to the staff about somatic troubles as well as a decrease in the number of unhappy, disturbed remarks in diaries. Pre- and post-interview ratings indicated that the participants felt less tense, depressed, apprehensive, and self-recriminating after the laboratory (Rothaus, Morton, Johnson, Cleveland, and Lyle, 1963).

A 9-month follow-up study (Johnson *et al.*, 1965) was conducted, which compared 76 patients from a conventional group therapy program with 114 PTL participants. The groups were closely similar on such psychiatric and demographic variables as age, intelligence, education, marital status, diagnoses, and times previously hospitalized. The results showed no differences between the programs in amounts of anxiety, depression, or other psychological symptoms reported. The group therapy patients reported significantly less somatic difficulty. The PTL showed significantly more men employed at the time of the follow-up, a longer mean time of employment, and a shorter period of time in the treatment program. Furthermore, laboratory participants showed a greater tendency to construe perceived change in interpersonal terms. The major advantages for the laboratory suggested by these results are economic; more men were working, they worked longer, and they spent a shorter period of time in a treatment program where fewer staff members were involved.

The PTL has spawned a considerable amount of research, some of it in the form of dissertations and theses. Henderson (1964) found that men who participate actively in group sessions change more favorably, as measured by the MMPI, than men who are comparatively inactive. Murillo (1965) used an extensive battery of tests and interviews before and after participation in the laboratory, and found a significant decrease in the amount of dependency, and anxiety and conflict about dependency. Sands (1965) studied problem-solving ability, using his Interpersonal Problems Attitude Survey in relation to behavior and psychological test changes of 60 PTL participants. The complex results were interpreted as showing an increase in group goals and a more cooperative attitude after laboratory training. Participants appeared to have more self-respect and self-concern, which formed the basis for more compassionate interpersonal concerns. Sands also found significant decreases in psychiatric symptoms.

Prospects for the Future

The versatility of the human relations training approach is being demonstrated in applications of the program in several other settings. Elements of the program, including the autonomous groups, are being used in a vocational rehabilitation program for chronically unemployed men at the Wadsworth, Kansas, VA Center. At the Topeka, Kansas, VA Hospital, a variation of the approach is being utilized with alcoholics. The group discussion procedures have been adopted in an institute for the severely hard-of-hearing in Chicago and at the Texas Institute of Rehabilitation and Research in Houston. Plans are being developed to establish human relations training for minority group children who are potential school drop-outs.

One of the most successful adaptations of the approach has been in training hospital personnel (Johnson, Rothaus, and Hanson, 1966). The combination of lectures, exercises, and the self-directed group discussions has been applied to the training of nurses, dietitians, hospital administrators, and other hospital personnel. The self-directed groups are especially successful since they allow free expression of ideas without the surveillance of an expert present. Personnel tend to reject discussions which appear to be forms of group psychotherapy because they do not want to be identified with the emotionally disturbed. In all of the many self-directed groups we have set up for hospital and other personnel, however, this has never been a serious issue.

Although the human relations training laboratory is still a newcomer to the field of planned behavioral changes in a hospital setting, its early success bodes well for the future. Should the approach be adopted as a mechanical technique applied to human misfits in production-line fashion, the outcome would be disappointing. The word "laboratory" is used in the title of the program to convey an attitude of experimentation and innovation. It is hoped that this attitude of experimentation will prevail.

References

BERZON, B. (1964), *The Self-directed Therapeutic Group: An Evaluative Study*, Western Behavioral Sciences Institute Working Papers.

BLAKE, R. R. and MOUTON, J. S. (1962), In Weschler, I. R. and Schein, E. H. (Eds.), *Issues in Human Relations Training*, NTL Selected Reading Series, No. 5.

BLANK, G. A. (1965), Effects of psychiatric language and a therapeutic program on patients' self-concepts, Unpublished Master's thesis, Univer. of Houston.

FAIRWEATHER, G. W. (Ed.) (1964), *Social Psychology in Treating Mental Illness*, New York, Wiley.

FRANK, J. D. (1964), In Bradford, L. P., Gibb, J. R. and Benne, K. D. (Eds.), *T-group Theory and Laboratory Method*, New York, Wiley.

GIBB, J. R. (1964), Mimeographed paper presented at the American Psychological Association annual convention, 1958, referred to in Bradford, L. P., Gibb, J. R. and Benne, K. D. (Eds.) *T-group Theory and Laboratory Method*, New York, Wiley.

HANSON, P. G., ROTHAUS, P., CLEVELAND, S. E., JOHNSON, D. L., and McCALL, D. F. (1964), *Ment. Hyg. N.Y.* **48**, 142.

HENDERSON, J. L. (1964), Factors related to amount of early participation in a development group, Unpublished doctoral dissertation, Univer. of Houston.

JOHNSON, D. L., ROTHAUS, P. and HANSON, P. G. (1966), *J. Hlth. Hum. Behav.* **7**, 215.

JOHNSON, D. L., HANSON, P. G., ROTHAUS, P., MORTON, R. B., LYLE, F. A. and MOYER, R. (1965), *Intern. J. Social Psychiat.* **11**, 188.

JONES, M. (1952), *The Therapeutic Community*, New York, Basic Books.

LUCE, R. D. and RAIFFA, H. (1957), *Games and Decisions*, New York, Wiley.

MORTON, R. B. (1965), In Schein, E. H. and Bennis, W. G. (Eds.), *Personal and Organizational Change Through Group Methods: The Laboratory Approach*, New York, Wiley.

MURILLO, N. (1965), Conceptual approaches to dependency assessment, Unpublished doctoral dissertation, Univer. of Houston.

ROTHAUS, P. and HANSON, P. G. (1965), *Community Ment. Hlth. J.* **1,** 29.

ROTHAUS, P. and MORTON, R. B. (1962), *J. Hlth. Hum. Behav.* **3,** 198.

ROTHAUS, P., HANSON, P. G., CLEVELAND, S. E. and JOHNSON, D. L. (1963), *Amer. Psychol.* **18,** 85.

ROTHAUS, P., HANSON, P. G., JOHNSON, D. L., LYLE, F. A. and MOYER, R. *J. Appl. Behav. Sci.* (in press).

ROTHAUS, P., JOHNSON, D. L., HANSON, P. G., LYLE, F. A. and MOYER, R., (1966), *J. Counsel. Psychol,* **13,** 68.

ROTHAUS, P., MORTON, R. B., JOHNSON, D. L., CLEVELAND, S. E. and LYLE, F. A. (1963), *Arch. Gen. Psychiat.* **8,** 572.

SANDS, P. M. (1965), Application of the interpersonal problems attitude survey in a patients' training laboratory, Unpublished doctoral dissertation, Univer. of Houston.

SZASZ, T. S. (1961), *The Myth of Mental Illness*, New York, Harper & Row.

22. Community Mental Health Services in the Thirteenth Arrondissement of Paris *

J. D. CHICK

THE structure and administration of French mental health services is somewhat similar to that in Britain, but in recent years the public authorities in France have not shown the same progressive spirit as those in this country. The rapid speed with which the 1959 Mental Health Act followed the report of the Royal Commission in 1957 contrasts with the frustrations which French doctors were experiencing during the same period.

In 1949, 150 years after Esquirol had condemned the conditions under which the mentally ill were detained in France, the Medical Council of Psychiatric Hospitals addressed a memorandum to the Minister of Health, stating that: "The inadequacy of nursing staff, in their numbers as well as in their training, the tragic overcrowding of the facilities, the decaying character and primitive equipment of most of the psychiatric hospitals, and above all, the pitiful number of doctors, do not allow the patients of those hospitals to be assured materially of the conditions of living and the care to which they have a right." A few years later, it was stated that: "The present state of affairs is due only to the inadequacy of funds devoted in general to public hygiene and health, and in particular to mental hygiene and health" (from Soubiran, 1965). In the debate on the 1953 Health Ministry Budget, it was stated that the mentally ill were still to be seen in chains in the province of Corsica, shackled to the floors of cells (*ibid.*).

In 1955 the State undertook to pay about 80% of the cost of extra-hospital consultations, which encouraged the development of more clinics outside psychiatric hospitals. But public expenditure on health and education has been limited because of defence costs, and this progress has been difficult to maintain. When the National Assembly discussed the 1965 Health Budget, there were demands that delinquents and criminals should no longer be sent to psychiatric hospitals and that the law on mental illness (of which the essential parts date from 1838) should be reformed.

French psychiatric hospitals are not part of a national hospital network, including all kinds of hospitals, as in Britain. The director of each psychiatric

* This report is included by permission of the Trustees of the Lazard Scholarship, Corpus Christi College, Cambridge.

Material in this paper is taken from the annual reports of the Association for Mental Health in the Thirteenth *Arrondissement*, and other local documents.

hospital (usually a doctor) is responsible to a section of the departmental Préfecture, which at a national level is responsible to the Ministry of Health. In 1963, for over 46 million people, France had 109 psychiatric hospitals with a total of 98,000 beds. There were also 5000 beds in private clinics and 1500 neuropsychiatric beds in general hospitals. This gave a total of 104,500 beds, or 2·3 per 1000 population. (Figures presented to the 1963 Conference of the European Association for Mental Health.) For a slightly smaller population, England and Wales had 216,602 beds (including mental sub-normality) or 4·7 per 1000 population. The number of doctors in French psychiatric hospitals, then, was 1 to 250 beds, compared with 1 to 135 beds in the U.K. and 1 to 140 in the U.S.A. (Jones, 1962).

Psychiatric out-patient clinics have been coming into existence in France since 1945 and there were 716 in 1961. They are run by a different section of the Préfecture from that dealing with mental hospitals (Service Départmental d'Hygiène Sociale), which in turn is responsible to a different section of the Ministry of Health. Since 1955, the State has provided 80% of the expenses of these clinics. There are a number of day hospitals, sheltered workshops and after-care hostels, but few in comparison with Britain.

Some regional general hospitals have neuropsychiatric services, but these are directed by doctors whose training differs from the medical staff of mental hospitals. Also, there is probably more private psychiatry practised in France than in Britain. The National Insurance Scheme (La Sécurité Sociale) finances hospitalization and reimburses about 80% of the cost of specialist consultations and of medication. Consultations at clinics run by the Préfecture are free.

Services for the mentally subnormal depend on yet another authority. At the departmental level, it is the Direction de la Population and within the Ministry of Health, the Direction Générale de la Population.

The Beginnings of the Project

Like many experiments in the arena of social change, the development of this project in the thirteenth *arrondissement* centres around one pioneer. In 1954, Dr. Philippe Paumelle was Assistant Medical Director of Le Service d'Hygiène Sociale de la Seine, which was responsible for psychiatric clinics and mental health services in that Département. His work included making urgent domiciliary visits at the request and in the company of social workers from clinics in Paris, whose consultants only worked part-time. It was this work which emphasized to him the possibilities of caring for psychiatric patients in their homes and in the community, thus avoiding unnecessary hospitalization.

After the Second World War, Dr. Paumelle believed that public opinion, sensitized by the existence of concentration camps, by the murder in the name of genetics of a large number of mentally sick Germans, and by the death from starvation, cold or tuberculosis of numerous patients in the mental hospitals themselves, could help to accomplish a real revolution in psychiatry. He wished to make a completely new start, free from all encumbrances, such as those caused by existing, but unsuitable premises, staff or administrative structure. The motive was not primarily philanthropic, but stemmed from Dr. Paumelle's belief that for the psychiatric patient, the psychiatrist may be the only person to whom his relationship difficulties with others can be expressed without danger. But if the first contact with the doctor is made under constraint, in an asylum setting; if the patient is confined; if the person of the doctor is confused with that of a custodian or gatekeeper, in charge of letting patients out; if admission to hospital simply confirms (by terminating it) the discomfort which the patient experiences in the world outside, then the doctor is perpetuating the maintenance of unsatisfactory relationships with his patients.

Dr. Paumelle had been asked by an elderly general practitioner, who treated alcoholics in the thirteenth *arrondissement*, to see some of his patients who had psychiatric problems. This doctor used a small room, lent by a tuberculosis clinic, and many alcoholics attended willingly, as they were keen to avoid the mental hospital. When he retired, Dr. Paumelle took over his consultations, and began to accept other psychiatric cases, referred by local organizations, such as family guidance centres. New patients came in increasing numbers, having been recommended by friends and acquaintances.

Thanks to his authoritative position within the Préfecture, Dr. Paumelle was able to recommend that as the tuberculosis clinic was becoming redundant, other rooms of the clinic should be taken over for the use of psychiatric patients. At first, this was as a kind of workshop, where his patients could spend the day under nursing supervision and with facilities for simple occupational therapy, such as rug making or basketry. Medication and E.C.T. were also available and there was a certain amount of group therapy. Most of the original patients were alcoholics, who used to come in for 3 or 4 days, to tide them over a crisis or period of detoxication, and to avoid admission to hospital. There were also some psychotic patients, who tended to come for about 3 months, and might also avoid hospitalization during relapses in this way.

Formation of the Association

In 1958, the Association for Mental Health and the Fight Against Alcoholism in the Thirteenth Arrondissement was founded. Its stated aims were to co-ordinate activities directed towards the preservation of mental health, and the treatment of mental illness and alcoholism in the area. It then received the support of the Ministry of Health, Préfecture, Sécurité Sociale, the

National Committee for Defence Against Alcoholism and the mayor and other prominent figures of the *arrondissement*. Finance was received from these sources and the association became entrusted with responsibility for all extra-hospital mental health facilities in the area. These included the child guidance clinic of the Ligue Fraternelle des Enfants de France, previously dependent on the Préfecture, and later the day hospital for children, opened in 1960 by the Rothschild Foundation. Although these latter two services have maintained their internal autonomy, they form part of the comprehensive mental health service for the *arrondissement*.

Although it is financed by public authorities, the association enjoys the status of a private organization and this has important consequences. The annual budget is agreed by the Administrative Council, whose members represent the supporting organizations and authorities. Within this budget, all decisions concerning policy, staffing, premises and equipment can be taken immediately by the Director, Dr. Paumelle. There is no need to refer these to any higher authority, such as the Préfecture (or Regional Hospital Board in Britain). The selection of staff is made entirely by the doctors, which is especially important because of the close degree of co-operation which is necessary between them. The independence enjoyed by the project is vital for an experiment which aims to obtain significant results quickly. This independence was derived firstly from the influential position of the original pioneer, and secondly from the strategy of waiting for the project to be functioning before seeking support from cautious public authorities.

Relationship of the Services

On the adult side, the service comprises seven teams. Each full team consists of a doctor, nurse, social worker, psychologist, psychotherapist and work counsellor, though some of the latter workers are shared between two or more teams. All the teams are based on the Medico-Social Centre, which is situated near the middle of the *arrondissement*, and each has responsibility for the 20,000–30,000 inhabitants of a subsector. (The association owns a small clinic in one subsector, where consultations are held.) The same team follows its patients through all forms of treatment and all facilities, including the psychiatric hospital, which is visited regularly by team members.

The types of treatment carried out on an ambulatory basis are as follows: firstly, E.C.T. and pharmacological treatments, which are administered by the doctors and nurses; secondly, relaxation therapy and "psychomotor re-education" (the association employs a physiotherapist and some part-time relaxation therapists, who treat patients with psychosomatic and psychomotor complaints (e.g. tics, stammering, writer's cramp), individually or in groups); thirdly, psychotherapy (all the doctors working with the association have had some psychoanalytical training and six part-time psychotherapists are employed). However, in 1964, only 10% of the association's clients were treated with individual psychotherapy on analytical lines. As well as psychotherapy with neurotics, there has been some experimental work with psychotic patients. Therapists have regular discussions with the other team members, to review patients' progress.

The work counsellors help patients to find suitable employment or training, particularly on leaving hospital. They are in regular contact with the post-cure workshop and keep in touch with patients who may subsequently fail at their jobs. Since unskilled and semi-skilled employment is scarce in France, the work counsellors try to maintain good relations with local firms; the attitude of employers towards former psychiatric patients has been found to constitute a problem. In 1964, out of 156 cases dealt with by the two work counsellors, 27 were directly placed in work by them. In the case of another 28, their intervention helped to retain a job or to change to another within the same firm. Smaller groups were referred to the association's workshop or to a sheltered workshop.

The psychologists, in addition to carrying out the usual psychometric testing, organize evening classes for a small group of adult patients at the centre. This followed findings by the work counsellors that patients of relatively high intelligence were too often being excluded from employment or professional training by an apparently low level of education. The classes help patients to take the entrance tests for training schemes, etc.

Except in cases of urgency, patients' first contact with the association is with the social workers, and it is they who keep in contact when patients leave the centre. They are responsible for liaison with other public or private services, with the community and with the family. In 1964, 1245 patients were seen and/or followed-up by the five social workers.

The staff of the centre includes four extra-hospital nurses, qualified in both general and psychiatric nursing. Their function at the centre itself is to administer physical and pharmacological treatment; this helps to emphasize the medical role of the centre. Their gradually evolving sphere of action in the community includes roles previously undertaken (but sometimes inadequately) by social workers. For instance, when urgencies arise at the patient's home, the experienced nurse is able to take immediate decisions. The fact that she is a nurse emphasizes the caring aspect of her role and helps to diminish the drama of the situation. She keeps up a fairly continuous therapeutic contact with long-term patients, particularly chronic alcoholics and psychotics; this may be done by a conversation with the concièrge (that corner-stone of Parisian society), by taking a cup of coffee with the patient or by regular administration of medication. The social worker is still too often treated as someone to whom the family can denounce the behaviour of a psychiatric patient, whereas the nurse's intervention may be both more effective and better tolerated by the family. The social worker tends to be invested with the function of protecting society.

The extra-hospital nurse is particularly useful in following-up those numerous patients who have stopped coming to the centre, and she is able to supply the other members of the team with objective information at assessment meetings. Finally, she helps former patients to re-establish their relations with the environment and may introduce them to associations or clubs, e.g. cultural, or those for adolescents or old people.

Each of the doctors in the association, as well as being the leader of a team operating in one of the subsectors, is also responsible for one of the association's establishments, which include two workshops and two hospitals. This organization ensures continuity of care and patients are not *transferred* from one service to another; referral to any particular facility is as a complement to the measures already being taken.

The Day Hospital

The day hospital has a psychiatrist attached to it approximately half-time and he is assisted by a doctor in training. There is also a nurse, a work supervisor and an occupational therapist. The nurse helps in the administration of physical treatments, cares for patients who may be temporarily too disturbed to be part of the group, and visits the homes of those who may be absent or have relapsed.

The majority of day patients would otherwise have to be admitted to a mental hospital, which in Paris would normally be of the closed type. The general principle of the daily programme is that it should be as near as possible to normal life. It is quite carefully structured, though varying somewhat from patient to patient, according to the recommendations of the team responsible for him. In practice, some of the time is spent in the workshops and the rest in more definite group activities. Occupations in the workshops include woodwork, weaving, pottery, and making rugs and dolls. In the day hospital, as in the psychiatric hospital, individual remuneration is not given for work performed. Money obtained from the goods sold goes partly towards the cost of materials, and the rest is used communally for extra comforts, excursions, etc.

Group activities include games, gymnastic sessions, and meetings (not attended by any of the staff) to take decisions about the group's activities. There is also a weekly group psychotherapy session, in which the doctor introduces a subject for discussion, such as "Happiness" or "Anger".

The Psychiatric Hospital (L'Eau Vive)

Instead of building a hospital with the nationally recommended figure (for 1970) of 3 beds per 1000 of the population, it was speculated that a therapeutically more efficient service could be provided by a hospital with only 1 bed per 1000, supplemented by community services. These would require little capital, but many staff and a substantial annual budget. It would be necessary for patients' stay in hospital to be as short as possible and for treatment to be intensive. There would also have to be maximum continuity of care; the sector teams, in fact, decide on admission and discharge, and see their patients in hospital very regularly. The doctors in charge of the various hospital villas are also leaders of sector teams. As far as possible, all admissions are voluntary.

The hospital is situated in the country, near to a large forest, the river Seine and a moderate-sized village; all these are often visited by the patients. Only two of the villas are ready so far, but each one is to have its own character. There are no large dormitories and bedrooms contain from 1 to 6 patients. Patients who require a similar régime are placed temporarily together under a single nurse, usually in groups of seven. Mostly, these units do not seem to develop very clearly and may mean little more to the patients than that the same nurse hands them their pills.

To achieve maximum therapeutic activity, the staff must be well above the traditional number, and at the moment, there are four doctors to 100 beds (excluding doctors of intern status). This is ten times the ratio for France as a whole, but each doctor here also has his team responsibilities. On the nursing side, the aim is to have one nurse *on duty* for every 7 patients. If a nurse works a 44-hour week, and if there are half as many on duty at night, then the total number of nurses must be a little more than one-third the number of patients. This is not unattainable, since the figure for France generally is one nurse to 4 beds, but nurses at L'Eau Vive are required to have both general and psychiatric training. It is hoped that the cost of this extra staff will be balanced by avoiding the financial consequences of prolonged hospital stay.

Most of the patients are encouraged to undertake work in the handicraft workshops, which include jewellery—a former professional jeweller works as a full-time work therapist. The director is always ready to try out new ways of involving patients in a therapeutic situation, and activities have included such things as dinghy sailing and group readings of Molière.

At present, there appears to be some degree of tension between staff and patients, partly resulting from the morning meetings of doctors and nurses, at which patients' condition and behaviour are discussed. This seems to have gained the reputation of a kind of session for police reports, and the difficulty might be overcome by opening the meeting to patients also. There is a weekly meeting for "group psychotherapy", which is led, rather than attended, by the doctor, and discusses matters of villa life. It did not seem to generate any feelings of community, and neither staff nor patients gave the impression of being accustomed to participate in a group decision. No doubt it will take time for a group feeling to form and for a tradition of group responsibility to develop.

The Therapeutic Workshops

The association believes that a period of re-adaption is often required between the prolonged idleness of illness and return to work. This should be in a working situation, where conditions approximate to those of normal factory life. There is, therefore, a Re-adaption Centre, where work is undertaken on contract for outside firms and is remunerated at piece-work rates. The working week is 35 hours.

The present centre has only room for 20 trainees and there is a waiting list. The maximum length of stay is 6 months and this is regarded as a very important rule. This centre does not have the role of a sheltered workshop; the ultimate objective of reintegration into normal life is never forgotten during the time each trainee is there. It resembles (on a smaller scale) the Industrial Therapy Organization at Bristol.

The permanent staff includes two female work therapists (one of whom has industrial experience), and a man with experience both in industry and as a work therapist in the day hospital. He takes the role of foreman of the workshop and is in continual contact with the doctor-in-charge, who divides his time between work with a team and this centre. The workshop is situated in a completely different part of the *arrondissement* from the other services and all the trainees live at home, except for a few who live in a hostel.

The two main problems are, firstly, the heterogeneity of the trainees, in terms of age, illness, and cultural and educational background, which makes it difficult to find suitable work for all, and secondly, the difficulty of finding enough work, particularly in times of economic recession.

Whilst it is difficult to evaluate the success of this kind of project, the following figures for 1964 show what became of the 22 trainees who left the workshop that year: 6 had taken jobs and were working on 31 December 1964; 2 were on professional training courses; 2 had tried to start work but suffered a relapse; 4 had relapsed and were in the psychiatric hospital; 6 had relapsed and were with their families; 1 had been hospitalized for a physical illness, and 1 had disappeared. Progress charts and assessments are discussed frequently by the foreman with each patient, and the objective of finding outside work is kept in view all the time.

Both therapeutic workshops operated by the association occupy former tuberculosis clinics and the structure of these premises has defined the size, site and situation of the workshops, relative to the association's other institutions. So far, there is no plan to incorporate residential facilities with either of the workshops.

The association's sheltered workshop has evolved as a centre for those who are no longer in need of hospital care, who are physically and intellectually capable of performing simple productive tasks, who have families to supervise them, but who are not able to take part in normal working life. The 22 patients include some of low intellectual ability, some who are elderly and some long-term psychotics. The work is of a simple contract nature, and the two full-time occupational therapists in charge maintain a protective atmosphere. Patients stay for at least a year and if they show signs of progress, may be transferred to the re-adaption centre. Separation of "long-term" patients in the sheltered workshop from "curable" ones in the re-adaption centre could be harmful, but the possible dangers of this distinction are well understood here.

The Mental Hygiene Services

The association works in an educative and advisory capacity, through various aspects of the life of the *arrondissement*. The aims have been to educate "key people" and the public in general to accept the existence of the problems of mental health.

Educative work has included parents' meetings (hitherto unknown at many schools), followed by the giving of private advice to anxious mothers. During 1964, workers from the association had a series of seminars with youth-club leaders and there has been regular contact with voluntary associations and with the press. The association has also organized, in collaboration with local authorities, a series of conferences on old age. These brought together representatives of a variety of public and private services in the area, and culminated in the creation of an Association for Gerontology. The Mental Health Association also co-operates with the Housing Association for the *arrondissement* in order to study sociological, economic and medico-social problems involved in urban renewal.

There is also a Parents' Film Club, which holds monthly showings of films of social interest in a local cinema. The committee is based on the association, but also includes representatives of the Union of Family Associations in the *arrondissement*, of the teaching profession and of social workers. Each film is followed by a discussion on some aspect of child care, which is led by a specialist in that particular field. The present membership is about 250 and this is one public activity of the association to which the population is certainly not indifferent though its reactions are varied.

These extensions of the association's work into community life have also been criticized from within the psychiatric profession. It is suggested that there is a tendency to try and take charge of problems which depend on factors outside the realm of psychiatry, and that this is a "face-saving process", representing the wish of the psychiatrist to be more integrated himself into society. The association should be aware of this point of view.

Le Club des Peuples

This club is a rendezvous for former patients treated by the service and aims to support them in social re-adaptation. Theoretically, it is run entirely by former patients, and the committee usually contains a high proportion of former trainees of the rehabilitation workshop. An attempt was made in 1965, with little success, to hand over to this committee the administrative responsibility for the production side of the therapeutic workshops.

There are about 80 enrolled members, most of whom are men. As well as the usual club activities, such as shows, talks, outing and parties, there are regular social group meetings of about 20 people, on evenings or Saturday afternoons. These are attended mostly by unmarried members.

Club meetings are held on the premises of the adult centre, and members are said to prefer this, so that their link with the centre is not completely severed. However, every effort is made to make the atmosphere as normal as possible, largely through the work of the club leaders (*animateurs*). At present, these are a husband and wife team of psychologist and social worker, who work at the centre but do not have any clinical contact with club members. They do not act as advisers; if help is required for any personal problem, discussion of it is encouraged amongst a group of members and from a non-psychiatric point of view. The members of the club—an extremely heterogeneous group (especially from the clinical point of view), of whom many share in common as a chief difficulty that of establishing successful relationships—seem to form a happy community here, which is strong enough to support its more vulnerable members.

Services for Children

Before they were incorporated into the association, the existing child guidance centres in the *arrondissement* consisted of a clinic, financed by the Ligue Fraternelle des Enfants de France and a day hospital, opened in 1960 by the Rothschild Foundation. It was relatively easy to incorporate both of these into the "sector" scheme. In 1963 Le Centre Alfred Binet was opened, and it is now the base from which the four sector teams operate— each team including a psychiatrist, a social worker, a psychologist and a speech therapist. Since it is independent from both medical and educational public services in the *arrondissement*, the association has been able to develop its children's section in accordance with the needs of the community. However, this freedom from restrictive ministerial or local authority structuring seems to have slowed up the establishment of close collaboration with schools, and with maternity and paediatric clinics.

Separation of adult from child psychiatry is particularly marked in the teaching of the Paris Faculty of Medicine. However, this may occur to a lesser extent in the thirteenth *arrondissement*, since the two services both depend on the same association. Children of patients attending the adult centre are often referred to the child section, and adolescents receiving psychotherapy at the child centre may be referred to the adult day hospital or one of the therapeutic workshops.

For a population of 165,000 in the *arrondissement*, there are the equivalent of six full-time psychiatrists or psychotherapists at the child centre. This is an unusually large ratio of qualified staff to population, which makes possible the impressive extent of the work of the child centre. By serving a well-defined geographical sector, each team gets to know the background of its patients well. As with the adult service, contact is maintained with key people in the life of the patient (teachers, employers, police, etc.), after the end of treatment. The social worker may then be an obvious figure for the family to turn to in a crisis. By operating directly in schools and maternity clinics, the teams see children in need of treatment, who would have been missed if special referral had been needed.

The Alfred Binet centre hopes to keep a balance between the growing needs of the community and the service's limited resources, by instruction of key people in the community, e.g. teachers, social workers, youth-club leaders and family doctors. This is done through case discussions and seminars, so that simple cases may be mostly cared for by non-psychiatric personnel. The work of the association's speech therapists in the schools constitutes a valuable link with teachers, and a starting point for discussion of educational and emotional disturbances in children. There is no equivalent in France of the British educational psychologist, who helps to secure liaison between child guidance clinics and schools.

Early on, attempts were made to secure collaboration between the association and local paediatricians. However, it has not been possible to develop these far, and paediatricians seem only able to take the role of a referring agent in the process. Many mothers have also been unwilling to proceed to a psychiatric consultation (40% of 60 cases referred by paediatricians in 1964).

The children's day hospital had a maximum attendance of 28 in 1964; all patients were aged between 8 and 14. The full-time staff comprises five teachers (of whom one is a nurse), a psychologist, a speech therapist and a housekeeper. About 80% of the children are regarded as suffering from severe emotional disturbances, with about equal numbers diagnosed as psychotic and neurotic during the last 2 years. Many cases also have motor disorders, such as dyslexia or dysorthographia, but the day hospital régime is not specially appropriate for these problems. Mental subnormality is not dealt with and the average I.Q. in 1964 was 96.

The daily life is on classroom lines, with the children divided into three or four small groups. Normal schoolwork is continued and the children also spend time individually with the more specialized members of the staff in psychotherapy, speech therapy or motor re-education. It is stated, however, that attempts to involve parents in the work of the day hospital have failed, and that they fail to realize that help is being offered to the family as a whole. It was thought at one time that referrals might be restricted to cases where the parents were clearly co-operative, but this would have involved too great a degree of selection.

Sociological Characteristics of the Arrondissement

The thirteenth *arrondissement* lies to the south-east of the Ile de la Cité and Notre Dame, and is separated from them by the fifth, which contains the Sorbonne and many of the university premises. Its eastern boundary is the Seine and its southern boundary forms part of the limits of Paris, with the district of Ivry beyond, characterized by older one- or two-storey houses. To the north are the tall, affluent office blocks of the boulevard Port-Royal, contrasting with the factories, warehouses and railway yards by the Seine.

From the way in which the inhabitants refer to the *arrondissement* as "our thirteenth" and the way in which other Parisians talk about the area, it seems that this part of Paris has some kind of unity, other than just administrative. But perhaps more important is the loyalty which each inhabitant seems to feel towards his own particular part of the *arrondissement*, with its own nucleus of social life—the bistro at the corner, the square shaded by poplar trees or containing its collection of little shops. The population is predominantly working-class; in 1954, 41 out of 100 of the working population were in the equivalent of classes IV and V of the British Registrar General's classification, compared with 31 for Paris as a whole. A growing proportion of the working population is North African, working chiefly in the larger industrial enterprises. The *arrondissement* contains a whole range of sizes and types of enterprises, from four firms employing over 6000 workers (including French Railways and Panhard), to several thousand with less than 2 salaried workers each.

On the whole, the housing problem is no more acute than in the rest of Paris. However, there are small pockets of serious overcrowding, such as "District four", where North African and (recently) negro immigrants have tended to settle in large numbers, and where living conditions have become very unhealthy. It is these districts which cause the thirteenth to have one of the highest death rates from tuberculosis in Paris, and one of the highest rates of juvenile delinquency. However, this is not true of suicide, for these districts are animated by an intense social life, with much group integration. The inhabitants seem to find a human way of living in an inhuman setting, and are very attached to their district, in spite of its discomforts.

What Has Been Achieved

The experiment in the thirteenth *arrondissement* is not regarded as constituting a blueprint for urban psychiatric services, applicable to the whole of France, but rather a means for trying out certain ideas, under conditions which are controlled to some extent. Therefore, a district was chosen which possessed a certain sense of community (as well as being an administrative entity), which could be divided easily into a number of subsectors and which, in its many-sidedness, represented much that was typical of other districts of Paris. The intention was to see to what extent the psychiatric team could be integrated into the population, i.e. to be accepted by them and to get to know them. This implies the creation of a working relationship with key people in the community, e.g. teachers, industrial leaders, local press, general practitioners. It also implies that the patient must be known in his social context.

The association has now been in existence for over 7 years, and it is appropriate to try and measure the extent to which its aims have been achieved, though this is extremely difficult to quantify. However, if the adult patients attending the centre are compared with those attending an out-patient clinic in Paris run on conventional lines, it is found that in 1964, 15% of the patients in the thirteenth made their first contact on their own initiative, compared with 5% at the clinic in the fourth *arrondissement*. This seems to indicate a greater tendency for individuals to seek contact with the psychiatric team spontaneously. Also, between January 1963 and July 1965, 60% of the patients aged 17–25 at the time of their first contact with the clinic in the fourth had been previously hospitalized, compared with 34% in the thirteenth. As the staff of the clinic in the fourth are overburdened by the care of large numbers of patients in the mental hospital to which they are attached, they are unable to do the same work with early cases. Dr. Paumelle believes that the process by which the psychiatrist and his team came to be regarded as therapeutic, rather than repressive, agents, is a first step in the recognition of the psychiatric patient as a sick person. This is likely to result in increased demands being made on the team, both by individuals seeking treatment for themselves and by others on behalf of patients. Such a trend has already been noticed by the association.

However, the project has not been encumbered by the need to accommodate many hundreds of chronic, institutionalized patients in its programme. This was because the patients of this sort belonging to the *arrondissement* were already hospitalized elsewhere. A few are gradually being referred to the centre from various psychiatric hospitals of Paris, and are being accommodated in the sheltered workshops or visited by community nurses. But the success of the association in the future is likely to be judged by the degree to which it has solved the problem of chronicity. The hospital (L'Eau

Vive) has been designed for short stay with intensive treatment, and the association has no accommodation for the long-stay patients. The question cannot yet be answered, whether the community-based, non-residential services will be able to provide adequately for the remaining "chronic" patients.

SECTION C
PSYCHIATRIC HOSPITALS

23. Needs and Beds: a Regional Census of Psychiatric Hospital Patients*

CHARLES P. GORE, KATHLEEN JONES, WALLIS TAYLOR and BRIAN WARD

ACCORDING to Ministry of Health policy, hospital beds for psychiatric patients in England and Wales will be reduced from about 3·4 beds per thousand population in 1960 to 1·8 beds per thousand population in the mid 1970s (Ministry of Health, 1961; Tooth and Brooke, 1961). Regional plans included in the Ministry's Hospital Plan have been compiled on this assumption. The estimate of 1·8 per thousand population assumes a 95% bed-occupancy rate, and covers all beds for psychiatric patients whether in mental or general hospitals. It is based on the hypothesis that the statistical trends established during 1954–59 will continue and is therefore a maximal rather than a minimal estimate. The official view is that clinical advances and the extension of community care may reduce the need for psychiatric hospital beds still further. In the past three years, however, a growing volume of evidence and expert opinion has suggested that this view may be too optimistic.

Norton (1961), Lindsay (1962), and P.E.P. (1963) have criticized the statistical basis of the Tooth–Brooke projection in some detail. Shepherd et al. (1961), Carstairs (1961), Weatherall (1962), and Hordern and Hamilton (1963) have stressed the limitations of the psychotropic drugs, attributing the decline in resident populations during 1954–59 to administrative policy and changes in attitudes to mental illness rather than to genuine chemotherapeutic advance. Catterson et al. (1963) are doubtful about the practicability of rehabilitating large numbers of long-stay patients, most of whom are schizophrenic. Gore and Jones (1961) and Hassall and Hellon (1964) have drawn attention to the social isolation and limited capacities of the long-stay populations in two hospitals, and the considerable expectation of life of many of the patients. Wing et al. (1964) have raised the moral issues implicit in the discharge of long-term schizophrenic patients and the effects of early discharge on both patients and their relatives.

The census we report in this paper was made in the Leeds region with the object of providing detailed, accurate, and up-to-date information on which a regional estimate of bed-demand might be based. We recognized that any long-range forecast can be no more than an attempt to balance probabilities, and to assess the effects of conflicting trends; but since regional boards must plan for the future, forecasts have to be made, and it is important that they should be based on realities.

* Reprinted from the *Lancet*, August 29, 1964, pp. 457–60.

The project was discussed with consultant psychiatrists in the region, and after revision, the questionnaire was sent to medical superintendents for their information, and then issued to matrons and chief male nurses, to be completed by ward administrative staff. The questionnaires showed the position at midnight on May 28/29, 1963. They were checked by senior nursing staff at the hospitals, and rechecked at regional headquarters.

The questionnaires were coded and transferred on to machine punch-cards. When the preliminary results were available, a validating sample, stratified by hospital, was constructed by the statistician (W. T.). The 488 patients included in the sample were visited and examined by one of the psychiatrists (B. W.) and the results of the sample were analysed and compared with those of the main survey. This comparison indicated that the questionnaires had been carefully and accurately completed.

The survey has provided a wide range of information about the characteristics and needs of psychiatric patients in the Leeds region; but the object of the present paper is to describe the population with particular reference to the short-stay and long-stay groups, and to give general assessment of bed needs in 1975.

Psychiatric Population

Table 1 sets out the psychiatric hospital population of the Leeds region on the survey date by sex and length of stay.

TABLE 1.

Total Population: Sex and Length of Stay

Patients	Male	Female	Total
Short-stay	515 (5·3%)	818 (8·4%)	1333 (13·7%)
Medium-stay	612 (6·3%)	903 (9·2%)	1515 (15·5%)
Long-stay	3096 (31·7%)	3818 (39·1%)	6914 (70·8%)
Total	4223 (43·3%)	5539 (56·7%)	9762 (100%)

Short-stay means continuous hospital residence for less than 3 months, medium-stay for between 3 months and 2 years, and long-stay for 2 years or more.

Females exceeded males in all three groups. Of the 9762 patients, 2007 (20·6%) were under the age of forty-five; 3865 (39·6%) were between forty-five and sixty-five; and 3890 (39·8%) were sixty-five and over. The female population was notably slanted towards the upper age-groups, 48·3% of women being sixty-five and over compared with 28·9% of men.

6317 patients (64·7%) had been admitted to a psychiatric hospital or unit for the first time, 1910 (19·6%) for the second time, and 716 (7·3%) for the third time. Less than 9% of patients were on their fourth or subsequent admission. There was no clear correlation between the length of stay and the number of admissions.

Length of stay did, however, have a clear correlation with three other factors—single status, a primary diagnosis of schizophrenia, and the absence of regular visits from relatives and friends (Table 2).

It is often assumed that patients who have been in hospital for less than 3 months are a homogeneous group for whom rehabilitation will be fairly easy. Thus paragraph 27 of the Hospital Plan says:

> It is now generally accepted that short-stay patients should be treated in units nearer to their homes than is generally possible . . . the majority of patients in such a unit will not require nursing in bed.

Our findings suggest that the short-stay group (1333 patients, 13·7% of all patients) has certain clear characteristics—a smaller proportion of single

TABLE 2.

Some Factors Varying with Length of Stay

	Under 3 mos.	3 mos. to 2 years	2–5 years	5–10 years	10–20 years	20 years and over
Single (%)	31·0	38·7	46·5	55·6	65·3	71·5
Schizophrenic (%)	23·3	30·7	31·3	50·7	62·4	68·0
Never visited (%)	8·5	16·7	18·3	25·9	36·7	53·3

patients than the other groups (less than one-third); fewer patients with a primary diagnosis of schizophrenia; and most patients have regular visitors; but further analysis shows that the group contains some very disparate elements. The term "short-stay" masks a considerable intake of geriatric patients and of "revolving door" patients, some of whom require only the lapse of time to convert them into long-stay patients. In our group 287 patients had psychoses associated with senile and/or organic brain disease, 509 had two or more previous admissions, and 5 were over seventy-five. Thus only 532, or 40·0% of the group, were short-stay in the commonly accepted sense of the term.

Analysis of the medium-stay group (1515 patients, 15·5% of all patients) suggests that this is essentially a transition group, without clear characteristics. It does not seem to require separate consideration in terms of policy. The long-stay group on the other hand is of great importance because of its size (6914 patients, 70·8% of all patients) and the known difficulties of rehabilitating long-term patients. Of the 6914 patients in this group, 5899 had been in hospital continuously for five years or more; 4731 had been in hospital continuously for ten years or more; 2896 had been in hospital continuously for twenty years or more. This huge chronic population dominates the work of mental hospitals.

The Menston survey (Gore and Jones, 1961) argued that the long-stay patient group in that hospital was not predominantly elderly, and that over 40% of the patients could be expected to be alive in sixteen years' time. Hardly any were used to occupations which would fit them for outside employment; few had marriage partners; half had virtually no visitors; and over two-thirds had advanced schizophrenia. It was concluded that "in this hospital at least, the Ministry's assumption that 'none will remain in sixteen years or a little more' is unlikely to be fulfilled". The Menston survey is not strictly comparable with the present regional survey, since it dealt only with those patients in hospital continuously for five years or more, and the figures necessarily refer to a longer period of projection; but an application of the same indices to the regional long-stay population in 1963 produces very similar conclusions.

The long-stay group shows a broad age-range. Though 2881 patients were aged sixty-five and over, 4033 were under sixty-five, the peaks coming in the 45–64 age-groups. On the basis of the Registrar General's English Life Tables 1950–52 No. 11, at least 54·4% of these long-stay patients, a total of 1814 men and 1949 women, can be expected to be still living in 1975, even if the higher mortality-rates for the East and West Ridings of Yorkshire are applied. If the rates for England and Wales as a whole are used as a standard, 58% would still be alive; and these rates may in fact be more applicable for people living in institutions, usually away from the main industrial areas.

The long-stay patients at present in hospital will not be eliminated by death alone by 1975. The question therefore arises as to how many can be rehabilitated, and in what circumstances.

In all 4389 patients (2285 men, 2104 women, 63·5% of the long-stay group) were single, and a further 1135 (268 men, 867 women, 16·4% of the long-stay group) were separated, widowed, or divorced. Only one-fifth of long-stay patients had a living marriage partner.

2708 patients (39·2% of the long-stay group) were never visited. A further 1272 (18·4%) were visited only annually. Thus less than half of all long-stay patients receive regular visits from friends and relatives.

4020 patients (58·2% of the long-stay group) had a primary diagnosis of schizophrenia. A further 1018 (14·7%) had psychoses associated with senile and organic brain disease, and 921 (13·3%) had a variety of conditions classified together, in which subnormality and severe epilepsy predominate. Probably less than 15% had a form of illness from which there is a reasonably good chance of adjustment to normal living.

2316 long-stay patients (33·5%) did no work. 1472 (21·3%) worked on the wards, 1788 (25·8%) on hospital utilities, and 1194 (17·3%) in the occupational therapy department or industrial workshop. Only 144 (2·1%) had employment outside the hospital.

Trends in the Treatment of Schizophrenia

Before a regional forecast is made, further consideration must be given to the schizophrenic patients. The validating sample indicated that their number had been underestimated in the census. The underestimate, amounting to perhaps 7%, occurred because some patients originally diagnosed as schizophrenic had lived on into the geriatric group and had been reclassified as

TABLE 3.

Patients with a Primary Diagnosis of Schizophrenia, Affective Disorders, and Senile Psychosis, by Date of First Admission

Date of admission	Schizophrenia	Affective disorders	Senile psychosis
1963[a]	105	285	296
1962	128	127	358
1961	77	95	250
1960	81	76	138
1959	91	72	139
1958	93	65	97
1957	96	59	85
1956	128	64	62
1955	129	45	66
1954	150	45	56
1953	180	42	47
1952	168	44	44
1951	153	27	29
1950	151	41	27
1949	138	37	29
1948	160	33	25
1947	125	23	22
1946	93	32	16
1945	121	24	18
1944 and earlier	2429	521	146
Total	4796	1757	1950

[a] Since the survey took place at the end of May 1963, the figures for that year represent only 5 months' admissions.

having senile psychosis. However, even the lower figures in the census indicate a variation in trends which is crucial to an estimate of bed-demand.

Over 87% of all patients were classified under the three main diagnoses—schizophrenia, affective disorder, and senile psychosis.

If the majority of patients with a particular diagnosis are being successfully treated and discharged, or if the majority die within a year or two of admission, there should be in hospital at any given time a relatively large number of patients recently admitted for the first time, and a very much smaller number of patients of long standing. This holds for the affective disorders (18% of patients) where many patients are discharged "relieved" or "recovered", and for the senile psychoses (20%) where the expectation of life is comparatively short, but it does not hold for the schizophrenics (49·1%) among whom there is a notable accumulation of cases first diagnosed twenty years ago or more.

Table 3 indicates that the number of schizophrenic patients remaining in hospital at the time of the survey from admissions in the years 1948–54 was about 150 a year, the highest number being 180 (1953 admissions) and the lowest 138 (1949 admissions). From 1955, however, the number declines steadily to 77 in 1961.

It is possible that the number of schizophrenic patients fell between 1955 and 1961 because the disease was being cured; or because, though the disease was not being cured, some schizophrenics who would previously have stayed in hospital were able to live in the community—because of the palliative effect of drugs, the increase in public tolerance, and the provision of community care. In either case, we can expect the residual number of schizophrenics to remain at least as low as in 1961—say at 75 a year. On the other hand, it is possible that the low figures of 1955–61 were due to overreadiness on the part of psychiatrists to discharge; if so, the residual number of schizophrenics may return to the level of the years before 1955, averaging about 150 again. Table 4 sets out two projections to illustrate these alternatives. In each the residual patients first admitted before 1964 (3105) represent the schizophrenics actually in hospital at the time of the survey, reduced by allowing for expected mortality from 1964–75.

TABLE 4.

Two Projections of the Number of Beds Required for Schizophrenic Patients in 1975

Projection (a):	
75 residual patients per year from 1964–75	900
Residual patients admitted earlier	3105
	4005
Less 10%	400
	3605
Projection (b):	
150 residual patients per year from 1964–75	1800
Residual patients admitted earlier	3105
	4905
Less 10%	490
	4415

Allowance has been made for a further reduction of 10% to cover possible discharges and deaths.

Community Care

Though the Ministry of Health's projection takes no account of the extension of the provision of community care, this must affect the demand for psychiatric beds in hospital. According to the Community Care Plan, which was published in 1963, community services in the Leeds region by 1972 will

TABLE 5.

Community Care Provision Forecast for Leeds Region, 1972[a]

	Additional	Total
Part III accommodation for elderly	4197	11,061
Psychiatric day centres	3	8
Hostel places	311	391
Home helps	683	2703
Social workers	162	421

[a] These figures are based on the proposals for Leeds, Hull, York, Bradford, Halifax, Huddersfield, Dewsbury, Wakefield, and the East and West Ridings of Yorkshire, which are shown in the plan as falling wholly within the area of the Leeds Regional Hospital Board. In fact the areas are not coterminous, about a third of the population of the West Riding being outside the board's area, while nearly half of the population of the North Riding falls within it.

be as shown in Table 5. A detailed study of the Plan makes it clear that local authority provision is likely to be very uneven.

For example, while the number of social workers needed in an area must vary with its size, density of population, and the provision of other services, there seems no logical explanation for the fact that York, with a compact area and good ancillary services, expects to have 0·23 social workers per thousand population by 1972, while the East Riding, with a large area of scattered population and less ancillary provision, expects to have only 0·06. If the York health and welfare services are not to be grossly overstaffed, one can only conclude that the East Riding (and Leeds, the West Riding, Bradford, Huddersfield, Dewsbury, and Wakefield, all of which envisage less than half the York rate of provision) are likely to be considerably understaffed.

The fulfilment of local authority plans depends on somewhat uncertain factors, such as the provision of money for capital expenditure from central government funds at a time when other needs, such as those of universities, technical colleges, and district general hospitals, are being given priority, and the recruitment and training of sufficient social workers in a known shortage. The targets in the Community Care Plan may not be reached by some authorities, and it is unlikely that they will be exceeded by any.

Assuming that the published plans are fulfilled by 1972, how far can local authorities be expected to allocate scarce resources to the mentally ill, in the face of other, and perhaps more pressing, needs? There will be 311 places in psychiatric hostels, plus perhaps 300 places for day-patients in psychiatric centres (assuming an average of 100 patients attending at some time during the week in each of the three centres planned). Places may be found for some borderline geriatric patients in Part III accommodation; but such accommodation is not intended for patients who require intensive nursing or other supervision, or who are likely to disturb the other residents. Since the Hospital Plan proposes to reduce geriatric beds in general hospitals in the region from 1·7 per thousand population to 1·4, we assume that the extra provision in Part III accommodation will be offset.

The effect of additional home helps and social workers on the demand for hospital beds is difficult to estimate, since it is not known what proportion of these extra workers would be devoted to the mental health services. 10%—i.e. an extra 68 home helps and 16 social workers—would be a reasonable guess.

Overall, the additional community care provisions may offer alternative care for about 1000 patients of the type now in long-term hospital care.

Planning for Future Bed Requirements

The number of psychiatric hospital beds required at any given time is affected by social and economic factors. Foremost among these is the "iceberg" effect, by which new provisions in mental health seem inevitably to reveal new dimensions in demand rather than relieving pressure on existing provision. Tooth and Brooke (1961) indicated the importance of certain other factors, such as the standard of public tolerance, the maintenance of full employment, and the possibility of major advances in treatment. Factors of this magnitude cannot be measured in advance, nor can we predict what their effects are likely to be. For the purposes of calculation, it must be assumed that what may be important variables remain constant.

For two factors, however, the effects can be calculated: the increase in the population and the apparent decrease in the length of stay in hospital.

The increase in the population forecast by the Registrar General (1963) affects the psychiatric hospital population in two ways: through overall population growth and through a change in the age-composition of the population. The risk of admission varies greatly with respect to age and sex, and the actual number of people of sixty-five years and over is expected to rise by 27%. On the basis of a detailed examination of trends, we have allowed for an increase of 11% on the present mental hospital population of the region—a total of 1074 beds.

Analysis of the evidence on length of stay (Registrar General, 1962) indicates that, although the median duration of stay fell between 1951 and

1959 from about 2·2 months to 1·6 months, this overall calculation masks the situation in the three length-of-stay groups. The median duration of stay for short-stay patients (here given as patients in hospital for less than one year) has fallen; that for long-stay patients is 3 % less for males, but 8 % greater for females: that for the medium-stay group (here 1–5 years) has risen slightly. It seems unlikely that the median duration of stay for short-stay patients can fall much below the 1959 figure of 1·38 months for men and 1·48 months for women. With these factors in mind, we have assumed that the overall length of stay will neither increase nor decrease further. But this length of stay is calculated only for "patients leaving by discharge or departure". A critical factor is the length of stay of those *not* leaving the hospital. If mortality-rates fall, they will "stay" even longer.

Table 6 shows the final estimate of bed-needs for the region. We have assumed that the treatment of the affective disorders on present lines has now reached its full effect (Table 3) and that the numbers of long-stay patients other than schizophrenic and senile patients will not be materially reduced. The known shortage of residential accommodation for severe epileptics and the severely subnormal indicates that this is a fair assumption.

TABLE 6.

Estimate of Bed-need in the Leeds Region in 1975

	Plus	Minus	Total
No. of beds occupied at the time of the survey	—	—	9762
Population increase in region and increased longevity in age-group 65 and over	1074	—	10,836
Extension of community care	—	1000	9836
On projection (*a*) (Table 4), reduce no. of beds for schizophrenics from 4796 to 3605	—	1191	8645
On projection (*b*) (Table 4) reduce no. of beds for schizophrenics from 4796 to 4415	—	381	9455

The total number of beds estimated as actually occupied in 1975 is between 8645 and 9455. If the figures are scaled on the basis of a 95 % bed-occupancy rate, the number of beds actually to be provided would be 9953 (plus 191 or 1·9 %) or 9100 (minus 662 or 6·8 %) in comparison with the actual number of beds on the survey date. Since these calculations can only be approximate, overall bed-need by 1975 will probably be 9000–10,000 beds.

According to the Hospital Plan the number of beds will be reduced to 5840 by 1975. Our calculations indicate that, if present admission and discharge policies are continued, the number of beds actually required is likely to be greatly in excess of this number. Patients can be discharged, and beds can be emptied, by administrative decision: but, in the absence of some substantial and favourable change in the situation, this can be achieved only at the cost of much hardship to patients and their families.

We wish to record our appreciation of the assistance and co-operation of the officers and staff of the Leeds Regional Hospital Board, and the medical and nursing staffs of the psychiatric hospitals and units in the region. The views expressed are our own, and do not necessarily represent those of the Board or of the people who helped us.

References

CARSTAIRS, G. M. (1961), *Practitioner* **187**, 495.

CATTERSON, A. G., BENNETT, D. H. and FREUDENBERG, R. K. (1963), *Brit. J. Psychiat.* **109**, 750.

GORE, C. P., and JONES K. (1961), *Lancet* **ii**, 544.

HASSALL, C. and HELLON, C. P. (1964), *Brit. J. Psychiat.* **110**, 183.

HORDERN, A. and HAMILTON, M. (1963), *Ibid.* **109**, 500.

LINDSAY, J. S. B. (1962), *Lancet* **i**, 354.

MINISTRY OF HEALTH (1961), HM(61) 25.

NORTON, A. (1961), *Lancet* **i**, 884.

P.E.P. (1963), Psychiatric Services in 1975, London.

REGISTRAR GENERAL (1962), *Statistical Review*, 1959, suppl. on Mental Health.

REGISTRAR GENERAL (1963), Quarterly Review for 1962, 4th quarter.

SHEPHERD, M., GOODMAN, N. and WATT, D. C. (1961), *Comprehens. Psychiat.* **2**, 11.

TOOTH, G. C. and BROOKE, E. (1961), *Lancet* **i**, 710.

WEATHERALL, M. (1962), *Brit. med. J.* **i**, 1225.

WING, J. K., MONCK, E., BROWN, G. W. and CARSTAIRS, G. M. (1964), *Brit. J. Psychiat.* **110**, 10.

24. The Growth of Mental Hospitalization: the S-shaped Curve*

J. A. BALDWIN

THE hospital plan for England and Wales (1962) assumes that the number of mental hospital beds required will fall from the present level of over 3 per 1000 population to about 1·8 per 1000 by 1975. The study on which the plan was based (Tooth and Brooke, 1961) assumed, *inter alia*, that admission rates to mental hospitals would not rise above their 1959 levels. In Scotland, the situation has always been rather different. Admission rates have tended to be higher than in England and Wales and there are about 4 mental hospital beds per 1000 population. Perhaps partly because of this, there is no comparable policy for Scottish mental hospitals and a more cautious attitude seems to have been adopted.

This "wait and see" approach has allowed time for detailed studies of the use of Scottish mental hospitals to be developed. One of these studies is being carried out in the North-east region, which is an area of some 4400 square miles containing 480,000 people in largely rural and coastal communities, with its natural centre in the city of Aberdeen. The whole area, which includes the Orkney and Shetland Islands, is served by a comprehensive and integrated system of mental health services consisting of a regional mental health centre (the Ross Clinic), two mental hospitals of 800–900 beds each, and one of about 200 beds, together with child psychiatric and mental deficiency services and hospitals (Baldwin and Millar, 1964). This setting provides an ideal "experimental area" for intensive research and the Department of Mental Health in Aberdeen University Medical School has been actively engaged in epidemiological research for some years (Innes and Sharp, 1962). In order to exploit its potential, a cumulative fund of data on all psychiatric patients has also been developed in the form of a case register based on the medical record (Baldwin *et al.*, 1965).

An aspect of mental hospital use which warranted early attention, in view of the hospital plan and apparent trends in England and Wales, was that of admission patterns. This paper discusses some salient features of admission, in relation to the difficulties of long-term planning.

* Based on a paper given at a post-graduate meeting at the Ross Clinic, Aberdeen, October, 1965.

Trends in Admissions to Mental Hospitals, 1956–64

Studies of admissions to mental hospitals generally make use of the distinction between "first admissions" and "re-admissions". A first admission is taken to reflect the onset of illness, whereas a re-admission is assumed to imply a recurrence of an old illness, or the onset of a new illness.

Since a patient can be a first admission on only one occasion, the class of first admissions must be composed of separate individuals. In contrast, the class of re-admissions contains only individuals who have been admitted more than once. Thus, in any time period, these individuals may be counted in both first and re-admissions, and more than once in the count of re-admissions, unless special precautions are taken. Many of the data used in this paper were not susceptible to the adjustments necessary to count individuals, so that analyses of them depict patterns of admission events rather than individuals admitted. For many operational purposes, analyses of events are satisfactory and all admissions may be considered together.

ALL ADMISSIONS

The national trend, which has been a consistent rise in admissions since the early 1940's (Baldwin, 1963), is largely reflected in the pattern in the North-east region (Table 1). With the exception of a slight fall in 1957, there was a rise in the number of admissions in each year of the period. Over the 9 years, the number of admissions almost exactly doubled.

The rise in numbers was not confined to any particular age or sex group, although by 1964 the largest rises were in the younger ages and in males. The steepest rise in admissions of the aged appears to have taken place in

TABLE 1.

All Admissions to North-east Scottish Mental Hospitals, 1959–64,
as Percentage of 1956

	1956		1959	1960	1961	1962[a]	1963	1964	
	N	%	%	%	%	%	%	%	N
Total	1041	100	116	133	143	—	181	200	2079
Males	452	100	102	127	136	—	172	206	930
Females	589	100	127	139	148	—	187	195	1149
Age 0–34	240	100	123	154	168	—	196	211	507[b]
Age 35–64	591	100	115	133	139	—	168	192	1135[b]
Age 65 and over	210	100	111	109	123	—	195	203	427[b]

[a] No comparable figures were available for 1962.
[b] Excluding 10 patients whose age was not known.

1961–3, the rate of rise falling off during 1964. Throughout the period, there were markedly larger numbers of women than men admitted and the middle-aged contributed over half of all admissions. However, the numbers of both young and aged admissions more than doubled over the 9-year period. The number of aged admissions remained notably lower than the number of young throughout.

Factors which appear to have contributed to the national picture were also operative in this region. The period was marked by the coming into general use of psychotropic drugs, a heightening of community awareness of the possibility of treatment rather than mere incarceration, a more active policy of early discharge and ready re-admission (perhaps in turn accelerated by the increased demand for admission), and in the last 2 years, the coming into effect of the Mental Health (Scotland) Act, 1960. Locally, two major factors were the opening of the Ross Clinic in 1959, and the appointment of a medical superintendent at the 200-bedded mental hospital in 1963.

Role of the Ross Clinic

The advent of the regional treatment centre in July 1959, with its small in-patient unit (38 beds), provision of improved regional out-patient and domiciliary and emergency services, and privileged staff position as the professorial teaching unit (Baldwin and Millar, 1964), is of special interest from both operational and service standpoints. Its possible effect on the use of existing services is important, because of the trend towards development of such centres as either adjuncts to, or substitutes for, traditional forms of service, particularly in the United States. Clinically, its new treatment policies could have a significant effect on the course of illness, which should be demonstrable.

Here, the repercussions on the regional picture can be outlined (Tables 2 and 3). The regional increase in admissions in the first year and a half of Ross Clinic operation was due in the main to the latter's in-patient unit.* There was also a smaller increase in admissions to the mental hospitals and a special study showed that this was not due to transfers from the Ross Clinic. This pattern was attributable to intake of females rather than males into the Ross Clinic. Thus there may have been an initial tendency to draw admissions away from the mental hospitals, but this was not sustained, and indeed, from 1961 to 1963, the burden of increase tended to revert to the mental hospitals. In 1964 the clinic again took a larger share of the increase, again also particularly of female admissions.

The mechanism is further clarified by the age distribution (Table 3). The early effect of the Ross was confined to the young and middle-aged, but was

---

* Prior to the opening of the Ross Clinic, there were 10 beds in the general hospital (Ward IV, Aberdeen Royal Infirmary), which took about 100 admissions per annum.

TABLE 2.

All Admissions to North-east Scottish Mental Hospitals, 1956–64, by Sex with Percentage Differences from Previous Year

	1956		1957		1958		1959		1960		1961		1962		1963		1964	
	N	%	N	%	N	%	N	%	N	%	N	%	N	%	N	%	N	%
Both sexes																		
Mental hospitals	1041	—	1023	98·3	1050	102·6	1103	105·0	1107	100·4	1210	109·3	?	—	1641	—	1789	109·0
Ross clinic	—	—	—	—	—	—	104[a]	—	283	272·1	276	97·5	254	92·0	238	93·7	290	121·8
Total N.E. region	1041	—	1023	98·3	1050	102·6	1207	115·0	1390	115·2	1486	106·9	?	—	1881	—	2079	110·5
Males																		
Mental hospitals	452	—	421	93·1	444	105·5	426	95·9	466	109·4	517	110·9	?	—	690	—	832	120·5
Ross Clinic	—	—	—	—	—	—	34[a]	—	107	314·7	96	89·7	109	113·5	90	82·5	98	108·8
Total N.E. region	452	—	421	93·1	444	105·5	460	103·6	573	124·6	613	107·0	?	—	780	—	930	119·2
Females																		
Mental hospitals	589	—	602	102·2	606	100·7	677	111·7	641	94·7	693	108·1	?	—	953	—	957	100·4
Ross Clinic	—	—	—	—	—	—	70[a]	—	176	251·4	180	102·3	145	80·5	148	102·0	192	129·7
Total N.E. region	589	—	602	102·2	606	100·7	747	123·3	817	109·4	873	106·8	?	—	1101	—	1149	104·3

[a] July to December only.

TABLE 3.

All Admissions to North-east Scottish Mental Hospitals, 1956–64, by Age with Percentage Differences from Previous Year

	1956 N	1956 %	1959 N	1959 %	1960 N	1960 %	1961 N	1961 %	1962 N	1962 %	1963 N	1963 %	1964 N	1964 %
Age: 0–34														
Mental hospitals	240	—	268	111·7	273	101·9	299	109·5	?	—	368	—	402	109·2
Ross Clinic	—	—	28[a]	—	98	350·0	105	107·1	105	100·0	103	98·0	105	101·9
Total N.E. region	240	—	296	123·3	371	125·3	404	108·9	?	—	471[b]	—	507[c]	107·6
Age: 35–64														
Mental hospitals	591	—	607	102·7	630	103·8	661	104·9	?	—	875	—	987	112·8
Ross Clinic	—	—	71[a]	—	157	221·1	162	103·2	137	84·6	120	87·5	148	123·3
Total N.E. region	591	—	678	114·7	787	116·1	823	104·6	?	—	995[b]	—	1135[c]	114·0
Age: 65 and over														
Mental hospitals	210	—	228	108·6	204	89·5	250	122·5	?	—	396	—	393	99·2
Ross Clinic	—	—	5[a]	—	25	500·0	9	36·0	12	133·3	14	116·6	34	242·8
Total N.E. region	210	—	233	110·9	229	98·3	259	113·1	?	—	410[b]	—	427[c]	104·1

[a] July to December only.
[b] Excluding 5 patients whose ages were not known.
[c] Excluding 10 patients whose ages were not known.

not sustained, while the mental hospitals took almost the whole increase in aged admissions. In 1964 the emphasis shifted, the Ross taking the whole of the increase in aged patients and the major share of additional middle-aged, while the increase in young admissions was practically confined to the mental hospitals.

In general, the role of the Ross Clinic in the regional pattern of admissions to in-patient services is quite specific. It caters mainly for young and middle-aged admissions, particularly females, but latterly has tended to absorb an increasing proportion of aged. Indeed, its admission picture tends to approximate more closely to that of the mental hospitals and vice versa. Its effect is materially to increase the overall number of regional admissions, but not at the expense of the mental hospitals. A question meriting further investigation is whether, in the absence of the Ross Clinic, the mental hospitals would have borne its contribution, or whether it is really admitting from a population which would otherwise have received no in-patient care.

Age distribution

The percentage distribution by age of all admissions in the region was quite constant over the period (Table 4). The most notable features were: (1) a modest but consistent increase in the proportion of admissions aged 35–44; (2) a decrease in the proportion of admissions aged 45–64; (3) an increase in the proportion of women aged 75 and over. In general, there has been a tendency for the sex differences in age distribution to become more emphasized over the period, namely higher proportions of early middle-aged males, and higher proportions of females in the age range 15–34 and the very old.

Diagnosis

Diagnostic breakdowns were obtained for the years 1956 to 1961 (Table 5). Over this period, there was a shift in the relative frequency of some diagnostic groups. The commonest in 1956 was manic-depressive reaction, but by 1960 neurotic depression was most common. It is not clear whether this represents a change in diagnostic usage or a change in the clinical features of depression, but the coincidence of the pattern with the development of the Ross Clinic should be noted. Neurotic depression replaced the diseases associated with ageing (the dementias and involutional depression) as the most common admission diagnosis among women, whereas among men, manic-depressive reaction was replaced by schizophrenia from 1959.

The proportion of admissions diagnosed as schizophrenic remained remarkably constant at about 16% over the period, though the proportion among males averaged 20% and among females about 13%. In contrast, the proportion

TABLE 4.

All Admissions to North-east Scottish Mental Hospitals, 1956, 1959, 1961, 1963, and 1964.
Percentage Distribution by Age Controlled for Sex

Age	Total					Males					Females				
	1956	1959	1961	1963	1964	1956	1959	1961	1963	1964	1956	1959	1961	1963	1964
0–14	0·1	0·2	0·3	0·4	0·2	0·2	0·4	0·5	0·6	0·3	0	0·1	0·2	0·3	0·2
15–24	7·0	9·5	9·7	8·9	8·3	9·7	10·4	9·3	8·6	9·9	4·7	9·0	10·0	9·1	7·0
25–34	16·0	14·7	17·2	15·7	15·9	18·8	18·3	17·1	16·3	17·8	13·9	12·6	17·2	15·3	14·3
35–44	17·8	19·2	20·0	20·4	20·8	18·4	19·1	19·2	23·3	21·6	17·3	19·3	20·6	18·2	20·1
45–54	21·3	19·5	19·3	16·0	19·4	19·4	18·0	20·1	15·3	19·3	22·8	20·3	18·8	16·6	19·5
55–64	17·7	17·5	16·0	16·5	14·4	17·3	18·5	20·6	19·0	15·0	18·0	16·9	12·8	14·7	13·8
65–74	12·1	12·3	9·4	11·2	10·8	8·0	8·5	7·3	8·3	7·5	15·3	14·6	10·9	13·2	13·4
75 and over	8·1	7·0	8·0	10·6	9·8	8·2	6·7	5·9	8·5	7·7	8·0	7·2	9·5	12·2	11·4
Not known	—	—	—	0·3	0·5	—	—	—	0·1	0·6	—	—	—	0·4	0·3
All ages N =	1041	1207	1486	1881	2079	452	460	613	779	930	589	747	873	1102	1149

TABLE 5.

All Admissions to North-east Scottish Mental Hospitals, 1956, 1959, 1960, and 1961.
Percentage Distribution by Diagnosis Controlled for Sex

Diagnosis	Total				Males				Females			
	1956	1959	1960	1961	1956	1959	1960	1961	1956	1959	1960	1961
Schizophrenia	16·2	13·8	16·8	16·5	20·6	18·5	21·8	18·9	12·9	11·0	13·2	14·9
Manic-depressive reaction	24·9	20·6	15·3	15·1	21·2	16·7	16·9	14·4	27·7	22·9	14·2	15·6
Other functional psychoses	6·3	7·3	5·8	6·1	7·1	7·2	4·7	7·3	5·8	7·4	6·5	5·3
Diseases of ageing	23·2	19·1	15·0	17·2	15·3	12·0	7·5	10·3	29·2	23·6	20·3	22·0
Neurotic depression	6·1	17·1	19·3	18·2	6·0	12·8	13·1	11·7	6·3	19·7	23·6	22·7
Other psychoneuroses	10·7	8·5	10·0	8·5	9·3	7·2	6·1	6·5	11·7	9·4	12·7	9·8
Alcoholism and drug addiction	3·8	5·1	7·4	8·0	8·2	12·8	16·2	17·8	0·5	0·4	1·2	1·1
Behaviour disorders	4·8	5·0	5·3	4·8	7·1	9·8	8·4	8·0	3·0	2·0	3·2	2·6
Other	3·9	3·5	5·1	5·6	5·3	3·0	5·2	5·1	2·9	3·7	5·0	6·0
All diagnoses $N =$	1041	1207	1390	1486	452	460	573	613	589	747	817	873

diagnosed as manic-depressive reaction fell from a quarter of all admissions in 1956 to 15% in 1961. Both sexes shared in this decline, though there was usually a higher proportion among females. There was a 6% fall in the proportion admitted with diseases of ageing up to 1961, but the proportion among women was at least twice that among men throughout. Both sexes shared in a threefold increase in the proportion of neurotic depressions, but the rise among females was considerably greater than among males. The proportions with alcoholism and drug addiction doubled in both sexes, but the great majority of cases were in males. Indeed, the rise in male admissions with alcoholism accounted for most of the rise in all male admissions, but this was entirely due to the rise in re-admissions. Thus, although alcoholics were being re-admitted much more readily for repeated treatment, there was no evidence of an increase in the number of new alcoholics coming into hospital.

FIRST AND RE-ADMISSIONS

The distinction between first and re-admissions to psychiatric in-patient services has been used for many years as an index of primary hospitalization, reflecting the incidence of morbidity. Its limitations for this epidemiological purpose are well known. Apart from the selective processes determining whether mentally ill people reach psychiatric treatment services, and additional selective factors determining whether those who reach treatment are hospitalized, there are usually ambiguities inherent in the definition of a first admission which further reduce the value of the distinction. For epidemiological purposes, a first admission would be defined best as the first psychiatric hospitalization in the patient's life or at least for the illness in question, but in practice, many hospitals define it as the first admission to the reference hospital, while others may define it as the first regional hospitalization. With a single hospital serving a defined and static population, the precise definition may be of little importance, but in a system of hospitals serving a common catchment area, and especially one containing a mobile population, fastidious adherence to exact definition would be essential to validity of the data.

The operational value of separating first from re-admissions without further information is also limited. From the point of view of availability of beds in any particular admission, it is of no consequence whether the user is in his first or nth hospitalization. Of much greater importance is the "stage army effect", whereby a relatively small number of individual patients can inflate admission and discharge figures by multiple hospitalizations. A further vital question is whether multiple hospitalization reduces the total time spent in hospital, compared with a single hospitalization over the whole period of a patient's illness (Brooke, 1963). Both these matters can be investigated adequately only by the register method, which accumulates data on all an individual's treatment experiences consecutively over an indefinite time period. At the time of this study, data on first and re-admissions were available for the period 1959 to 1961, and are presented as rough indications of the extent to which multiple hospitalization is of operational importance in this region.

Multiple hospitalization

The proportion of re-admissions rose from one-third to one-half of all admissions between 1959 and 1961 (Table 6). First admissions exceeded re-admissions in both sexes, all age groups and all major diagnostic groups in 1959, but by 1961 only among females, the young and the elderly, and diseases of ageing and psychoneuroses. Multiple hospitalization was therefore most prevalent among males, the middle-aged, functional psychoses and the group of "other" diagnoses, which comprise mainly alcoholism and behaviour disorders. First admissions declined between 1959 and 1961 in both sexes, all ages except the young and all diagnostic groups except psychoneuroses, while re-admissions rose in all sex, age and diagnostic categories by from 43% to 185%. The importance of multiple hospitalization as a major influence on the utilization of hospital facilities can hardly be overestimated, but much more information is required for proper investigation than the simple distinction between first and re-admissions. Continuation of the trends which occurred in the period 1959–61 seems likely, further emphasizing a tendency to multiple, short treatment periods for a decreasing number of most categories of patient.

CONCLUSIONS

What conclusions can we draw from this brief look at the salient features of the pattern of admission to mental hospitals in North-east Scotland? The most noticeable is, of course, the growth in the total number of admissions in the year. In terms of rates per 1000 total population, it represents an increase from 2·10 in 1956 to 4·34 in 1964—that is, the rate more than doubled in 9 years. This fact alone should be enough to make administrators and planners sit up and boggle, and give clinicians cause to consider what is happening. If the same sort of thing is happening in England and Wales, the assumption of a steady admission rate in the hospital plan is, to say the least, unrealistic.

However, the data also indicate very strongly indeed that by far the greater part of this growth is due to multiple hospitalization, rather than to any real rise in the rate of person morbidity in the community. Indeed, the few, and rather unreliable, figures we have indicate that the number of new *people*

TABLE 6.

First and Re-admissions to North-east Scottish Mental Hospitals, 1959 and 1961.
Percentage Changes by (A) Sex, (B) Age, and (C) Diagnosis

A. By Sex	Total			Males			Females		
	1959	1961	%±	1959	1961	%±	1959	1961	%±
First admissions	66·5	49·3	91·3	67·2	43·9	87·0	66·1	53·1	93·9
Re-admissions	33·5	50·7	186·4	32·8	56·1	227·8	33·9	46·9	161·7
Total N =	1207	1486	123·1	460	613	133·3	747	873	116·9

B. By Age	0–34 years			35–64 years			65 and over		
	1959	1961	%±	1959	1961	%±	1959	1961	%±
First admissions	69·2	51·5	101·5	62·1	42·6	83·4	76·0	67·2	98·3
Re-admissions	30·8	48·5	215·4	37·9	57·4	183·6	24·0	32·8	151·8
Total N =	296	404	136·5	678	823	121·4	233	259	111·1

C. By Diagnosis	Functional psychoses			Diseases of ageing			Psychoneuroses			Other		
	1959	1961	%±	1959	1961	%±	1959	1961	%±	1959	1961	%±
First admissions	59·6	39·7	74·3	73·6	65·9	98·8	74·1	60·3	104·4	63·4	37·6	99·0
Re-admissions	40·4	60·3	166·5	26·4	34·1	142·6	25·9	39·7	196·2	36·6	62·4	285·0
Total N =	503	561	111·5	231	255	110·4	309	396	128·1	164	274	167·1

being hospitalized is tending to fall, and with a slightly falling regional population, this probably means a more or less constant or possibly slightly falling first admission rate. In other words, while statistically the use of these mental hospitals in terms of total admissions has risen dramatically, actually fewer people are using them more often. This is, of course, merely the numerical expression of the clinical experience of early discharge and ready re-admission rather than prolonged incarceration, and the next part of this paper presents some data on outcome of hospitalization which substantiate and quantify this trend.

Patterns of Outcome of Admission to Mental Hospital*

One of the most useful ways of investigating admission patterns is to describe what happens to patients after they have been admitted to hospital. Such straightforward information, as how long they stay and how they leave, whether by discharge to the community or transfer to other forms of care, or by death, should be readily available for a variety of purposes. Operationally, changes in the rate of leaving hospital must have a profound effect on the use made of the facilities. Clinically, knowledge about patients' expectations on entering hospital is prognostically vital, and an important indication of how treatment methods and policies work out in practice. From the point of view of the patient and his relatives, it is most important that some idea of what is likely to happen should be available. Yet, to the author's knowledge, no systematic information about the outcome of admission to Scottish mental hospitals has ever been published. Work in other countries, particularly England and Wales, and the United States, has proceeded along these lines for many years, so that it is possible to give quite detailed predictions about such factors as the probability of discharge or death, time out of hospital between admissions and re-admissions for various age, sex and diagnostic categories of patient (Brooke, 1963; Kramer *et al.*, 1957; Bahn and Bodian, 1963). Similar studies of out-patient and other forms of psychiatric care are also being undertaken (Bahn and Chandler, 1961).

The cohort method

The most generally used method of longitudinal research of this kind is that of the cohort. A cohort is simply a class of subjects having one or more characteristics in common, and the objective is to describe differences within the class occurring over time. In present context, the class of subjects is admissions to mental hospitals, and the common feature is the year of admission.

* The assistance of Miss Mhairi Russell in the preparation of analyses for this section is gratefully acknowledged.

Three cohorts were selected: (1) all admissions in 1956, (2) all admissions in 1959, and (3) all admissions in 1963. The year 1956 was chosen since it was the earliest year for which data were available, thus providing a suitable baseline against which to compare later years, and the longest period for follow-up, i.e. the 5 complete years to the end of 1961. The year 1959 was chosen because it was the latest year for which data were available which would permit follow-up for 2 complete years, the minimum period which, at the commencement of the study, seemed useful. The year 1963 was chosen later in the study because there was evidence from the general pattern of admissions that important changes were taking place in the outcome of admissions subsequent to 1959, particularly in the first months of admission. 1963 was the most recent year on which follow-up could be made for a full year.

It will be noticed that in taking admissions over a whole year, the assumption is made that admissions in one part of the year will not differ materially from admissions in another part. Admissions throughout the year are treated as if they were all admitted on the same day. This assumption is necessary in order to yield large enough numbers for analysis. A further point is that the cohorts consist of all admissions, regardless of whether they were first or re-admissions. The reasons for ignoring this distinction have been given, and for the purpose of this study it was not required. However, a consequence of taking all admissions is that individuals admitted more than once in a year will be counted more than once. Strictly speaking, therefore, the cohorts are not of individuals, but of admissions, or admission events. Only where the duration of stay exceeds 1 year can it be assumed that the analyses are of individuals. Moreover, the same individual could have been admitted and discharged in each of the 3 years, and thus appear in two or even all three cohorts.

Presentation of results

The analyses to be presented are of uniform type. Intervals of time since admission were selected on the basis of previously known duration-of-stay patterns. The numbers remaining resident in hospital after each interval were calculated and the mode of separation in each interval tabulated. From these figures, percentage decrements of the cohort were calculated, together with percentage accumulations of separations. An example of the calculation is shown in Table 7. For simplicity of interpretation, results are shown graphically. Figure 1 gives an example of the chief types of curve used. The cohort decrement curve, for instance, shows clearly that loss of admissions from the cohort was very rapid in the first 9 weeks, but also goes on at a progressively smaller rate thereafter. It should be noted that the sudden change in rate after some intervals is a consequence of choice of intervals. Smaller intervals would

TABLE 7.

All Admissions to North-east Scottish Mental Hospitals in 1963 by Outcome

Intervals in weeks	Starting cohort		Outcomes after each interval			Cumulative interval outcomes as % admissions					
			Discharges	Deaths	Separations	Discharges		Deaths		Separations	
	a		b	c	d = b + c	$\frac{b}{a} \times 100$		$\frac{c}{a} \times 100$		$\frac{d}{a} \times 100$	
	N	%	N	N	N	N	%	N	%	N	%
0	1881	100·0	—	—	—	—	—	—	—	—	—
1	1749	93·0	127	5	132	127	6·7	5	0·2	132	7·0
2	1624	86·3	114	11	125	241	12·8	16	0·8	257	13·6
4	1309	69·5	297	18	315	538	28·6	34	1·8	272	14·4
9	710	38·0	577	22	599	1115	59·3	56	3·0	1171	62·6
26	313	17·0	376	21	397	1491	79·2	77	4·0	1568	83·3
52	195	10·3	98	20	118	1589	84·5	97	5·1	1686	89·6

have yielded more rounded curves and it cannot be assumed that changes occur at the precise intervals chosen. The curve of discharges* as a proportion of admissions, in conjunction with the death curve, shows the extent to which discharge and death play a part in reducing the cohort. It is sometimes also useful to present deaths, discharges, and separations after each interval as a proportion of all separations.

Comparisons of outcome between the three cohorts in the first year of hospitalization are discussed first, followed by further data on the longer durations from the two earlier cohorts.

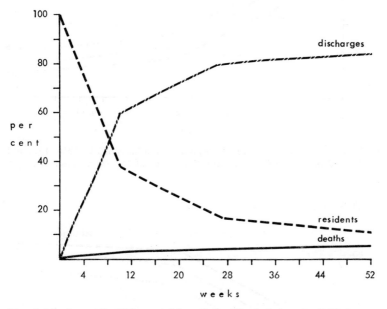

FIG. 1. North-east Scottish mental hospitals. All admissions in 1963. Outcome after specified intervals as proportion of starting cohort.

OUTCOME IN THE FIRST YEAR

There are three general features of outcome in the first year of admission to mental hospital which emerge from preliminary examination of the accompanying figures:

1. The rate of separation from hospital in the first 2 months or so of hospitalization was relatively high, considerably less in the third to

---

* In all the cohort analyses, transfers to other psychiatric in-patient care were included in discharges, since their numbers in each case were extremely small (between 5 and 10 per annum).

N.A.M.H.S.—P

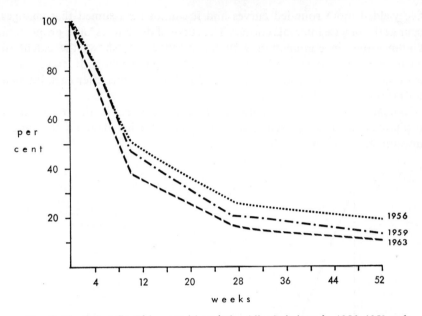

FIG. 2. North-east Scottish mental hospitals. All admissions in 1956, 1959 and
1963. Proportion of starting cohort, retained after specified intervals.

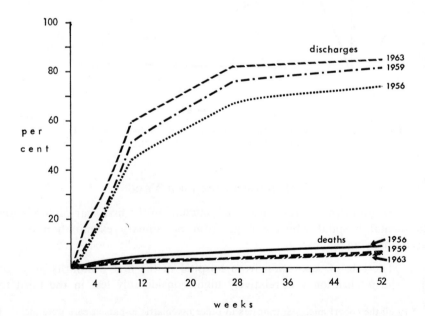

FIG. 3. North-east Scottish mental hospitals. All admissions in 1956, 1959 and
1963. Outcome after specified intervals as proportion of starting cohort.

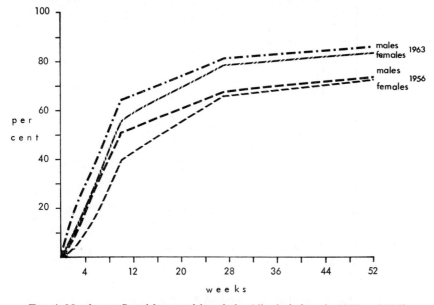

FIG. 4. North-east Scottish mental hospitals. All admissions in 1956 and 1963, by sex. Discharges after specified intervals as proportion of starting cohort.

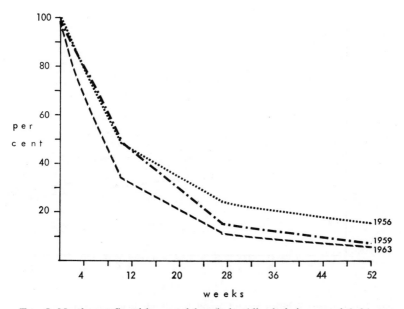

FIG. 5. North-east Scottish mental hospitals. All admissions aged 0–34 years in 1956, 1959 and 1963. Proportion of starting cohort retained after specified intervals.

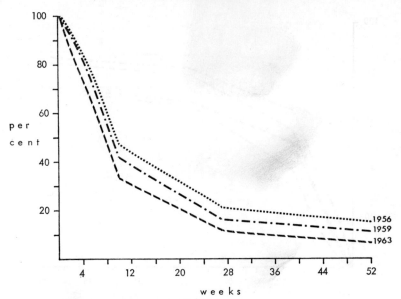

Fig. 6. North-east Scottish mental hospitals. All admissions aged 34–65 years in 1956, 1959 and 1963. Proportion of starting cohort retained after specified intervals.

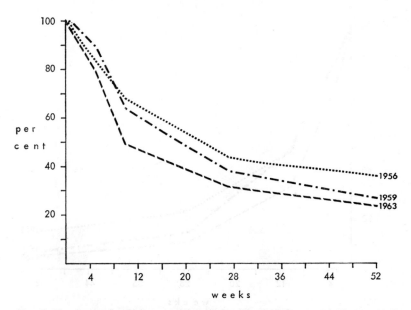

Fig. 7. North-east Scottish mental hospitals. All admissions aged 65 years and over in 1956, 1959 and 1963. Proportion of starting cohort retained after specified intervals.

sixth months and still less to the end of the first year (Fig. 2). This generalization applied regardless of age or sex (Figs. 4–7). Thus, the longer a patient remained in hospital, the smaller his chances of being discharged.

2. Throughout the period, males had a higher expectation of discharge than females, particularly in the first 2 months (Fig. 4). This generalization applied, with only minor exceptions, to young, middle-aged and elderly (Fig. 9).

3. Patients aged 65 years and over had a much smaller expectation of discharge, and of course, a higher expectation of death, than younger patients. Among elderly admissions, the chance of dying was highest in the early weeks of hospitalization but *decreased* thereafter.

Over the period 1956 to 1963, there was a fall in the proportion retained more than 2 months from 51% to 38%, but the rate of separation in subsequent months actually decreased, so that the proportion retained after 6 months and 1 year fell by only 10%. This change in the pattern of outcome was mostly due to a higher proportion of discharges in the first 2 months, but also due to a fall in the death rate, especially in the remainder of the year (Fig. 3). The change was shared almost equally by males and females (Fig. 4).

The young, middle-aged and elderly all experienced improved expectations of discharge in the first 2 months, though to varying extent (Figs. 5, 6 and 7). For patients up to 34 years old, the most marked improvement was in the first 2 weeks, whereas there was no greater chance of release after the second month in 1963 than there had been in 1956. The same was broadly true also of patients aged 35–64. Among patients aged 65 and over, the picture is complicated by the part played by death* (Fig. 8). While the over-all separation rate changed little in the first month between 1956 and 1963, the proportion of deaths in the first month fell remarkably, and continued lower thereafter. Almost the whole of this change was in males in the first 4 months, but there was a less marked reduction of death rates among females in the later months of the year (Fig. 10). For those who survived to the second month, the expectation of discharge rose considerably. From the third to the sixth months, the expectation of both discharge and death was lower in 1963 than it was in 1956. In the last half of the year, there was little difference between 1956 and 1963 with respect to total separations, but the chance of death continued about the same as in the third to sixth months.

The expectations of discharge by age and sex in 1963 are shown in Fig. 9. Among patients up to the age of 64, there were slight differences, with males usually experiencing higher rates than females. Aged men did slightly better

* The expectation of death in the first year in hospital among patients up to 34 years was 0·4% and for those aged 35–64 1·8% in 1963.

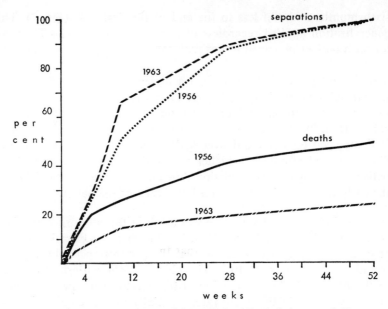

Fɪɢ. 8. North-east Scottish mental hospitals. All admissions aged 65 years and over in 1956 and 1963. Separations and deaths after specified intervals as proportion of all separations.

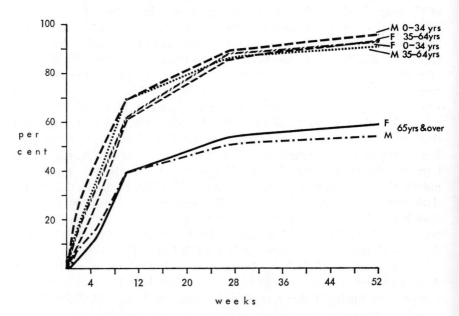

Fɪɢ. 9. North-east Scottish mental hospitals. All admissions in 1963 by age and sex. Discharges after specified intervals as proportion of starting cohort.

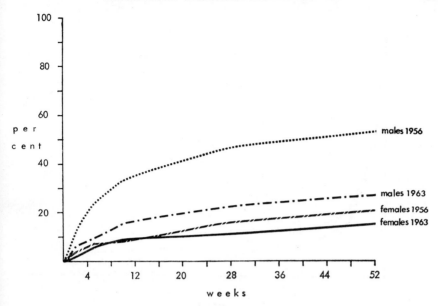

FIG. 10. North-east Scottish mental hospitals. All admissions aged 65 years and over in 1956 and 1963, by sex. Deaths after specified intervals as proportion of starting cohort.

than aged women in the first 2 months, but thereafter there was a slightly better chance of discharge among aged women.

OUTCOME IN THE SECOND AND SUBSEQUENT YEARS

Data from the 1956 and 1959* cohorts, which could be followed beyond the first year of hospitalization, confirmed the main trends observed in the first year. The expectation of separation from hospital continued to decline at least up to the fifth year (Fig. 11). This applied to both sexes, and young, middle-aged and elderly patients (Figs. 12–15). The association between increasing age and decreasing expectation of separation was also confirmed. A notable finding was that the increased proportion of deaths among aged admissions with increasing length of hospitalization did not decrease the proportion retained at a uniform rate (Figs. 15 and 16). In the fifth year, the rate of loss from the 1956 cohort was reduced to almost nil. The greater expectation of death among males than among females remained unchanged after the first year, but the sex differences in expectation of discharge were reversed between 1956 and 1959.

The differences between the 1956 and 1959 cohorts noted in the first year of hospitalization were also observed in the second year. The smaller

* The Ross Clinic was excluded from this cohort.

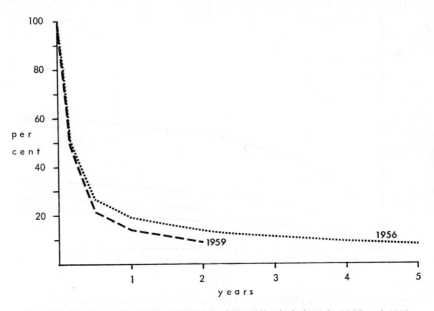

FIG. 11. North-east Scottish mental hospitals. All admissions in 1956 and 1959.
Proportion of starting cohort retained after specified intervals.

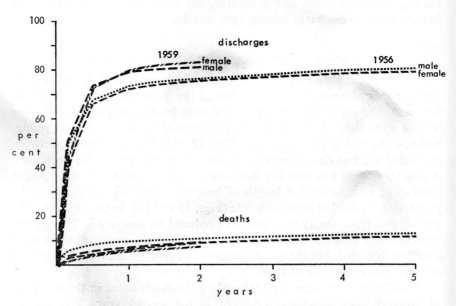

FIG. 12. North-east Scottish mental hospitals. All admissions in 1956 and 1959,
by sex. Outcome after specified intervals as proportion of starting cohort.

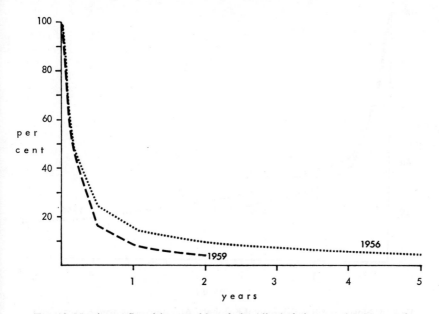

FIG. 13. North-east Scottish mental hospitals. All admissions aged 0–34 years in 1956 and 1959. Proportion of starting cohort retained after specified intervals.

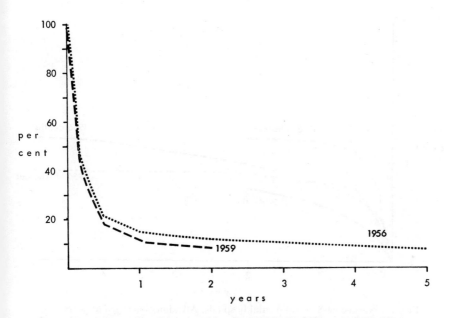

FIG. 14. North-east Scottish mental hospitals. All admissions aged 35–64 years in 1956 and 1959. Proportion of starting cohort retained after specified intervals.

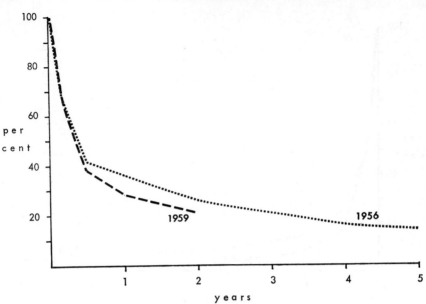

Fig. 15. North-east Scottish mental hospitals. All admissions aged 65 years and over in 1956 and 1959. Proportion of starting cohort retained after specified intervals.

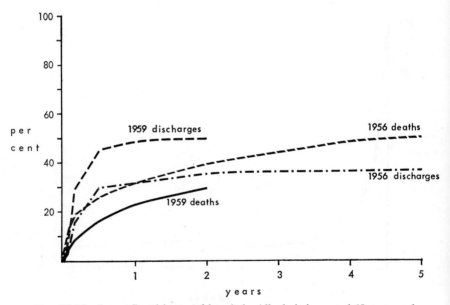

Fig. 16. North-east Scottish mental hospitals. All admissions aged 65 years and over in 1956 and 1959. Outcome after specified intervals as proportion of starting cohort.

proportions remaining in hospital in both sexes and all age groups were maintained but not increased in the second year.

The remarkable fall in the proportion of deaths among aged admissions in the first year of hospitalization is further illuminated in Fig. 16. Whereas in the 1956 cohort, deaths exceeded discharges after the first year, in the 1959 cohort there was a large preponderance of discharges over deaths. The earlier discharge in 1959 admissions of the elderly was accompanied by a fall to nil in the expectation of discharge in the second year. Among 1956 admissions, this did not occur until the third year. Thus for elderly admissions, the only way of leaving hospital after the second or third year was by dying.

DIAGNOSTIC OUTCOMES

Analyses of outcome by diagnosis on admission were obtained for the 1956 and 1959 cohorts, and a selected group of diagnostic outcomes, comprising 80% of all admissions, is reported here. Figure 17 shows the broad differences in the proportions retained after various intervals in the 1956 cohort. Although there were large differences between the diagnostic groups, it will be seen that all also conformed to the general pattern described for age and sex groups. Expectation of separation from hospital was lowest for schizophrenia, somewhat higher for diseases associated with ageing, and considerably higher for manic-depressive reaction and psychoneuroses. The differences appeared in the first 2 months of hospitalization in all groups and were maintained thereafter. However, it was notable that there was about the same chance of separation after the first year in all the diagnostic groups. On the other hand, the proportions retained after 5 years of manic-depressives and psychoneurotics were very small, but about 10% and 20% for ageing and schizophrenics, respectively. Discharge accounted for almost all separations in all groups except ageing (Figs. 18–21).

Schizophrenia (Fig. 18)

The increased expectation of discharge in the early months of hospitalization between 1956 and 1959 admissions was particularly marked among schizophrenics. In the second year, however, there was little difference in the two cohorts. The importance of this group as a major contributor to the long-stay population should be noted in terms of both numbers, and the relatively low expectation of separation after the first year.

Manic-depressive reaction (Fig. 19)

The marked contrast with schizophrenia in this group of psychoses in the higher expectation of discharge in the first year of hospitalization has been

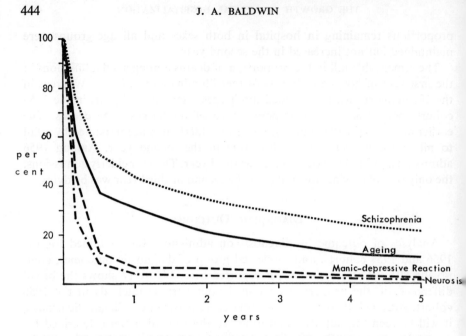

FIG. 17. North-east Scottish mental hospitals. All admissions of selected diagnoses in 1956. Proportion of starting cohort retained after specified intervals.

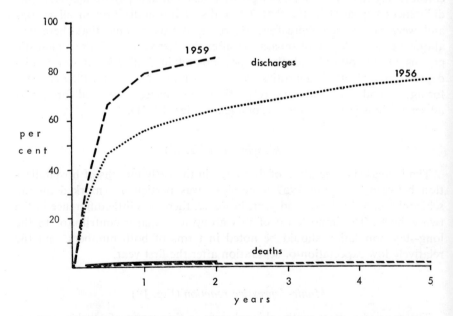

FIG. 18. North-east Scottish mental hospitals. All admissions of schizophrenia in 1956 and 1959. Outcome after specified intervals as proportion of starting cohort.

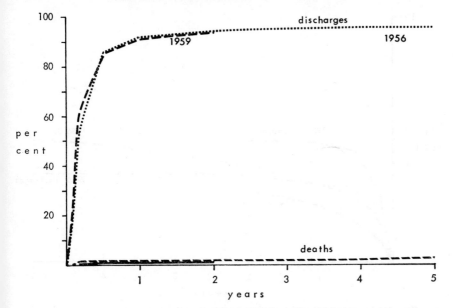

FIG. 19. North-east Scottish mental hospitals. All admissions of manic-depressive reaction in 1956 and 1959. Outcome after specified intervals as proportion of starting cohort.

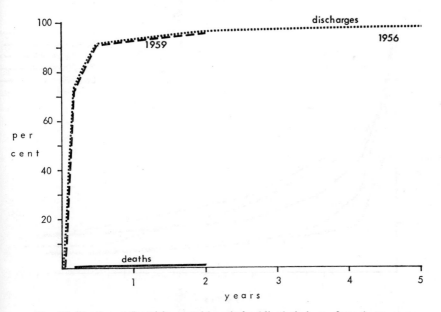

FIG. 20. North-east Scottish mental hospitals. All admissions of psychoneuroses in 1956 and 1959. Outcome after specified intervals as proportion of starting cohort.

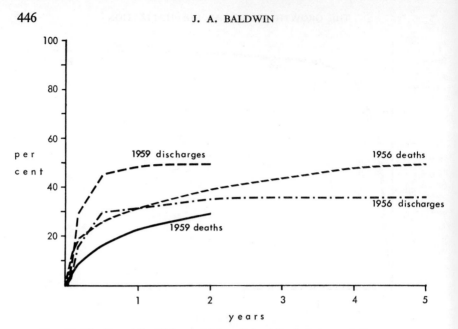

FIG. 21. North-east Scottish mental hospitals. All admissions of diseases associated with ageing in 1956 and 1959. Outcome after specified intervals as proportion of starting cohort.

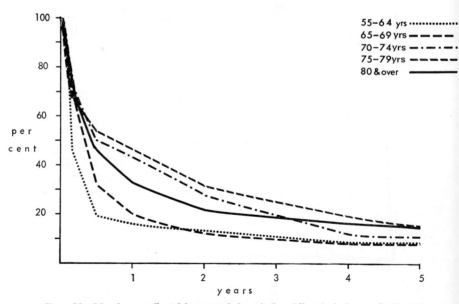

FIG. 22. North-east Scottish mental hospitals. All admissions of diseases associated with ageing in 1956 by age. Proportion of starting cohort retained after specified intervals.

noted. Furthermore, there was very little difference between the 1956 and 1959 cohorts in this respect. Thus, the pattern of treatment outcome for manic-depressives showed no marked changes in the period studied.

Psychoneuroses (Fig. 20)

The similarity in outcome between psychoneuroses and manic-depressive reaction has been noted. A further similarity is that there was also little change in expectation of discharge between 1956 and 1959.

Diseases associated with ageing (Figs. 21–7)

The increased expectation of early discharge, and much-reduced expectation of death between 1956 and 1959 admissions aged 65 years and over can be seen to apply exclusively to patients admitted with diseases associated with ageing. Although the total proportion separated by the end of the second year did not differ appreciably between 1956 and 1959, the mode of separation altered in important ways. The increased chance of discharge in the first year was accompanied by a much-reduced chance of death, particularly in the first 2 months. On the other hand, the expectation of discharge for those retained for more than a year was virtually nil in both cohorts, and the expectation of death after the first 2 months was little lower in 1959 than in 1956. Thus, separation from hospital after the first year was almost entirely by death, and death accounted for the continued fall in the proportion retained.

Because of the importance of this group of admissions in terms of its use of facilities, the analysis was carried further. Differences in proportions retained from the 1956 cohort are shown by age in Fig. 22. With the exception of those 80 years old and over, the expectation of separation decreased with increasing age. There was a definite difference in the proportions retained after 6 months between patients under 70 years and those over 70 on admission.

For patients under 65 years old, the chance of discharge in the first 6 months was high in 1956, and rose further in 1959, although the probability of discharge was low in both cohorts thereafter (Fig. 23). Death played a very small part in reducing the cohorts of this age group. The age groups 65–9 and 70–4 years (Figs. 24 and 25) experienced rather similar outcomes of admission. In spite of some rise in the proportions discharged in the early months of hospitalization between 1956 and 1959, the maximum was about 50% in both age groups. In the 1956 cohort, the proportion of admissions who died was nearly equal to the proportion discharged by the end of 5 years in both age groups. Of those aged 65–9 years, a lower proportion died in the later cohort, but among admissions aged 70–4, the expectation of death in the first year was rather higher in 1959 than it had been in 1956.

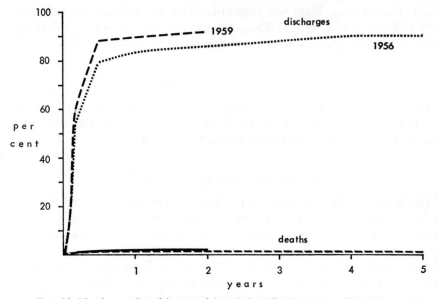

FIG. 23. North-east Scottish mental hospitals. All admissions of diseases associated with ageing aged 55–64 years in 1956 and 1959. Outcome after specified
intervals as proportion of starting cohort.

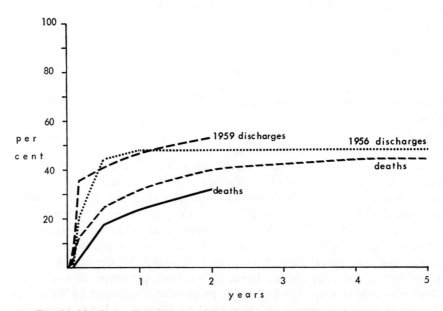
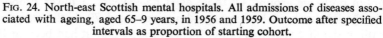

FIG. 24. North-east Scottish mental hospitals. All admissions of diseases associated with ageing, aged 65–9 years, in 1956 and 1959. Outcome after specified
intervals as proportion of starting cohort.

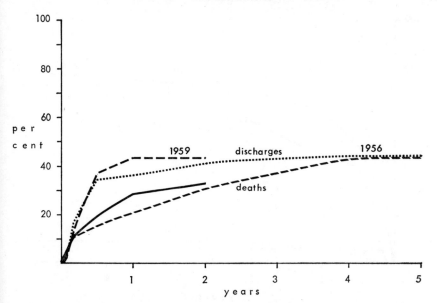

FIG. 25. North-east Scottish mental hospitals. All admissions of diseases associated with ageing, aged 70–4 years, in 1956 and 1959. Outcome after specified
intervals as proportion of starting cohort.

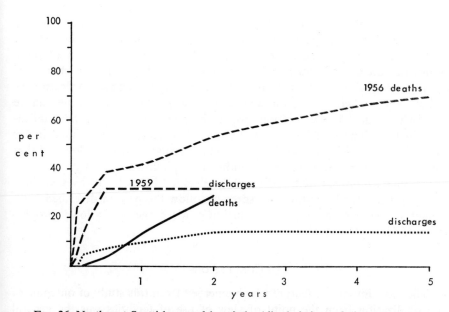

FIG. 26. North-east Scottish mental hospitals. All admissions of diseases associated with ageing, aged 75–9 years, in 1956 and 1959. Outcome after specified
intervals as proportion of starting cohort.

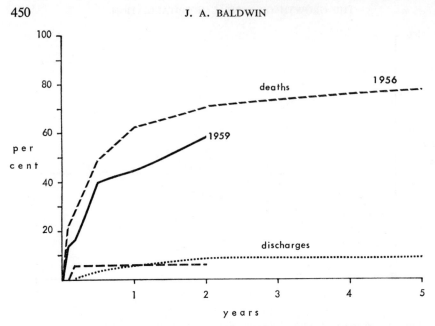

Fig. 27. North-east Scottish mental hospitals. All admissions of diseases associated with ageing, aged 80 years and over, in 1956 and 1959. Outcome after specified intervals as proportion of starting cohort.

It should be noted that the expectation of death in the first months of admission is high in this age group, but decreases with increasing survival in hospital.

Admissions with diseases of ageing, aged 75–9 years, experienced quite different patterns of outcome in 1956 and 1959 (Fig. 26). The chance of early discharge was very much higher in 1959 and the chance of death very much lower. Whereas there was a high expectation of death and a low chance of discharge in 1956, the position reversed in the first 6 months of hospitalization in 1959. The experience of patients aged 80 years and over was similar in both cohorts (Fig. 27). The expectation of discharge was very low and that of death, especially in the first 6 months of hospitalization, very high.

Although numbers were too small for detailed breakdowns by sex, there was a general tendency for both sexes to follow the pattern described, with females experiencing a higher proportion of discharges and a lower proportion of deaths than males.

CONCLUSIONS

The most important feature which emerged from this study of outcome of hospitalization from the point of view of use of facilities was the general reduction in the proportion of admissions in most age, sex and diagnostic categories who were retained after the first few months of hospitalization. Of

1963 admissions, 60% were separated in the first 2 months, and about 80% by the end of the first 6 months. Although there was little evidence of any major change in the rate of loss from the cohorts studied for longer periods, and in general the expectation of discharge (and, with the exception of the very old, of death also) was much lower in the second and subsequent years, three main implications may be suggested.

1. *Non-replacement of long-stay population.* The early attrition of admission cohorts results in a smaller proportion of patients retained for long-term care. Thus, even though the rate of attrition in the second and subsequent years did not increase, the time required for complete elimination of a cohort from the hospital population probably has been progressively reduced. Hence, the residues of cohorts remaining in the total mental hospital population are unlikely to accumulate to such a great extent as in the past, and the long-term part of the population is not being replaced fully.

2. *Concentration of therapeutic effort.* It was not the purpose of this descriptive study to seek explanations of the observed trends. However, it is permissible to suggest some of the possible explanations as general areas for further inquiry. The early attrition of admission cohorts, together with the policy of early discharge and ready re-admission, may imply a concentration of therapeutic effort on the new admission, with relative reduction of effort on the long-term patient. The much smaller chances of discharge in the later years of hospitalization tend to support this suggestion. Several mechanisms could be operative to bring about this situation, such as staff shortage coupled with increasing demand for admission and overpopulation of available long-term beds.

3. *Classification by duration of stay.* Classification of patients according to length of stay is necessary as a guide to the numbers of beds and the size of wards required for different purposes. At present, most mental hospitals have a small proportion of beds available for short-term admissions, in which nearly all turnover takes place, while up to 85% of beds are occupied by very long-term patients, who are the residues of cohorts of admissions dating back to the turn of the century. In the last 20 years or so, the increasing tendency towards early discharge of some of the patients, who used to be retained continuously for many years, has brought out the need for a third category—the medium-stay patient. Standard definitions of short-, medium- and long-stay patients in use at this time are:

Short-stay: 0–3 months;
Medium-stay: 3 months–2 years;
Long-stay: over 2 years.

The early attrition of admission cohorts in recent years necessitates redefinition of these categories, if hospitals are to be planned for current and future rather than past patterns of patient movement, since the huge population of very long-term patients will eventually disappear, if much more slowly than originally thought (Tooth and Brooke, 1961). Short-stay admission wards, with a high staff–patient ratio and rapid turnover, will be required for evaluation and intensive treatment of perhaps the majority of admissions. Medium-stay wards, with facilities for active treatment and rehabilitation over longer periods, will be needed for a further large segment of admissions. Long-stay provision will be necessary for a very small proportion of admissions of mainly aged senile and infirm patients. Accommodation for these patients would probably be concerned mainly with providing a high standard of amenities and nursing in "care and protection" units. Using the major points of change in the rate of separation of current admissions as a guide, an appropriate duration of stay classification would be:

> Evaluation and treatment: 0–2 months (60% admissions);
> Continuous treatment and rehabilitation: 2–12 months (30% admissions);
> Care and protection: over 1 year (10% admissions).

The Pattern of Growth of Hospitalization

These changes in the use of mental hospitals raise some very important questions and point to some rather interesting implications. It is best to begin by taking a longer and broader look at the growth of admissions to mental hospitals by going back in time and taking in the whole national picture. The dramatic rise in total admission rates to mental hospitals began suddenly in 1942 in Scotland, and has gone on steadily ever since. Although we do not have data, there is no reason to suppose that the regional pattern was very different. Moreover, it has not been peculiar to Scotland. With some readily explainable differences, it has occurred in both England and Wales, and in the United States. Also, the experience of England and Wales and Scotland has been broadly similar with respect to the influence of multiple hospitalization on these rates.

The most obvious questions to ask about this extraordinary picture are, "How long is this going on for?" and "Why is it happening?". It is suggested that the answer to the first question may lie in the answer to the second. What we have here is essentially the first part of the so-called logistic or *s*-shaped growth curve (Fig. 29). This well-known and exceedingly common phenomenon has recently been discussed at length by J. R. Platt (1965), Professor of Biophysics at Chicago University. He points out that the change from the straight part of the curve to gradual levelling out is always a consequence of diminution of the original cause of growth, or reaching of a natural limit, and gives many examples of current growth (Table 8).

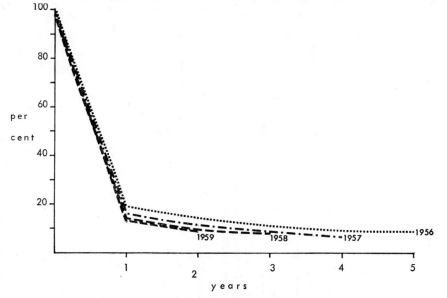

FIG. 28. North-east Scottish mental hospitals. All admissions in 1956, 1957, 1958 and 1959. Proportion of starting cohort retained after annual intervals.

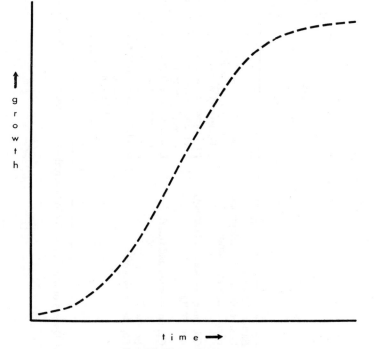

FIG. 29. The growth curve.

TABLE 8.

Examples of the Growth Curve[a]

Subject	Growth rate	Limiting factor
1. Bacterial colony	Varies	Nutrient
2. U.S. research and development	Now in steady state at 3% national income	Money
3. High energy accelerators	10^5 energy increase in 35 years; ×10 in 7 years; ? the next 35 years	Money
4. Computers—speed and capacity	10^5 increase in 20 years—not much room left for further increase	Speed of light
5. Leisure time	Enormous increase in 100 years (any further change cannot be so revolutionary)	?
6. Communication and travel	Limits being approached even in space—next 20 years may be limit for 100s years.	
7. Bombs	6 orders of magnitude increase in 10 years	Overkill (limit reached)
8. Population of world	Doubling every 30–40 years i.e. 6 billion in 2000 / 50 billion in 2120 = ×20 present level	? Space ? Food ? Other

[a] Dozens of other examples in "normal states"—e.g. animal growth, cities, etc.

The growth of mental hospitalization is analogous. The lowest rate for all admissions to Scottish mental hospitals was 0·66 per 1000 in 1941. The rate doubled in 10 years to 1·30 in 1950, and doubled again in 12 years to 2·62 in 1961. Thus we are, as in Platt's examples, in the midst of the most rapid phase of growth. How long can it go on?

Before discussing some of the reasons why it is unlikely to go on for ever, one projection of the current trend is presented, which assumes that the rate of growth will slacken off from now on and reach stability in about 1984. The projection involves a further increase in admissions in the North-east region, again doubling the rate in the 10 years from 1963 to 1972, when it would be 8·19 per 1000. Stability would be reached at a rate of 12·00, giving an increase of eighteen times in the 44 years from 1941 to 1984.

Projection and prediction

One of the chief reasons for carrying out this projection was to estimate the way in which the residues of annual cohorts of admissions may build up a resident population in the mental hospitals. This is a matter of great importance to planners and administrators, and was one of the main reasons for instituting the operational research programme 3 years ago. Before discussing the projection itself, it is important to clarify the general problem of prediction. The first point is that there is a critical distinction between a "projection" and a "prediction". A projection is a legitimate calculation of the continuation of a trend complex. No claim is made for it, other than that it is an estimate of what *would* happen in the future if events conform to the assumptions on which it is based. On the other hand, a prediction is a much more categorical, even imperative statement of what *will* happen in the future. A prediction may make use of projections, but may also take into account expected events which alter the projection in important ways. Predictions are also legitimate in certain circumstances, such as standard experimental procedures, where the objective is to predict the outcome of a causal sequence and improve the chances of controlling it.

The behaviour of mental hospitals, or for that matter mental health services in general, is not susceptible to this kind of prediction. The reason why they are not predictable in this sense is not that they are not subject to identifiable causal sequences or outside human control. Indeed, the reason is just the opposite. Because they are so much under our control, and only a very little subject to impersonal forces, we cannot predict their behaviour *and* act as if we wanted to bring the prediction true, without actually bringing it true. This is precisely the problem with the psychiatric hospital plan for England and Wales. The *projective* study on which it was based was used to *predict* events which were then *planned* to happen. The circularity of Merton's "self-fulfilling prophecy" is now well known, but a simple analogy helps to make the point. If you observe someone's behaviour carefully, you may detect certain regularities in it and eventually reach a point where you can predict with considerable confidence that he will put his hand in his pocket in 5 seconds from now. If, however, he tells you that *he predicts* that he will put his hand in his pocket in 5 seconds from now, you will rightly think he has gone daft, because the word "predict" is correctly applied only in circumstances where we do *not* have direct control over events. Predicting mental hospital behaviour is logically and semantically daft for the same reason that someone predicting when he will put his hand in his pocket is logically and semantically daft. We do have control of the mental hospital system, collectively as a community, and as will be argued, in large measure collectively as a profession. Indeed, in the same way, we have a large measure of control over all our professional services, just as we have a large measure of control over our own behaviour.

Why then make projections? What use are they if they cannot predict what is going to happen? The answer is that unless you know what is happening and what the consequences of your activities are, you are not in a position to exert intelligent control over them. If one is not aware of voluntarily controlling the movements of one's hand, one is in the same position as the predicting experimenter who only experiments on things he cannot understand and control. One function of operational research is thus to bring awareness to the mental health services. However, it should be noted that even if it is the consciousness, in no sense is it the conscience!

PROJECTION OF ADMISSIONS, 1964–84

Although the rate of separation from hospital is relatively low in the second and subsequent years, there is a gradual attrition of each cohort of admissions, so that eventually none will be left. If the rate of attrition for each cohort was known, it would be possible to calculate quite accurately the composition of the hospital population resulting from the specified admission cohorts, at any period in the future. However, several factors contribute to an alteration of the attrition rate, some of which can be worked out fairly reliably and some of which are quite unknown. The age, sex and diagnostic composition of each cohort is likely to differ slightly from year to year, leading to differences in the pattern of outcome. For instance, a marked increase in the proportion of very old admitted might inflate the figures for patients retained in the first 5–7 years, but because of the high death rate among these patients, few might remain thereafter. Changes in treatment policies and methods could radically change the expectation of separation from hospital at any point. In particular, it is known that changes in clinical and administrative staff can have a profound effect on patients' expectations (Astrup and Odegard, 1960). On the other hand, a high admission rate can lead to a concentration of available manpower on the new admissions, result-ing in an increase in expectation of early separation and re-admission, and reduced expectation of separation in the second and subsquent years.

Because of these uncertainties, a rational approach which may have operational utility is to make specific assumptions about them and carry out projections based on defined criteria. Thus, values which seem reasonable at the time can be assigned to each of the variables. If it should prove impos-sible to arrive at only one set of values, then the projection can be repeated for one or more different sets, leading to a range of projections. One of the several sets will eventually be seen to be more realistic as time goes by. Put another way, any projection will be less reliable the further into the future it reaches and adjustments to accord with events must be made repeatedly.

One such projection is presented here as an example. Taking data from the admission cohorts of 1956, 1959 and 1963, and supplementing with similar information from the intervening years, the main trends were abstracted and quantified. Values were then calculated for outcome in the years following those for which data were available. It should be noted that this calculation does not represent the true state of affairs in the hospitals, even during the period for which the facts are known, since no allowance is made for the spread of admissions over each year. However, it is a rough approximation, which illuminates some important features of the accumula-tion of long-stay patients in the period from 1956, and illustrates the implica-tions of the observed trends, should these continue beyond the present time.

The assumptions

The projection was based on the following assumptions:

1. The rate of attrition of the 1956 cohort remains unchanged after the 5 years for which data were available. There was no evidence from the data that any large change can be expected.
2. The rate of attrition of admission cohorts in the years 1957 to 1959 will follow substantially the pattern of the 1956 cohort in the period following that for which data were available. From the available data, it will be seen that rates in the second and subsequent years did not differ greatly from 1956 (Fig. 28).
3. The rate of attrition of annual admission cohorts in the first year of hospitalization will continue to increase up to 1967, and will remain stable thereafter. It seems reasonable to assume that the well-established trend from 1956 to 1963 will continue, but there will probably be a limit to the proportion of patients who can be discharged or who die in the first year of hospitalization. The assumption here is that $9 \cdot 0\%$ retained after 1 year is the most likely point of stabilization.

4. The rate of attrition of annual admission cohorts from 1964 on, after the first year of hospitalization, will follow a similar pattern to that observed from 1956 to 1959.

5. The number of admissions will continue to rise in the years 1965 onward, but the rate of rise will be reduced gradually, so that there will be no further rise after 1984. This assumption is, of course, speculative but not entirely arbitrary, since there is some evidence of a deceleration in the period 1959 to 1964.

Since no figures were available for admissions in 1962, an intermediate position between 1961 and 1963 was adopted, in order to complete the picture.

The results

Part of the results of this projection are shown in Fig. 30 and Tables 9 and 10. It will be seen that:

1. The number of patients in hospital at the end of most years would increase, but each annual increment would be smaller than in the previous year, and in a few years there would be a slight decrease. Carrying the projection to its limit, the long-stay population would reach a maximum of 1034 in 1986 and then fall to a stable level of 1022 about 1990.

2. The long-term effect of reducing the proportion of each cohort retained after 1 year is demonstrated. The 1956 cohort would not be eliminated until about 1990, but successive cohorts would disappear after progressively shorter periods up to 1967, when the maximum period of stay would fall to 6 years.

Although this projection does not take account of the already existing mental hospital population composed of the residues of admission cohorts prior to 1956, there are clear implications in the operational field. The large effect of a reduction in the proportion of admissions retained beyond the first year, on the length of hospitalization of the residue, is striking, and implies a quite different kind of hospital organization than exists at present. The virtual absence of very long-term patients would have profound effects on the clinical character of the hospital, while the reduction in total numbers to about two-thirds of the present long-term population would necessitate large structural and administrative changes. The advent of such changes might in turn produce further effects on the population structure. At the same time, the very great increase in the total number of admissions would have a marked effect on the number and size of admission wards, in relation to long-term accommodation.

Outcome of All Admissions to North-east Scottish Mental Hospitals, 1956–1964,[a] and Projections to 1970

	1956	1957	1958	1959	1960	1961	1962	1963	1964	1965	1966	1967	1968	1969	1970
% change from previous year	—	98·3[a]	102·6[a]	115·0[a]	115·2[a]	106·9[a]	113·2	111·7	110·5[a]	110·0	109·5	109·0	108·5	108·0	107·5
No. of admissions in year	1041[a]	1023[a]	1050[a]	1207[a]	1390[a]	1486[a]	1683	1881[a]	2079[a]	2287	2504	2729	2961	3198	3438
Intervals in years															
1	201[a]	170[a]	151[a]	159[a]	174[a]	180	187	195[a]	202	206	228	246	266	288	309
2	147[a]	117[a]	102[a]	106[a]	107	108	106	103	102	91	108	115	124	134	144
3	112[a]	87[a]	87[a]	88	88	88	82	77	73	69	73	76	83	89	96
4	96[a]	67[a]	67	65	61	59	50	41	33	27	25	25	27	29	31
5	94[a]	64	64	62	57	55	45	36	27	21	17	16	18	19	21
6	91	61	61	58	53	50	40	30	21	14	10	8	9	10	10
7	87	58	58	54	49	46	34	24	19	7	2				
8	84	55	55	51	44	42	30	19	12						
9	81	52	51	47	40	37	25	13	6						
10	78	49	48	43	36	33	20	7							
11	75	46	45	40	32	28	15	2							
12	72	43	42	36	28	24	10								
13	69	40	39	33	24	19	5								
14	66	37	36	29	19	15									
15	62	34	33	25	15	10									
16	59	31	29	22	11	6									
17	56	28	26	18	7	1									
18	53	24	23	14	3										
19	50	21	20	11											
20	47	18	17	7											
21	44	15	14	4											
22	41	12	11												
23	38	9	8												
24	35	6	5												
25	32	3	2												

[a] Figures in these cells only based on real data.

TABLE 10.

Projected Outcome of All Admissions to North-east Scottish Mental Hospitals, 1971–84

	1971	1972	1973	1974	1975	1976	1977	1978	1979	1980	1981	1982	1983	1984	Total no. in hospital after each interval
% change from previous year	107·0	106·5	106·0	105·5	105·0	104·5	104·0	103·5	103·0	102·5	102·0	101·5	101·0	100·5	
No. of admissions in year	3679	3918	4153	4381	4600	4807	4999	5174	5329	5462	5571	5655	5711	5740	
Intervals in years															
1	331	353	374	394	414	433	450	466	480	492	501	509	514	517	201[a]
2	154	165	174	184	193	202	210	217	224	229	234	237	240	241	317[a]
3	103	110	116	123	129	135	140	145	149	153	156	158	160	161	380[a]
4	33	35	37	39	41	43	45	47	48	49	50	51	51	52	444[a]
5	22	23	25	26	28	29	30	31	32	33	33	34	34	34	528[a]
6	11	12	12	13	14	14	15	15	16	16	17	17	17	17	597
7															660
8															715
9															755
10															782
11															803
12															835
13															854
14															870
15															884
16															887
17															885
18															886
19															884
20															911
21															929
22															945
23															961
24															980
25															995

THE TERMINATION OF GROWTH

How long will this growth in admissions go on and why is it taking place at all? In asking these questions, we move from the strict concept of "projection" to the concept of "explanation", and close to the idea of "prediction", entering very speculative territory. The projection was based partly on trends inherent in real data, but the precise rate of reduction in the growth rate cannot be projected very adequately on this basis and it could be a very long way out. Nevertheless, it is legitimate to hypothesize about the mechanisms involved in the growth process, since they are still genuinely unknown to us. And if we knew why there was this growth in admissions, we would also know what would stop it, and perhaps even when. (There are obviously self-limiting factors inherent in this growth pattern, such as 100% hospitalization of psychiatric patients, but such improbabilities do not warrant serious consideration.)

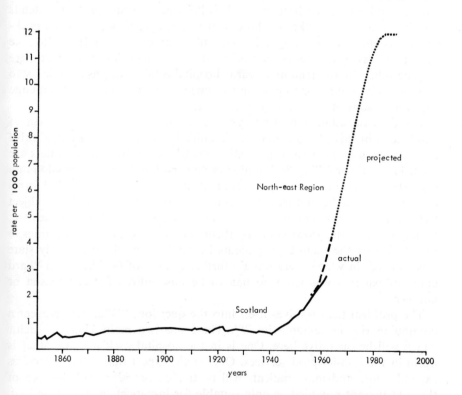

FIG. 30. Total admissions to Scottish mental hospitals. Rates per 1000 population, 1850–1964 and projected to 1984.

Possible causes of growth

The usual approach to the study of this phenomenon has been to seek explanations in the legal and social events which have a direct bearing on the use of mental hospitals. The trouble with this sort of thing is that, for the period of most rapid growth at least, it simply does not work. Many of the major contributory events are unrelated to changes in the admission rate. We must look elsewhere. The most sensible place to look would be at the decision point which determines an admission to mental hospital. Who determines who will be admitted, when, and for what reasons? This is clearly an area warranting much more study, although we do have a certain amount of information about it already. It seems most probable that the psychiatrist working in out-patients, and in domiciliary and emergency work is the most potent force in the eventual process of hospitalization. Naturally, he is under certain social and professional pressures when he takes action, but we still need to know a lot more about the reasons why he admits some patients and does not admit others. It is known, for instance, that he tends not to admit those he likes or those of the same age, or sex, or social background as himself, according to his particular personality—preferring to take these patients on for one-to-one treatment on an out-patient basis. But there may be other factors tending towards hospitalization, such as a tendency to take the safest course or to pass on to someone else patients he cannot cope with for reasons of time, ability or interest.

The data on admissions lend support to the argument. The growth of admissions in this phenomenal way is unlikely to be simply a quantitative change; it must represent a qualitative change in the way the hospitals are used. The static or falling *first* admission rate and the rising re-admission rate suggest rather that more new patients are being taken into non-hospital forms of treatment than heretofore, whereas those who are hospitalized are subject to the rapid turnover conditions which are so well known. If this is the case, we might expect the growth of out-patient and other non-hospital facilities to reduce further the number of patients hospitalized until some steady state was reached, in which there was no further growth of facilities, or a "hard core" of patients was left who had to be hospitalized for one reason or another.

The problem then resolves itself into the question, "What will prevent a continuing rise in re-admissions?". There are two main kinds of factor which will be operative here. One is in the hospital itself and the other is again in the non-hospital services. One would expect that as these services expand, more and more patients will be treated outside hospital—even of those at present regarded as only suitable for in-patient treatment. Indeed, many of those currently inflating the "stage army" might be treated in other ways, if staff and facilities were available.

The factors in the hospital are more complex. There is little question that the current, huge, very long-stay population is slowly being reduced, largely by death, but to some extent also by discharge, and is not being completely replaced. This will result in more accommodation becoming available and the question will be whether it will simply be filled by increasing the duration of stay of new admissions (and so reducing the proportion of readmissions), or whether the number of available beds will be reduced, as has happened in some places. There may be a strong tendency to fill all available beds, particularly with geriatric patients, but against this there will be a large rebuilding programme, developing in about 15 years' time, and it is doubtful whether such large numbers of beds as we now have will be replaced. Economics are against it, and perhaps not fortuitously, the psychiatric and cultural fashions are against it. But above all, being aware of the possibilities enables one to take active decision one way or the other.

Paradoxically, therefore, the limiting factors in the growth of mental hospitalization, complex though they are, lie in the growth of the psychiatric services themselves and their changing character in response to economic, social and, to some extent, professional pressures.

Summary

Examination of admission patterns to North-east Scottish mental hospitals showed that, in common with the national picture, admissions continued to rise, and in fact doubled in numbers between 1956 and 1964. National and local reasons for this are discussed and the role of the Ross Clinic regional treatment centre analysed. Age, sex and diagnostic distributions are examined.

It is shown that by 1961, re-admissions constituted half of all admissions and were most prevalent among males, the middle-aged, functional psychoses, alcoholism and behaviour disorders. The number of first admissions declined between 1959 and 1961, emphasizing a tendency to multiple hospitalization for a decreasing number of most categories of patient. Limitations of the simple distinction between first and re-admissions are discussed, and it is pointed out that the register method is a more satisfactory approach to the study of multiple hospitalization.

The cohort method is discussed and results of analyses of cohorts of admissions in 1956, 1959 and 1963 presented. The chief findings were:

1. The longer a patient remained in hospital, the smaller his chances of discharge.
2. Males had a higher expectation of discharge than females.
3. Elderly admissions had a much smaller expectation of discharge than younger patients. Among aged admissions, the chance of dying was highest in the early weeks of hospitalization, but decreased thereafter.

4. There was a marked fall in the proportion retained more than 2 months, between 1956 and 1963, but the rate of subsequent separation declined over the same years. This change was shared by both sexes and all age groups, in varying degrees. It was most marked among schizophrenics and patients with diseases associated with ageing.
5. The expectation of death among aged admissions, particularly those with diseases associated with ageing, declined markedly between 1956 and 1963.

The main implications of these findings are: (a) the current long-stay population of the mental hospitals is not being fully replaced; (b) the early attrition of admission cohorts may be partly a consequence of concentration of therapeutic effort on admission wards and a policy of early discharge and ready re-admission; (c) the planning categories of short-, medium- and long-stay patients require redefinition, to accord more closely with hospital use.

An attempt is made to project the outcome of admission cohorts from 1956 to 1984, in order to illustrate the accumulation of long-stay patients resulting from admissions over this period. The projection is based on specific assumptions, and the difficulties in obtaining a reliable set of assumptions (so that such projections can be used for planning purposes) are stressed. It is suggested that, in common with other growth phenomena, mental hospitalization is following the normal growth pattern, and will eventually be curtailed by the development of other kinds of mental health service and by economic and social pressures.

References

A Hospital Plan for England and Wales (1962), London, H.M.S.O.

ASTRUP, C. and ODEGARD, O. (1960), *Acta Psychiat. Neurol. Scand.* **35**, 289.

BAHN, A. K. and BODIAN, C. (1963), A Life Table Method for Studying Recurrent Episodes of Illness or Care. Presented at 91st Annual Meeting, American Public Health Association, Statistics Section, Kansas City.

BAHN, A. K. and CHANDLER, C. A. (1961), *J. chron. Dis.* **15**, 71.

BALDWIN, J. A. (1963), *Scot. med. J.* **8**, 227.

BALDWIN, J. A. and MILLAR, W. M. (eds.) (1964), *Community Psychiatry*, Boston, Mass., Little, Brown.

BALDWIN, J. A., INNES, G., MILLAR, W. M., SHARP, G. A. and DORRICOTT, N. (1965), *Brit. J. prev. soc. Med.* **19**, 38.

BROOKE, E. M. (1963), *Studies on Medical and Population Subjects*, No. 18. London, H.M.S.O.

INNES, G. and SHARP, G. A. (1962), *J. ment. Sci.* **108**, 447.

KRAMER, M., PERSON, P. H., TARJAN, G., MORGAN, R. and WRIGHT, S. W. (1957), *Amer. J. ment. Def.* **62**, 481.

PLATT, J. R. (1965), *Science*, **149**, 607.

TOOTH, G. C. and BROOKE, E. (1961), *Lancet*, **i**, 710.

25. The Current Place of Therapeutic Communities in Psychiatric Practice

Maxwell Jones

THE concept of a therapeutic community implies that trained staff and all other sources of potential help interact optimally with patients and their families or other interested persons to bring about an improvement in the patient's state of health. Such a concept can be applied with equal relevance to both the intra- and extramural dimensions of treatment. In the past, I have been associated with the development of treatment communities in an intramural setting. During the past 25 years, I have had the opportunity of playing a leadership role in seven different therapeutic communities in the U.K. and U.S.A., including a large mental hospital, a psychiatric unit in a community hospital, a psychiatric unit in a university teaching hospital, special units for selected patients and now a small psychiatric hospital of 400 beds. Since coming to Dingleton Hospital I have been concerned with the concept of the therapeutic community in both the intra- and extramural dimensions, but will only concern myself here with the former. I mention these factors because it is important to get away from the commonly held misconception that therapeutic communities are relevant to special units, such as the one at Henderson Hospital which treats character disorders, and not to psychiatric hospitals in general. It is commonly held that a therapeutic community is practicable only in a small hospital or unit, but it has been demonstrated particularly in America (Garcia, 1960; Jackson and Smith, 1961) that large mental hospitals can be decentralized into relatively small treatment units serving discrete geographical areas. This arrangement allows for a state of affairs which can be compared with the advantages of a small hospital with a clearly defined local area to serve.

Many hospitals in Britain and America have tried to develop a therapeutic community and several of them have been described in book form (Jones, 1952, 1962b; Greenblatt, York and Brown, 1955; Wilmer, 1958; Rapoport, 1960; Martin, 1962; Clark, 1964). There is also a growing literature on day hospital practice (Bierer, 1951; Farndale, 1961) and to the practice of psychiatry in the community, making use of the various community resources (Freeman and Farndale, 1963; Bellak, 1964). The concept of a therapeutic community can be applied to any of these areas with equal facility, provided there is a consistent attempt on the part of the leader or leaders to analyse the nature of the staff–patient interaction on a day-by-day basis, with a view to assessing the value of the methods being used. It is easier to illustrate what is meant by using the psychiatric hospital model than the practice of psychiatry in a community setting, but the same principles apply in both areas. Quantitatively at least, the major psychiatric practice is still carried out in the wards of psychiatric hospitals, which is also the area where most training is available for both doctors and nurses, and to an increasing extent for the other disciplines associated with psychiatry as well. A fairly typical psychiatric hospital unit would be the admission ward of, say, thirty beds. For such a unit to operate as a therapeutic community, it is necessary to have some examination of what is occurring between staff and patients on any one day. Perhaps the simplest device used is the ward meeting, where there is a face-to-face confrontation of all patients and staff associated with that particular ward. Such a meeting characteristically lasts about an hour and the nature of the interaction will depend upon many variables, including the type of patient, their length of stay and the psychiatric orientation and psychodynamic skills of the staff. Intimately associated with the ward meeting, and essential for the training and evolution of the staff, is the review. This meeting, ideally, should follow immediately after the ward meeting, in order that the impressions and feelings engendered by the ward meeting should still be uppermost in people's minds. Sometimes the review is left to some period later in the day. This is probably a mistake, as in the interim, all kinds of rationalizations and defences may have occurred and the feelings can no longer be revived in their original form. The review session is essentially a learning situation. All staff present at the review have been exposed to a similar experience, but will have perceived it in ways which are subjectively different, depending on the personality, training and current mood of the individual concerned. The ward meeting and review session are of such importance that I think that they ought to be considered in greater detail.

The Ward Meeting

SHORT-STAY WARDS

It goes without saying that when a group of patients live together on a ward, their behaviour makes manifest many of the problems which have obtruded in the world outside and which are repeated in their relationships with other patients and staff on the ward. The nurses come into closest contact with the patients in their ward life but, in general, they are not seen as having the same psychotherapeutic training or skill as the doctor, and what happens to them in their relationships with the patients may not even be of interest to the doctor. The doctor's interaction with the patient alone in his office tends to be seen as the essential part of a patient's treatment. This psychotherapeutic period, including the prescription of drugs or physical treatment, is the corner stone of the treatment programme. When, however, the daily ward meeting (Jones and Hollingsworth, 1961; Jones, 1962a, b) is instituted, the doctor is brought into much closer contact with the ward life and, even although the ward meeting affords a somewhat artificial setting, the doctor is still brought closer to the characteristic behaviour and feelings of the patients and staff in the ward life. The extent to which the patients can communicate their feelings and talk about current problems will depend to a large part on the skill of the psychiatrist in charge of the ward. Often, he has had no training in group work and will tend to be didactic. If growth is to occur, there should be a training psychiatrist or supervisor who is experienced in group work and can establish a model for his staff to follow in the ward meeting. Without such skills, nothing much may be achieved by a meeting of the staff and patients on the ward and they will soon lose interest. An experienced group therapist should have little difficulty in making patients and staff aware of what lies behind behaviour and helping them to express some of the feelings which in the past they have denied even to themselves. It takes weeks before patients can convince themselves that the doctor really means what he says, when he encourages them to express their feelings, no matter how anti-social these may appear to be. There is an understandable fear of the authority of the doctor and of the nursing staff, while the possibility of reprisals and the abuse of power looms large. After all, people do not criticize their more senior associates in the world outside and if they do, they can usually expect to be punished for their behaviour. The ward meeting offers a setting in which patterns of a lifetime, modelled on the early family constellation, can be modified in the direction of more spontaneous communication than has been possible in the past. The patient has to be shown that such free communication serves a purpose before he is willing to go against his established patterns of behaviour. For a patient to realize that his animosity towards a parent may not arouse censure from his peers, and that relief can follow such an expression of feeling and analysis of content, opens up new opportunities for learning. So much goes on in the life of the ward that reflects the past personality and problems of the patient that one can be concerned almost wholly with the present. The analysis of problems of relationships and their resolution has at times been referred to as sociotherapy. With the mixed psychiatric conditions which characterize the average admission ward, there is little opportunity, or even justification, for psychoanalytical group therapy. To begin with, the size of the ward precludes such a methodology as one can only be fully aware of eight or ten people at any one time. Moreover, for psychoanalytical work one needs to be confident that the subject has the ego strength, motivation and intelligence to justify such an approach. The aims of the ward meeting are much more modest and are concerned primarily with looking at what lies behind current behaviour and limiting oneself to "here and now" situations. I think that such an approach is much more allied to learning new approaches to situations which in the past have proved difficult or overwhelming, than to the analysis of latent content. That a certain amount of uncovering work and insight may be involved is probably true, but the major purpose of a ward meeting would seem to be the examination of problems in a setting where there are certain psychodynamic skills and a population which is motivated by a desire to help.

LONG-STAY WARDS

It is possible for a ward of even sixty long-stay patients who have the capacity to communicate and learn from social interaction to discuss their daily problems of living, with demonstrable change in their behaviour and in the ward life. In such a long-stay ward, the patients can come to discuss their responsibility towards each other and the need to share with the staff their concern when sexual excesses, etc., may be occurring. They may come to talk about their attitudes towards "normality", e.g. whether they want ordinary people to make use of the canteen and mix with them in much the way that occurs in life outside. They may discuss what getting well means and whether they really feel that they can face the outside world after many years in hospital. They can discuss the significance of the selection of patients to make use of single rooms, which changes the role of the patient and the expectation of the staff regarding his future. They frequently discuss the role of the staff, as well as of the patient. The doctor may be told about his ineptness, as perceived by the patients; many delusional ideas about his aims and personality may be expressed. He may be told that he gets a bonus for the number of patients discharged to the outside world, or that he has a vested interest in the profits of the patients' canteen. At the very least, he will become aware of many of the attitudes and beliefs of patients which would find little or no place in the formal interview in his own office. He may be faced with problems of social distance and to what extent he should dispense with an office altogether and come closer to the role of the nurse on the ward. Perhaps, like the nurse, he will come to feel that even the ward life represents only a very small part of the patient's day and that he should be much more involved in the patient's work programme or in the highly significant interaction which occurs at mealtimes or at bedtime. The ward meeting throws up problems inherent in the patient as an individual, as a social organism, and in his relationships with the various staff members. Opportunities for treatment in the familiar models of psychotherapy abound, but in addition, one cannot escape the greater awareness of one's significance to patients, in terms of role and role relationships. It is from the study of such problems and the better use of the psychotherapeutic opportunities afforded by the ward meeting, that the review session becomes imperative if better treatment of the patient is to develop and a more therapeutic climate and social organization evolve.

The Review Session

It is assumed that all staff working on a ward will be able to attend the ward meeting. In my experience, even in an admission ward, it is exceptional that a patient or patients will be unable to attend. If the meetings are in the morning, it may be that several patients have had E.C.T. or there may be some serious physical illness. Even in a hospital with a turnover of 3000 new admissions a year, it was possible to get the patients to attend daily ward meetings with relatively few exceptions. In general, it is the psychiatrist who acts as the leader in the ward meeting and the same applies to the review session. This seems to be more determined by the fact that the doctor is finally responsible for patients, while the fact that other disciplines such as social work, psychology or nursing may have greater skills in group work is frequently overlooked. The important thing is that the review session should have sufficient skilled personnel, so that any abuse of authority or defensive manipulation can be recognized. Much as in the ward meeting, the initial stages of a review session may be fraught with difficulty. Nurses are traditionally shy about speaking, and their training all too frequently implies a passive recipient rather than an active role. They are frequently content to let the doctor or other disciplines with higher educational standards do most of the talking (Jones, 1963). The fact that social workers and psychologists have a university training seems to overawe most nurses at the present time. However, a day-in-day-out confrontation with these other disciplines in a review setting following a ward meeting can work wonders, even with the most insecure and inhibited nurse. This, however, calls for skilled leadership and a willingness on the part of the doctor to face an examination of his own behaviour and skill. Nothing impresses the staff more than the willingness of the doctor or leader to practise what he preaches and to admit that he has misconstrued a situation or overlooked an important detail. If he is willing to have his own feelings analysed and to admit that he has learnt from such scrutiny, then he represents a much more human and understandable model than the doctor who plays the traditional role of the individual who knows best. This is not to say that the skills of the various disciplines are unimportant, quite the contrary—they are all essential to the teaching and evolutionary process. Each discipline has its own contribution to make and this applies to the most junior nurse who, given the confidence and encouragement, may frequently come closer to understanding the feelings of patients than the more highly trained staff members. There is no desire to devalue the role of the doctor, social worker, etc., but rather to stress the inadequacy inherent in any one training at the present time. The doctor is trained to see himself as the leader of the team and as the individual who prescribes treatment which the nurses, in particular, are expected to carry out. The idea that the doctor will frequently learn from other disciplines, and even the most junior staff, is a relatively new one. This applies even more to the patients, who frequently have a great deal to contribute to the treatment of other patients, and is one of the best arguments in favour of ward meetings. It would be foolish to expect that the patients, meeting daily in a ward meeting, would be able to resolve their difficulties and get adequate treatment without trained staff being present. In a somewhat similar way, review sessions will tend to get into pointless arguments and unproductive discussions, unless there is considerable skill and familiarity with group dynamics in at least one of the staff members. The great value of the review (Jones, 1962a, b) is that it allows teaching to occur, based on what has happened in the ward meeting or what is happening currently in the review session itself. The treatment that has occurred in the ward meeting has much in common with the training that occurs in the staff meeting, and both are liable to be abortive unless adequate trained personnel are available. Therapeutic communities have failed not infrequently and the failure been put down to the inappropriateness of the approach. It would, I think, be much more accurate to attribute these failures to the lack of staff skill. Perhaps one of the most important aspects of the review session is the analysis of roles and role relationships which inevitably occurs.

Social Structure, Roles and Role Relationships

We have talked briefly about the social organization of a ward and its relationship to treatment and training. The patient's life and activities are not limited to the ward. However, there is a great need to evolve a social structure which will maximise the value of the relationships formed by the patient in the hospital as a whole and in the outside community (Menzies, 1961; Jones, 1962a). What is needed is a communication network which embraces the total hospital population in a two-way communication system. In the past, relatively little attention has been given to the social organization in a psychiatric hospital. As a result, the social structure has tended to copy the lines of the general hospital, where doctors and nurses have their primary training. This gives a rigidity to roles and role relationships, which would seem to be most inappropriate to the functioning of a psychiatric hospital. Much depends on the personality, training and skills of the leader. If he welcomes open communications and sanctions the examination of roles and role relationships, the social organization will, through time, reflect the needs and wishes of the staff and patients. A flexible social structure seems to be highly desirable, so that with changing personnel and increasing insights, the social organization can be modified to make maximum use of the potential of the new staff members or the new insights. In this way, the enthusiasm and positive motivation which many people arrive at when they start psychiatric work can be retained and developed, and not lost in the frustrations of rigid conformity, all too often found in psychiatric hospitals, day hospitals, or throughout psychiatry in general. One of the difficulties at the present time is the lack of basic training in the behavioural sciences which applies to most, if not all, personnel working in psychiatry. Until the training of psychiatrists and others in this field is adequate in this dimension, there is no alternative but to develop social sensitivity and skills as part of the in-service training. Every hospital will develop a social structure appropriate to its own requirements, as perceived by the administration, which should be influenced by the other staff members and patients. In order to illustrate this, I would like to use the present social organization of Dingleton Hospital as an example. This hospital has 400 beds and serves the mental health needs of a population of approximately 100,000. In 1965 there were 343 new admissions and 180 new out-patients were seen. Altogether there were 904 out-patient attendances and 74 domiciliary visits were carried out. Most of the out-patient work is carried on at the hospital, which is in the centre of our catchment area, but we have a weekly out-patient service at the largest town and an out-patient club in the second largest town in our area. The medical staff consists of the physician superintendent and one other consultant, one assistant psychiatrist, one registrar and one senior house officer. There is a position for a clinical psychologist, but this is at present vacant. There is a staff of three fully qualified psychiatric social workers, while another psychiatric social worker is based at Dingleton, but is employed by the local authority and serves as an invaluable link between Dingleton and the community. We have a strong work therapy programme. This is headed by a rehabilitation officer, whose chief concern is to supervise an activity programme, covering work therapy, work placements in the outside community and a carefully graduated pay incentive scheme. In addition, he is responsible for the evening activities and an important programme which will be discussed in greater detail later, under the heading of "New Roles". There are approximately 96 nurses, but a considerable number of these are part-time. There are three training programmes for pupil nurses, student nurses and postgraduate nurses. The latter is for general trained nurses who take a psychiatric training, recognized by the General Nursing Council, in 12 months as opposed to the more usual 18 months. When high priority is placed on communications and social organization, one expects a large number of meetings. These can be divided roughly into administrative meetings and clinical meetings, but these tend to overlap considerably and both serve a useful training function.

Administrative Meetings

The day starts officially at 8.30 a.m. with a meeting of the matron, hospital secretary and superintendent together with other senior staff, so that all disciplines are represented. This meeting deals with immediate practical administrative problems and when anything is raised which bears on patient welfare, it is fed back to the next meeting, which is concerned primarily with clinical matters and patient well-being. This meeting, at 9 a.m., is called the Senior Staff Committee and comprises the 5 senior nurses, the 5 doctors, the 3 psychiatric social workers, the rehabilitation officer and several of his staff. Minutes are kept, and this ensures that matters raised for discussion are recorded and that action formulated is actually carried out. The physician superintendent acts as chairman of this committee and as far as possible, all matters of policy and patient care are processed through this committee and decisions arrived at by consensus. If there is no general agreement, it is usually taken to infer that the Senior Staff Committee (S.S.C.) is not yet ready to arrive at a decision and that the matter would be better postponed if possible. This meeting embodies some of the concepts of administrative therapy touched on by Clark (1964) in his book. As far as possible, we try to be aware of a hidden agenda when this is present, and if it seems that the discussion is dragging on because of tension between two staff members, some attempt will be made to look at the underlying conflict. If necessary, we may focus on this conflict and postpone any decision on a practical issue until such time as the conflict is resolved. These two daily meetings represent an attempt to keep the senior staff informed of all important current events, and the feed back of decisions and plans formulated at the S.S.C. is mediated through personal communication by the various disciplines represented to the lower echelons or through a news letter, which is made available to all staff members and to the wards each week. Each discipline has its own meetings at least weekly, where matters concerning that particular department are dealt with in an informal discussion and any policy decisions or new programmes fed back to the S.S.C. for approval. The physician superintendent and senior nursing staff have weekly meetings with each of the nursing categories, charge nurses, staff nurses, student nurses and assistant nurses. These are informal seminars where every effort is made to get the nursing staff to express feelings and to create a living–learning situation where information is exchanged and attitudes modified, both on the part of the administration and of the nurses. Again, a feed-back of relevant material is made to the S.S.C. It is clear that we are talking about meetings which are both administrative and training, and that the skills learnt in the formal group treatment programme and in the review sessions which follow the groups have a profound effect on the use made of the administrative meetings under discussion.

Clinical Meetings

Under this heading are included the daily ward meetings (Jones 1961, 1962a, b) followed by a review session which are characteristic of the short-stay wards and the less frequent ward meetings which are held on all the long-stay wards in the hospital. There is also the familiar clinical meeting once a week for discussion of a difficult case by the staff who can be spared from other activities, and monthly case conferences with the local authority personnel when they often present a problem which has been a matter of concern to both services. There are also admission and evaluation sessions thrice a week on the male side of the hospital, when new patients are screened by representative staff members with a view to admission, out-patient care or other disposal. Nurses from the various possible admission wards take part in the discussion as to where the patient would be best placed. In this way, the patient and his family are brought into contact with the staff they are likely to meet; everyone is indoctrinated with the problems presenting not only to the patient but to his family. They are then much better aware of these individuals than would be the case if they were merely to read the case notes or hear a verbal account from the doctor. Sometimes the one-way screen is used so that a more intimate contact between the doctor, the patient and his relatives can be accomplished. This is an example of where the model of general medicine should be accepted if patients expect a confidential situation with the doctor alone. In our experience, this concept can be modified readily with the majority of new patients, but it is important that the family doctor should also be helped to understand the advantage of such a group process at induction.

New Roles

From what has already been said, it is clear that there are many meetings when the overall functioning of the hospital, its administrative difficulties and clinical problems are discussed and analysed. Such a process of social analysis carried out daily inevitably raises the question of the specificity of roles and the need for new personnel to cover areas which are neglected or which have been entirely overlooked in the past. One of the inherent problems is that nurses have in the past been trained to a rather passive, repetitive role, but things are improving and nurse trainers are becoming very well aware of the need to stimulate spontaneity and more original thinking (Orlando, 1961; Royal College of Nursing, 1963; Clark and Jones, 1965). Much of the blame for this state of affairs can be placed legitimately on the doctors, who pay far too little attention to the potentialities of nurses in developing new skills and new roles for themselves. In the meantime, many new disciplines have emerged, such as occupational therapy, recreational therapy and industrial therapy (Early, 1960). How far nurses should participate in these roles is a matter for conjecture, but the trend is for nurses to become increasingly involved in such programmes. The development of new roles is to some extent hampered by the rigidity of hospital administration and of the administrative aspects of the National Health Service. There are no categories in the Whitley Council Scales for such new personnel as industrial therapists and these have to be paid from nursing or other funds. Some movement in this direction has been made by the creation of an unqualified social worker category, which allows individuals with a good general education and suitable personalities to work without meeting the formal requirements for social work in hospitals. I would like to describe some of the new roles which have emerged under the heading of "Work Therapy", to illustrate how the creation of a new role may have certain advantages in short-circuiting the time and effort required to extend, say, the nurse's role. It seems to me that nurses face a very real challenge to their versatility at the present time, and unless they are willing to accept this challenge, they may find that activities which might reasonably be part of their own function will be taken over by the establishment of new roles. So far as Dingleton is concerned, we would like to see nurses filling as many of these roles as possible but at the present time, find it necessary to look outside, to university graduates and others, who have as yet greater potentialities for developing a new programme. At present, we have seven relatively new appointments, and a description of these roles will help to clarify what has already been said. The head of this work therapy department has already been mentioned and he is given the title of Rehabilitation Officer, although his activities include much beside formal rehabilitation and he supervises all the following programmes.

1. *Activity therapy*. This post is filled by a young woman who has a training both as a psychiatric nurse and as an occupational therapist. She works with the patients on an entertainments committee, which seeks to find an active programme for the patients, particularly after working hours. She uses volunteers from outside, links up with outside clubs, social organizations, etc., so that the patient activities are brought in to contact with the outside world as far as possible.

2. *A patient occupational therapy* or *P.O.T. programme*. This programme is headed by a trained occupational therapist, who was given a month when she first arrived to look round the hospital and decide for herself what would be the best way to use her skills. She was impressed by the great need in the geriatric wards for a more active programme, and felt that to reach her rather isolated department on the second floor was an impossible physical feat for many of the people who would like to use it. In concert with nursing staff and other personnel, she decided that it would be much better to try to

establish an occupational therapy team amongst the younger and more able patients, who would go to her department for early morning sessions and then go as a team with prepared work to the geriatric wards during the later part of the day. This programme has proved a great success and has changed the whole function of the O.T. department. There is no longer any attempt to make articles for sale or to recover the money spent on materials, nor is there the same emphasis on handicrafts and finished products. A great variety of indoor games, outside activities and simple craftwork have replaced formal O.T. The aim of this group is to involve the less strong and less severely mentally handicapped patients in any form of activity which they are capable of entering into.

3. *The patient assistant nurse* or *P.A.N. programme.* This is headed by a trained nurse who takes about twelve patients and supervises them in the feeding and simple care of the bed patients and severely incapacitated patients. They have their daily meetings, like all the other work therapy groups, at which they discuss any problems which may arise in the course of the day's work.

4. *The heavy cleaning group.* This group is headed by a trained nurse and contains about ten or twelve patients. They are mostly from the long-stay population, and are able to do much of the polishing, moving of beds and heavy cleaning which would be impossible for the staff and patients to do in the geriatric wards. Again, the nurse has a daily seminar to look at the problems which have arisen during the working day.

5. *The canteen group.* An assistant nurse is seconded to one of these work therapist roles, while a girl with a domestic science diploma is given the other supervisory role. These two girls look after the different shifts in the canteen, which is open daily from 8.30 a.m. to 9.30 p.m. In addition to supervising the patients who do the serving and cleaning of the canteen and adjoining social centre, they are there as social therapists to help with the intermixing of patients, their relatives and outside visitors. This is a very demanding job, requiring group work skills as well as business competence.

6. *The laundry group.* The work therapist in this group was previously the hospital hairdresser, but she showed such competence and skill in group work that she was successful in competing with other applicants for this job. She is in charge of twelve patients who work with the paid staff in the laundry which serves the other hospitals in the Borders area. Like all the work therapists, her function is to ensure that the patients have a meaningful social and therapeutic experience and that they are not exploited. It is made quite explicit that the patients' rehabilitation comes first and the job performance second.

7. *Dining hall group.* The dining rooms employ about twelve waitresses and waiters, trained by a work therapist who came to us from the local tweed mills. She helps the waitresses to become competent in serving, laying

tables, etc., and several of the patients have been successful in getting employment in local hotels.

The above brief descriptions of new roles indicate how, as a result of increasing awareness of the gaps in our patients' day, we have been trying to use the patient potential. Our aim is to develop roles compatible with their interests and abilities and to create a greater feeling of self-respect, independence and possible rehabilitation to the outside world. All the work therapy groups have daily meetings with their patients in which problems of inter-relationship, accepting authority, time-keeping and so on, are discussed. Increasingly, the work groups are linking up with the ward groups, so that the feedback from the work situation to the ward situation is implemented. The work therapists go to all the ward groups and each is identified with one ward. In their work therapy staff groups, they then are able to feed back from the ward group what is relevant to each individual work therapist about their own particular patients. An interesting recent trend has been the growing awareness on the part of the doctors and nurses that their ward group, which they want people to attend, must pay increasing attention to the rights and needs of the work therapy group. This is an example of an evolutionary process, whereby doctors and nurses are being made increasingly aware of the importance of the patients' work situation and the potential within that situation for treatment. The in-service training of the work therapists is met by having their own supervisor, by involvement in the group treatment programme, and by a weekly training seminar taken by one of the psychiatrists.

Activity Assistants

For the past year, we have experimented with the use of school-leavers to help geriatric and long-stay patients to participate in various activities. In Scotland, Cadet Nursing Schemes which cater for this age group ($16–17\frac{1}{2}$) are not permissible, and we set out to offer the girls hospital work which did not involve formal nursing. We felt that by exposing girls to most aspects of hospital work they would come to have some idea about their suitability for future training in a hospital occupation such as occupational therapy, catering, office work, social work, hairdressing, etc. Our main hope was that they would ultimately tend to gravitate towards nursing. Marsh and Wilcox (1965) have studied the problem of nurse recruitment in Mansfield. They found that only 1 in 7 of the nurses had been to grammar schools, and this state of affairs was not uncommon in other parts of the country. They point out that areas which have to rely on secondary modern schoolgirls have inevitably to tackle the problem of bridging the gap between the school-leaving age and the age of entry to the nursing profession. They feel that there can be no doubt that during these years, girls inevitably drift into other jobs and lose the initial interest which many of them have in nursing. They feel that there is a strong case for carefully controlled and evaluated experiments in recruitment at an earlier age. Quite understandably, a scheme employing girls between the ages of 16 and $17\frac{1}{2}$ arouses a great deal of anxiety, and in our case, various strictures have been imposed by the employing authorities to ensure that these young girls were not exposed to any adverse influences. Moreover, the scheme has been put on a trial basis and will be re-evaluated at the end of its second year. From the start, the activity assistants have had the full-time services of a university educated supervisor and at the end of each day, they have a 45-minute seminar to discuss what have been their experiences and problems during the day. I have been present at most of these seminars, and it is fascinating to see how young people come to use the seminar to express anxieties and learn to deal with problems with increasing skill. Instead of being exposed to formal training and the memorizing of class work, they are invited to discuss emotional problems in which they are involved. It could be said that the first objective of all education is to develop the capacity to inquire, to learn how to find out, to become better at asking questions or to practise how to tackle problems. In this context, learning is a social process designed to enhance this ability. The response of these girls to this approach to learning has been highly gratifying. They have become much more confident and articulate and have learned a great deal about the problems of relationships and how to handle them. They talk freely about the difficulties they have met in the various activity areas. Their work with patients is limited to activities such as feeding and bathing, and social activities such as walks, visits to the canteen, and various forms of music and movement. They are not assigned to the admission wards, but have confined their activities largely to the geriatric patients. In addition, they have worked in the Ladies Hairdressing Department, the Catering Department, Occupational Therapy, Administrative Office and the Laundry. They have also played a very important role in complimenting the work of the P.O.T.s and P.A.N.s (patient occupational therapy and patient assistant nurse programmes). It is in music and movement and simple games like dominoes, skittles, darts, etc., that the activity assistants have filled a much-needed gap in the daily activity of the older and long-stay patients. The sense of rhythm and general vitality of these young people seems to awaken latent potentialities within the patients. Inevitably, there have been difficulties in role relationships between the activity assistants and the nursing staff. At times, the nurses have criticized or laughed at them, and at such times the activity assistants have felt embarrassed and inadequate. On the whole, however, the nursing staff have been extremely supportive, more particularly as their work is considerably lightened by the help given by these young people. After a year of this scheme, there are five of the original eight activity assistants left. All five have decided that they want to take up psychiatric nursing, and they represent a type of recruit one would like to see more often. They already have a year of exposure to hospital work and are in a much better position to know exactly what they want than had they spent this year working in mills or offices. Moreover, the hospital authorities are in a very good position to assess these girls from the point of view of their potential for nursing. We are attempting to get permission for day release, so that further formal education can be undertaken by those girls requiring more O-levels to meet the requirements for student nurse training. It may be, however, that such an approach has equal validity for pupil nurse training when O-levels are not required. It is as yet too early to talk about this experiment in any final terms, but all the indications are that given adequate selection and supervision, and a programme which does not expose young people to traumatic situations on the ward, it might be possible to overcome many of the difficulties of nurse recruitment for psychiatric hospitals by a procedure such as this.

Living–Learning Situations

We have already talked about ward meetings followed by a review and how these two meetings represent important aspects of both treatment and training (Jones and Hollingsworth, 1961; Jones, 1962a, b). These are regularly scheduled meetings on wards and may occur daily or less often. We have also touched on administrative meetings and the daily meetings which all work therapy groups have, to discuss the interactions which occur within the work group. There are also the non-verbal meetings, such as the music and movement carried out by the activity assistants, primarily on patients who suffer from organic states or are so deteriorated that they cannot communicate verbally. At all meetings so far described, there is the possibility of current emotional problems being used as a basis for a learning situation. In a therapeutic community, there is a tendency for groups to emerge in any situation where the analysis of problems and examination of roles and role relationships is called for. Thus, even in an administrative meeting, it may be that the formal agenda gives way to the hidden agenda if some obvious tension between staff members calls for immediate attention. In such a situation, the analysis of the emotional problem will be seen as a desirable preliminary to any administrative decision. Any form of group therapy would appear to be countenanced, provided the new development is subject to examination as to what people were doing and why they were doing it. Thus, if a ward wishes to initiate a family group once a week, the form that this group should take would be a matter for staff and patients to decide by discussion and then decision by consensus. However, the formally constituted, regularly scheduled group may not meet the requirements created by a crisis situation, which may involve people from different wards or different aspects of the hospital life. A crisis arising between say, the engineering staff and some of the patients who had been interfering with work and equipment might call for an immediate confrontation, so that the problem could be looked at while feelings were still high. The postponement of a confrontation till a few days later, or the decision to refer it to several different groups in which the patients are involved is less effective than constituting it immediately round the individuals directly concerned. To turn such a crisis into a living–learning situation calls for considerable skill on the part of one, or preferably several staff members. The patients concerned may have a much greater awareness of group processes than do the engineering staff, and it may be difficult to reconcile the two groups. It may require repeated confrontations, or better still, a training group built round the engineering department to get across to the people involved the meaning of the learning situation, as opposed to usual arbitrary judgement made by an authority figure. This situation could be compared with the problem of "teach-ins", which seem to offer so much hope in the national sphere, particularly in relation to political issues. A chairman, to cope with such a situation, would require considerable political, social, military and other knowledge, plus a capacity for leadership, a knowledge of group dynamics and a sensitivity to social situations. Even then, it would seem to be a long process of education before the real possibilities of "teach-ins" became apparent to both politicians and academicians, let alone the general public. As used here, the concept of the living–learning situation implies nothing new and is implicit in all the meetings already described. It is mentioned here under a separate heading, in order to draw attention to the fact that formally constituted meetings may not be enough and that it may be necessary to have a face-to-face confrontation as soon as possible after the development of some crisis situation.

The therapeutic community programme, as outlined, seems to offer possibilities for the development of learning situations which apply to both patients and staff and for the development of treatment and training in the social dimension. The emphasis is on utilizing current situations for learning. In this way, it is felt that not only do the patients benefit by the process of maturation, giving them greater capacity than before to meet the problems of the outside world, but the process also leads to a more mature staff. Sociotherapy would seem to be more linked with education than with psychoanalytical concepts or psychotherapy. However, there is no intention to devalue the latter, which should be used whenever appropriate, and there seems to be no reason why individual psychotherapy should not be seen as complimentary to sociotherapy as described.

References

BELLAK, L. (1964) (Ed.), *Handbook of Community Psychiatry*, New York, Grune & Stratton.
BIERER, J. (1951), *The Day Hospital*, London, H. K. Lewis.
CLARK, D. H. (1964), *Administrative Therapy*, London, Tavistock Publications.
CLARK, M. A. and JONES, MAXWELL (1965), *Nursing Mirror* 120, 45, 64.
EARLY, D. F. (1960), *Lancet* i, 754.
FARNDALE, J. (1961), *The Day Hospital Movement in Great Britain*, Oxford, Pergamon Press.
FREEMAN, H. and FARNDALE, J. (1963) (Eds.), *Trends in the Mental Health Services*, Oxford, Pergamon Press.
GARCIA, LEONARDO B. (1960), *Mental Hospitals* 30–1, November.
GREENBLATT, M., YORK, R. H. and BROWN, E. L. (1955), *From Custodial to Therapeutic Patient Care in Mental Hospitals*, New York, Russell Sage Foundation.
JACKSON, G. W. and SMITH, F. V. (1961), *Mental Hospitals* 5–7, January.
JONES, MAXWELL (1952), *The Therapeutic Community*, New York, Basic Books.
JONES, MAXWELL (1962a), *Amer. J. Psychiat.* 118, 705.
JONES, MAXWELL (1962b), *Social Psychiatry*, Springfield, Illinois, Charles C. Thomas.
JONES, MAXWELL (1963), *Lancet*, ii, 1108.
JONES, MAXWELL and HOLLINGSWORTH, S. (1961), in *Proc. Third World Congress of Psychiat.*, Montreal, 1, 252.
MARSH, D. C. and WILCOX, A. J. (1965), *Focus on Nurse Recruitment*, London, Nuffield Provincial Hospitals Trust.
MARTIN, D. V. (1962), *Adventure in Psychiatry*, Oxford, Cassirer.
MENZIES, J. E. P. (1961), *The Function of Social Systems as a Defence Against Anxiety*, Tavistock Pamphlet No. 3, London, Tavistock Publications.
ORLANDO, I. J. (1961), *The Dynamic Nurse–Patient Relationship*, New York, G. P. Putnam's.
RAPOPORT, R. N. (1960), *Community as Doctor*, London, Tavistock Publications.
ROYAL COLLEGE OF NURSING (1963), *Role of Psychiatric Ward Sisters and Charge Nurses in the Rehabilitation of Patients*, London.
WILMER, H. (1958), *Social Psychiatry in Action*, Springfield, Illinois, Charles C. Thomas.

26. The Modern Role of the Psychiatric Hospital

HUMPHREY KIDD

MENTAL hospitals entered a dark period with the advent of the Industrial Revolution, and between 1870 and 1930 many of the insights and ideas of earlier writers and practitioners of psychiatry were lost. The mental hospital then became a closed institution for the custody rather than treatment of psychotics. It had few links with the community, and was often in an isolated situation. After discharge, patients had little or no further contact with the hospital. The organization of the hospital was a monolithic hierarchy, presided over by the medical superintendent. But since the 1930's, and with gathering momentum after the war, the nature and function of the progressive psychiatric hospital has changed radically. Although some of the ideas of the nineteenth century have been rediscovered, the hospital has progressed far beyond the hopes of these early writers. Yet many of them would no doubt see the progressive hospital as one that had built upon their early ideas.

In this later period, the psychiatric hospital began to take a wider view of its responsibility to the community, and was no longer a custodial repository for severe psychotics. The first step in this change was the establishment of Out-patient Clinics, either in the hospital itself or in a neighbouring general hospital. Later, came the provision of more adequate admission wards for the treatment of a wider variety of psychiatric illness, including neurosis.

Many factors brought about this change. The Mental Treatment Act of 1930 made provision for voluntary treatment. The introduction of E.C.T. and insulin therapy brought a wave of therapeutic enthusiasm. The National Health Service gave a fresh impetus to this change from isolation to integration, by bringing mental hospital administration more into line with that of general hospitals. In many cases more adequate funds were made available for the modernization of buildings. But above all, the professional status of psychiatry was raised by making the terms of service of consultant psychiatrists equal and identical with those of consultants in other fields. This had the effect of attracting a better type of doctor. Because the consultant was of equal clinical status with the medical superintendent, a very necessary and desirable change towards a more democratic and less hierarchical organization of the hospital became possible. Unfortunately, the trend was stubbornly resisted by many superintendents, and this resulted in a struggle for power in many hospitals, to the detriment of its efficiency.

481

Further advances in the treatment of psychiatric illness—including new and more active drugs, the awareness of group psychodynamics leading to the whole hospital being seen as a therapeutic community (Martin, 1962), and the emphasis given to both social and family factors in the development of psychiatric illness, have led to the mental hospital becoming in some cases the active centre of a comprehensive psychiatric service to its community. It then offers a full range of treatment for out-patients, day-patients and in-patients, as well as community care services in close co-operation with the local authority. However, the greatest success and progress in changing from an isolated to an integrated role has been achieved in urban areas served by former county borough mental hospitals. The reasons for this are many, but the compactness of the area served is the most important. This means there is no real problem of transport for the patient or his relatives in coming to the hospital as an out-patient or day-patient, or in visiting or going on leave. Also, the provision of an efficient domiciliary service by doctors, social workers, etc., has been easily achieved. In such compact areas, the hospital has become part of the community it serves. On the other hand, the larger and more isolated country hospitals, where patients may live up to 70 miles away, encounter greater difficulties. This isolation has made the recruitment of adequate staff very difficult. It is this problem of the large and badly sited mental hospital that has led to the present policy of planning to close these hospitals, and to replace them by psychiatric units in general hospitals. The whole policy was summed up by Mr. Enoch Powell in his speech to the N.A.M.H. (1961): "For the great majority of mental hospitals there is no appropriate future use, and I for my own part would resist any attempt to foist another purpose upon them, unless it could be proved to me in each case that such a building would have had to be erected in that or some similar place to serve the other purpose if the mental hospital had never existed." In other words, unless a mental hospital in its present position can cater adequately for the psychiatric needs of the population it serves, it must go.

It is inevitable that just as the psychiatric hospital has had to change radically its organization and use, so it will eventually be replaced by com-prehensive psychiatric units at district general hospitals. Eventually, each district general hospital will have accommodation and treatment facilities for all types of psychiatric patients, and the mental hospital will cease to exist.

However, for many reasons (not least financial) the majority of psychiatric hospitals will continue to exist for at least a further half-century. What in the meantime? They must be organized efficiently to care for the community they serve, and where only small psychiatric units for acute admissions are built in existing general hospitals (particularly in country areas) they must be served by the staff of the area mental hospital. "The essential foundation of a good psychiatric service is based on a continuing doctor–patient relationship—

in other words the patient is always under the care of the same consultant whether in the hospital or in the community. This continuity is an essential condition to the maintenance of the doctor-patient relationship and should take priority in every form of treatment" (Balier, 1964).

The psychiatric hospital must not be only a place for the treatment of psychotic disorders. It must not become, as are so many state hospitals in the U.S.A., the end of the line for secondhand cases passed on by others. If this is allowed to happen, its morale sinks and staff shortages become inevitable.

What follows below is an account of how a psychiatric hospital serving a compact urban area of 270,000 people, with a small rural area of 90,000 also, has been organized so that it can fulfil its modern role efficiently, within the framework of the following principles.

(1) The provision of a full range of psychiatric treatments for all types of adult psychiatric patients, both in hospital and at home.
(2) Full independent responsibility to consultants and absolute continuity of care throughout treatment.
(3) The provision of an open-door, flexible, therapeutic community, summed up in our patients' booklet as follows: "This hospital has very few rules, because we find by experience that if our patients' requests and feelings are treated with respect and understanding, a long list of 'Do's and Don'ts' is unnecessary. The basic rule underlying all human relationships in this hospital is consideration for the needs and feelings of the other person."

In 1959 the Towers Hospital was predominantly a locked hospital (although a few wards were open) run on conservative lines. That is, separate male and female divisions, two locked admission wards, parole cards, etc. The medical superintendent still exercised overall control.

Architectural remodelling had only just begun. The senior medical staff then had a series of discussions to decide how the efficiency of the hospital could be raised. The decision was reached that whatever the practical difficulties, whatever compromises might have to be made, and however long it might take to put into complete practice, the basic organization must be three independent clinical teams (Kidd, 1961). Each team must be able to give treatment to any type of case, of either sex, and yet at the same time, the teams must be linked by an overall policy, because the hospital is administered as one, and many essential services such as catering, occupational therapy, etc., are shared. The appointment of a new chief male nurse, medical superintendent and group secretary within a few months was most fortunate in this connection. Although problems were solved step by step in a pragmatic way, and the upheaval and tensions caused by this radical reorganization of the hospital were at times very severe, the secret of success was giving ample time for full consultation with all members of the staff. Considerable patience and tact had to be exercised, so that all decisions were group decisions, and not those of one person.

Buildings

The basic physical facilities required for each team included accommodation for admissions, out-patients, day-patients, geriatric and long-stay cases, and some security provision. It will be realized that the provision of ideal buildings is impossible where one has to use a nineteenth-century hospital, however well modernized. This means that the architectural solution requires compromise, and must be dictated by the existing structure. Therefore, solutions will vary from hospital to hospital.

In the early stages, whilst the ward modernization programme was being formulated, it was felt that the clinical team concept must be implemented without delay. The two existing admission wards, which were overcrowded, were allocated to one team, and the further four units were created temporarily out of existing chronic wards. This, in fact, meant transferring patients, aggravating overcrowding, and having a proportion of better chronic patients on admission wards as a temporary expedient. The three detached villas became a mixed unit for better patients. Originally, it was intended that these villas should be used as admission wards for neurotics, but this never materialized, it being decided that all types of patients should be admitted to the same admission ward. The two closed wards (now semi-open) and the psycho-geriatric wards were shared by all three teams. The rest of the wards were divided equally between each team, so that although they were often inconveniently sited, each team possessed one male and one female admission ward, one mixed villa, an equal number of male and female long-stay wards and a share in the closed and psycho-geriatric wards.

During the past 4 years, radical modernization of the hospital has allowed us to develop the old female side as the active treatment section (the hospital never had a separate admission unit). This is on three floors—one for each team. The wards were the old L-shaped gallery type, radiating out on either side of what was once the medical superintendent's house. This house is now a long-stay ward for active patients, many of whom go out to work. It is hoped that it will eventually become the medical and nursing administrative centre of each team. At the end of the L-shaped ward is a column of what are best described as the old barn-type square ward. This whole area of the hospital has been completely gutted and redesigned to a very high standard. The success of the modernization has been due to the fact that all architectural plans have been critically reviewed at all stages by medical, nursing and administrative staff, before being passed by the Management Committee and Regional Hospital Board. Male and female wards are adjacent, so that social mixing is facilitated. The old male side has been modernized, although less radically, to take male and female long-stay, semi-closed accommodation, and psycho-geriatric accommodation. The closed wards are now in process of becoming open, and it is believed that such security as is required for a tiny minority of patients should be by good nursing rather than locks. One hundred per cent open doors should eventually be the norm in a psychiatric hospital. Day-patients use either the mixed villas or the admission wards. As overcrowding is further reduced, it will be possible to provide a day ward for each team, although from the therapeutic point of view, if not from the point of view of ward administration, mixing day-patients with in-patients has distinct advantages.

A new occupational therapy unit has been built and the old male unit converted into a factory-type industrial unit to accommodate 150 patients. A further 100 patients do industrial therapy on the wards, although it is expected that part of the new occupational therapy unit will also be used for industrial therapy in due course.

Each team has its own out-patient sessions in the detached clinic, and out-patients are also seen at the Leicester Royal Infirmary.

Medical Staff

It will be clear from the above that a planned modernization programme has allowed us to transform an old, inconvenient hospital in such a way that groups of patients can be concentrated under the care of their own consultants. Ideally, there should be one consultant in sole charge of a comprehensive group of patients, because treatment in psychiatry should include his philosophy, with which he imbues his staff. But this is not always possible.

The consultant staff of the hospital is six, and the provision of twelve admission wards was an administrative impossibility. Therefore, as the division of the hospital into three units was the only feasible answer, each team has two consultants, and this has proved workable. In fact it has positive advantages, because it means that teams can make their own arrangements for leave; when one consultant is away, the other can exert overall responsibility for the team.

Step by step, the junior establishment has been increased. It was felt early on that if an active treatment programme was to permeate the hospital, it was essential to have at least eight young trainee psychiatrists. In order to recruit such people, serious attention had to be given to provide a proper stimulus to learning. This has been done in the following ways: firstly, by the provision of an adequate and expanding library, which has a budget of £250 per annum. Secondly, by regular seminars and case conferences. Thirdly, by encouraging doctors to attend lectures at the Department of Psychiatry at Sheffield.

Fourthly, by developing a close liaison with the Departments of Psychology and Sociology of Leicester University; both these provide regular courses of lectures. Fifthly, by proper supervision of their work with both out-patients and in-patients. Junior staff should never be seen as just a pair of hands.

The proposed medical establishment for each team is two consultants, one senior registrar or medical assistant, two registrars, one general practitioner and, it is hoped, one senior house officer.

It has been encouraging that notwithstanding the shortage of doctors, we have been able to fill all our training posts with the right sort of men. The junior medical staff rotate throughout the teams in order to get a variety of experience. It has been interesting to note that although in theory each team is on weekly "take", and accepts the full range of psychiatric problems, nevertheless, the special interest of the various consultants results in some differences in the type of patients treated. For example, team 1 admits more schizophrenics and affective disorders, team 2 more young patients and psychopaths, and team 3 more organic cases and psychoneurotics. These differences reflect the special interests of the consultants (Milner *et al.*, 1963). For example, the rather odd combination of more organics and psycho-neurotics on team 3 is explained by the fact that one consultant is in charge of the E.E.G. Department, and has a strong interest in the organic side of psychiatry, and the other has had special experience and interest in the treatment of psychoneurotics.

Nursing Staff

When the team system was introduced, a very severe strain was put on a depleted nursing staff, particularly as a consequence of creating four more admission wards and dividing old large wards into two separate ones. However, as the result of the new approach, the recruitment to the nursing school has increased satisfactorily. The system has made nurse-training more efficient, varied and interesting, as student nurses also rotate throughout the teams.

One assistant chief male nurse and one assistant matron are allocated to each team. The fact that the old separation of male and female patients has been abolished has made the perpetuation of male and female services archaic. Therefore, the appointment of a principal nursing officer is being made, and in due course full integration of nursing services will come about, with a mixed nursing staff on most, if not all, wards.

Administration

In this process, problems arose regarding the overall administration of the hospital. Firstly, the development of the independent clinical teams tended to lead to the hospital becoming three independent hospitals. This had the effect initially of producing tension between the medical superintendent, who as chief officer of the hospital is responsible for its overall policy and direction on the medical side, and consultants. It also led to difficulties with the group secretary. Similarly, the matron and chief male nurse, who are responsible for all nursing throughout the hospital, found the situation confusing. The absolute freedom and autonomy of the clinical teams to run their own affairs was naturally a radical swing away from the old hierarchical system. It led them to try and deal with the lay and nursing administration on an entirely independent basis, so that, for example, the hospital secretary might get requests for new equipment from each team on different days or weeks, which obviously led to inefficiency. The problem then was how to devise a system of administration which did not interfere with the clinical freedom of the teams and yet co-ordinated them so that they could see themselves as part of one hospital. It should also lead to smooth integration, so that "common services" were efficiently deployed without prejudice to team freedom. This began to become even more vital as departments such as physiotherapy, industrial therapy and occupational therapy were developed to a high degree of efficiency.

The essentials of good administration in a psychiatric hospital can be summed up in one word—"communication". Even though final executive decisions and responsibility for the efficiency of the hospital may lie with the medical superintendent, chief nursing officer, chairman of management committee or group secretary, it is vital for the morale of the hospital that no decision is taken without full consultation in an atmosphere of free discussion, and that members of staff at all levels should feel that their voice can be heard. Therefore, a network of meetings was evolved throughout the hospital. At team level, meetings which include all nursing, medical, social work and local health authority staff, discuss the problems of the team. Anything arising at these meetings that cannot be solved immediately is referred on to higher level meetings, which are under the informal chairmanship of the medical superintendent. These include all medical staff meetings and senior medical staff meetings, which are held on alternate weeks, However, the most important meeting of all is the Senior Officers' Committee. This meets once a month, and is composed of all the consultant staff, group secretary, hospital secretary, finance officer, matron and chief male nurse. This committee really decides the overall policy of the hospital and it can discuss and co-ordinate medical, nursing and administrative problems. Its vital contribution is to allow the medical superintendent, whether dealing with the Management Committee or Regional Hospital Board, to present the unified views of the hospital. Similarly, the group secretary, when dealing with the Management Committee or Regional Board on administrative matters, is in an equally strong position. It is essential that there should also exist a close working relationship between the chairman of the Hospital Management Committee, group secretary and medical superintendent. There is no doubt that with this network of meetings and committees, tension in the hospital has been reduced to a minimum, and that there is a general feeling of confidence that no decisions will be taken without consultation.

The Group Medical Advisory Committee, which also represents the staff of the Mental Subnormality Hospital within the Group, serves a useful function, especially because it includes representatives from the general hospitals, and also the medical officer of health. The chairman of the Group Medical Advisory Committee attends the Hospital Management Committee meetings, and a member of the consultant staff is a member of the Management Committee.

It is in my view essential that medical superintendents should remain. It is difficult to define their role precisely, within the more democratic system of a modern psychiatric hospital. But because he is a permanent officer, he is able to act at times with greater confidence and decisiveness than an elected chairman of a medical committee. In addition, he is responsible for presenting the image of the hospital to the public, and is able to devote important time to developing links with the local community, and to representing the hospital at national level. Furthermore, as the senior lay administrator and senior nursing officer are permanent appointments, an elected chairman would be in a position of weakness, whereas a medical superintendent has time to develop close personal working relationships with these senior officers.

Community Links

Dichotomy in treatment—hospital or home—is false; treatment should be hospital and/or home. The open-door should allow flexible two-way traffic between hospital and community. The essentials of treatment include absolute continuity of care, so that the patient relates not only to the same psychiatrist, but also to the same social worker or mental welfare officer who, like the nurse, shares his philosophy of treatment. To this end, therefore, with the co-operation of the medical officer of health, the Mental Health Department has been divided into three teams. Five mental welfare officers are attached to each hospital team, and have their own team offices in the Mental Health Department. Team mental welfare officers attend the hospital team meetings, out-patients and ward rounds, and keep in close touch with their patients, both inside and outside hospital.

In an integrated community service, the role of the hospital social worker is significantly affected. Social workers were added to the staff of psychiatric hospitals some 25 or more years ago, when hospitals began to realize that they had a continuing responsibility for their patients in the community.

This was at a time when the local authority's duly authorized officers were generally untrained in social work, and limited their activities to the ascertainment of the mentally ill and conveying them under order to hospital. However, since the Mental Health Act, they have increasingly become community social workers. It is becoming clear, as more and more recruits to the service have social science qualifications or are trained psychiatric social workers, that much of the work formerly done by hospital social workers will be taken over by the local authority Mental Health Department. In a sense, the artificial division between hospital social workers and mental welfare department is created by the administrative organization of the National Health Service, which arbitrally places responsibility for in-patient and community care respectively under two separate divisions of the Mental Health Service. Where the local authority co-operates and integration is achieved, the roles of the two become merged. Possibly, the hospital social worker will only continue to exist so long as there is a shortage of adequately trained mental welfare officers. But this post could only disappear when the quality and number of mental welfare officers is such that they have the time and skill to undertake the more time-consuming casework, and are able to spend a greater proportion of their time in the hospital.

In practice, at the Towers Hospital, the hospital social workers are used primarily for those patients who come to out-patients or to the hospital direct from their homes. They also do the more time-consuming casework with neurotic patients. The hospital social workers have developed a special interest in public relations, i.e. lecturing or taking groups round the hospital, and they are able to pick up social problems arising in the hospital, and deal with them on the spot. In an ideal arrangement the social work services should be hospital-based, reaching out into the community, rather than community-based, reaching into the hospital. However, we have found no real difficulty in practice in overcoming the problem of the M.W.O. being technically under a different administrative control.

When considering community links, the role of the general practitioner is a vital one (Kidd, 1963). At the present stage of development in psychiatry, the majority of general practitioners tend to hand over their psychiatric patients to the psychiatrist with relief. This is partly due to the fact that many general practitioners today have had little training or experience in dealing with psychiatric problems. Nevertheless, our experience over the last 5 years, due to our policy of screening all new patients together with the general practitioners, is that the latter is becoming increasingly aware of the valuable part they can play. At the same time, the psychiatrist has become increasingly accepted as a valuable colleague. There is no doubt that in future, the general practitioner and mental welfare officer working together will be able to manage and treat successfully an increasing number of psychiatric patients, bringing in the hospital team with greater discrimination. Treatment of psychiatric illness is often an intuitive art and continuing process. The team system allows this principle of continuity to be carried to the family doctor, because the consultant accepts that he keeps his patients at all times when they are ill.

There is also the role of the psychiatric nurse. As yet, we have only tentative plans for using nurses to supplement, or perhaps complement the work of mental welfare officers or hospital social workers. Three of our nursing staff have in fact become mental welfare officers, and have proved themselves to be most effective in this respect. In other areas, psychiatric nurses have been employed full-time on community visiting, but this would seem to be unnecessary, as they are visiting patients not previously known to them. This could be done as well by a social worker or health visitor. The justification for a nurse visiting in the community is to maintain a relationship already made in hospital. For there is a small proportion of patients, particularly perhaps the more chronic schizophrenics, who value highly the trust that they have built up with a particular nurse during their stay in hospital, and who, because they find it difficult to make new relationships, will be helped more by visits from someone they know than from a new person. However, the administrative aspects of this may present difficulties, until the present shortage of nurses has been lessened.

The team system developed at the Towers Hospital does not operate on a basis of geographical areas. At one point, consideration was given to dividing our catchment area into sections, each cared for by a team. This was abandoned, because we felt that in such a compact urban area, general practitioners should have the right of choice of consultant, if they so wished. Since the lines of communication are so short, there is no real loss of time or efficiency in team mental welfare officers operating in all parts of the catchment area. Clearly, this would not be satisfactory in rural areas, but there is no reason why a hospital team, linked with the community services, cannot operate these on a geographical basis, as has been described by Barker (1964).

Treatment Programmes

The old-type mental hospital was primarily a custodial institution. The number of patients receiving active treatment was minimal; the number of patients actively occupied was small, and these were predominantly serving the needs of the institution itself.

During the past decade, there has been a sustained effort to change the hospital from a static to a dynamic community. But it is possible to see the psychiatric hospital as fulfilling two roles at the present time. Firstly, it is an active treatment centre for all types of acute psychiatric cases, offering them the full range of treatments, whether as in-patients, out-patients or day-patients. Secondly, it is a therapeutic community, especially for the long-stay patients who form the majority of its population. For this reason, it is important to separate these two groups if possible.

There is not very much controversy at present concerning the treatment of acute cases. But there is a growing concern that psychiatric hospitals are discharging too many chronic patients into the community, without adequate thought. In its understandable anxiety to reduce overcrowding, and to raise the standard of its care and see itself more and more as an active treatment centre, the psychiatric hospital is under great pressure to discharge anyone who appears not to need treatment. But a treatment responsibility also exists to the long-stay, and although the goal must be resettlement in the community, it must be realized and accepted that for many, the leading of an active and useful life within the hospital is the limit of their resources.

There is no doubt that the development of industrial therapy units has been one of the most powerful weapons in raising morale, dignity and sense of purpose in large numbers of otherwise aimless psychotics. Through it, some are rehabilitated, others are able to go out to work in the community from the hospital, and still more feel themselves to be human beings with some use and purpose in life.

The team system in itself prevents thoughtless discharge, because it insists on continuity of treatment and care, whether in hospital or community. It means that the general practitioner and mental welfare officer have access to the consultant, who cannot evade this personal responsibility, rather than just to an impersonal doctor at the hospital.

The Future

Rightly or wrongly, official policy in this country is to transfer the active treatment of the mentally ill to psychiatric units in general hospitals. This is an imaginative and laudible proposal. There is little doubt that good psychiatry can be done within the general hospital, but it can only be done if these units are large enough to provide a full range of treatment for patients who may need to be in hospital for at least 2 years. Furthermore, these units must have sufficient autonomy to be able to resist any pressure from the more rule-ridden régime of the general hospital, and be strong enough to exert a beneficial psychiatric effect on the attitudes of the general hospital staff.

It is significant that in the U.S.A. locks are sometimes retained, in deference to general hospital staff, and that psychiatric floors of general hospitals tend to be over-selective in what they have admitted. This means that the state hospital does not do comprehensive psychiatry, but is left to take only the more severe psychotics. It is therefore important that during the next 25 years, when this transition from mental hospital to general hospital is slowly taking place, general hospital psychiatric units should be comprehensive and have their own catchment areas. It is imperative that they should not act as acute "creaming" units, taking only new admissions away from mental hospitals. During this transitional stage, the mental hospital must remain an active comprehensive psychiatric unit, the only difference between the two being that the mental hospital will necessarily retain a large number of long-stay patients for many years to come. But it is quite essential that it too should be a balanced unit, having its own catchment area and offering the full range of psychiatric services to everyone living in its district. In a sense, it is unfortunate that the revolution in psychiatry has come so fast, at a time when many out-dated mental hospitals with low morale were struggling to change. This has resulted in the mental hospital being inadvisedly written off. It is also unfortunate that many influential psychiatrists, working in teaching units, have not appreciated the difficulties of out-dated psychiatric hospitals or the tremendous potential residing in them, once properly reorganized and upgraded. For the forseeable future, the Towers Hospital will remain an active treatment hospital, and we claim that it can provide efficient treatment for all its patients. As the hospital continues to develop, it should offer all the same advantages as a psychiatric unit in a general hospital. It is sometimes maintained that to go to a psychiatric hospital involves a stigma, which will be removed by having psychiatric units in general hospitals. However, with a younger generation growing up, the climate of change may show this to be an unfounded fear.

Conclusion

A psychiatric hospital is able to give a first-class, comprehensive psychiatric service, equal to that of general hospital psychiatry, if organized along the following lines: sited close to its catchment area; with modernized buildings; adequately staffed; organized as an open-door therapeutic community; organized on a team basis, so that a consultant has continuing responsibility for his patient; and linked with the local authority community services. It may be right and inevitable that the mental hospital will one day disappear, and that all psychiatry will be done in general hospitals. Until that far-off day, mental hospitals must maintain a high standard of psychiatry for all, and receive encouragement and support from the professional as well as the lay public.

References

BALIER, C. (1964), *World Hospitals* **1**, 43.
BARKER, J. C. (1964), *Nursing Mirror* **119**, 285.
KIDD, H. B. (1961), *Lancet* **ii**, 703.
KIDD, H. B. (1963), *Medical World* **98**, 292.
MARTIN, D. V. (1962), *Adventure in Psychiatry*, Oxford, Bruno Cassirer.
MILNER, G., *et al.* (1963), *Brit. Med. J.* **i**, 389.
POWELL, E. (1961), in *Emerging Patterns for the Mental Health Services*, London, N.A.M.H.

27. Administration of Psychiatric Hospitals

B. M. C. GILSENAN

ALTHOUGH there is general agreement that the aim of hospital administration should be to create and maintain the best conditions for the efficient treatment of patients, there is far less agreement as to how this can best be achieved in psychiatric hospitals. The Bradbeer report (1954) advocated strongly that hospital administration should be regarded as essentially tripartite—medical, nursing and lay (or business), on the basis of a functional partnership between these three. Although, on the evidence available to it at that time, it saw no reason to depart from the medical superintendent system traditional in psychiatric hospitals, the need was recognized for experiment in hospital administration generally. The opportunity for such experiment arose, not only from the administrative changes consequent on the introduction of the National Health Service in 1948, but from the considerable legal, clinical and social changes in psychiatry that have occurred since then.

It may not be generally recognized that in the early stages of discussion in this country, there was, according to Dr. W. Rees Thomas (1965), a wide diversity of view as to the desirability of including the psychiatric services within the scope of the new National Health Service. When it was finally decided to establish a fully comprehensive hospital service, the decision was of first importance to psychiatry, and one which was to have far-reaching effects on the administration of psychiatric hospitals. In the first paragraph of the National Health Service Act, 1946, reference is made to mental health in these terms: "It shall be the duty of the Minister of Health to promote the establishment in England and Wales of a comprehensive health service designed to secure improvement in the physical and mental health of the people of England and Wales, and the prevention, diagnosis and treatment of illness."

A Central Health Services Council was set up to advise the Minister on general matters relating to the services provided under the Act, and the Minister was empowered, after consultation with this Council, to set up Standing Advisory Committees in the Ministry of Health. A senior principal medical officer, a psychiatrist, is responsible for the Mental Health Division. The National Health Service Act transferred all hospitals, both voluntary and local authority, to the Minister with the exception of a small number of hospitals which were "disclaimed".

Regional Hospital Boards were set up to administer the hospital and specialist services on the Minister's behalf. These boards have twenty to thirty members, medical and non-medical. They provide the hospital management committees with their budgetary allocation. Their duties include the appointment of officers to hospitals and the maintenance and equipment of these hospitals, "subject to the exercise of functions by Hospital Management Committees". The teaching hospitals were placed under the management of Boards of Governors, and were charged with the additional duty to "provide for the University with which the hospital is associated such facilities as appear to the Minister to be required for clinical teaching and research". In Scotland the arrangement differs somewhat, in that the regional hospital boards have administrative jurisdiction over both teaching and non-teaching hospitals, and the hospital management committees are known as Boards of Management. Many of the functions of the medical officer of health in regard to the Hospital and Specialist Service were transferred to a senior administrative medical officer, appointed to each regional hospital board.

Until the Act came into operation, the psychiatric hospital was unique, in that its organization was governed in some detail by the law, as stated in the Lunacy, Mental Treatment Acts and Mental Deficiency Acts. The hospital authority was the Visiting Committee, appointed by the local authority, and composed of members of its Council. In addition to their managerial function, members were invested with legal powers under the Lunacy and Mental Treatment Acts, and were required, under the Lunacy Act, to draw up rules and regulations for the hospital staff which required the sanction of the Board of Control. The following extracts from these rules and regulations provide perhaps the most effective commentary on the great changes that have taken place in the administration of psychiatric hospitals in the past 20 years.

6. Visitors to any of the Staff are not allowed without special permission from the Medical Superintendent.
7. . . . Should any patient express a wish to see a Minister of Religion, the nurse must without fail acquaint the Medical Officer of the fact.
26. . . . The nurse in charge of a patient who may escape renders himself liable to repay the whole of the expenses incurred in the attempt to recapture.
32. The Visitors to Patients must not be allowed to give them any intoxicating liquors; and if, after being informed that it is contrary to the Rules, they persist in doing so, one of the Medical Officers must be sent for immediately; nor are the nurses permitted to bring any into the hospital, whether for themselves, for any other members of the staff, or for the patients. A violation of this rule renders the nurse liable to immediate dismissal.
53. The electric lamps are to be lighted in all day-rooms and corridors at the approach of dusk, and to be turned off immediately the Patients retire to bed, excepting those lights which are allowed to remain on for the night. The Nurses are not allowed to have the light in their own rooms except when they are off duty, and it must be turned off not later than 10.30, at which time all nurses are required to be in bed. Should their rooms open off a dormitory or a gallery, they must be careful to make as little noise as possible, and proceed direct to their rooms. Every nurse must be in his own room by 10.15 p.m. and lights out by 10.30 p.m. . . .

56. At the time of their engagement, or subsequently, they (Nurses) are not to bring any clothing into the hospital, except their own personal clothing and effects, without the express sanction of the Medical Superintendent. All boxes, packages, etc. before entering or leaving the hospital to be seen by the Chief Male Nurse or Matron.
[and finally]

68. No nurse is allowed to get married without the sanction of the Medical Superintendent. The marriage certificate must in all cases be submitted to the Medical Superintendent.

Dr. David J. Vail (1965) says that the advent of the National Health Service infused a new life into the mental hospitals and enabled British mental hospital psychiatry to move into a leading world position. He adds that one effect of this is that in British psychiatry, the hospital psychiatrists are at the top of the professional heap and not at the bottom, as is the case in the United States.

Psychiatric Representation at Regional Hospital Board Level

A review carried out by Stead (1961) showed that there were mental health committees or sub-committees in fourteen of the fifteen regional hospital boards in England and Wales. These committees consisted of members of the boards, reinforced by consultant psychiatrists and sometimes medical officers of health, and met at monthly, or 2- or 3-month intervals.

In addition to these principal committees, there were, in thirteen of the boards, regional psychiatric advisory committees, variously organized.

The Hospital Management Committee

The Hospital Management Committee is the governing body of the institution. It dispenses to the hospital the funds provided for it by the Regional Hospital Board. Vail (1965) stresses the importance of the personality, ability and interest of the hospital management committee chairman, since it is he who is consulted on day-to-day matters of policy, in between meetings of the hospital management committee.

The National Health Service Act describes the function of the hospital management committee in these words:

> It shall be the duty of the Hospital Management Committee of any hospital or group of hospitals, subject to and in accordance with the regulations and such directions as may be given by the Minister or the Regional Hospital Board, to control and manage that hospital or group of hospitals on behalf of the Board, and for that purpose to exercise on behalf of the Board such of the functions of the Board relating to that hospital or group of hospitals as may be prescribed.

The National Health Service effectively broke up the tight hierarchy surrounding the medical superintendent, by superimposing hospital management committees to take over general control of functions in all areas of management, especially those relating to finance and personnel (Vail, 1965).

Hospital management committees have twenty to thirty members, who are appointed by the regional hospital boards after statutory consultation with certain bodies and organizations, and such others as are thought appropriate, and are selected for the contribution it is felt they can make to the management of the hospitals within the Group by reason of a wide variety of experience and interests. Although there are a number of psychiatrists who are members of hospital management committees, this is largely fortuitous, and members of management committees are not appointed for their specialized medical knowledge only. The management committee receives advice on psychiatric matters affecting the medical administration of its hospital from the medical superintendent and/or from the medical advisory committee, through its chairman. These, it should be emphasized, are not members of their management committees, but act in an advisory capacity.

Many large psychiatric hospitals constitute a Group in themselves, so that they have their own management committees. Others are constituent members of a Group with other general or special hospitals and consequently share a management committee. When a psychiatric hospital has its own management committee, it has certain advantages in the way of relative financial autonomy, and better facilities are available for effective communication between staff and management.

There has been an increasing tendency in some regions to amalgamate hospital management committees, so that psychiatric hospitals are brought into larger mixed groups. The reason advanced for this is that integration at management committee level is appropriate to the concept of hospital services being grouped round a district hospital, providing a full range of facilities, including in most cases a short-term psychiatric unit. Doubt has been expressed as to whether the special needs of psychiatric hospitals will be sufficiently appreciated by members of hospital management committees who are traditionally orientated to the requirements of general hospitals, and there is a fear that psychiatric hospitals may come to occupy a position at the end of the financial line. Vail shrewdly comments that since power derives from the hospital management committee, access to it is an issue of great importance in the hospital organization.

Tripartite Administration

To function efficiently, an administrative system requires:

(1) *Adequate delineation of role.* The more tenuous the inter-personal relationships are between administrative heads, the more concise must this delineation be, whereas a considerable blurring of role boundaries is permissible where inter-personal relationships are good.

(2) *Adequate communication.* In a large hospital, this can be very difficult to achieve, and considerable judgement is necessary to strike the

desirable balance between the time required for the staff meetings necessary to achieve this, as against the time required by staff members for their other professional commitments.

The Porritt report states that:

> Under the National Health Service and particularly since the introduction of the recent Mental Health Act, the position of the Medical Superintendent has changed radically. Medical policy is no longer the prerogative of the Medical Superintendent alone, since the Medical Staff Committee is vitally concerned and should have an effective voice in determining it. Furthermore, the other consultants on the hospital's staff, as Responsible Medical Officers, have become as answerable as the Superintendent for the proper admission, treatment and discharge of the patients under their care. At the same time, the general administration of the hospital has passed into the hands of the lay Secretary and there has been a healthy trend towards giving the heads of the nursing services more direct access to the Hospital Management Committee (Board of Management).

The members of the Bradbeer Committee considered that hospital administration could be subdivided into (a) medical administration, (b) nursing administration, and (c) lay, or business administration. While they recognized that the borderlines between these could not be sharply defined, they were

> fully persuaded that the conception of partnership between the three parts of the whole administration should be regarded as fundamental, and should determine the lines of all future developments, whatever variations of superficial pattern may be necessary to give expression to varied circumstances.
>
> Partnership is the important word. None of the three parts can do without either of the others, each has its own set of functions, which it is better adapted to perform than the others, and none should regard itself as superior to the others. Co-operation alone is not enough; it must be willing co-operation, springing from a consciousness of fellowship in a shared desire to serve.

On the allocation of functions between the three parts, three general principles were advanced:

(1) that all administration must always be carried out within the general policy of the governing body;
(2) that because of the inevitable interaction of their duties, all who are doing administrative work must work together, as a team;
(3) that neither a medical man nor a nurse should as a rule do work which a layman could do equally well.

Lay Administration

In some large hospitals which themselves constitute a group, the secretary holds two offices, that of group secretary and that of hospital secretary. The secretary is appointed by the hospital management committee and is its agent.

Prior to the introduction of the National Health Service, there was a Clerk to the Visiting Committee, as well as a Clerk and Steward to the Hospital (who might also be Clerk to the Committee) and a Treasurer. In practice, the clerk to the committee often acted also as the lay officer in the hospital and was often on the legal staff of the local authority. His function was to execute the committee's business, pass on its directions, and advise it legally. The clerk to the hospital was often responsible for the business management of the hospital under the medical superintendent, but might answer direct to the committee. The relations of these officers with the medical superintendent and medical, nursing and other staff were governed by the rules and regulations made by the visiting committee.

The effect of the National Health Service Act was to break up the separate administrative system for mental and mental deficiency hospitals, and to place them on the same footing as other hospitals. The administrative functions of the board of control were transferred to the Minister of Health, and the visiting committees gave way to hospital management committees.

When these committees were set up in 1948, a Ministry Circular provided for a full-time secretary for each committee to be the principal administrative officer, responsible for the administration of the group as a whole, and normally also for one hospital in it. A saving clause was included in the National Health Service Act, to protect the position in the psychiatric hospital of the medical superintendent, who by Statutory Instrument 1948, No. 419 (described later), was designated the chief officer of the hospital.

Where the psychiatric hospital was part of a Group, the group secretary could at one and the same time be principal administrative officer responsible for the administration of the Group as a whole, and the subordinate of the chief officer (the medical superintendent), within a psychiatric hospital, in which he acted as hospital secretary. A subordinate of the Group officer working in a psychiatric hospital might find himself under contrary instructions from the medical superintendent, who had powers to suspend him. Doubts about the respective functions and authority of group officers and their subordinates in the hospitals *vis-à-vis* the superintendent, with his general and unspecified powers, could and did produce impossible situations.

The Association of Hospital Management Committees was mainly concerned with the problems of authority created by S.I. 419, when read in conjunction with the Ministry's circular. Committees wished to rely on one principal officer appointed by them, and responsible only to them for the administration of their hospital or hospitals, and this was provided for them by the Circular. S.I. 419, however, interposed between secretary and hospital a superintendent, charged with the general management of a psychiatric hospital, and thus enjoying some degree of independence of the principal officer. Moreover, the medical superintendent was a doctor of consultant status, and as such, not only appointed by but also in contract with a superior body.

It was felt that these difficulties might be met by the drawing up by the Ministry of Health of model standing orders, to take the place of the rules and regulations previously prescribed under the Lunacy Act. The governing body could be left free, taking the model into account, to frame such standing orders, definining the functions of its officers, as it thought fit. To produce a desirable degree of uniformity, these standing orders could be made subject to the approval of the Minister, in the same way as the rules and regulations under the 1890 Act were subject to approval of the Board of Control. A more appropriate solution would appear to be the replacement of the concept of precedence, inherent in a hierarchical structure, by that of partnership in a tripartite system, as advocated in the Bradbeer report.

Vail feels that the rise of the hospital administrative profession has so far had less impact on the total power shift than have the medical staff changes and hospital management committee influences which he describes.

Nursing Administration

It is the matron and her nursing staff, who, according to the Bradbeer report:

> create the comfort, the content, and the atmosphere of the hospital and (who) can most influence the feelings of the general public with regard to it. The Matron is the personal link between the community and its hospital.
>
> Whilst it is of great importance that the Matron should not be burdened with responsibilities which can equally well be undertaken by lay staff, or which are more properly the concern of specialized talents, it is also of importance that her position, as an equal partner in the scheme of tripartite administration, should be fully recognized.

The report, quoting the memorandum of evidence of the Royal College of Nursing, states that "the position, scope, and responsibility accorded to the Matron of today affect the calibre of new entrants to the profession, and so the calibre of the matrons of tomorrow and their contribution to the hospitals' administrative efficiency". As head of one part of the tripartite administration of her hospital, the matron must be regarded as directly responsible to the governing body of the whole group.

The Bradbeer report recognizes a duality in the position of a matron. In her professional functioning, she should be responsible to the governing body direct, and in what may be called her non-professional duties to the chief administrative officer in the first instance, rather than directly to the governing body. Failure to recognize this duality has been suggested by the King Edward's Hospital Fund for London as a common cause of lack of understanding between the matron and the chief administrative officer.

The Bradbeer report recommended that the medical superintendent's supervision over matters within the matron's or chief male nurse's jurisdiction should be both discreet and minimal. Reference was also made to possible neglect of consideration of the status of the chief male nurse, and to the need to recognize the importance of his joint responsibility with the matron for nurse training.

Under a tripartite administrative arrangement, the heads of the nursing services undoubtedly have more responsibility, and more scope for initiative and imagination than under the medical superintendent system.

Medical Administration

MEDICAL SUPERINTENDENCY

In 1828 the Metropolitan Commissioners of Lunacy Act stipulated that every madhouse of more than 100 beds in the London area should have a resident medical officer, and the provision by which the medical officer or one of the medical officers of the asylum was to be its superintendent was made in 1853. Authority was given to the medical man, in order that the function of the asylum as a place of treatment should be emphasized and its work co-ordinated from this point of view.

Many hospitals appointed medical superintendents, but their powers were not fully defined until the Lunacy Act of 1890. This and subsequent Acts required the visiting committee to appoint a medical superintendent, who should be a resident medical officer unless the board of control otherwise agreed. The board of control insisted that the medical superintendent should be paramount in the hospital, with power to suspend any member of the staff. The medical superintendent was the person responsible to the medical officer of health for the whole administration of the hospital. He had considerable clinical and statutory powers which, when the National Health Service was introduced, were preserved by Statutory Instrument 419, which made him chief officer of the hospital. Such powers as his deputy and assistant medical officers possessed were derived by delegation from him.

Since 1948, medical superintendents are no longer appointed by the visiting committee, nor its successor the hospital management committee, but by the regional hospital board.

The Bradbeer Committee (1954) heard evidence in favour of medical superintendents from the Medical Superintendents Society, the Royal Medico-Psychological Association and the British Medical Association, and the opposite view from the Institute of Hospital Administrators, the Association of Hospital Management Committees and the National Federation of Hospital Officers. It decided to recommend that, because of their special characteristics, mental and mental deficiency hospitals should have medical superintendents.

Statutory Instrument 1948, 419, paragraph 4, provided as follows:

> The Superintendent shall be the Chief Officer of the hospital or institution, and he shall be responsible for the general management thereof in accordance with any

directions which may be given by the Regional Hospital Board or the Hospital Management Committee.

This Statutory Instrument was revoked with effect from November 1960, and H.M. (60) 66 later removed the need to appoint a medical superintendent to a psychiatric hospital, leaving this to the discretion of the hospital management committee and the regional hospital board.

The Bradbeer report, having declared in favour of the retention of medical superintendents in psychiatric hospitals, recommended a financial inducement to make these posts more attractive, and the Royal Commission on doctors and dentists remuneration (1960) recommended this. However, when this recommendation was accepted as part of the "package deal", it became necessary for the Ministry of Health to define the conditions of the award. This they did in H.M. Circular (61) 105, as follows:

> An allowance of £250 per annum shall be paid to a medical officer . . . who holds an appointment as Medical Superintendent of one or more psychiatric hospitals or an appointment the duties of which require him to be the Chief Officer of such hospital or hospitals for the whole of the therapeutic sphere. . . .

The qualification, as here described, has some resemblance to the defunct Statutory Instrument 419, and is open to the similar criticism that it describes a role inconsistent with that of the responsible medical officer, described in the following section.

Vail says that in America, where, as in Minnesota, the chief medical officer has surrendered authority in purely administrative areas, he still retains hierarchical power and discipline over the medical staff. This, he points out, is no longer the case in Britain, where, whatever he may retain in the way of a little prestige and an extra £250 (now £285) per annum for his pains and influence over the whole milieu of the institution, he does not retain this kind of clinical decision-making authority over his colleagues.

According to information received from regional hospital boards in November 1966, medical administration was carried out by the chairman of the medical staff committee in fourteen of the 108 psychiatric hospitals in England. Four of these were in the Metropolitan regions. In Scotland, the medical superintendent is purely an administrator.

The Psychiatric Consultant

The National Health Service Act, 1946, having taken the critical step of recognizing the importance of psychiatry, took the further logical step of recognizing the importance of senior psychiatrists. The consultant psychiatrist was no longer appointed by the visiting committee of the hospital, but by the regional hospital board. For the first time, he was placed on terms of financial and clinical parity with the medical superintendent.

Notwithstanding the provisions of the National Health Service Act, the medical superintendent retained considerable power by reason of Statutory Instrument 419 and where this power was exercised, it could and did limit the clinical freedom of the consultant. Although it was held that these statutory powers were not necessarily incompatible with the autonomy of other consultants in purely clinical matters, the final responsibility in certain semi-clinical matters was declared as lying undoubtedly with the medical superintendent. These were mainly matters dealing with leave, absence or discharge of patients. The medical superintendent's legal responsibility to the patient and the public was considered to be such that his decision would be final in any question affecting the general welfare of any patient under detention, and of allocating patients to a particular part of the hospital. If, therefore, in the judgement of the medical superintendent, it became necessary to transfer a patient from the wards of one consultant to another, he could do so. But there was not considered to be any medical reason why a consultant should not continue his interest in such a patient, even though he was no longer responsible for the treatment. While absolved from responsibility for the clinical treatment of patients of other consultants, a medical superintendent, if dissatisfied with the kind of treatment administered, would have his remedy in a report to the management committee, who had confirmed the allocation of beds. Although the view was expressed that wise administration would enable the medical superintendent to maintain close contact with all his patients, it was difficult to see how this situation could be realized in a hospital of 2000 or more patients.

The Mental Health Act, 1959, designated the consultant as the "Responsible Medical Officer", defined by Mr. D. Walker-Smith (1959), the then Minister of Health, as

> the medical practitioner in charge of the treatment of the patient, by which was meant the doctor who was in clinical charge and not answerable to any other doctor; the doctor who could put up the notice said to have been put up by President Truman in his office, "the buck stops here". The test was not day-to-day attention but ultimate supervision. It was the Consultant who had the ultimate responsibility of supervision, and not the junior doctor who gave the day-to-day treatment.

Vail points out that this is in marked contrast to the situation in the U.S. hospitals, where the medical superintendent can intervene, if he desires, in the treatment of any patients, if need be by overruling the patient's physician. Such a system, he adds, prevailed in British mental hospitals prior to 1948, and, indeed, in many local authority hospitals administered by medical superintendents. He says that the capable and independent-minded physicians coming into the mental hospitals after 1948 did not take kindly to this kind of dictation in clinical matters, and it was this discontent that led to the establishment of the responsible medical officer provisions. Is it not, however, possible that the change was determined by social changes generally and by the return from the Services of many psychiatrists whose status had been enhanced by their enlarged opportunity and experience there?

The Medical Advisory Committee

Although Medical Advisory Committees have long existed in teaching hospitals, they are a comparatively recent innovation elsewhere. Each hospital group, and below that, each hospital of appropriate size in the group, should have its own medical committee, for which there is a model constitution described in Circular R.H.B. (53) 91, drawn up by the Ministry, in consultation with the Joint Consultants Committee. This model applies equally to both psychiatric and general hospitals.

Although the importance of an actively functioning medical advisory committee to a hospital has been repeatedly stressed, there is evidence to suggest that, in some psychiatric hospitals, their role as an advisory body has yet to be fully realized. An investigation by Tetlow (1957) showed that of thirty hospitals which replied to a questionnaire, the medical staff of only five were satisfied with the working of the medical advisory committee. Similarly, an inquiry made in 1959 by Middlefell showed that in fifty psychiatric hospitals, only twenty-five felt that the liaison between the medical advisory committee and the hospital management committee was good.

Based on 87 replies to a questionnaire sent out to 102 psychiatric hospitals, Hutchinson (1963) contrasted the practice in these hospitals with that obtaining normally in general hospitals.

TABLE 1. *Medical Advisory Committees in General Hospitals*

Membership	All senior staff + group secretary + chairman of hospital management committee
Frequency of meetings	Monthly
Change of office bearers	Regularly by elections
Frequency of reports to hospital management committee	Monthly
Representation to hospital management committee	Representative member(s) attend hospital management committee

TABLE 2. *Medical Advisory Committees in Eighty-seven Psychiatric Hospitals*

Membership	All staff + M.O.H. + G.P.(s)	59
	Senior staff only	28
Frequency of meetings	Monthly	62
	Infrequently	25
Status of medical superintendent	Not office bearer	53
	Office bearer	34
Change of office bearers	Regular elections	63
	No elections	24

Attendance of group secretary	No	59
	Yes	28
Attendance of chairman of hospital management committee	No	80
	Yes	7
Frequence of reports to hospital management committee	Monthly	51
	Infrequently	36
Representation to hospital management committee	By medical superintendent only	51
	By medical superintendent and others	36
Minutes typed and circulated to members	Yes	69
	No	18

Recent Developments in Medical Administration of Psychiatric Hospitals

A PSYCHIATRIC HOSPITAL WITHOUT A MEDICAL SUPERINTENDENT

In 1962 the Group Medical Advisory Committee of Shenley Hospital decided to recommend to the Hospital Management Committee that when the medical superintendent of the hospital retired in May 1963 he should not be replaced, and that the medical administration of the hospital should be carried out by the chairman of the Medical Advisory Committee in conformity with the requirements of paragraph 3 of H.M. (60) 66 (Administration of Psychiatric Hospitals).

In March 1963 the acting chairman of the Group Medical Advisory Committee wrote to the group secretary informing him of this opinion. He pointed out that there was an active Group Medical Advisory Committee at Shenley Hospital, composed of the consultant staff and the group secretary, with power of co-option. This met at least once a week at that time. It was proposed that the chairman of the Group Medical Advisory Committee would express the collective point of view of this committee. He would deal with matters of day-to-day medical administration, and, in matters of urgency, might act without formal consultation with his committee. In these circumstances, he would act as far as possible in conformity with the declared policy of his committee. The chairman would have responsibility to ensure that where "a committee adopt a policy which needs to be applied uniformly throughout the hospital, that policy is carried out" (H.M. (60) 66, para. 3).

The Group Medical Advisory Committee declared their acceptance of the principle of tripartite administration, as recommended in the reports of the Bradbeer and Porritt committees. While making these recommendations to the Hospital Management Committee, they drew the latter's attention to H.M. (60) 66 (Administration of Psychiatric Hospitals) and R.H.B. (53) 91 (Medical Committees in Hospitals and Hospital Groups). The North-West

Metropolitan Regional Hospital Board and Shenley Hospital Management Committee accepted these recommendations, and since May 1963 the medical administration of the hospital has been carried out by the chairman of the Group Medical Advisory Committee. A similar system of medical administration has been in operation at Cane Hill Hospital since early in 1962 (Hutchinson, 1962).

These changes were foreshadowed a few years previously by Shaw and Samuel (1959), who described an experiment in medical administration at Belmont Hospital. Following a statement of some of the arguments for and against medical superintendents, they described the ideal structure of medical administration in a psychiatric hospital as follows:

(1) An adequate number of senior medical staff, who enjoy complete clinical independence.

(2) An active and fully representative Medical Advisory Committee, with a chairman and secretary who are preferably not the medical administrator or his deputy. This committee should have direct access to the Hospital Management Committee.

(3) A medical administrator and his deputy nominated by the medical staff and fully acceptable, both to the Hospital Management Committee and the Regional Hospital Board, and appointed by agreement among all three bodies, with a period of office of four or five years, renewable if desired.

(4) The medical administrator should be regarded as a representative of the medical staff committee as well as the representative of the Regional Hospital Board and the Hospital Management Committee.

They added that as far as (3) was concerned, it worked in practice and had many advantages, but unfortunately, (4) had not been achieved. Although the administrative arrangement described by Shaw and Samuel differs in important respects from that described first by Hutchinson (1962) and now in existence at Shenley and other psychiatric hospitals, it is, nevertheless, of importance in that it broke new ground at the time in the administration of psychiatric hospitals. It stressed the importance of the Medical Advisory Committee, and in placing a limit on the tenure of office of the medical administrator, departed from the traditional authoritative-hierarchical administrative structure of psychiatric hospitals.

The transition in Shenley Hospital was not a difficult one. In many ways, it could be regarded as a logical development of the medical administrative system that had been in operation there for many years. Not only was there an effective medical advisory committee, but the medical administrative structure was based on the firm system, pioneered there in 1947.

Since 1947 there have been three firms or divisions—two female and one male—each enjoying a considerable amount of autonomy, but this system is now in process of modification, so as to allow each division to admit and treat patients of both sexes, and to provide a psychiatric service for a specific part of the total catchment area. Until recently, there has been one consultant in charge of each division, but the increased consultant establishment now allows for two consultants for each division. The eventual medical establishment (Platt Committee recommendation) of each division will be two consultants, two registrars—of whom one may be a senior registrar—two medical assistants, and two senior house officers. Each division has its own nursing officers, psychiatric social workers and secretaries.

The Group Medical Advisory Committee consists of the consultants, the senior hospital medical officers and the group secretary. The inclusion of the group secretary is considered to be most important, and greatly facilitates a satisfactory working relationship, not only with the lay administration generally, but with the Hospital Management Committee. The committee now meets once a fortnight, and more often if the occasion demands it. The proceedings are formal and minuted.

An arrangement which has proved very satisfactory in practice is for the Group Medical Advisory Committee's chairman's secretary to attend, and record the proceedings. This means that one of the members does not have to act as secretary.T he matron and chief male nurse are invited to attend meetings when matters concerning the nursing services arise. It will be noted that the group secretary of the hospital has a double role in the hospital administrative arrangement. He is not only a member of the Group Medical Advisory Committee, but is one of the partners in the tripartite administrative system—medical, nursing and lay.

The former medical superintendent's office, renamed the "Central Medical Office", has been redesigned and refurnished as a small board room, to serve a double function. Firstly, to act as administrative office for the chairman of the Group Medical Advisory Committee, and secondly, to act as a meeting place for formal functions, e.g. meetings of the Medical Advisory Committee, or the reception of visitors to the hospital.

The chairman of the Hospital Management Committee is invited to attend meetings of the Medical Advisory Committee once a month, and his attendance is so timed as to allow of discussion with him of appropriate items on the Hospital Management Committee agenda. He is invited to be present at other times, as the occasion demands, and this arrangement has done much to facilitate a good working relationship with the Hospital Management Committee.

There is a Ways and Means Committee, composed of the Group Medical Advisory Committee and representatives of the Hospital Management Committee which meets when items of special interest or administrative difficulty arise. These meetings provide the opportunity for a free exchange of opinions, and do much to prevent misunderstandings, and to ease any tension in the life of the hospital. The entire medical staff also meet periodically with their own chairman, not a consultant, to discuss matters affecting their work and interests.

In addition to the above meetings, the chairman of the Group Medical Advisory Committee holds monthly informal meetings, to which representatives of the various interests in the hospital are invited in addition to the doctors, the matron, chief male nurse and the group secretary. This occasion serves to welcome officers newly appointed to the hospital, and to introduce them to their future colleagues. The chairman of the Group Medical Advisory Committee attends meetings of the Hospital Management Committee, some of the sub-committees, and meetings of the Joint Consultative Committee of the Whitley Council. Prior to the monthly meetings of the Hospital Management Committee, the consultants meet the House Committee of the Hospital Management Committee, and accompany them on a tour of a part of the hospital.

The object of a scheme such as this is to provide a communication system in which the tripartite administrative arrangement, as described in the Bradbeer and Porritt reports, can work.

The change from an authoritative to a democratic administrative structure is bound to impose strains on those who have to take on new roles and develop new relationships. The ease with which the administrative partners adjust to the new situation depends to a large extent on their personalities and attitudes, but in all circumstances requires goodwill.

It has been said that a system works just as well as those operating it wish it to work, and there has fortunately been in this hospital goodwill on all sides. There has been criticism, and this has come from the lay side, where the opinion has been expressed that more power should be vested in the office of the chairman of the Group Medical Advisory Committee. It is perhaps not sufficiently recognized that this increase in power could only be obtained at the expense of the consultants, whose unique statutory obligations appear to preclude this.

All hospital administration must, in the last analysis, serve patients' needs. The onus of giving administrative expression to these rests mainly on the psychiatric consultant, on whose competence more than anything else the reputation of the psychiatric hospital depends. In an administrative system such as is here described, the consultant has, individually or through the medical advisory committee, power commensurate with his great responsibility.

I conclude by two final quotations from Vail's recent book on the *British Mental Hospital System*, which I found stimulating and well informed.

> In the final analysis, the real secret of power within the hospital organization remains elusive. The chances are it rests with the medical staff, though not necessarily the chief medical officer, by whatever title he may be known.

One could spend a long time discussing Great Britain and the British people. Related to the theme of this monograph are two aspects of the British character and the British style that are important. One is their way of going about things through deliberation, discussion, compromise, working things out, "getting on with it". This is tangential, but related to their phobia (the word is used deliberately) of the written document as a way to clarify and resolve subtle relationships. The other is the diversity of the British, their ability to tolerate varying points of view. Diversity has a very important bearing here: just as the "typical Englishman" is a myth, so it is impossible to state that any one method is the way the British run their mental hospitals. Each hospital is different; each hospital is organized differently; each one has a different configuration; a different history, a different tradition, its own flavour and personality.

References

DAINTON, C. (1961), *The Story of England's Hospitals* (*London*), London, Museum Press.

HUTCHINSON, J. T. (1959), Medical notes in Parliament, *Brit. Med. J.* i, 867.

HUTCHINSON, J. T. (1962), *Royal Medico-Psychological Association*, Maudsley Bequest Lecture.

HUTCHINSON, J. T. (1963), *Lancet* i, 314.

Medical Staffing Structure in the Hospital Service, report of the Joint Working Party, 1961, London, H.M.S.O.

MIDDLEFELL, R. (1959), *Brit. Med. J.* (supplement), ii, 4.

MINISTRY OF HEALTH, Central Health Services Council, Report of the Committee on the Internal Administration of Hospitals, 1954, London, H.M.S.O.

National Health Service Act, 1946, London, H.M.S.O.

REES THOMAS, W. (1965), Personal communication.

Review of the Medical Services in Great Britain (1962), London, Social Assay.

Report of the Committee of Inquiry into the Recruitment, Training and Promotion of Administrative and Clerical Staff in the Hospital Service (1963), London, H.M.S.O.

Royal Medico-Psychological Association's Memorandum of Evidence to the Royal Commission on Mental Illness and Mental Deficiency (1954).

Royal Commission on Doctors and Dentists Remuneration (1960), London, H.M.S.O.

SHAW, D. and SAMUEL, A. (1959), *Lancet* ii, 170.

STEAD, J. S. (1961), A Summary of the Committee Structure of Regional Hospital Boards in Relation to Mental Health (unpublished).

TETLOW, C. (1957), *Lancet* i, 89.

VAIL, DAVID J. (1965), *The British Mental Hospital System*, Springfield, Illinois, Charles C. Thomas.

28. Psychiatric Nurse Training and its Implications for Patient Care

UNA V. BUDGE

IN ENGLAND, psychiatric nurse training began in 1891, when the Royal Medico-Psychological Association decided that their staff of attendants needed some instruction to help them to "a due understanding of the work on which they are engaged".

It is interesting to note that the prescribed 2 years' training consisted of:

(a) Lectures;
(b) Clinical instruction in the wards by medical staff;
(c) "Exercises" under the Head and charge attendants in the wards, in the practice of nursing and attendance upon the insane;
(d) Study of the *Handbook* issued by the association;
(e) Periodical examinations, at least one in each year.

In later years, the rise of tutorial departments tended to divorce theoretical from practical teaching, a mistake which was not made by the pioneers of nurse training.

It is, however, true that when practical skills are learned (as is desirable) where they are carried out, the learner is at the mercy of the person demonstrating. If senior staff provide indifferent care, or are unskilled and unsympathetic, those who learn from them will develop the same bad habits and poor skills. The provision of a specialist who has time to teach nursing skills well, having no other duties and carrying no responsibility for the ward administration, seems a reasonable idea, and has been developed by training tutors, and latterly clinical instructors (i.e. nurse instructors who teach students in the wards), whose whole responsibility lies in training students.

To those who trained in the 1920's and 1930's it seems that nurse training today, with its introductory courses designed to orientate students to their work, and its block or study day systems, which do not interfere with time off or ward work, must be a pleasant and easy experience. We forget that sickness of mind or body is not pleasant to suffer or to watch, and that nursing can never be without strain for those who do it. In particular, the mentally sick person needs the constant company of others who can understand and support, and help him to bear or solve his problems. It is the ability to give this kind of help that is the measure of the success of any training in psychiatric nursing.

509

The Syllabus

An examination of the syllabus shows how ideas are changing. In 1923, the R.M.P.A. considered that the nurse should know:

(a) First aid (this included some elementary anatomy and physiology);
(b) General features and varieties of mental disorders;
(c) Ordinary requirements of basic nursing;
(d) General symptoms of physical disease.

Thus, out of four main headings, three were concerned mainly with bedside care and physical disorders, though the greater majority of the patients were physically healthy and up and about, many working in the kitchens, gardens, farms and laundries in the hospital. The words "occupational therapy" had not yet been heard, but those patients were certainly occupied, some would say exploited, as they were virtually unpaid.

The G.N.C. syllabus in 1946 included quantities of anatomy and physiology and a subject known as "hygiene", full of such useful knowledge as "the disposal of refuse by the water carriage system", "sources of water", and "methods of lighting and heating". Sick nursing and physical disorders occupied three pages in the syllabus. Instruction in purely psychiatric matters, however, had also expanded to fill three pages, though several of the headings were purely physical nursing, one being the recording of temperature, pulse and respiration.

Sickroom cookery was also taught. No space was devoted to pharmacology, though at this period large quantities of drugs were widely used in all mental hospitals, and in particular such substances as aperients, sedatives and hypnotics.

By 1950, psychology had appeared for the first time in the preliminary syllabus for all student nurses. (For many years, this examination was the common portal of entry to all the registers maintained by the General Nursing Council.) By 1952, giving and safe keeping of medicines had been added to the preliminary examination syllabus. In the final (mental) examination, four of the six subject headings had now become entirely concerned with psychiatry and psychology.

In 1957, the experimental mental syllabus appeared, and with it the common preliminary examination vanished unregretted. The long-sought policy of a common portal of entry was at last seen to be unrealistic and psychiatric training was free to expand and develop along lines more suited to the changes that were to come about in psychiatric hospitals as a result of the Mental Health Act.

This syllabus envisaged training along three broad lines of study:

(a) A systematic study of the human individual, both mind and body, relating normal development and behaviour with the effects of mental disorder and physical illness;

(b) The various skills in dealing with mental disorder and bodily diseases, associated with or occurring in psychiatric patients;

(c) Concepts of mental disorder, psychiatry and psychopathology.

A bid was made to get rid of the preliminary examination which had always been taken at the end of the first year of training, but it was retained under a new title—the Intermediate Examination. At the present time, the general training has been re-aligned to a similar pattern and has succeeded in removing the preliminary examination. So it is that psychiatric hospitals, having led the way in the planning of a new syllabus and in the move to get rid of the restrictions imposed by having to prepare for an examination in the first year, find themselves at present having to retain it, whilst general hospitals have managed to break free.

What Nurses Do

In recent years, a good deal of attention has been paid to the work of the mental nurse. In 1955, a committee was set up under the leadership of Mr. G. C. Goddard, to investigate the "character and scope of the work of the Ward staff" and the "training and role of the mental nurse" in the Manchester region. They were concerned mainly about the shortage of qualified mental nurses in their region and with the need to deploy more usefully those who were available. Not the least interesting part of their findings was the type of work that occupied most of the nurse's time. One may perhaps compare the work done with the work the nurses were trained for. In 1955, the syllabus of instruction covered these headings:

Preliminary
- Anatomy and physiology
- Personal and communal health (the former "hygiene")
- First aid
- Bacteriology and principles of asepsis
- Principles and practice of nursing (geared to the bedfast) but including normal psychology and ward management (cleaning, etc.)
- Theory and practice of invalid cookery

Final
- Principles and practice of nursing (more advanced technical skills)
- Bodily diseases and disorders
- Legal and administrative aspects (including admission and discharge of the mentally ill)
- Psychology (normal and abnormal)
- Psychiatry—including the management of the mentally ill as well as the study of mental illness.

Let us now look at the headings under which Mr. Goddard's team examined the work of the nurse in eight wards of a mental hospital:

Administration and organization   27 items
Basic nursing   19 items including meal service
Technical nursing   19 items
Supervision   13 items
Domestic   6 items
Sundries, including lectures, meetings and mealbreaks.

The survey reveals that although most mental nurses considered they spent large amounts of time doing *domestic work*, in none of the eight wards was more than 14% of time spent on these activities, and in one it was less than 2%. Curiously enough, the highest percentage of domestic work was done by nurses in the convalescent ward, where it might be thought that some help might have been persuaded out of the patients, if only under the guise of occupational therapy.

Supervision occupied also a low percentage of time, except in the disturbed ward, where over 40% of the time was spent by nurses on this task. The next highest amount was only 14%. Supervision included such social tasks as taking patients to entertainments, clinics, and on walks, also seeing that they washed, dressed and performed such personal and social duties as were considered suitable. This can therefore be said to be one of the tasks for which mental nurses are specifically trained, and in the performance of which they can make face-to-face relationships of a highly therapeutic nature with patients, if they understand fully how to do so.

Technical nursing varied from 24% to just over 1%, basic nursing from 42% to 10%, though wards where a large amount of technical nursing (giving injections, treatment, etc.) was done did not necessarily spend as long on basic nursing (beds, washing, feeding, etc.). In one, for example, 23% of the time was spent in basic nursing and just over 1% in technical nursing. Other wards showed less wide variations.

Administration accounted for over 30% of the time in one ward, and was not less than 16% in any ward examined. Under this heading is included the giving of reports, clerical duties, official conversations with staff, ward rounds, inspections, etc. It also includes putting away stores, checking linen, changing uniform, looking for other staff and lost property, and answering the telephone.

Trained for the Job

In this survey, approximately one-third of the nurse's time was spent in basic and technical nursing, for which the syllabus adequately prepared her. Another third was spent in administration and domestic tasks, many of which were unskilled. However, the syllabus included instruction in such items as ward cleaning, care of kitchen, bathroom, etc., and also in some of the skilled aspects of administration such as giving reports, and clerical duties such as charting.

The final third of the nurse's time is accounted for by the delightfully named "sundries", which do not occupy less than 20% of the time in any ward, and the supervisory duties already referred to, which can be used therapeutically by nurses if they are sufficiently skilled and interested. In this survey, "sundries" includes lecture time—obviously no study day or block system of training existed in this hospital at the time—and staff meetings, which would now be regarded increasingly as an administrative necessity.

Thus it seems that the accusation sometimes levelled at training syllabuses, that they are not geared to the actual work done by nurses, was not very valid, even in 1955 with the old common portal of entry, though it is true that a number of items taught seem not to be needed by the nurse in the ward. Nevertheless, some extra background material is necessary in all training to support, enlarge, and make clear the work that actually has to be learnt.

How Much Skill?

What does emerge very clearly from this study is that a great deal of the work done by nurses is semi-skilled or totally unskilled, and could certainly be learned in less than 3 years. Also, it seems that many of the tasks performed, even if necessary, should not be done by people who, if they have benefited from training, should be utilizing their skills more fully than many of them seem to have been doing. Audrey John remarks (1961): "If the nurse is not contributing as fully as possible to the recovery of her patients, she has failed to fulfil her function."

Broadly speaking, it would appear that in this survey, very little time was spent doing any task for which any high degree of specific training was required. For example, in "administration", the only tasks requiring training were those involved in reports and charting. Most of the other tasks would have been equally well performed by any reasonably sensible person; it needs no training to count linen, check stores, move furniture or search for lost property.

Though many mental nurses complain that their syllabus is overloaded with nursing (i.e. physical care of patients), we have seen that at least a third of the time spent on duty was used for performing nursing tasks. However, these were in the main of a very elementary nature and required little more skill than that developed by an affectionate and adequate mother of young children; weighing, bathing, cutting nails, doing hair and serving meals are examples of this. Some require both skill and insight, such as lifting and moving helpless people, conversing with worried, distressed ones, or hand-feeding those who are unco-operative, whilst all of the technical procedures carried out in this survey require a considerable depth of know-ledge, understanding, conscientiousness and skill. When talking to nurses, both trained and in training, it often seems that they themselves are unaware of the importance of the work they do, and miss many opportunities of using and developing their skills. For example, they may spend less time in super-vising patients, with its unrivalled opportunities for observation and contact, than they do in so-called administration, which largely consists of duties not directly involving patients at all.

The Effects of the Mental Health Act

With the passing of the Mental Health Act, a number of changes which had been developing in the whole climate and policy of psychiatric hospitals began to take shape. The old custodial attitudes are slowly breaking down and more therapeutic ones beginning to prevail. But this is a slow process, since it involves more than the surface changes of "open doors" and informal admission. It is of no value to open the doors of the hospital if its policy is still being formulated and carried out by closed minds, and minds are difficult to open, reacting vigorously against changes which seem to threaten them. Maxwell Jones, talking of his early experiments with a therapeutic community during the Second World War, remarks: "These early changes in the community structure threw a considerable strain on the Ward Sister who felt that her authority was being undermined; in fact, the whole develop-ment almost broke down as a result of the anxiety aroused in the senior nursing group." It seems clear that the more patients are encouraged to make decisions for themselves and to function as full members of the com-munity, the greater the need for training that will fit the nurse to abandon her supervisory and controlling role and to function more as an equal participant in treatment. She will have to learn to sit back and watch patients struggling to work through their own problems, and only suggest solutions when it becomes clear that help is needed. She will need to abandon her belief that nurses are there to tell patients what to do because "they can't help themselves", and find ways of assisting them to make their own decisions. Yet in the immediate past, the training of nurses and the requirements of the hospital combined to make it impossible for therapeutic attitudes to exist. Russell Barton (1959) says: "The nurse is taking the patient out of her own life by doing everything and making all decisions for her. The nurse often has no option but to do so because of the way many mental hospitals have been run."

The Urge to Improve Training

The present syllabus of training, while including the preparation of the student in the basic and technical nursing skills she is likely to need, also offers ample opportunity for enabling her to develop an understanding of her own behaviour, fears and attitudes and how these may affect her ability to be relaxed, accepting and helpful towards patients, without desiring to rob them of independence. Nevertheless, the inculcating of such understanding depends very largely on the climate of the hospital, and to some extent upon the intelligence and personality of the student. The nursing world in England has recently been presented with the Platt Report, which proposed that the time has come to limit the number of students training for registration, and to abandon the apprenticeship system of training which has become traditional in this country. This report has aroused considerable opposition, yet its recommendations are in line with findings made previously, for example by World Health Organization (1961): "A reorientation in the thinking of those concerned with nursing education and practice is required", and Audrey John (*ibid.*): " . . . the need for distinguishing between the duties of the skilled nurse and those of the semi-skilled, and the desirability of more careful recruitment, selection and training".

The Nurse Assesses Her Skills

The W.H.O. report (*ibid.*) asked what duties are rated as "extremely important" for trained psychiatric nurses, and came up with the following:

(a)   Preparing, serving meals, etc.
(b)   Group therapy
(c)   Habit training (of deteriorated patients)
(d)   Giving and receiving reports
(e)   Basic nursing care
(f)   Case conferences
(g)   Contact with relatives.

But asked what they thought would *ideally* be considered the most important work of such a nurse, they left out meal service altogether, rated habit training and group therapy lower in the scale, and gave precedence to basic nursing, reports, contact with relatives and doctors, assisting with technical procedures and occupational therapy.

Nevertheless, much basic nursing care can be done by semi-skilled personnel under some degree of supervision, and many of the other "ideal" tasks listed above remove the nurse for long periods of time from the vicinity of the patient, who might be considered to need skilled persons functioning around him.

As early as 1943, the Nursing Reconstruction Committee of the Royal College of Nursing had stated that: "The first essential in the establishment of true nursing education is the clear separation between the training of nurses and the obligation to provide nursing services for hospital patients."

This was reiterated in 1960: "the need to reduce intake of student nurses—experience planned in the interests of students and not to solve staffing problems". The Platt Report comes 21 years after the first R.C.N. report, and in spite of alterations in the syllabus and considerable advances in the régime of psychiatric hospitals, little advance has been made towards planning a training that will fit the psychiatric nurse for the part she should be playing in the care of the mentally ill, both within and outside hospitals.

Enrolment

One recent advance may pave the way to a real "reform of nursing education" in the psychiatric field. We have shown that "the majority of the recorded activities (in the ward) are such as lie well within the ability of staff less highly trained than the registered nurse" (1955). In this country, enrolled nurse training was devised for just this purpose. The enrolled nurse is not an inferior, half-qualified S.R.N.; she is a fully trained person, capable of carrying out many, if not most, of the routine ward duties concerned with basic and technical care and administration. Her role is not one of "general dog'sbody" to the S.R.N., who is too proud to perform simple nursing tasks, but is to provide continuing day-to-day care efficiently and with understanding. Unfortunately, the attitudes of registered nurses to their enrolled colleagues have resulted in S.E.N.s being treated and regarding themselves as inferior, and trainees for the Roll have not been forthcoming in the numbers that are needed. Now, psychiatric training schools have been given the opportunity to undertake training for the Roll, and it will be interesting to see whether the psychological preparation and training in social skills, which are a part of the R.M.N. syllabus, will make it easier for the trained psychiatric nurse to accept her enrolled colleague. Will the S.E.N. fit into the psychiatric hospital in her proper place, and can the present gap in relations between enrolled and registered nurses be bridged?

Training Today

Today, a student entering a psychiatric hospital can expect to find a planned system of training, with ample time for learning. She will have days or weeks in the classroom at regular intervals and will be encouraged to question, discuss and search. There will be a good library, qualified teachers, visits, films and lectures. On the wards, she will meet well-qualified people, a relaxed atmosphere, and problems vastly different, more interesting but more difficult than those faced by the first groups of "Attendants upon the insane" who received their lectures in the board rooms of the county asylums so many years ago. Then, the patients were likely to stay in the hospital for life; it was their home, and the staff acted very much as parents. The entire structure was authoritarian—benevolent or otherwise, as determined by the individuals concerned. Life was bounded by many rules, both for patients and staff; it was secure, enclosed, entirely detached from the normal community, a world in itself. Today, the tendency is to open out, and to try to retain the mentally ill within the normal community as far as possible, and where this is not possible, to provide in the hospital an environment as nearly like the normal as can be tolerated by patients—and indeed by staff! It is hoped that in future, the closed community will become less and less necessary and that patients will need hospitals for a shorter time. Quicker response to treatment may mean that patients can be treated in clinics, or day hospitals, or even as out-patients, and followed-up by community services. Most existing mental hospitals have had for years their own out-patients clinics—usually operating in general hospitals—while many have their own day hospitals and hostels, and provide follow-up care in conjunction with the local authority.

Nowadays, there is a desire to avoid hospitalization and the loss of contact with working life, which arises when people are prevented from making a contribution to the community for long periods. They develop a tendency to retreat into the belief that "work is not possible for me", and this adds to the difficulties of rehabilitation.

Rehabilitation

Noticeable in the reports we have quoted of the work of nurses is the absence of the word "rehabilitation". It does not occur in any of the syllabuses of training until 1957, where it is mentioned both in conjunction with after-care and indirectly in this telling phrase: "Psychological rewards and penalties associated with recovery of function and return to family, industrial and community life." Most nurses have had experience of the patient who has lost the habit of fighting life's battles and learned to expect four square meals a day, clothing and shelter, for little or no return, yet they seldom realize that this is inevitable if the hospital environment is too secure, too "mothering".

If people are to be kept in the community, we must think in terms of training workers to support them in their family and work situation. Present syllabuses of nurse training are only scratching the surface of this problem; even the Platt Report still assumes that we are training hospital nurses, and has not turned its attention to producing a worker who could be as capable in the patients' homes or factories as in the hospital wards and departments. Yet perhaps this is asking too much of any training, and nurses should be prepared to think in terms of further study and specialization after registration, and continuing acquisition of knowledge and skill, far more than is at present the case. Perhaps in the psychiatric hospital, there is greater scope for the nurse as a "social therapist". Is it the title "nurse" that holds us back in developing the kind of person we need to help the mentally ill? "Nurse" suggests beds, medicines, washing, hot drinks; yet the mentally ill seldom require any more skilled degree of nursing than is carried out by the average housewife for her family. If they do, the nearby general hospital is often enlisted to carry out operations or investigations, and to cope with serious casualties. It is possible today for mentally ill people who have a physical illness to be nursed in a normal general ward, without causing distress or anxiety either to staff or patients. What the mentally ill *do* need is encouragement to talk, to discuss their ideas and problems, to occupy themselves in interesting ways, to feel wanted and useful—to reach out for life instead of retreating from it. There is still too little time, either in the patients' daily life in hospital, or in the nurses' training, devoted to learning how to communicate with one another. Much "occupational therapy" still consists of helping with the ward housework; too many staff-hours are spent filling in forms and tidying cupboards—an escape from the frustration of trying to help patients without proper instruction in techniques for doing so. By and large, the psychiatric hospital remains a place where patients improve simply as a result of being removed from the environment that has exacerbated their problems, as a blister will disappear when a tight shoe is removed. Similarly, when the victim is returned—"relieved" as the quaint old terminology has it—to his environment, he will more often than not break down once more, simply because his problem has not been solved, but only temporarily shelved.

In the future, the comprehensive hospital may provide basic and specialized trainings for nurses based in a nearby independent school of nursing, attached perhaps to a university. Can we hope for a training for the psychiatric nurse that will reflect more understanding of how to communicate with and assist patients and other workers; less of the ability to bath people competently and see their hair is tidy and free from lice—valuable and necessary as these skills are—and more of how to encourage, support, sustain and guide patients into taking up the challenge of living fully?

References

A Comprehensive Mental Nursing Service (1960), London, Royal College of Nursing.
BARTON, R. (1959), *Institutional Neurosis*, Bristol, John Wright.
BOARD OF CONTROL (1925), *Nursing Service in Mental Hospitals*, London, H.M.S.O.
FREEMAN, H. L. and FARNDALE, W. A. J. (1963), *Trends in the Mental Health Services*, Oxford, Pergamon Press.
GENERAL NURSING COUNCIL, *Syllabus of Training from 1923 to 1964*.
JOHN, A. (1961), *A Study of the Psychiatric Nurse*, Edinburgh, Livingstone.
JONES, M. (1952), *Social Psychiatry*, London, Tavistock.
MANCHESTER REGIONAL HOSPITAL BOARD (1952), *Work of the Mental Nurse*.
Nurse in Mental Hospital Practice (1961), Geneva, W.H.O.
Reform of Nursing Education (1964), London, Royal College of Nursing.
ROYAL-MEDICO-PSYCHOLOGICAL ASSOCIATION (1902), *Handbook for Attendants on the Insane*, 4th edn., London.

29. Psychiatric Hospital Services in the South-West Metropolitan Region

E. G. Braithwaite

This Board, appointed in 1947, found that the population of the region at this time was 4,308,805, in an area consisting of Dorset (except Lyme Regis), the Isle of Wight, the county boroughs of Bournemouth, Croydon, Portsmouth and Southampton, the counties of Hampshire, Surrey and West Sussex, a part of Wiltshire, and the south-west sector of London. The western area of the region, administered after the initial years in almost every respect by its own committee, became in 1959 the Wessex Regional Hospital Board. The area now served covers most of Surrey, West Sussex, a small part of Hampshire, and in Greater London, the new London boroughs of Croydon, Kingston upon Thames, Merton, Sutton and Wandsworth, and parts of Richmond on Thames, Hammersmith, Kensington and Chelsea, Westminster, Lambeth, and Southwark, and the population in the region is 3,244,000. For the purpose of this article, the psychiatric hospitals in the area now forming the Wessex Region have been excluded.

Early Years

During the early years, there was a mass of detailed administration, partly imposed by the National Health Service Act itself and partly arising from the accumulated arrears of the war years. Since then, it has been necessary to modify the original plan when later experience showed it to be desirable. In addition, during the middle of the period covered in this report it was possible, because of additional funds made available to the board, to plan extensions in establishments and buildings, and to provide better psychiatric facilities. However, it is only intended to deal with broad changes and larger trends in this article.

At the beginning of this period, the Mental Health Committee decided that each of the large mental hospitals should be given its own Hospital Management Committee. When it is considered that the board had virtually 9 months to organize the administrative structure of the region, it is greatly to their credit that the pattern set up at that time, although modified since, has remained fundamentally the same and has worked extremely well. Modifications of the original plan for the grouping of hospitals were made when later experience showed them to be desirable. The public assistance institutions presented a major problem, because of the mixed population to be found in them. Chronic cases of physical illness, psychotics and mental defectives were often found together in the same institution, with such medical care as could be provided by a busy local practitioner. As far as possible, those institutions coming to the Mental Health Committee were divided between its two principal branches, and each public assistance institution was then transferred to an appropriate group. In each case, the institution was made an annexe to the parent hospital, so that transfers between them (up to the commencement of the Mental Health Act, 1959) could be made without statutory formalities. The final stage of this arrangement, in an attempt to segregate the different types of patients, has been a slow process and is not yet complete. Most of these patients are old and have been in their institutions for a long time, so that to up-root them from familiar surroundings would not be in their best interests.

Allocation of Beds

In considering the allocation of beds, the Mental Health Committee found that the situation in London was a little complex, particularly in the case of mental hospitals. In Epsom and not far from it were assembled more London County Council hospitals than the other three metropolitan regions possessed together, and within the south-west part of London stood Springfield and Tooting Bec. After a joint study of the problem by the four metropolitan regions, certain hospitals were alienated to other regions for all practical purposes. Cane Hill was to serve the south-east, and Long Grove went to reinforce Claybury in the north-east. Horton served areas in the north-west and Springfield too was made available to that region, since it previously belonged to the Middlesex County Council. These arrangements proved satisfactory and have remained much as they were. Tooting Bec, because of its unusual arrangements for the admission of older patients, has been made available in equal shares to all four regions. It is, however, appropriate to mention here that following the Hospital Plan, it is now considered desirable and necessary to provide a local or district service for psychiatric patients. In the circumstances, negotiations are taking place between the four metropolitan boards, so that the original arrangements made in 1948 should cease, as soon as the other three metropolitan boards are able to accept responsibility for their own patients at hospitals in their own region.

The board then proceeded to a further subdivision of the hospitals retained to serve the south-west part of London. Each psychiatric hospital left to it was allocated a definite area to serve with out-patient illness in that area, and it was intended that the hospital should come to regard itself as standing in the same relation to its catchment area as the county hospital to its own county. It proved possible to make this division of catchment areas largely in terms of whole boroughs, except where the Minister himself had divided them by regional boundaries. Thus, Banstead serves the former metropolitan boroughs of Battersea, Chelsea, Fulham, Hammersmith, Kensington, and Westminster, as far as these lie within the region.

The board decided not to set up any form of bed-finding organization and the hospitals passed overnight to a state of local autonomy when the National Health Service Act came into force. In the counties and in Croydon County Borough, catchment areas have remained much as they were. Separate arrangements were made in the case of special hospitals such as Belmont, the Cassel, Holloway Sanatorium and Roffey Park.

It will be seen from the appendices that the increase in resident population was already slowing up in 1954. In 1955 a decrease occurred for the first time, and has continued since then.

The Mental Health Act

The period under review has been marked by the coming into force of the Mental Health Act, whose main aims were to shift the emphasis from hospital admission to community care, and to encourage such admissions as are necessary to be on an informal basis. The board may well congratulate itself on having anticipated the latter object by several years, as most of its hospitals were already accepting informal admissions. In some it was already the rule rather than the exception when the Mental Health Act came into operation in November 1960. On 1 April 1953, parts of four mental hospitals, namely Graylingwell, Netherne, St. Ebba's and Warlingham Park, were de-designated from the provision of the Lunacy and Mental Treatment Acts, to enable patients to be admitted directly without any formality. These experiments were the basis of the board's Evidence to the Royal Commission on Mental Illness.

The Worthing Experiment was begun in January 1957 under the direction of Dr. Joshua Carse, and combined visiting of patients in the home by a consultant team with the provision of day hospital facilities at The Acre, Worthing—a separate building in the town attached to Graylingwell, the parent hospital. The experiment was later extended to the Chichester area. The venture aroused tremendous interest, not only in this country but also internationally.

Mental Subnormality

In the case of mental deficiency institutions, the problem was peculiar. In disposing mental hospitals in London, the board had been able to look at London alone, but in the case of mental deficiency this was impossible. As a number of local authorities had provided no accommodation of their own, it was necessary for the available institutions to be divided equally throughout the region. After the London County Council colonies had been allocated mainly between the four metropolitan regions, catchment areas were drawn up as in the case of mental hospitals. Later on, it was necessary to alter the original arrangements, and accommodation is now distributed on the basis of population and estimated needs. Until recently, provision was made for patients from other metropolitan regions, and Hampshire and Portsmouth in the Wessex Region, but these arrangements have now ceased, except that accommodation is made available at St. Lawrence's Hospital for patients from the London part of the north-east region.

Various small schemes in the early years produced additional accommodation, and the board has recently arranged for a change of use at St. Ebba's Hospital, previously a psychiatric hospital, in order to provide much-needed accommodation for subnormal and severely subnormal patients. The number of out-patient clinics has increased considerably since 1948 and the medical staff at these hospitals are thus enabled to decide which cases on their waiting lists are in most urgent need of admission.

The Minister of Health accepted the Royal Commission's recommendations on informal admissions to mental deficiency hospitals in advance of the Mental Health Act, and issued a circular in January 1958 about their implementation. The circular was put into effect with varying enthusiasm by hospitals, but it is appropriate to record that the Fountain Hospital was able to de-certify all their patients, and become the first mental deficiency hospital in the country to be wholly de-designated.

As mentioned previously, the reduction in the number of in-patients in hospitals for the mentally ill has continued since 1955. Between 31 December 1956 and the end of 1964, the resident population has fallen by 3348, i.e. from 21,490 to 18,142. This shows an average yearly reduction of just over 400, but indications are that this rate is likely to decrease. Overcrowding is being eliminated slowly and it is pleasing to note that at the end of 1964, the over-all situation showed little or no overcrowding at more than half of the hospitals concerned. The situation in the subnormality field is not so encouraging, as the resident population has remained much the same, including a large measure of overcrowding. It seems likely that improvement in this branch of the service will not take place for a number of years, or until such time as new hospitals are provided. The change of use at St. Ebba's Hospital has helped to alleviate the position slightly, but it was never anticipated by the board that this would solve the problem in the region.

One hospital in the region, the Fountain at Tooting, provided accommodation for about 500 subnormal and severely subnormal patients, most of whom were children, and had done excellent clinical work in appalling conditions, in buildings erected temporarily in 1890 to meet the emergency of a fever epidemic. At the same time, the occupancy of Queen Mary's Hospital for Children, Carshalton, had been steadily falling, to about a third of its capacity. The board in October 1959 took this opportunity of establishing the first comprehensive children's hospital at Queen Mary's by evacuating the derelict building at Tooting and rehousing the subnormal children at Queen Mary's and the remaining patients at St. Ebba's. The merger has been a great success, and the comprehensive hospital at Carshalton may well prove to be a pattern for the future.

Integration

Since the establishment of the comprehensive hospital at Carshalton, the board turned its attention to the problems created in this region by the large number of psychiatric beds (28,000), as compared with the general beds (14,000). The outstanding trend of the past few years has been the attempt to integrate psychiatric services with the work of the general hospitals. In the past, this amounted to little more than a small observation unit, with the subsequent transfer of patients needing psychiatric treatment to the separate psychiatric hospitals. The only active treatment, as such, in general hospitals occurred in one or two small units in teaching hospitals.

With the inception of the 10-year plan, although progress in this region has been severely hampered by lack of money (as indeed throughout the country), each plan for a district hospital includes a psychiatric unit of at least 60 beds. As the carrying-out of this work in this region is somewhat remote in time (with one exception), the board has felt it necessary to establish psychiatric units immediately in existing general hospitals by adaptation, and by new building of light construction. The first of these will be opened in 1966 and will probably be followed by others, as soon as finances permit.

The problem, however, remains with the large percentage of psychiatric patients for whom medium-stay treatment or long-term custodial care is appropriate, and numerically, this amounts to a very high percentage of the present patient population.

Although the establishment of these units is a progressive and desirable step, it clearly has immediate repercussions upon those psychiatric hospitals which had made a special point of increasing their active psychiatric treatment. Reference has already been made to this and to the early attempts in this region at de-designation, which rapidly became the general pattern. The board was anxious that by establishing special units, it would not be putting the clock back in terms of the standard of care for those patients who would remain in the psychiatric hospitals. Accordingly, an attempt was made to offset this by a process of administrative amalgamation with general groups.

Apart from the comprehensive children's hospital already mentioned, the board has brought into effect six amalgamations, of which five are between general and psychiatric hospitals. It is too early to assess what importance this move will have, but there is no doubt that already it has fostered a closer understanding of the problems between the staff, both medical and lay, serving each hospital, as well as ensuring that a single management committee, in recommending capital expenditure to the board, does this on a basis of comparative need between hospitals previously isolated. Although there is a feeling that this might have been to the detriment of the psychiatric hospital, in fact, in some cases the reverse has been the result. Quite clearly, amalgamation succeeds more easily where the hospitals are not separated geographically by too great a distance, and it is in these groups that the beneficial effects will no doubt first develop.

Conclusion

In conclusion, although much progress has been made, and the standard and quality of treatment in the psychiatric hospitals is very different today from when the board took over in 1947, much yet remains to be done. Future developments will centre around a re-organization of the catchment areas, where possible, to bring the psychiatric hospital closer to the area which it serves, so that the links with the local community, encouraged in the Mental Health Act and by the Ministry of Health, can be extended. Although there is a popular belief, borne out by some figures, that the bed population is falling, in actual fact there is an increased demand for psychiatric treatment, which is revealed by the greater turnover.

Another important factor in the metropolitan area is the increasing interest which is being taken by the teaching hospitals, not only in the shorter-stay patient but also in the care of the long-term patient, in connection with rehabilitation and return to the community. The medical schools are increasingly interested in teaching their students on the community as a whole, and discussions at present taking place with the teaching hospitals will have this trend very much in mind.

Great as the change has been in the past 18 years, the two outstanding problems which the board will need to face to continue the improvement, are firstly, an increase in the amount of money available for providing services, both in terms of building and staff, and secondly, the establishment of closer and more realistic links with the other authorities responsible in the health field. Ultimately, it may be possible to serve the psychiatric needs of a district hospital catchment area of 200,000 population, largely by the psychiatric unit in the district hospital, but with the large number of beds in our region serving communities outside, it will be many decades before this is realized. A promising start has, however, been made and it will be interesting to see how quickly the new conception can take root.

Appendix 1

(a) PATIENTS ADMITTED TO MENTAL HOSPITALS AND RESIDENTS ON 31 DECEMBER OF EACH YEAR 1949–64

Year	Total admitted per year	Total resident on 31 December	+ or − on total resident in previous year
1949	9,418	20,482	
1950	9,385	20,623	+ 141
1951	10,294	20,992	+ 369
1952	10,846	21,405	+ 413
1953	12,388	21,718	+ 313
1954	12,510	21,858	+ 140
1955	12,913	21,771	− 87
1956	13,691	21,490	− 281
1957	14,702	21,003	− 487
1958	15,305	20,756	− 247
1959	15,934	20,226	− 530
1960	16,444	19,706	− 520
1961	16,809	19,379	− 327
1962	17,079	18,754	− 625
1963	17,418	18,416	− 338
1964	17,085	18,142	− 274

(b) MENTAL HOSPITAL BEDS AT 31 DECEMBER 1964

Hospital	Available beds
Banstead	2,005
Brookwood	1,740
Cane Hill	2,231
Graylingwell	1,210
Holloway	637
Horton	1,605
Long Grove	1,850
Netherne	1,847
St. Ebba's	125
Springfield	1,910
Tooting Bec	2,002
Warlingham Park	1,121
West Park	1,975
Total	20,258

Appendix 2

(a) PATIENTS RESIDENT IN MENTAL SUBNORMALITY HOSPITALS ON 31 DECEMBER IN YEARS 1949–64

Year	Residents on 31 December	Year	Residents on 31 December
1949	6201	1957	6593
1950	6310	1958	6645
1951	6410	1959	6694
1952	6528	1960	6651
1953	6596	1961	6584
1954	6648	1962	6603
1955	6607	1963	6612
1956	6596	1964	6665

(b) MENTAL SUBNORMALITY HOSPITAL BEDS ON 31 DECEMBER 1964

Hospital	Available beds	
Botleys Park	1222	
Murray House	255	
Brook House	23	
Royal Hostel	23	
Sherborne House	25	
	———	1548
Queen Mary's	320	
South Side Home	82	
Ellen Terry Home	40	
Osborne House	47	
Brooklands	16	
The Turret	20	
St. Ebba's	390	
	———	915
Royal Earlswood	675	
Forest	322	
Farmfield	174	
	———	1171
St. Lawrence's	2180	
	———	2180
The Manor	1130	
	———	1130
Total		6944

30. The Work of a Junior Doctor in a Psychiatric Hospital

ROGER MORGAN

THIS article contains an account of a time study of the work of a Senior Registrar during a period of 3 weeks in August 1960 at a large mental hospital.

"In 1894 it was calculated that if each State hospital physician in Massachusetts worked ten hours a day and moved from patient to patient with the speed of light, he could perhaps give ten minutes daily to each patient" (Greenblatt, York and Brown, 1958). Under the same conditions, a doctor in an English mental hospital in 1960 would probably have been able to give some twenty minutes daily to each patient. The writer, who usually moves at about three miles per hour, felt that it would be interesting to discover how much his pedestrian pace kept him away from his patients, and to measure the amounts of time that he allocated to the various commitments of his job.

It seemed that the techniques of job analysis and time study would be appropriate to such an investigation. They have been used to study the work of general nurses (*The Work of Nurses in Hospital Wards*, 1953), and mental nurses (Manchester Regional Hospital Board, 1955), but so far as is known, they have not previously been applied to the work of doctors. "In recent years some attempts have been made, though to our knowledge none have been published, to estimate the amount of time which psychiatrists in mental hospitals actually spend in the care of patients. Psychiatrists are understandably reticent on this score. As professional men, they feel that the allocation of their time is their own personal responsibility, and that their work cannot be adequately measured by the number of minutes spent on this duty and that" (Jones and Sidebotham, 1962).

The present writer, who would probably have declined any invitation to become the subject of a time study organized by someone else, was perfectly willing, however, to act as a guinea pig in his own experiment. The aims of the investigation were formulated as follows:

1. To discover how much time the subject spent with his patients;
2. To establish whether long-stay patients received from the subject less medical attention than short-stay patients;
3. To measure the amount of time that was wasted.

The Setting in which the Study was Carried Out

The subject was a Senior Registrar working at Severalls Hospital, Colchester. At the time, the hospital had 1650 available beds and there were 1546 patients in residence. A new Physician Superintendent had taken office 7 months before. There were altogether fourteen doctors on the staff. Their case-load was approximately as shown in Table 1.

TABLE 1.

	Number of wards	Number of patients
Physician superintendent	—	—
Deputy physician superintendent	—	—
Consultant psychiatrist	2	58
S.H.M.O. 1	2	84 (inc. short-stay)
S.H.M.O. 2	2	103
S.H.M.O. 3	1	48 (all short-stay)
S.H.M.O. 4	1	61
Senior registrar	5	160
Registrar	3	197
J.H.M.O.	4	155
Locum J.H.M.O. 1	4	248
Locum J.H.M.O. 2	4	234
Locum J.H.M.O. 3	3	154
Locum J.H.M.O. 4	1	50 (+ holiday relief)

There was no organized system of consultant supervision, no organized firms, no ward rounds, no case conferences or clinical meetings, no formal teaching (or learning) and little continuity of ward tenure. There was, in fact, little difference between the roles of senior and junior doctors. The traditional daily 10 o'clock office meeting, attended by all the doctors, had been abolished 15 months earlier. Three months earlier, the system of days off for doctors had been changed; previously, one could take off any one of the 7 days of the week, in the assurance that one's wards would be "covered" by the duty doctor, but the change introduced Sunday as the day off for all but two of the medical staff. After the first week of this study, the system for admitting patients was changed; previously, they were seen first at the Centre by the duty doctor, who filled in the statement of particulars and allocated them to a ward. The change involved their being admitted in a pre-arranged ward by a nurse, and the duty doctor was thus freed to do other work.

The subject had 6 years' experience in psychiatry and had been on the staff of the hospital for 16 months. Under nominal consultant supervision, he was in medical charge of five wards, all of them in the main building, and containing 160 patients. He had worked in one of these wards (housing women patients) for 15 months and in the remaining four wards (for men) for 13 months. He therefore had a working knowledge of his patients at the time of the study, and had assembled most of the available information about them. The length of time that the patients had been in hospital is shown in Table 4. Detailed information about the patients, their diagnoses, the patterns of ward management, their staffing arrangements and medical equipment, and the distances between them and other departments visited by the subject, were all recorded at the time and are available on request; shortage of space forbids their publication here.

The following miscellaneous items of information about the hospital are relevant to an understanding of the findings described later. The subject had a particular interest in a "factory", founded 8 months earlier in the hospital, in which 25 long-stay male patients manufactured wooden toys, and in addition to visits to this factory, he attended the weekly meeting of the staff concerned in its management. He acted as general practitioner to the resident nurses, and was committed to visiting the male and female staff sick bays, at or soon after 9 a.m. each day. The Centre was the term used by staff and patients to describe the front entrance to the hospital and the adjoining telephone switchboard, Committee Room, Medical Superintendent's office, Medical Secretaries' office and (upstairs) the doctors' quarters and dining room. Each Monday afternoon, the subject worked at the psychiatric out-patient clinic at the general hospital in Colchester. On Tuesdays at 2.30 p.m., he attended the Forum, which was a meeting of doctors, nurses and other staff from all sections of the hospital. On Wednesdays at 12 noon, he attended a meeting of patients and staff of the women's ward, which was followed by lunch and a meeting of the staff of the same ward. Each third Wednesday at 7 p.m., there was a meeting of the combined staffs of three of the four wards for men. During the second and third weeks of the study, because another doctor was on holiday, the subject was given two of his wards to look after, containing 85 male patients.

Emergencies and admissions were the responsibility each day of two doctors "on duty". It was the custom in this hospital for the duty to be shared equally by all doctors of Senior Registrar status and below, though the numbers available would vary according to the staff situation and people on holiday. It was the subject's responsibility to arrange the duty rota. Each week during the study, six doctors were available, which represents an average number, and the share that fell to the subject was as follows:

Each Tuesday, he was on duty from 9 a.m. until the following morning at 9 a.m., with responsibility for the male side of the hospital. Each Friday, he was on duty from 9 a.m. until 6 p.m. (or later if duty commitments were not completed by then), with responsibility for the female side of the hospital. On the third weekend, he was on duty at the hospital on the Saturday from 9 a.m. to 1 p.m., on call at home from then until 9 a.m. on the Sunday, and then on duty at the hospital until 9 a.m. the following morning. This represents an average cycle of duty commitments, and it was because weekend duty came round every three weeks that this length of time was chosen for the study. Full details of the duties of the duty doctor were recorded at the time, but the only item out of ten recorded that requires mention here is the obligation to "do a tea round". This could be done at any time after 5 p.m., and involved visiting three specified wards, as well as any other wards where one might be asked to call.

Method of Study

The first stage in the planning of this study was an analysis by the subject of his working day. Experience gained during a preliminary observation period showed that the general lines of the analysis were sufficiently realistic, but a few alterations and additions had to be made. The outcome of this was a list of 38 elements (full specifications of these are available on application to the author). These 38 elements fall into eight groups, as follows:

A. Time spent in the presence of patients.
B. Time spent discussing patients with other people.
C. Paper work.
D. Other commitments which reduce the time available for hospital patients.
E. Personal.
F. Miscellaneous.
G. Time spent on duty between 8 p.m. and 9 a.m. when not required to do anything.
H. Time-wasting activities.

These groups of elements will not be elaborated at this point, but will be discussed in the next section. (See also Fig. 1.)

Having completed the preliminary job analysis and made a provisional plan for carrying out a time study of his work, the subject obtained the services, as observer, of a young, intelligent male staff nurse. Discussions began between the subject and the observer, who quickly showed his energy and enthusiasm, and made several contributions to the final plan.

Six days were available for practice before the study began. Equipped with a home-made study board, the observer soon gained experience with a stop-watch, having never handled one before. Six days is a short time to achieve perfection with an instrument that is said to need 3 weeks to master, but we were dealing with comparatively long periods of time, and it is felt that in these circumstances, an adequate degree of accuracy was obtained.

During the 6-day preliminary study, the opportunity was taken of explaining to everyone that we saw, the method and purpose of the study. Discussion was encouraged, and in view of certain prejudices, suspicions and misapprehensions known to exist about time and motion studies, we were not satisfied to leave the topic until two points in particular had been established. Firstly, that the task was self-imposed and the subject was not in need of any well-meaning help, with which to frustrate some attempt from "higher up" to spy on him. Secondly, that everyone would help most by being as natural as possible, as slow or brisk, as chatty or as relevant as they were accustomed to be. The nurse who "just put on the blood pressure cuff this time to help you with your time study, Doctor" was one who needed a little further explanation.

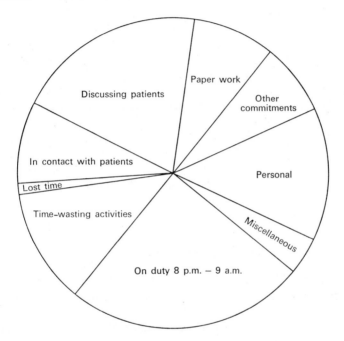

FIG. 1. Proportions of time spent in all activities.

We wondered if senior nursing staff would be inhibited by, or resentful of the presence of a junior nurse in their discussions with the doctor of hospital or personal matters. We found no evidence of this, which was probably due to the respect for his nursing and personal qualities which the observer had earned previously, and to the tact and discretion with which he succeeded in his deliberate attempt to efface himself at such times. The patients showed remarkably little reaction to the presence of the observer; this may have been due partly to the subject's usual (but not invariable) habit of interviewing patients in the company of a nurse anyway, and partly to the preliminary explanations that had been given.

It was not practicable for the subject and observer to remain together throughout the working day and they separated at meal times. In all cases, the meal time was recorded as such and no record could be kept of the clinical discussions, etc., that are a usual feature of such gatherings. The observer did not sit in at the Superintendent's meeting on Tuesday mornings, but waited outside. Again, when the subject read medical books and journals (which were kept in the doctors' sitting room), this passed unrecorded. The study has been less comprehensive on this account, but so long as it is appreciated that these additional activities do occupy some of one's time, it was felt neither necessary nor practicable to measure them.

The specimen time sheet in Appendix 1 shows the form in which the observer recorded the events. Each day, the recorded times had to be transferred to another sheet, on which were listed the 38 elements. This was done sometimes by subject and observer in the hospital, if a suitable opportunity arose, and otherwise by the subject at home. The daily sheets had to be compiled, added up and balanced, and each week the daily totals in each category were transferred to a weekly sheet, and these similarly onto a final sheet at the end of the study. Each sheet had to balance, and all this took between 2 and 3 hours each day. This work was done in the hospital only when the subject would otherwise have been doing nothing, e.g. after a meal or in the evening on duty, and the time spent on it in the hospital has been recorded as "doing nothing". When it was done at home, it has not been recorded at all.

It was the subject's aim during the course of this study to work at his normal pace, to disregard completely the fact that he was under observation, and to carry on the same pattern of activities to which he had become accustomed over many previous months. He started the preliminary 6-day period with the deliberate intention of avoiding an exhibition of quite unusual energy. This study was not devised as a way of demonstrating the subject's long hours of unremitting application to duty, and indeed, the figures quoted later give no particular indication of this.

It was realized that nothing remains quite the same under observation, but it was hoped that awareness of this would minimize any tendency to deviate in either direction away from the habitual pace. In fact, it was found on the first morning of the preliminary period that as much had been done in the first hour as it usually took an hour and a half to get through. This effect became less marked as the 6 practice days went by, and it seems that it had settled down to the irreducible minimum by the time the 3-weeks study began, for it appeared to be no more and no less at the end than at the beginning of that period.

In fact, it was felt that this study would be of value only to the extent that it gave accurate and realistic measurements of the time spent in various activities during 3 *normal* working weeks.

Analysis of Recordings

The total times recorded over 3 weeks under each element are shown in Appendix 2. The 38 elements fall into eight groups, and the total times divided by three give the average time (to the nearest minute) spent each week in the various activities, as shown in Table 2.

TABLE 2.

		Time		% of total
A.	In direct contact with patients	5 hr	35 min	8·6
B.	Discussing patients with other people	12 hr	31 min	19·4
C.	Paper work	5 hr	27 min	8·4
D.	Other commitments	5 hr	10 min	8·0
E.	Personal	9 hr	26 min	14·5
F.	Miscellaneous	1 hr	55 min	3·0
G.	On duty between 8 p.m. and 9 a.m.	16 hr	9 min	24·9
H.	Time-wasting activities	7 hr	50 min	12·1
I.	Lost time		41 min	1·1
Total		64 hr	44 min	100

If, however, one omits "Personal activities" and all time spent "On duty from 8 p.m. to 9 a.m.", and "Lost time", the times and percentages are as shown in Table 3, and the proportions of time are shown in Fig. 2.

TABLE 3.

		Time		% of total
A.	In direct contact with patients	5 hr	35 min	14·5
B.	Discussing patients with other people	12 hr	31 min	32·6
C.	Paper work	5 hr	27 min	14·2
D.	Other commitments	5 hr	10 min	13·4
F.	Miscellaneous	1 hr	55 min	4·9
H.	Time-wasting activities	7 hr	50 min	20·4
Total		38 hr	28 min	100

These times will now be amplified and considered, group by group.

A. IN DIRECT CONTACT WITH PATIENTS

Of the 5 hours 35 minutes per week spent in contact with patients, half was spent in routine examinations at the statutory intervals prescribed by the

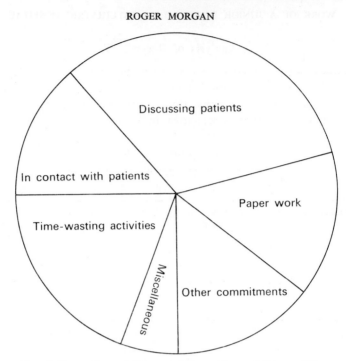

FIG. 2. Proportions of time spent in positive activities omitting
"Personal" and "On duty 8 p.m.—9 a.m.", and "Lost time".

Board of Control,* 2 hours 33 minutes being devoted to interviews and 13
minutes to physical examinations. However, another 1 hour and 15 minutes
were spent in interviewing patients at times other than the statutory intervals,
and this amounts to almost exactly half as much again. To anyone who assumes
that psychiatric treatment consists largely of listening and talking to individual
patients, it may seem rather surprising that no more than 3 hours 48 minutes
were spent each week in this way. A further 37 minutes per week, however,
were spent in a group situation at the patients' meeting in the women's ward.

Physical examinations, demanded by the appearance of symptoms or signs
(as opposed to routine examinations called for only because a year had
elapsed since the last one), occupied only 19 minutes per week, but this was
half as much again as the routine examinations took. Special treatments
occupied only 10 minutes in the 3 weeks, and they figure here only because
the subject had to deputize for a sick colleague in the administration of three
electrical treatments.

Admitting patients at the centre took 26 minutes in the first week, after
which, as previously explained, the system was changed. This is counted
(somewhat fallaciously) as 9 minutes per week. Examinations in the admission

* Since the Mental Health Act came into force on 1 November 1960, these have become
obsolete, but they were in force at the time of the study.

wards of newly admitted patients occupied 26 minutes per week. This was another duty commitment, and as none of the junior doctors sharing the duties worked at the time in the admission wards, it always happened that they had no further contact with the patient in question during his or her stay in hospital, unless the patient was at some later stage transferred to one of their wards. At the end of this study (but not as a result of it), this system was also changed, so that patients admitted in the mornings or afternoons were examined by the doctors working in the admission wards who would be responsible for their further treatment. This administrative change (1) established continuity of patient–doctor relationship, (2) eliminated a duplication of physical examinations (a brief superficial one by the duty doctor on the patient's arrival and a fuller one the next day), (3) avoided a day's delay in the institution of treatment, and (4) saved the duty doctor from performance of a disagreeably impersonal task. (See Fig. 3.)

B. Discussing Patients with Other People

This group of activities could have been classified in several ways. Elements 13–19 suggested themselves as obviously definable and discrete activities, with an individuality in terms of the other people present, and in most cases of the topics of discussion also. There remains the mass of less formal discussions

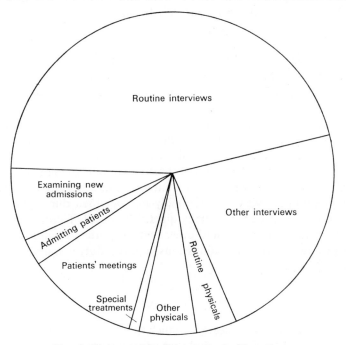

Fig. 3. Time spent in direct contact with patients.

held with a great number and wide variety of people. It seemed best to classify these basically according to the topic of discussion, and they are contained in elements 9–12.

Reading the nurse's daily report is a clearly defined activity but it may be interrupted by questions to the nurse, and items in the report may give rise to brief discussions of patients, both as individuals and in groups, the topic changing rapidly from one to another with a speed that makes accurate recording very difficult. It was decided to include such discussions arising out of the report in the same category with the report itself, to avoid this difficulty, and it was found that the exchange of information on matters contained in the report usually ended at the moment when the report book was closed. This exchange took 1 hour and 15 minutes each week. At this time, daily reports tended to be somewhat perfunctory and to contain information of greater administrative than psychiatric interest or importance. This is not to be wondered at, because each evening, the daily report had to be copied onto a separate piece of paper and taken to the Matron's office or the Chief Male Nurse's office. This system has certain advantages, but it discourages lively or detailed reports.

"Discussing individual patients" was the largest item in this group, and amounted to 2 hours and 24 minutes per week. "Discussing a group or ward of patients" occupied 61 minutes per week and "matters of general hospital interest" were discussed for 1 hour and 16 minutes per week. These totals, of course, exclude the time spent discussing similar topics at formal meetings, which will be listed shortly.

The discussions included in elements 9–12, just described, were held with a variety of people, as follows: nurses, doctors, occupational therapists, social workers, secretaries, and people in charge of hospital workshops and departments where patients work.

The remaining items in group B "Discussing patients with other people" can now be listed. Staff meetings occupied 54 minutes per week, involving only ward nursing staff. The Forum lasted for 52 minutes per week. Meetings with the Physician Superintendent occupied 63 minutes. Seeing relatives took 37 minutes; this activity varied in amount quite markedly from week to week, and a representative view was probably not obtained during the 3 weeks, which in this respect were unusually quiet. The weekly factory meeting went on for 78 minutes per week, and other factory matters occupied another 71 minutes per week. Arranging admissions (a purely duty commitment) took 40 minutes per week. (See Fig. 4.)

C. Paper Work

This occupied each week nearly as much time as was spent in direct contact with patients, and bearing in mind that some note-taking was carried out in the course of interviews, it is probably true to say that the subject spent more time on paper work than in actual conversation with patients.

The total time under this heading was 5 hours and 27 minutes per week. The largest item (taking 1½ hours) was the writing of summaries of long-stay patients' notes. This activity was used by the subject to occupy afternoons on duty when nothing was happening but, for example, an admission was expected, which would require prompt attention and prevented work in the distant wards or in the factory, where there was no telephone.

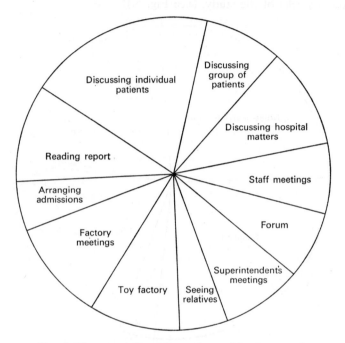

Fig. 4. Time spent discussing patients with other people.

Writing notes in the casepapers occupied altogether nearly 2 hours per week, 84 minutes of this being after interview and the balance of 30 minutes (a surprisingly high figure), without a previous interview. The sort of note written without interview was the final note after a patient had been discharged, a record of an interview with a relative, a change in the dose of a drug based on a nurse's report, etc.

The writing and signing of all manner of forms and cards took 38 minutes per week. This was less than might have been expected, probably because wherever possible, the forms were made out by the nurse, leaving only clinical details and his signature for the doctor to insert. When planning this study, it was felt that the completion of leave passes wasted time, and this was kept in a separate category for that reason, but in fact, it occupied only 3 minutes per week.

Item 24, "Daily correspondence", is also to do mainly with patients' leave but deals in addition with a wide variety of other matters, familiar to all working in mental hospitals. It occupied 70 minutes per week and the subject's habit was to write longhand replies for subsequent typing. Reports on discharged patients, however, were dictated, and the time taken for this was 12 minutes per week; there happened to be fewer discharges than usual during the 3 weeks of the study. (See Fig. 5.)

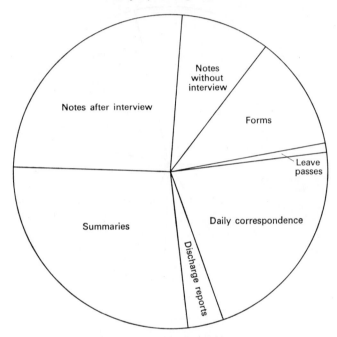

FIG. 5. Time spent on paper work.

D. OTHER COMMITMENTS

Attention to sick resident staff took 52 minutes per week. The study was done in August, and it is probable that the time recorded is shorter than it would have been at other times of the year. The subject had between 70 and 80 staff on his list at the time.

The weekly out-patient clinic occupied an average of 3 hours and 38 minutes on Monday afternoons. It was not relevant to the purpose of the study to analyse this time at all, which included the time (about 12 minutes) taken to travel to the clinic. The observer took an afternoon off on this day, and the time of finishing the clinic was noted by the subject. The total time was recorded only to measure its contribution to the working week and to assess the time it occupied that would otherwise have been available for in-patients.

No secretary was provided at the general hospital, and letters were dictated the following day at the mental hospital. This and other business arising from the out-patient clinic occupied 40 minutes per week. One large item which has inflated this figure was the need to study a casepaper (44 minutes), received from another hospital, in which one of the out-patients had previously been an in-patient.

E. Personal Affairs

These were recorded under one heading but have been analysed subsequently. Meals (including morning coffee, lunch, afternoon tea and, on duty days, supper also) occupied 8 hours and 25 minutes per week. All other personal affairs occupied 61 minutes per week and consisted of the following activities: reading personal correspondence (mainly advertisements from drug firms), buying cigarettes at the canteen, talking to other people about personal matters, reading notices, going to the toilet, telephoning the subject's wife, and changing coats and leaving hospital at the end of the day. There was also a large item of 43 minutes spent at a committee meeting of the hospital cricket club.

F. Miscellaneous

Miscellaneous activities occupied 115 minutes per week. Of this total, 22 minutes per week were spent on what were called "Conventional courtesies" (see Appendix 2). Five minutes per week were spent washing hands, and 35 minutes per week walking inside wards. This was regarded as unavoidable if there is a need to visit wards at all (as opposed to work places), and it has been differentiated from "Walking in corridors and grounds" which, unless some administrative effort is made to keep it to a minimum, is very wasteful of time (see elements 33 and 36 in Appendix 2).

"Other miscellaneous" items occupied the balance of 53 minutes per week. The only large item here was a visit one afternoon, lasting 1 hour, to a number of patients working in open employment in the local town (this 1 hour in 3 weeks contributes 20 minutes to the weekly average). The remaining items are all small, none amounting to more than 5 minutes per week as follows: telling telephone operator one's whereabouts while on duty, looking at the admission book to see how many admissions were expected, arranging the doctors' duty rota, first-aid to staff casualty, escorting a solicitor acquaintance to visit another doctor's patient, borrowing another stopwatch when the original one broke, arranging to give lectures to nurses, examining physically a nurse who had newly joined the staff, seeing a drug traveller, obtaining drugs from the dispensary in the evening, filling pen and trying to make a torch work.

G. ON DUTY 8 P.M.–9 A.M.

The author has found it very difficult to decide how best to treat this part of the working week. One consideration that had to be taken into account was that the observer was not available, so there could be no detailed recordings. Time spent in bed, getting up and having breakfast could conveniently have been classified under "Personal affairs" in Group E, and all other time could have been classified under "Time-wasting activities" in Group H, but this did not seem altogether satisfactory. If one is at the hospital only because of being on duty, it seems legitimate in the late evening to relax and do what one pleases, in the intervals of duty commitments. "Doing nothing" at this time of day is a different matter from "doing nothing" in working hours, which suggests either laziness or some fault in personal or administrative arrangements. One purpose of this study was to identify such faults. The inactivity that they caused would have been obscured if late evening inactivity had not been separately classified here.

Similarly, there seemed to be good reasons for presenting under "Personal affairs" only those activities which figure there now because they occur in the ordinary working day. If hours of sleep had been included under "Personal affairs", this category would have lost any precision that it may have.

For these reasons, it was decided to fix arbitrary time-limits (8 p.m.–9 a.m.), and to allocate to this special category all time spent in activities that were not obviously to be classified elsewhere. Sixteen hours and 9 minutes per week are shown in this category, which is almost a quarter of all the time spent at the hospital in one average week. It is this figure which inflates the total time of the working week somewhat misleadingly to 64 hours 44 minutes. Four nights were spent at the hospital on duty during the 3 weeks. A simple calculation shows that, between the hours of 8 p.m. and 9 a.m. on the 4 duty nights, a total of 3 hours 33 minutes was spent working, and this has been classified elsewhere.

H. TIME-WASTING ACTIVITIES

Walking in corridors and grounds occupied 2 hours 53 minutes per week. The tea round involved a long walk, of course, which could be shortened sometimes if a telephone call established that nothing was required. However, this amounted to only 17 minutes per week. The remainder of the time was spent walking between the subject's own wards and other places he was bound to visit during the ordinary day's work. A car was used very little during the 3 weeks; because of the geography of the hospital and the positions of the wards in question, it usually did not help at all. It is likely that other doctors, especially those with outlying villas to visit, spent more time than the subject in walking, though in their case, a car might have been of more use.

There were 28 minutes' delay per week. Altogether in the 3 weeks, there were 75 episodes of delay. On 26 occasions, the delay was because the subject had to wait for the key to an office; 17 times, the delay was while a patient was fetched (unavoidable, and one would prefer to wait longer or more often rather than have patients lined up or brought to interview at the double); 13 times a nurse had to be found (apart from the 26 times above), and 6 times it was a matter of waiting for a meeting to begin.

The author was surprised to find that "Delay" occupied so little of his working time. The minor frustrations of daily work (calls to a distant telephone, waiting for instruments to be fetched, problems of convening patient, nurse, notes and medicine card, etc.) had loomed much larger in his estimation than the records show to be justified.

During an average week, 4 hours and 29 minutes were spent "doing nothing". As explained earlier, some work on this study was done at the hospital and recorded as "Doing nothing". Two hours 49 minutes per week while on duty with nothing particular to do were spent in this way. Another 1 hour and 22 minutes per week is the sum of short periods, when for example, there was time to spare before or after a meal, and the opportunity was taken of getting on with the same transposing and balancing of figures. Had the subject not been occupied on this special project, he might have had something else in hand and been working on that at these times, but would almost certainly have spent a substantial proportion in conversation, reading the newspaper, etc. In fact, during the 3 weeks, he was so unusually busy with the additional work connected with this study that only the balance of 18 minutes per week was spent in the latter way.

I. Lost Time

Finally, there is a small item of 41 minutes per week called "Lost time". If one times with a stopwatch and records a series of brief activities for say an hour, the sum of all the small periods of time never quite adds up to the hour, because a second or two is lost each time one stops and restarts the stopwatch. Lost time is the sum of all these seconds that passed by during manipulation of the watch (see Specimen Time Sheet in Appendix 1). The observer was using a watch so constructed that one click stopped it, the next click returned the hand to zero and the third click started it again; he would read the time between the first two clicks and record it after restarting the watch.

Patient–Doctor Time

One of the aims of this study was to obtain data from which could be calculated the amount of time that the average patient spends with his or her doctor. On the middle day of the 3 weeks (19.8.60), there were 160 patients in the subject's own wards and this number has been taken as constant throughout the 3 weeks. He spent 4 hours and 20 minutes per week on interviews and physical examinations (elements 1–4); 44 minutes of this were spent on patients other than his own (i.e. patients in the two wards belonging to other doctors who were away on holiday during part of the period, or patients in other people's wards whom he was asked to see while on duty), and this time has been deducted. This leaves 3 hours 36 minutes that he spent with individual patients of his own per week. This is about 1⅓ minutes per patient per week or 70 minutes per patient per year. This, however, is only a crude figure, which pays no regard to the patient's length of stay in hospital. When it is analysed, it will be seen that patients spent progressively less time with their doctor at individual interview the longer they had been in hospital (see Table 4).

TABLE 4.

	Length of stay in hospital in years				Totals
	< 1	1–10	11–20	> 20	
Time spent with individual patients in 1 week	137	54	15	10	216
Numbers of patients	43	50	22	45	160
Calculated time per patient per year	165	56	35	12	—

Times are in minutes to the nearest whole number.

Few people would contend, perhaps, that the limited time available for chronic patients is most profitably spent entirely on individual interviews. One's approach and contact is likely to be in part non-verbal or one may seek to form a therapeutic relationship over any one of a number of concrete topics. Equally, there is so much to be done in a hospital where modern methods are something of a novelty, in the way of reorganizing ward life and encouraging a different attitude in the nurses, that it may be felt one can make a more useful contribution by concentrating on such things as these and waiting for their indirect impact on the patients. This aspect of the work is contained in elements 6, 9–11, 13, 16, 20–26 and 31 in Appendix 2, including routine ward administrative work, staff meetings, all paper work, "conventional courtesies", group meetings of staff and patients and seeing relatives. These activities occupied the subject for 12 hours and 7 minutes per week. If this time had been spent on matters concerning every patient equally, it would amount to 236 minutes or nearly 4 hours per patient per year. It is not possible from the nature of several of the activities, and hence from the records that were kept, to break this figure down according to the patients' length of stay in the hospital.

Again, the discussions of matters of general hospital interest with individual colleagues and in the Forum and at the Superintendent's meetings and at factory meetings, ultimately make an impact on the patients, though the connection is less direct than in the case of the previous items. They (elements 12, 14, 15, 17, 18) occupied altogether 5 hours and 40 minutes per week, or in other words, 110 minutes per patient per year.

Viewed in this way, the average patient may be said to receive nearly 7 hours of medical attention per year, made up as follows:

Individual interview with doctor	70 min.
Doctor's contribution to treatment by team	236 min.
Indirect impact of community methods	110 min.
	416 min.

Conclusion

It must be emphasized that the findings of this study relate to conditions in 1960.

In an average working week of nearly 65 hours (if one includes meals and nights on duty) or 38½ hours (if one excludes these), the subject spent only 5 hours and 35 minutes in direct verbal contact with his patients.

The amount of time spent with individual patients varied according to their length of previous stay in hospital. It is calculated that the average patient admitted within the previous year would have received from the subject 165 minutes per year of his individual attention. The calculated amount of time devoted to the average individual patient becomes progressively less the longer he or she has been in hospital, and is only 12 minutes per year for the patient who has already been in hospital for over 20 years.

Such figures call for an examination of the way in which the subject spent the remainder of his working week, and in particular, of those parts of it which appear to have been spent wastefully. Nearly 3 hours were spent each week in walking in the corridors and grounds, from one to another of the wards and other places that the subject had to visit. His wards were all in the main building, so presumably other doctors spent even more time in walking if they were responsible for patients in outlying villas. This would seem to offer one justification (there are no doubt others too) for the administrative changes that would allow a doctor to work in a group of wards that are as close together as possible.

There was an average of nearly half-an-hour's "Delay" each week. Though irritating, this appears to be unavoidable. It could be reduced, however, if the doctor had a key to each ward office door, or if it was no longer felt necessary to keep these doors locked.

Four and a half hours have been recorded as "Doing nothing", but in fact all but 18 minutes of this time per week was spent on prompt analysis of the recordings of this study. This was felt at the time to be essential, for fear that the material would accumulate and become unmanageable if left any longer, but it now appears unfortunate that the findings should have been contaminated in this way.

The above findings relate only to the way in which the particular subject of this study occupied himself during 3 working weeks in 1960, in a particular hospital at a particular stage in its evolution. It may be that other doctors in the same hospital at the same time spent either more or less time in activities directly concerning their patients. The subject would have felt happier had the findings appeared more creditable than they do. It was a surprise to him that extraneous activities took up so much of his time, as they have been shown to do. It is to be hoped that other studies along similar lines will be conducted, that may lend support or otherwise to the findings reported here, and may indicate medical administrative arrangements that encourage more profitable use of a doctor's time.

Acknowledgements

This study has depended on the help of many people and the author would like to thank Mr. J. Goodlad, R.M.N., the observer, for his helpful contributions and accurate records; Dr. Russell Barton, Physician Superintendent of Severalls Hospital, for encouraging this investigation and allowing the results to be published; Mr. H. Kniveton, Chief Male Nurse, for the loan of his staff nurse; Mr. F. Glen, Senior Psychologist, for technical advice and help; Mr. D. J. Hooton, Group Secretary, for advice and for making available the resources of his department; Miss Wendy Steward and Miss R. M. Orme for secretarial help; and all nurses and other staff who helped by being natural and unaffected under the trying ordeal of being observed and timed.

References

GREENBLATT, M., YORK, and BROWN (1958), *From Custodial to Therapeutic Care in Mental Hospitals*, New York, Russell Sage Foundation.
The Work of Nurses in Hospital Wards (1953), London, Nuffield Provincial Hospitals Trust.
MANCHESTER REGIONAL HOSPITAL BOARD (1955), *The Work of the Mental Nurse*, Manchester University Press.
JONES, K. and SIDEBOTHAM, R. (1962), *Mental Hospitals at Work*, London, Routledge & Kegan Paul.

Appendix 1

SPECIMEN TIME SHEET

DATE: Wednesday, 24.8.60   TIME: 9 a.m.–10 a.m.

Place	Time (min)	Activity	Element no.
Corridors	2·32	Walking	36
Ward A	·05	Sick nurses	27
Corridors	1·05	Walking	36
Stairs	·20	Walking	33
Ward 7	1·40	Discussing summaries	12
Ward 7	·45	Reading and discussing report	9
Ward 7	·05	Signing medicine card	22
Ward 7	·35	Daily report—oral	9
Ward 7	3·44	Filling in D.P.1(U) (Gold)	22
Ward 7	·57	Discussing Gold	10
From 7 to 8	·21	Walking	33
Ward 8	·20	Delay (key)	37
Ward 8	1·10	Ward in general	11
Ward 8	·18	Signing prescriptions	22
Ward 8	·38	Talking about number of tablets sent from pharmacy	12
Ward 8	1·00	Report	9
Ward 8	·47	Looking at weights book	9
Ward 8	1·40	Discussing patients on pass	11
Ward 8	1·45	Discussing ward patients (individually)	10
Ward 8	·27	Walk to side room	33
Ward 8	4·01	Routine physical (Pugh)	3
Ward 8	·15	Walk to wash bowl	32
Ward 8	·55	Washing and drying hands	32
Ward 8	·39	Walk back to office	33
Ward 8	3·45	Reading casepaper, writing notes (Pugh)	20
Ward 8	13·23	Interviewing Cuppitman—routine mental	1
Ward 8	13·35	Interviewing Ericstrop—routine mental	1
Ward 8	2·02	Writing notes on Ericstrop	20
Total	58·58		
Lost time	1·02		
Total	60·00		

Appendix 2

TOTAL TIMES RECORDED UNDER EACH ELEMENT DURING PERIOD OF 3 WEEKS

Group	No.	Element	Totals for 3 weeks (min and sec)		Average per week to nearest min	
A In direct contact with patients	1	Interviewing patients—routine	458·12		153	
	2	Interviewing patients—not routine	224·24		75	
	3	Routine physical examination	39·12		13	
	4	Other physical examination	56·11		19	
	5	Special treatments	10·16		3	
	6	Patients' meetings	110·51		37	
	7	Admitting patients at Centre	26·00		9	
	8	Examining admissions to ward	77·24		26	
				1002·30		335[a]
B Discussing patients with other people	9	Reading and discussing report	225·59		75	
	10	Discussing individual patient	433·11		144	
	11	Discussing group of patients	184·20		61	
	12	Discussing matters of hospital interest	228·06		76	
	13	Staff meetings	161·28		54	
	14	Forum	155·34		52	
	15	Superintendent's meetings	190·44		63	
	16	Seeing relatives	111·01		37	
	17	Toy factory	212·36		71	
	18	Factory meetings	233·01		78	
	19	Arranging admissions	119·05		40	
				2255·05		751[a]
C Paper work	20	Writing notes after interview	250·47		84	
	21	Writing notes not seeing patient	90·49		30	
	22	Writing and signing forms	113·21		38	
	23	Signing leave passes	10·15		3	
	24	Daily correspondence	209·26		70	
	25	Reports on discharged patients	35·58		12	
	26	Writing summaries	270·00		90	
				980·36		327
D Other commitments	27	Attention to sick resident staff	155·19		52	
	28	Out-patients	655·31		218	
	29	Letters about out-patients	120·28		40	
				931·18		310
E Personal	30	Personal	1697·55		566	
				1697·55		566

[a] These figures are the sum of the averaged elements in the previous column. They are not exactly one-third of the group totals for 3 weeks.

Appendix 2 (*contd.*)

Group	No.	Element	Total for 3 weeks (min and sec)		Average per week to nearest min	
F Miscel- laneous	31 32 33 34	Conventional courtesies Washing hands Walking in wards Other miscellaneous	65·00 15·03 105·10 159·38	344·51	22 5 35 53	115
G On duty	35	Between 8 p.m. and 9 a.m.	2906·44	2906·44	969	969
H Time- wasting activities	36 37 38	Walking in corridors and grounds Delay Doing nothing	519·55 83·42 806·37	1410·14	173 28 269	470
Lost time			121·47	121·47	41	41
Total				11651·00		3884

31. The Education of Children in Hospitals for the Subnormal: a Survey of Admissions

PETER MITTLER and MARY WOODWARD

EACH year about 1300 children are admitted to hospitals for the subnormal in England and Wales. Very little is known about their previous educational history and still less about the educational facilities available for them in hospitals. No guidance on educational matters has come from the Ministry of Health and there is no evidence of any official interest in the work of hospital schools. The Scott Report (Ministry of Health, 1962) indicated that over 80% of supervisors and deputy supervisors had no qualifications of any kind.

It seems important, therefore, to collect information on the intelligence and previous educational history of a sample of children admitted to hospitals for the subnormal and to enquire about the educational facilities available.

This was the aim of a survey carried out by a working party of the British Psychological Society's English Division of Professional Psychologists; this survey was intended to complement a previous inquiry on adult admissions Castell and Mittler, 1965). A questionnaire was sent to each head of the psychology department of all twenty hospitals for the subnormal admitting children and employing psychologists. The first part of the questionnaire requested, for each child admitted in 1962, details of official classification, assessment procedures with test results wherever possible, and details of previous education. The second part was concerned chiefly with qualifications of teaching staff, pupil : teacher ratios and the work of the schools.

Of the twenty hospitals approached, seventeen sent the data requested; two could not obtain the necessary information because the psychologist worked part-time and the other hospital was unwilling to co-operate. As in our adult survey, the sample cannot be considered representative of the country's subnormality hospitals as a whole, since it excluded most of the smaller hospitals, the larger hospitals in the south-west and north of England, and all those without psychology departments. Comparison of the size of our sample with figures available for all hospitals in England and Wales (General Register Office, 1964) suggests that the 403 children described in this report represent approximately a 30% sample of all admissions under 16.

The seventeen hospitals investigated were far from uniform in respect of the kind of patients admitted and the provisions made for them. In particular,

548

one had a special unit for psychotic children, while another, at least during the year of the survey, admitted adolescents with behaviour problems to a special unit. Finally, the survey hospitals appear to be well above the national average in respect of the proportion of teaching staff with formal qualifications, as suggested by comparison with the figures published in the Scott Report (Ministry of Health, 1962).

Survey of Admissions to Seventeen Hospitals

CHARACTERISTICS OF THE SAMPLE

Data were received for 403 children, all of whom were admitted during 1962 to seventeen hospitals. One hospital sent data only for alternate admissions. Fifty-nine per cent were boys and 41% were girls.

AGE AND CLASSIFICATION

The ages and classifications of these children are summarized in Table 1. It will be seen that only 15% of admissions were under 5 years of age, a further quarter were under 8 years, and one-third were between 13 and 15 years. The age distribution varied considerably between hospitals, some catering for all age-groups, some mainly or entirely for adolescents.

Those classified as Severely Subnormal (SSN) comprise nearly three-quarters of the sample; 53% of these were under 8 years of age, and 19% between 13 and 15. On the other hand, four-fifths of those classified as Psychopathic Disorder (PD) and four-fifths of the Subnormal (SN) were in the 13–15 year age-range. A classification of Mental Illness (MI) was not found below the age of 5 years, and most of the younger children described as "withdrawn"

TABLE 1.

Classification and Age of 1962 Admissions (N = 403)

Age (yr–mos.)	Classification							
	SSN	SN	PD	MI	U/C	No Inf.	Totals	%
0–1 to 4–11	55	1	0	0	4	0	60	14·9
5–0 to 7–11	95	4	0	1	4	0	104	25·8
8–0 to 10–11	55	4	1	1	1	1	63	15·6
11–0 to 12–11	26	3	4	2	1	2	38	9·5
13–0 to 15–11	53	48	22	4	6	5	138	34·2
Totals	284	60	27	8	16	8	403	100·0

For meaning of abbreviations see text.

or "inaccessible" were unclassified (U/C). All but 17 of the sample were admitted informally.

PHYSICAL AND BEHAVIOUR DISORDERS

Table 2 shows the frequency of physical and behaviour disorders in the sample; 23% of the total were reported to have at least one motor, visual or auditory handicap; the motor handicap most frequently reported was cerebral palsy.

TABLE 2.

Frequency of Reported Physical and Behaviour Disorders in 1962 Admissions (N = 403)

Physical Handicaps		Behaviour Disorders	
	N		N
Motor handicap	51	Psychotic	34
Visual handicap	14	"Inaccessible",	
Auditory handicap	14	"unco-operative", etc.	40
Multiple handicaps	14	"Hyperactive", etc.	26
Total	93	Total	100

"Behaviour disturbance" is used merely as a blanket term for the three categories shown in Table 2; no specific questions about behaviour disturbance had been included in the questionnaire, but many respondents referred to a medical diagnosis of psychosis, and some also commented on the child's lack of social response or his inaccessibility in a test situation.

These comments have been classified into three categories, as shown in Table 2. Children were included in Category 1 only if they were described as psychotic or autistic. In addition, 10 children in Category 2 were described as inaccessible, mute, withdrawn or as making no social response; the remaining 30 children in this category could not be given a test because of limited co-operation. Those in Category 3 were described as hyperactive, destructive, negativistic, restless, or as showing poor concentration.

The reported incidence of behaviour disturbance must be regarded as a minimal estimate, since not all psychologists offered information on this point. Nevertheless, even this minimal estimate suggests that at least 10% of the total sample of admissions (34 in Category 1 and a further 10 in Category 2) were described as psychotic, autistic or withdrawn in a test situation, and that up to 25% of the sample could not be tested because of limited co-operation or disturbed behaviour.

PSYCHOLOGICAL ASSESSMENTS

Ninety per cent of the children were seen by a psychologist, but only 155 could be given a standardized intelligence test, e.g. a Wechsler or Binet-type scale. In another 120 cases other means of evaluation had to be used, including Gesell's developmental scale (Gesell, 1954), the Vineland Social Maturity Scale (Doll, 1953) and pre-school tests used for children below the "floor" of the Wechsler or Binet. Results of these assessments could often be given only in approximate form and will not be tabulated in this paper. A further 87 children were seen by a psychologist but could not be assessed, either because of limited co-operation or for lack of a suitable test. Finally, 41 children were not examined because they were not referred or because they were in hospital for too short a time.

Table 3 presents data only on the 155 testable children who were given Wechsler, Binet or Merrill–Palmer tests. Data are presented as frequency distributions, and results on similar tests, e.g. different versions of the Binet, have been combined to simplify the presentation. The 155 testable children include 24 who were physically handicapped or emotionally disturbed.

It will be seen that 98 (24%) of the total sample of admissions had IQs over 50; of these, 57 (14% of the total sample) had IQs over 70, and 15 (4%) had IQs over 100.

TABLE 3.

IQs of Testable Children Admitted to Subnormality Hospitals in 1962 (N = 155)

Scales	IQ Range	< 50	50–59	60–69	70–79	80–99	100+	Totals
Wechsler	46–140	6	10	10	13	10	8	57
Binet	18–108	49	8	9	7	11	6	90
Other	40–112	2	3	1	1	0	1	8
		57	21	20	21	21	15	155

Because of the limited scope of the survey, we could not obtain information on the reasons leading to the admission of these children. Nevertheless the fact that so many children are admitted to hospital with IQs over 50—a range of intelligence within which children are commonly considered suitable for education in schools—raises a number of questions concerning the educational provision available in hospitals for the subnormal.

Educational Facilities in Seventeen Hospitals for the Subnormal

The second part of the questionnaire inquired about the previous educational history of the children admitted in 1962, and also asked for information on the organization of schools, qualifications of teaching staff, and staff: pupil ratios.

PREVIOUS EDUCATION OF ADMISSIONS

Of the seventeen hospitals, sixteen were able to provide information under this heading for a total of 359 children. Of these 135 (38% of the total sample) had attended a school within the educational system at some time before their admission, 16% had gone to primary schools, 10% to schools for the educationally subnormal, and 12% to other forms of special education, such as remedial classes attached to normal schools, units for partially hearing children, etc. A further 23% had been to Junior Training Centres; 39% had not attended either schools or training centres. Details of the time spent at these schools could not be classified, as information was not available in enough cases, but a period of 2–3 years was commonly mentioned.

HOSPITAL SCHOOLS

All the hospitals in the survey had school facilities of various kinds and two had more than one school each. Of the nineteen schools reported, eight were described as "purpose-built" and the remaining eleven as "converted wards".

The administrative responsibility for all the schools lay with the hospital management committee, but two of the hospitals reported a "consultative relationship" with the local education authority. This usually took the form of informal consultations on questions concerning salaries and allowances of Burnham-scale teachers. One with a subunit for psychotic children was about to have the school in this unit administered by the local education authority; the other reported a close liaison with their authority's Further Education Department, who provided teachers for evening classes attended by adult and adolescent patients over school-leaving age.

TEACHING STAFF

The seventeen hospitals taking part in the survey employed 100 teachers, whose qualifications are shown in Table 4, with comparable figures from the Scott Report (Ministry of Health, 1962) showing the qualifications of supervisors and deputy supervisors found in a nation-wide survey carried out in 1959 of all subnormality hospitals, and local health authority training centres in England and Wales.

Comparison of the seventeen survey hospitals with those reported by the Scott committee shows that the present sample appears to be well above the national average both for hospitals and training centres, at least by 1959

TABLE 4.

Qualifications of Teaching Staff in Hospitals and Junior Training Centres (by percentage)

Qualifications	Survey Hospitals	Scott Report	
		Hospitals	Councils
NAMH Diploma	22	3	15
Qualified teachers	13	1	2
Other	8	14	18
None	57	82	66

standards. Thus, (1) the seventeen survey hospitals contain a higher proportion of staff with the appropriate training provided by the National Association for Mental Health; (2) a smaller proportion of their staff are working without any stated qualification; and (3) the survey hospitals are employing many more qualified Burnham-scale teachers. In these respects, therefore, these hospitals seem to enjoy a comparatively favoured position.

The thirteen qualified teachers were employed in a total of five hospitals; it was impossible to judge whether these catered for more intelligent pupils. But considering only the test results of the 1962 admissions, no clear connection emerges between the tested intelligence of children and the number of qualified teachers employed.

STAFF:PUPIL RATIOS

Table 5 summarizes the main findings of the present survey on size of classes and staff:pupil ratios for the 1284 children being regularly taught for at least half the day.

Some hospitals have to cater for much larger numbers than others, but this is not clearly reflected in either the number of teachers available or the type of child admitted. The staff:pupil ratio is lowest in the hospital that admitted the highest proportion of adolescents with IQs over 70. No clear pattern of relationships between needs and facilities is thus apparent.

LINKS WITH LOCAL EDUCATION AUTHORITY SCHOOLS

Inquiries were made as to how many children from subnormality hospitals were discharged to schools within the educational system in the year of the survey. Only 9 left hospital to attend normal schools in 1962; there does not, therefore, appear to be a high rate of transfer of those children of higher intelligence who were presumably admitted to hospital for social or medical reasons. An additional 15 children attended local education authority schools while still resident in hospital. These all came from the two hospitals that reported a working relationship with the local educational authority. Eleven of them attended a secondary modern school, one a junior school and the remaining three a school for the educationally subnormal.

TABLE 5.

*Size of Classes and Staff:Pupil Ratios in
Seventeen Hospital Schools*

No. of children regularly taught (range per school, 28–145)	1284
Median no. of classes per school (range 2–10)	4
Average no. of children per class (range 10–23)	15
Average staff : pupil ratio (range 1 : 28–1 : 9)	1:13

Discussion

This survey shows that out of 403 children admitted to subnormality hospitals in 1962 there were 24% with IQS over 50, 23% with a physical handicap, and 25% with emotional disorders or behaviour disturbances of various kinds.

Only 10 of the physically handicapped and 14 of the psychotic children were among the 155 testable children. It follows that the intelligence of a large number of children was not known, and that the admission to hospital of the majority of children with IQS over 50 cannot be accounted for by the need for special treatment resulting from physical handicap or severe behaviour disturbance.

This raises the question of why these children, whose intelligence test results suggest that they might in certain circumstances be suitably educated in schools within the educational system, were admitted to subnormality hospitals, where they are likely to be taught by staff who, even if they have the appropriate qualifications to teach in hospital schools, are specifically trained to work only with the severely subnormal. It may be assumed that these children either had no home, or that they needed residential care for a variety of social reasons which made it impossible for their families to look after them. They may also present behaviour problems which makes their education in ordinary schools difficult.

It may, however, be questioned whether a hospital for the subnormal can be regarded as a suitable educational establishment for such children under present conditions. The suggestion has been made (Tizard, 1964) that many children would be more appropriately placed in residential schools for educationally subnormal or maladjusted children than in hospitals where educational facilities are inadequate to meet their needs. At present it is difficult to avoid the conclusion that a number of children who cannot remain at home are admitted to hospitals for no better reason than that there are apparently no other places to which they can be sent. The current Wessex subnormality survey (Kushlick, 1965) indicates that one-third of all children in subnormality hospitals are continent, ambulant and free from major behaviour disorders. On the other hand, it is likely that a small proportion of children are so severely disturbed that hospital treatment is necessary and unavoidable. In such cases, however, it seems imperative that the quality and range of educational facilities provided by the hospital authorities should be commensurate with the children's intellectual and educational needs, that the hospital school should be staffed by qualified teachers with special training and experience with retarded and disturbed children, and that the schools should be under the aegis of the education authorities, who, in conjunction with the hospital staff, would then provide educational services and facilities in the same way as those already available to normal children in long-stay and other children's hospitals.

It is, however, important that concern for the educational needs of the more able children should not divert attention from those who, at least under the present system, might be regarded as "unsuitable for education in school". They are the largest group in subnormality hospitals, and their education has not received any official consideration.

We do not know how many subnormality hospitals in the country as a whole have educational facilities, nor can we know the proportion of children who are not receiving training or education, even though they might benefit from them. Nothing short of a national system of inspection could provide reliable information on the quality of educational services at present available.

The needs of children in subnormality hospitals are not, of course, to be seen entirely in terms of education, however broadly the concept of education is interpreted. Recent work has demonstrated the need for a carefully planned programme of social and intellectual stimulation on the wards and outside school hours. The Brooklands experiment (Tizard, 1964) exemplified ways in which the verbal and social development of severely subnormal children could be accelerated by placing them in a small family-type unit, run as far as possible along the lines of a residential children's home. There is a growing body of evidence (e.g., Clarke and Clarke, 1966) that the development of mentally subnormal children can be further retarded by adverse environmental factors, and, specifically, by unstimulating surroundings and poor methods of child care. Moreover, those who show autistic features—at least 10% of admissions in the present survey—are thought to be particularly vulnerable to unstimulating environments.

The Ministry of Health is now taking a more active interest in the living conditions of patients in hospitals, but there is still no evidence of any serious concern with education. There has been no guidance to mental subnormality hospital schools or junior training centres on educational methods and techniques, and there is no means of keeping the staff informed on current research in the relevant aspects of mental subnormality. Hospital schools and training centres are, through no fault of their own, isolated from the main stream of education. There are no channels of communication between staff of such centres and schools within the educational system. There is little awareness of relevant developments in education or psychology, and any experimental work in progress may well suffer from the absence of the kind of informed guidance and help that can often be given by an experienced headmaster, educational psychologist or inspector of schools.

For these reasons, we would favour the implementation of policies designed to bring the educational work of hospital schools within the framework of the education authorities. As a preliminary measure, arrangements might be made to encourage educational psychologists and inspectors of schools to visit hospital schools, to advise the staff on educational methods, and to keep them in touch with important developments in the field.

Acknowledgements

We should like to thank the medical superintendents and clinical psychologists of the hospitals for their co-operation and assistance in collecting the information reported in this paper, and Prof. Alan Clarke for help in its preparation. The other members of the working party were Mr. J. H. F. Castell, Dr. A. T. Ravenette and Mrs. D. Stern.

Summary

A survey is reported of 403 children under 16 admitted to seventeen hospitals for the subnormal in 1962. These hospitals varied greatly in the type of child admitted and the range of provisions made. Three-quarters of the admissions were classified as severely subnormal, of whom just under half were under 8 years of age. About one-third of those admitted were over 13 years, and these were mostly classified as Subnormal or suffering from Psychopathic Disorder. Most children were admitted informally.

About a quarter of all admissions had a motor, visual or auditory handicap, and between 10 and 25% showed behaviour disturbance amounting at times to psychosis.

Of the 155 children who could be given a standard intelligence test, 98 (24% of the total of 403 children) had IQs over 50 on any test; 14% had IQs over 70, and 4% had IQs over 100.

An investigation of educational facilities available in these hospitals showed that, of the 100 teaching staff employed, 22% had the appropriate National Association of Mental Health qualification, 13% were qualified teachers, and 57% had no stated qualification. These figures are much above the national average for hospital schools, as given in the Scott Report. There was no evidence that children with higher IQs were being taught by better qualified staff or in better conditions than those with lower IQs. Only 9 children were transferred from hospital to schools within the educational system in 1962.

These findings are discussed in relation to recent proposals for increasing the contribution of the education authorities to the work of schools in hospitals for the mentally subnormal.

Résumé

L'ÉDUCATION DES ENFANTS DANS LES HÔPITAUX POUR SUBNORMAUX: UNE ENQUÊTE SUR LES ADMISSIONS

L'enquête décrite porte sur 403 enfants de moins de 16 ans admis dans 17 hôpitaux pour subnormaux en 1962. Ces hôpitaux varient beaucoup quant au type d'enfant admis et l'étendue des soins. Trois-quart des enfants admis ont été classifiés comme sévèrement subnormaux, parmi ceux-ci juste un peu moins de la moitié avaient au-dessous de huit ans. Un tiers environ de ceux admis avaient plus de 13 ans; ils étaient surtout classés comme subnormaux ou souffrant de désordres psychopathiques. La plupart des enfants ont été admis sans formalités.

Environ un quart de tous les enfants admis avaient un handicap moteur, visuel ou auditif reconnu, et entre 10 et 25 pour cent présentaient des troubles de comportement atteignant parfois la psychose.

Parmi les 403 enfants, 155 étaient capables de subir un test d'intelligence standard. Quatre-vingt-dix-huit de ces enfants (24 pour cent du total) avaient un QI supérieur à 50 à tous les tests; 14 pour cent avaient un QI supérieur à 70 et 4 pour cent avaient un QI supérieur à 100.

Une enquête sur les facilités d'éducation disponibles dans ces hôpitaux a montré que, parmi les 100 éducateurs employés, 22 pour cent avaient les diplômes N.A.M.H. appropriés, 13 pour cent étaient des instituteurs diplômés, et 57 pour cent n'avaient pas de diplômes officiels. Ces chiffres sont très supérieurs à la moyenne nationale pour les écoles d'hôpitaux indiquée dans le Rapport Scott. Il n'y avait aucune évidence que les enfants d'un niveau d'intelligence plus élevé recevaient une instruction par un personnel plus qualifié ou dans de meilleures conditions que ceux ayant un QI plus bas. Neuf enfants seulement ont été transférés des écoles des hôpitaux aux écoles ordinaires en 1962.

Ces résultats sont discutés en relation aux récentes propositions pour augmenter la contribution de l'éducation publique au travail des écoles d'hôpitaux pour les subnormaux.

Zusammenfassung

DIE BILDUNG DER KINDER IN KRANKENHÄUSERN FÜR DIE GEISTIG
UNTERENTWICKELTEN: EINE AUFNAHMEN-ÜBERSICHT

Es wird von 403 Kindern unter 16 Jahren berichtet, die in 17 Krankenhäuser
fur die geistig Unterentwickelten in 1962 aufgenommen wurden. Diese
Krankenhäuser variierten beträchtlich in den aufgenommenen Kinder-Typen
und in dem Umfang der getroffenen Vorkehrungen. Dreiviertel der Aufnahmen wurden als „schwer zurückgeblieben" eingestuft; etwas weniger als die
Hälfte davon waren jünger als 8 Jahre. Ungefähr ein Drittel der aufgenommenen Kinder waren über 13 Jahre alt, und diese wurden meistens als
„zurückgeblieben" oder „psychopathische Störung" klassifiziert. Die meisten
Kinder waren zwanglos aufgenommen worden.

Bei ungefähr einem Viertel aller Aufnahmen war motorische, visuelle oder
auditorische Beeinträchtigung angegeben und zwischen 10 und 25 Prozent
wiesen emotionale Störung auf, die sich bisweilen zu Psychose entwickelte.

Von den 403 Kindern konnten 155 ein Standard-Intelligenztest gestellt
werden. Neun und neunzig dieser Kinder (24 Prozent der gesamten Gruppe)
wiesen Intelligenz Quotas von über 50 bei allen Tests auf; 14 Prozent hatten
IQ über 70 und 4 Prozent IQ über 100.

Eine Untersuchung der diesen Kindern zur Verfügung gestellten Bildungs-
möglichkeiten erwies, dass von dem 100 Personen starken Lehrkörper 22
Prozent die angemessenen N.A.M.H. Qualifikationen hatten, 13 Prozent
qualifizierte Lehrer und 57 Prozent ohne angegebene Qualifikationen waren.
Diese Zahlen stehen bedeutend über dem nationalen Durchschnitt für
Krankenhausschulen, wie sie im Scott-Report dargelegt sind. Es liegt kein
Beweis vor, dass Kinder mit höherem Intelligenz-Niveau von besser qualifi-
zierten Lehrern oder in besseren Umständen unterrichtet würden als solche
mit niederen Intelligenz-Quotas. Nur 9 Kinder wurden innerhalb des
Unterricht-Systems 1962 von Krankenhäusern in Schulen versetzt.

Diese Befunde werden besprochen in Beziehung zu kürzlichen Vorschlägen,
den Beitrag der Unterrichts-Autoritätsstellen für Arbeit in Krankenhausschulen der geistig Unterentwickelten zu erhöhen.

Resumen

LA EDUCACIÓN DE NIÑOS EN HOSPITALES PARA LOS SUBNORMALES:
UNA REVISTA DE LAS ADMISIONES

Se presenta una revista de 403 niños menores de 16 años admitidos a 17
hospitales para los subnormales en 1962. Había muchas variaciones entre
estos hospitales con respecto al tipo de niño que admitían y a las facilidades

que proveían. Tres cuartos de las admisiones se clasificaban como gravemente subnormales, y un poco menos de la mitad de éstos tenían menos de 8 años. Cerca de la tercera parte de los niños admitidos tenían más de 13 años, y la mayor parte de éstos se clasificaban como subnormales o afectos de un trastorno psicopático. La mayor parte de los niños entraron sin formulismos.

Se halló que cerca de la cuarta parte de todas las admisiones tenían un impedimento motor, visual, o auditivo, y entre el 10 y el 25 por ciento mostraban un disturbio emocional que a veces llegaba a ser una psicosis.

De los 403 niños se podía dar a 155 un test corriente de inteligencia. Noventa y ocho de estos niños (el 24 por ciento de la muestra entera) tenían un cociente intelectual de más de 50 según cualquier test que se les diera; el 14 por ciento tenían un cociente intelectual de más de 70, y el 4 por ciento tenían un cociente intelectual de más de 100.

Una investigación de las facilidades educacionales provistas para estos niños reveló que, entre un personal docente de 100, el 22 por ciento tenían la calificación apropiada de la N.A.M.H., el 13 por ciento eran maestros calificados, y el 57 por ciento no tenían ninguna calificación declarada. Estas cifras son muy elevadas sobre el promedio nacional para las escuelas en hospitales, según el informe de Scott. No había evidencia de que los niños cuyo nivel de inteligencia era más alto tuviesen maestros cuyas calificaciones eran mejores, ni que disfrutasen de mejores condiciones que los niños cuyo cociente intelectual era más bajo. En 1962 solamente 9 niños se transferieron de hospitales a escuelas dentro del sistema educacional.

Se dicuten estos hallazgos con relación a sugestiones recientes que las autoridades educacionales debieran aumentar su contribución a las escuelas en hospitales para los niños subnormales.

References

CASTELL, J. H. F. and MITTLER, P. J. (1965), Intelligence of patients in subnormality hospitals: a survey of admissions in 1961, *Brit. J. Psychiat.* **111**, 219.

CLARKE, A. M. and CLARKE, A. D. B. (Eds.) (1966), *Mental Deficiency: The Changing Outlook*, 2nd edn., London, Methuen (in the press).

DOLL, E. A. (1953), *The Measurement of Social Competence*, Minneapolis, Educational Test Bureau.

GENERAL REGISTER OFFICE (1964), *The Registrar General's Statistical Review of England and Wales for the Year 1960, Supplement on Mental Health*, London, H.M.S.O.

GESELL, A. (1954), *The First Five Years of Life*, London, Methuen.

KUSHLICK, A. (1965), *Community Services for the Mentally Subnormal*. A plan for experimental evaluation, *Proc. roy. Soc. Med.* **58**, 374.

MINISTRY OF HEALTH (1962), *The Training of Staff of Training Centres for the Mentally Subnormal*, Standing Mental Health Advisory Committee, Report of the Sub-Committee, Chairman, J. A. Scott, London, H.M.S.O.

TIZARD, J. (1964), *Community Services for the Mentally Handicapped*, Oxford Medical Publications, London, Oxford University Press.

SECTION D
EXTRAMURAL SERVICES

32. The Newham Community Mental Health Service

J. H. KAHN

COMMUNITY mental health services are the responsibility of the health departments of local authorities in Britain, and fit into a wider framework of mental health services (Freudenberg, Harding and Kahn, 1965). The *clinical* treatment of psychiatric illness is the responsibility, first of the family doctor, and next of the hospital system—whether in-patient or out-patient. The local authority is responsible for *supportive* and *rehabilitative* services, and for fulfilling the statutory requirements, whenever a patient is to be admitted to hospital under some form of legal compulsion. The diagnosis of mental illness has ceased to be the decision to take an individual from his work and his home, and place him in some remote institution. The 1959 Mental Health Act redefined mental illness and marked the progress which had been made in treatment and changes in public attitudes.

I propose to describe a particular scheme, inaugurated in 1960 in the County Borough of West Ham and now extending to an enlarged area—the London Borough of Newham, created by the amalgamation of the two previously independent areas of East Ham and West Ham. The amalgamation took place in April 1965 as part of a major reorganization of local government in the London area. Prior to the amalgamation, the community mental health service in East Ham was less developed than its counterpart, and, at the time of writing, the service for the new borough is the old West Ham service spread a little more thinly than before the amalgamation.

The Setting

West Ham itself, although part of the great Metropolitan area, has had a long tradition and history which is separate from its neighbours. Although only 8 square miles in extent, it had a population of over 300,000 before the Second World War. This was reduced to approximately 80,000 by bombing and evacuation, and gradually built up again to 160,000, where it had remained static. The population is regarded as uniformly working class and those who advanced financially and socially tended to move out of the borough. This uniformity has been a twentieth-century phenomenon, and the borough had in the past been composed of separate minor townships, each with its own shopping centre and own individuality, including Stratford (the "Stratford-Atte Bow" of Chaucer) and Forest Gate, which in the nineteenth century

563

was the residential area of fairly prosperous commercial families. Canning Town, Silvertown, Custom House, and Albert Docks are districts close to the River Thames, and here there are some small residential pockets between the various docks, isolated except for swing bridges, from the rest of the area. These, and many other parts, have their separate level of social esteem. Many of the nineteenth-century substantial terraced houses have been sub-divided without structural alteration into homes for a number of families. Houses, factories and docks are intermingled.

The southern part of the old Borough of West Ham is mainly dockland, occupied by families who have lived in the locality for many generations. The northern part, with mixed heavy and light industry, includes a proportion of transient and immigrant population, and an increasing proportion of these are of West Indian origin.

Slum clearance, and rebuilding into flats, has broken up some of the continuity of the older communities in the area. Nevertheless, the inhabitants in general remained conscious and proud of the borough's separate existence. The Council has been responsible for many pioneer social projects; and it was part of West Ham that returned Keir Hardie, the first Labour M.P., to Parliament. There is no division between the decisions of the Council and the wishes of the population. New modern flats and schools represent a corporate spirit, and are worthy successors to the well-designed public buildings erected at the turn of the century. A long tradition of social progress, and a certain degree of geographical isolation from other parts of the Metropolitan area, is expressed, surprisingly, by a conservatism in the culture.

In spite of a vigorous housing programme, the shortage of accommodation remains acute, and recommendations for favourable treatment in the alloca-tion of a Corporation house or flat on grounds of threats to mental health are likely to be met with the uncontrovertible statement that other families on the waiting list are in worse plight.

Stereotypes: Legend and Reality

Newcomers to local authority employment are presented with a stereotype of large families congregated around a surviving grandmother (a West Ham "Mum"), and of neighbourhoods each having a cohesion which is represented by informal support for families in trouble. Voluntary organizations, such as are well represented in middle-class areas, are thin on the ground, since the Borough Council itself is felt to represent the population. There are, however, a number of charitable "Settlements", and, in the past, the area was a practis-ing ground for many voluntary social workers coming in from outside.

Few of the senior administrative staff of the local authority live in the borough. Even the family doctors mostly live at a distance, in more salubrious areas, and have lock-up surgeries; and very few teachers have homes in the area. In some of the local authority departments, members of the staff (many of whom had risen in the employment of the local authority from the post obtained immediately after leaving school) claimed that they knew the population, having followed families sometimes through two or three generations. It was implied that those who used the local authority services felt either that they were being forced to do something which they did not wish to do (and therefore resisted it), or that they wanted something that the local authority did not wish to give them (and therefore insisted upon having it). There was none of the middle-class familiarity with social work, where worker and client accepted a joint aim.

East Ham with its population of 100,000 is contiguous with West Ham and has a briefer history. Much of its building of houses took place between 1890 and 1910. The streets are neat and regular, and industrial buildings are few.

Although the population is largely working class, there is a significant middle-class element, and the whole area has been considered socially superior to West Ham. Some of the professional people who work in West Ham, but could not consider living there, have found residence in East Ham. Some have moved on to the still more desirable residential areas in the rapidly growing commuter towns in once-rural Essex. Newham suffers, in common with other large working-class Metropolitan areas, in having no unbuilt rural fringe in which new suburbs can be developed.

The impressions described above have been found to require considerable correction. All the stereotypes have their embodiment, but the majority of the inhabitants are not represented by them. A school welfare officer, for example, may know a few hundred families intimately and consider that he knows the town. Some surnames are recognized at once by the staff of the Children's Department, which is responsible for children deprived of parental care, and the same names may be familiar to a host of other statutory and voluntary agencies. The health visitors, whose work includes the visiting of homes and families, have a wider range, and meet inhabitants who never come to the notice of services which deal with the materially deprived. Many families, however, are not numbered amongst the consumers of any of the local authority social services. Some are unknown even to the family doctor on whose list they are registered. There is an invisible middle class, which has only just begun to reveal itself to professional staff, as the image of the local authority service gradually alters.

The Planning

Most local authorities have based their community mental health service on the existing provisions for the psychotic patient. The "Duly Authorized

Officer" (who had remained responsible for the legal processes of emergency admission to mental hospital since the 1946 National Health Services Act came into operation in 1948) was given social work functions with psychiatric and mentally subnormal patients without any formal training for that work. Many new entrants to the renamed posts of "Mental Welfare Officer" are being recruited from those who have taken the (Younghusband) General Social Work Training Course.

For theoretical concepts, many local authorities have turned to psychiatric hospitals. Some consultants who are appointed to psychiatric hospitals have been allowed to devote part of their time to advisory and consultative duties in the local community mental health service. These contributions vary in the same way as psychiatrists and psychiatric hospitals vary. The primary concern of psychiatric hospitals is the medical treatment of mental illness, and the thinking in clinical categories, which is meaningful in a hospital context, needs to be translated into other terms before it becomes relevant for social care in the community (Querido, 1963).

Child guidance, in contrast, has developed somewhat differently from adult psychiatry in that its multidisciplinary system (Kahn and Nursten, 1964) is based upon the principle of simultaneous investigation by a team of at least three highly trained professional workers. It is recognized that the identified patient who requires treatment is a *child*, who is living and growing *within a family* and *within an educational framework*. If account is taken of the *adult's occupational life*, and his *family and social interaction*, it would follow that a similar multidisciplinary approach to the mentally disturbed adult also, would have advantages. Moreover, although medical treatment is usually best focused on the individual, there are many instances when the family structure can be looked upon as the unit of pathology, and in these cases, treatment is directed to the family interaction, rather than to separate individuals. This kind of concept allows intervention into the problem at an earlier stage than when an individual has been singled out as carrying the illness, and could also provide a basis for preventive services.

The Medical Officer of Health for West Ham, Dr. F. R. Dennison, chose the system of child guidance as his model for the community mental health services for the borough. For over 3 years before any plans were formulated, discussions took place between the Medical Officer of Health and his staff, consultants of the psychiatric and general hospitals in the area, representatives of family doctors, an officer of the Regional Hospital Board, and a consultant from the Tavistock Clinic.

When the principles of the services were agreed, the first step was to construct an appointment jointly between the regional hospital board and the local authority, for a psychiatrist who would be both the Medical Director of the Child Guidance Clinic and Consultant Psychiatrist in charge of the community mental health service.

The next step was to find skilled family case-workers to work in the com. munity service, which was to be integrated with the child guidance clinic- It was decided to try to recruit qualified psychiatric social workers, who would be prepared to accept the statutory duties of mental welfare officers (including the night emergency rota) as well as the more familiar functions in the child guidance clinic. The remaining mental welfare officers, who were experienced but untrained, and whose numbers had been reduced by retire- ment, were to be integrated with the newly appointed psychiatric social workers into a single team and share the title "Mental Health Social Worker". Well before the Mental Health Act of 1959 came into operation, this outline scheme was accepted by the Health Committee of the West Ham Borough Council and also by the Education Committee, which was concerned with the administration of the existing child guidance clinic.

Pilot schemes, including discussion groups with health visitors and medical officers in the Health Department were introduced, and the first consultant psychiatrist took up his appointment on 1 January 1960. The early stages of the service were described previously (Kahn, 1963).

How the rapid growth of the service was achieved remains somewhat of a mystery. Planning of the service still continues, and any description of the procedures actually being undertaken becomes rapidly out of date. Conflict, disillusionment and frustration alternate with pride of achievement.

The first and main obstacle was the unavailability of qualified psychiatric social workers. A trainee scheme was set up, under which holders of degrees or diplomas in social science were appointed and later released, on full salary, to university training courses for the Mental Health Certificate. Four such trainees were appointed in 1960, and the first to become qualified returned to the service in 1962.

Other newly qualified psychiatric social workers were then recruited, and it was discovered that the more a service has, the more it can attract. A surprising number of qualified and experienced psychiatric social workers showed a courageous readiness to expose themselves to the unstructured and uncertain demands which come from professional workers in a variety of services for something called "community care".

There are at present fourteen qualified psychiatric social workers and two trainees. The establishment at present allows for the number to be increased gradually, in stages approved by the committee.

The staffing in the other disciplines has not shown the same growth. Psychiatrists, psychologists and psychotherapists are under-represented in relation to social workers.

Functions

The obligations of the local authority with regard to mental health were originally discussed in planning under five headings.

1. Statutory Obligations

(a) *Compulsory admission* of mentally ill patients to psychiatric hospitals, and "after-care" of patients discharged from hospital. In this field, it was hoped that a continuous process of family case work, given in advance of hospitalization, might sometimes avert it.

(b) *Residential care* of patients discharged from hospital who are not yet able to live unsupported in the community. This was first thought of in terms of hostels for different categories of patients—emotionally disturbed children, mentally handicapped children and adults, elderly patients with minor degrees of psychiatric disturbance, and patients who have had clinically recognized psychiatric illnesses but who do not require hospital treatment at that particular time. This provision is now being thought of on lines of functional need, rather than the above categories.

(c) *Training centres* for subnormal children and adults. Training centres for the partly recovered and partly disabled mentally ill adults were also envisaged.

2. The Child Guidance Clinic

This was operated on traditional lines. Its function includes case-work with parents, as well as treatment of the children on whose behalf intervention was sought in the first place. Treatment was based upon recognition of family interaction and the co-existing life in school. There was an existing establishment for psychiatrists, psychologists, psychiatric social workers, and a part-time psychotherapist.

3. In-service Training Schemes

These were for health visitors and assistant medical officers of health, to be extended to professional workers in other departments of the local authority.

4. A Consultative Service

This was for many types of local authority staff including health visitors, school medical officers, welfare officers, probation officers, and for voluntary workers in organizations such as the Marriage Guidance Council. This service was designed to help in dealing with mental health problems which became apparent in the course of the work of non-psychiatric services.

5. A Co-ordinating Committee

This consisted of workers from different local authority departments and voluntary bodies, which had been in existence for a considerable time. This committee discussed problem families whose social and economic needs called for attention, and whose psychiatric problems may be relevant to their situation.

The Mental Health Social Workers

The original conception was of an all-purpose team of social workers, practising family case-work in all the different areas of the service. With the expansion in the size of the team and the extension of its range of activities, a steady increase in specialization became inevitable. However, the principle of one integrated service has been maintained, with each social worker appointed to the service as a whole, and becoming identified with the total service rather than any particular part of it. Specializations are developed, but no specialization is exclusive. Each social worker continues to work with the family allocated to him or her, drawing upon the total resources of the service, however diverse and shifting the areas of need might be.

The starting point, still the central core, was the statutory services that must be provided: the emergency admission of patients to mental hospitals, the social after-care following discharge, and the child guidance service. The aim has been to bring these into a family case-work service, which has gradually extended its activities as areas of need have been uncovered, and as the special interests and abilities of different members of the social work-team have permitted. To a considerable extent, the service has been shaped by special interests and abilities.

The psychiatric social workers state that they all feel untrained for much of the work that they do. Their training as psychiatric social workers gives a basis, but is not enough. They have to draw on other resources in themselves. They need replenishment through conferences and discussions within the department and elsewhere and the support of an administrative structure whose growth keeps pace with theirs.

The aim of the integrated service is to provide for a flexible matching of community provision and patient's needs, with a minimum of administrative lets and hindrances. To quote Caplan (1962),

> ... all treatment services and institutions should be viewed as interlocking parts of a programme which is designed to meet the needs of the patient, rather than to try to fit the patient into institutions in order to satisfy administrative needs or the vested interests of professional groups.

Boundaries between different parts of the service must exist, but they are divisions of convenience rather than barriers to be surmounted. It is hoped to make the service a preventive one by making it a better service, finding that where a disability is seen to be given better provision, it attracts less stigma. Access to the service is made easy, so that families at risk can approach us before the difficulties become acute or became crystallized into some form which is difficult to resolve. Attempts are made to create links with other professional workers, in order to find ways of working together in areas of mutual concern, joining resources so that all can extend the range of their work.

When the total family situation and the needs of all the family members are considered, the work has a *preventive* aspect.

The use of qualified psychiatric social workers for statutory duties concerned with admission of patients to hospital is an unusual feature, but it is the essence of the scheme. The aim is to start work with families before admission to hospital of a family member becomes necessary, with the hope that it may be forestalled. Even if hospitalization should occur, the dynamically trained worker may take the drama out of the situation and thereby prevent division in the family, which leads to alienation of the patient.

The family may be helped to hold its sick member through the acute stage of his illness, and to allow admission to hospital to be arranged later and at leisure. This process has been helped by good communication with psychiatrists at the hospital which serves West Ham. Admission to psychiatric hospital is looked upon by them as mainly a medical decision of the family practitioner, and they are ready to visit the homes of patients, in consultation with the patient's doctor. Patients themselves learn that it is not necessary to be violent before they can be acknowledged as in need of psychiatric treatment. The mental health social worker is ceasing to be the officer who responds to an emergency call by removing a troublesome individual to a psychiatric hospital, in order to oblige the doctor or members of the patient's family.

The convenience of the emergency service provided by the old D.A.O. (Duly Authorized Officer) is missed by some people. An *officer* responds to a call on the terms on which it is made. A *professional worker* redefines the terms, and this redefinition may not always be welcome.

It is necessary to establish a new image of a service in which calls are dealt with in the context of long-term needs of the patient, the family, and the community. All this has to be carried out in association with the psychiatric hospital, family practitioner, ambulance driver and, sometimes, the police.

A new development is that two mental health social workers are on duty during office hours for emergency calls and to see members of the public who may call in without appointment. This "walk in" service has been formulated to cater for the increasing number of people who were calling at the offices. This was when it was noticed that the type of client and type of problem was becoming more varied. Professional workers, university students and grammar-school leavers entering employment, not previously thought to be typical of the borough, were coming for help with severe emotional problems.

At this point, it becomes possible to realize that *all the patients and clients seen previously were also atypical.* A common language exists as a ready-made medium of communication between the professional worker and the middle-class client. Even here, there are some differences of vocabulary which need translation, but a basis for communication is present. Difficulties of communication are greater with those whose language is restricted by lower levels of intelligence, class barriers, and absence of identification with the educational system. When, however, the range of understanding of the worker increases, so does the range of individuality of his clients!

Young People's Consultation Service

This was established a year ago to cater for those whose needs are not met by adult psychiatric services, and who would not consider attending a child guidance clinic. Young people are encouraged to approach the service directly, and where, as usually happens, an introduction is in fact made by another worker, the young person is invited to get in touch with the service himself, to arrange his first appointment. The age group has not been defined. It could perhaps be looked on as a service for people who have begun to break away from the primary family group, but have not yet become identified with an independent adult role. The youngest client was a boy of 13, who was in fact transferred to the child guidance clinic. The oldest person to approach the service was a man of 29 years, who wrote asking for a consultation because of the difficulty he had in making friends, particularly with women. More than one married couple has been referred to the service, and the majority of cases have been concerned with problems of interpersonal relationships.

Special interests of individual psychiatric social workers have provided the service with growing points. One or more have assumed some personal responsibility for the work in the areas described below.

1. PSYCHIATRIC HOSPITALS

Although there is no joint appointment of social workers between local authority and the psychiatric hospital serving the area, individual social workers are attached respectively to the medical "firms" in the hospital. They attend ward meetings and the discharge conferences. They have links with the psychiatric out-patient clinics. They are responsible for *after-care* which, when it is an extension of the primary relationship, becomes *continuing care*.

2. THE CHILD GUIDANCE CLINIC

Four of the social workers spend a major part of their time in the clinic. There are no full-time psychiatric social workers in the clinic. Child guidance is brought into relation with other parts of the service by those workers of all disciplines whose duties overlap.

3. LIAISON WITH CHILDREN'S DEPARTMENT AND PROBATION DEPARTMENT

This is mainly a function concerned with the child guidance clinic, but other parts of the community mental health service may be involved. One psychiatric social worker has been allotted special responsibilities where these departments are concerned, and arranges contacts and communications on behalf of, or together with, other members of the staff.

4. MATERNAL AND CHILD WELFARE CLINICS

There are nine of these, spread out strategically over the borough. Each clinic looks to a particular social worker for regular contacts.

5. HANDICAPPED CHILDREN

A Development Clinic has existed for some time under the direction of one of the medical officers, who works with health visitors and a visiting consultant paediatrician. Mothers of infants with suspected physical, sensory, or mental defects are invited to attend regularly for investigation of the child and for the preparation that is necessary for the next stage of training or education.

Social workers interested in this field will be introduced in turn, and each will build up a case-load for long-term counselling of families.

6. JUNIOR TRAINING COURSES FOR THE MENTALLY SUBNORMAL

This will be referred to later. One of the social workers attends parent–teacher meetings, and also has her own group of parents needing special counselling or case work.

7. THE NATIONAL ASSISTANCE BOARD, THE INDUSTRIAL REHABILITATION UNITS, HOUSING DEPARTMENTS, WELFARE DEPARTMENTS

The staff of these departments are all confronted with problems of a psychiatric nature in the people whom they serve. Sometimes, this necessitates transferring a client to the community mental health service from the service where the problem is first recognized. At this stage, he becomes a patient. This transfer is not always appropriate, and an individual who has some mental abnormality may not desire nor be responsive to psychiatric procedures.

Many people show symptoms of mental illness, yet live reasonably normal lives and have no wish to receive psychiatric treatment. Others appear to need treatment on account of the damage or distress that they cause to others. They may deny the fact that they are in any way mentally ill and yet their disturbance may not be of a nature which makes them subject to a compulsory order. These individuals may demand (and need) other types of social service, and in these cases, the non-psychiatric services may require help in the form of consultations in the absence of the client.

8. ADULT MENTALLY SUBNORMAL INDIVIDUALS

These present a special problem that increases in magnitude with the longer expectation of life that some of these individuals may now enjoy. In addition to the severely subnormal, this group includes those who have attended schools for the educationally subnormal. Although in this case the mental handicap is of a moderate degree, they may still have difficulty in fitting into occupational or social life.

Mentally subnormal adults are not a statutory responsibility of the Health Department under present-day legislation if they and their families can manage their own affairs efficiently, but at the time of school leaving, a conference of Education and Health Department staff is held and some may be recommended for supervision by the Health Department.

Here, the new service seems to fail in comparison with the traditional friendly visiting by the former Duly Authorized Officer. His range of work was somewhat narrower than that expected of the psychiatric social worker, but some areas were dealt with more intensively. Supervision of the adult subnormal (formerly "defective") was undertaken in-between other duties. He might call at the home and pay a doorstep visit, or would be invited into the house. Problems of the "defective's" behaviour would be discussed and, at times, he might have even been invited to give the young man or woman "a good talking to". In a paternalistic society, such service is valued. Trained social workers are unwilling and, in fact, unable to do this kind of work.

Those who withdraw a previous service must face criticism if they do not provide something that can be seen to be even better. The solution must be a long-term one, which will mean establishing a case-work relationship with the family *at the earliest point of recognition of the handicap* in infancy. On this basis, the handicapped member of the family would not be expected merely to conform to some rigid and restricted pattern of behaviour, but would continue to receive some encouragement for development of his intellectual and emotional potentials, even in his adult life.

The above list by no means exhausts the separate functions that are distributed amongst the social-work staff at present, nor does it include those in preparation.

Reference has been restricted so far almost entirely to the social-work function. The service was planned on a multidisciplinary pattern. Growth in function and numbers has, however, been mainly in psychiatric social-work staff.

One additional maximum part-time consultant psychiatric post in community mental health and child guidance has been approved and is about to be advertised.

The psychological contribution has been mainly the inspiration which has come from Dr. Ravenette, the Senior Psychologist, who has duties in the School Health Service in the child guidance clinic, and also has a function directly under the Education Department in the School Psychological Service. He has no formal connection with the Health Department, but has made himself freely available in individual consultations and in the broad planning.

The amalgamation of West Ham with East Ham to form the Borough of Newham has provided a new beginning and an opportunity to review the staffing needs and to face shortcomings. Fresh recruitment and re-appraisal of concepts and techniques have to go hand-in-hand.

The Community Psychiatrist

The psychiatrist's function in the service as a whole presents difficulties. The function of a medical director of the child guidance clinic has its established pattern. He is the leader of a professional team, which has traditions of separate areas of competence and of shared responsibilities. Conferences are held weekly at the former West Ham clinic for case discussion and development of diagnostic and therapeutic concepts, which provide a common language for the team. The clinic itself provides a base in which the work with patients *within the clinic* gives its professional members the confidence to *go out beyond the clinic walls* and meet teachers, nurses, and doctors, who are dealing with the child guidance patients at other levels and with other aims.

The community psychiatrist's function in the other sections of the community mental health service is more ambiguous. He has to maintain contact with psychiatrists at whatever hospital is providing clinical treatment for mentally ill patients. The hospital consultant himself carries clinical responsibility for all patients receiving in-patient or out-patient hospital treatment. The psychiatric social worker who is attached to the particular hospital consultant keeps in contact also with the family doctor, and may become the focus for unifying the work with the family as a whole.

Formulations of conjoint family therapy are being built up wherein a group of workers (psychiatrists, psychiatric social worker and psychologist) carries out joint therapeutic interviews, in selected cases, with whole families rather than distribute the therapy of different individuals among the different therapists.

In the community mental health service generally, the psychiatrist leads a conference, which originally was designed to deal with the intake of new referrals to the service. The social-work team has recently been provided with its own principal, and its own case-work supervisor, but the psychiatrist has had to take the lead at times in laying down limits and saying what should *not* be done. The service has sometimes been the victim of its own propaganda and of expectations which have been raised too high.

Psychiatric Social Workers—Conflicts of Role

A psychiatric social worker is often called upon to act as a pacifier to a person justifiably distressed by unsatisfactory housing conditions, by poverty, or illness. The individual is suffering from emotional disturbance, and the psychiatric social worker is therefore expected to make a relationship that will lead the patient to accept case-work in lieu of his material necessities. Sometimes the skill of the psychiatric social worker can in fact be directed to the confronting of an individual with realities of his situation, but there are illusions about the ability to make a relationship in order to carry out later some subtle modifications in the attitudes of a patient or his family. Medical specialists sometimes expect a psychiatric social worker to be his eyes and ears, and "*take a social history*". If the psychiatric social worker does this, it does not save the specialist any time—it opens up new dimensions of the problem to be dealt with; sometimes a psychiatric social worker is expected to be the legs of some other worker and "*take a message*"; sometimes, to be the heart, and "*make a relationship*" in order to induce the patient to accept some unpalatable decision.

It sometimes happens that during the process of extending the range of community mental health service, requests which come from other agencies have to be refused. The refusal should not be made without a redefinition of the problem, in a way which enables the original agency to handle the problem at a new level within its own service. The intake conference is sometimes used to discuss a problem with workers from other services, or to decide upon a consultation process, in which the psychiatrist and a psychiatric social worker pay a visit to the other agency. Consultation is not always as acceptable as the taking a patient off someone else's hands would be, but frequently, the psychiatric service is less well equipped to deal with the problem than the referring agency. It seems easier to accept a referral, and fail, than to provide acceptable alternative formulations in conjunction with another profession; to accept an unsuitable referral is the line of least resistance.

There are natural and understandable resistances to the idea that psychiatric personnel have anything to add to existing methods of working or to existing diagnostic formulation by others. All professional workers face the problem of insufficient time to deal with present tasks. They naturally resent any attempts to modify their role. Their acceptance of any addition to the range of their work will depend upon their own perception of some need which they cannot fill at present, within what they consider to be their own field.

The psychiatrist and psychiatric social worker have their own professional field, and they also have problems with regard to the extension of their role when they go outside that field. They may have attributed to them a claim to a superiority of their methods over those of workers in a different setting.

People believe that the psychiatrist is itching to take over the work of other professions or to tell them how to do their work. The psychiatrist or the psychiatric social worker may frequently be invited to enter into the field of work of others, who are confronted with problems of behaviour. They face criticism when they accept the invitation, and criticism when they refuse. They are asked to take responsibility for altering the behaviour of some individual and then to hand him back, or to keep him secluded, even when the law does not allow this to be done.

The psychiatric contribution to other fields can never be a higher level of knowledge of someone else's work, but it is a method of approach to problems which includes an examination of the basic assumptions used when dealing with the problems.

Professional Boundaries and Hostility

The exploration and examination of basic assumptions and of personal attitudes is always accompanied by the release of hostility, whether it be in the clinical setting with patients, or in the professional setting with colleagues. Hostility can be tolerated when there is clarity about respective roles. Hostility is, however, damaging to the recipient, and the one who expresses it, if it finds expression outside the boundaries of defined relationships.

In the clinical setting, any psychiatric worker has the protection of professional traditions, the knowledge of the role boundary on both sides, and the support of the clinical team. A clinical base is a support to the psychiatric workers in community care, when going out into other professional fields. It is also the setting in which professional and personal development and progress in the psychiatric worker takes place after initial training. The spread in the range of work with patients and other professional workers should be expected to increase the degree of tensions which the worker experiences.

Psychiatric Formulation

The consultant psychiatrist has been expected to provide some continuity of clinical and theoretical concepts of psychiatry, throughout the process of building up a practical working system of community psychiatric social work.

His task is to develop and communicate the medical or psychiatric contribution to the treatment of social problems, and to make himself familiar with the thinking of other professional workers sharing this field.

The main difficulty in this role is the absence of relevant formulations. The classical medical model is that of investigation leading to a diagnosis, and the prescription of some treatment appropriate to the category of disorder which has been diagnosed. This system has been responsible for the tremendous progress in the treatment of physical illness in the last hundred years, and the extension of this progress into the field of mental illness has resulted in recent years in what has been described as a therapeutic explosion. The treatment of established psychosis remains the main contribution of the medical man to the field of mental illness, and the psychiatrist is first and foremost a clinician. When the psychiatrist enters the field of social services, and becomes involved with the creation of systems of prevention, he needs new levels of thinking. Medical *treatment* depends upon *diagnosis*; *prevention* is based upon *aetiology*—we must know the cause of what we try to prevent. In social medicine, however, the clinical diagnostic categories seem irrelevant, and the aetiological concepts of psychiatry are not sufficiently well established for them to become the basis of large-scale preventive measures.

The making of a diagnosis of schizophrenia, for example, is an essential preliminary to the provision of medical treatment. How relevant, however, is the same label to the industrial procedures which are used in rehabilitation, or to the consideration of the way in which a partly recovered mentally ill parent will affect the emotional stability of children? Additional dimensions of diagnosis are required in terms of function and in these considerations, other individuals are going to be involved. Employers want information about men and women returning to work. Health visitors ask about the effect that the discharged patient is going to have on the marital partner or the children. Child care officers are concerned about the way in which children move in and out "of care", as mothers enter and leave psychiatric hospital. National Assistance Board and National Insurance officials want to know whether pressure should be applied to compel some former mental hospital patient to return to work, when he appears unwilling, or to return to hospital in order to become cured. They all believe that the answer is in the possession of the psychiatrist, and that it can be transmitted by the psychiatric social worker. The psychiatric worker has to confess that it is the non-psychiatric field worker who has access to most of the knowledge of the way in which the mentally ill patient fits into family, occupational and social life. We need this knowledge to add new dimensions to the *clinical* diagnosis.

The *social* diagnosis is the dimension in which the competence of an individual to deal with his external affairs is described; the *family* diagnosis is in terms of family interaction; an *occupational* diagnosis is in terms of his limitations, capacities, and the resources available in the community for them to be used and developed. These other dimensions of diagnosis are not at present within the orbit of psychiatric training—which is for clinical work—although many psychiatrists have made contributions to the knowledge of these factors (Clark, 1964; Early, 1960; Martin, 1962). Some psychiatrists have, for example, developed ideas of the therapeutic community within the hospital. Others have developed industrial units up to a level of importance at which the wards serve merely as a dormitory, for patients whose therapy takes place in the workshops and who begin their rehabilitation at the moment of admission to hospital.

These processes have not yet been professionalized within psychiatry, and in many cases, they do not survive the transfer of some pioneer worker to another post.

We need new formulations, in which to relate the clinical findings with the standards by which we prescribe some of the present-day procedures, such as industrial therapy, social clubs, and group discussions. It may sometimes seem that we prescribe them merely because someone has developed a unit in which these facilities exist. Many of such processes are at present quite fortuitously under the direction of medical men of different specialist training, or of non-medical personnel from any one of a variety of professions.

Multidisciplinary Processes

It would seem that the professionalization of social and industrial techniques will need the kind of multidisciplinary approach that exists in the child guidance clinic where psychiatrist, psychologist, and psychiatric social worker represent three areas of the child's life, each with the maximum competence in just one area, but with some knowledge of the other two. Within the community mental health field, the psychologist could contribute to both the diagnostic assessment and the therapeutic process, with occupational factors forming the counterpart of the educational factors in which he is the expert as regards the child.

The psychologist's role has not been adequately represented in the developments in West Ham, nor in Newham, and the multidisciplinary nature of the scheme is incomplete, except in so far as the child guidance clinic provides a clinical base.

Intradepartmental Communication

The medical officer of health, in addition to being the originator and chief designer of the scheme, has remained an active participant in the conceptualizations of methods of professional work, and in providing administrative machinery to make the work possible. He has made himself available to members of professional and administrative staff at all times. He holds weekly sessions with each of the senior staff separately to discuss problems, and the different sections of the department have their own consultation committees, which meet regularly. Joint meetings are held at regular intervals, and whenever one of the frequent crises occurs.

The John F. Kennedy Centre

Planning of each new development is always a joint affair. One example is the Junior Training Centre for Mentally Handicapped children—now called the John F. Kennedy Centre. For some years, this had been housed in pre-fabricated buildings that were disused army huts. Good work was being carried out in unsuitable premises. Before plans for the new buildings were drawn up, a number of conferences were held with the borough architect's staff, and these were attended by the medical officer of health, his deputy, the principal of the centre, a health visitor and the consultant psychiatrist. A member of the architect's staff visited the existing centre, watching the activities and asking members of the staff what they would like in the new premises. They were ready to give answers, once they knew that they were being taken seriously. At the conferences, an attempt was made to see how the building could be adapted to the kind of activities that were intended to take place. The assumption was made that the defect in mentally handicapped children is not static. The children are all subject to emotional disturbance as a result of failure to fit in with inappropriate expectations. They may deteriorate intellectually, if given insufficient stimulus, and they have a capacity for intellectual growth, if given a level of education appropriate to their developmental stages. This requires all the usual nursery-school equipment (Tizard, 1964), adapted to children older than the usual nursery-school age. They can also accustom themselves to domestic equipment, such as electric washing machines, cookers, sewing machines and all the fittings of a modern home; and to craft work, using machinery for making articles in wood, metal and ceramic materials. They can acquire social skills, recognize the words in public notices, go on outings to shops, cafés, cinemas and clubs. Above all, they can learn to play and enjoy themselves, alone and with one another. They also need psychotherapy.

The model for a building for all these purposes could not be taken from any existing institution, and something had to be abstracted from the concepts of a home, a school, a workshop, a social centre, and a child guidance clinic. The architect took note of the activities that were to take place and provided a structure that has an artistry of its own.

The building contains its assembly hall, classrooms, work rooms, playground, indoor swimming pool and a special care unit for the emotionally disturbed, with built-in sand and water pits and space in which over-activity can be legitimized. The classrooms have cranked walls, to allow nooks for dividing a small class into still smaller groups. The plans captured the imagination of the committee, who authorized an expenditure greater than was first contemplated, and when the building was approaching completion, at the time of the assassination of John F. Kennedy, it was decided to give the centre his name.

The move to the new building provided a challenge to the staff that was undertaken with mixed feelings. Would they miss the homely atmosphere of the old building? Would they be equal to the opportunities offered by the new one?

The challenge came from an unexpected quarter. The new building attracted many professional visitors from this country and abroad. The staff find themselves faced with questions about their work to which there is no ready answer, and with compliments that are difficult to live up to. Visitors do not hesitate to ask about their salaries and about their private lives. Some have questioned whether mentally defective children would appreciate, or merited, such a fine building or such devoted work.

The justification for the building came from the parents, who are proud that their children are thought worthy of facilities which help them to develop. The children are dressed better, look prettier, and seem more intelligent than before. Even mentally handicapped children don't look "silly" when carrying out activities that interest them.

Sometimes visitors say, "But of course you don't have those of lower level of intelligence"; sometimes, "Of course, this is a *showplace*". The answer to these statements was first that it was the *only* provision, and therefore it is the *standard* provision and not a showplace, and next, that the children were not specially selected, but covered the whole range of those children in West Ham who are severely subnormal. The Education Department provides a special school within the educational system for those with less severe handicaps, who are designated educationally subnormal.

Adult Centres

A shortcoming in the provision is made apparent when the children leave the centre. The adult provision for mentally handicapped and for those with chronic mental or physical illness is still in the process of reorganization. Two adult centres exist at present in the part of Newham that was formerly West Ham, and a combined centre (children and adults) in former East Ham. A comprehensive scheme for the borough is being worked out, in order to provide several different kinds of centre to serve different functional needs.

Adaptation to Changing Patterns

Dissatisfactions, frustration, and disappointments with the performance of the community mental health service have been experienced by the staff of other departments. Those who alter traditional methods of working have to justify the changes by successful results, and these are not always obtainable. Change is not always seen as an improvement and is not acceptable unless some dissatisfaction has been felt with previous methods. The professional and lay population of the West Ham part of the new borough has made its contribution to the development of the service, and has given expression to its own brand of resistances to the new image of community mental health. There was no reason to expect that a ready-made system would be acceptable to the East Ham part, which had had no share in the preliminary thinking and rethinking.

Much heartaching among the senior administrative staff had been experienced throughout the local government services in the Greater London area when the corresponding departments of two or more separate boroughs became united into single departments. The amalgamation of East Ham and West Ham was seen as a take-over, one way or the other. West Ham was the larger of the pre-existing units, but not always the leader. In the mental health field, it was the West Ham pattern which was to prevail, and which would therefore remain suspect in the eastern part of the new borough.

Difficulties within the staff of the mental health team exist and have increased when new members are recruited, who have not had to survive previous turmoil and disappointments. The service as a whole is one which is much visited by professional workers from many parts of the world. The staff develop a patter, which is a mixture of accounts of actual practice and of aspirations. We sometimes deceive ourselves by our own patter. Prospective recruits to the service are encouraged to pay visits before making a formal application for an advertised post. They are warned about the deficiencies in the service, but they pick up the enthusiasm and the excitement of those working in the field. The enthusiasm frequently wanes, in old and new staff alike. A staff that is larger and more highly qualified than that of many other similar areas finds itself, nevertheless, stretched beyond its capacity by demands that grow faster than the number of its personnel.

Fulbright Scholar

Many short-term and long-term visits of observation have been made to the service. During the academic year 1964/5, a Fulbright Professor was placed with us. We were fortunate in that the one chosen was Henry Maier, Professor of Sociology at the University of Washington, Seattle. He had had experience of studying "the helping process" in social work, particularly with families which included handicapped children. He participated in case conferences, staff discussions, and planning meetings. He conducted seminars with the staff of the community mental health service, and with the staff of other departments. He proved a source of strength, at times when the reorganization of a rapidly growing service was creating tensions within the department.

Community Care Centre

The latest phase has been the provision in December 1965 of a building to act as "Community Care Centre" for the whole Borough of Newham. Up to this time, the social workers had used offices in one wing of the administrative office block which housed the West Ham Health Department. There was insufficient accommodation for the social-work staff, and interviews with patients were apt to be interrupted by office routine. The new community care centre is an old-fashioned building, with bare steel girders across a large central hall, and industrial glazed bricks lining the inner walls. With very little redecoration, it has acquired a welcoming appearance, and there are a number of small rooms in which interviews can be held comfortably.

It is intended that it will provide experience on which to plan a purpose-built centre sometime in the future. Individual and group therapy, and social club activities, can take place there, and it will be the home for the young people's consultation service. It is hoped that diagnostic assessments for comprehensive and integrated treatment will be carried out there, including those for the consideration of placement in one or other of the specialized training centres. This will have advantages over the present practice of holding interviews at the centre at which placement is being requested, as the interview then appears to be for the purpose of acceptance or rejection—rather than for choosing the most suitable placement. It will also allow for a diagnostic conference of all the different professional contributors to the diagnosis, which is a decision for action.

The community care centre will also provide facilities for group meetings and group discussions with professional workers from the Health Department and other services.

Integration or Fragmentation

An integrated, comprehensive, or multidisciplinary approach need not become an ideology. The purpose of diagnosis is to separate off the relevant aspects of a problem, and no diagnosis can ever be total. In many cases, intervention in just one area of living is sufficient, and one should not uncover more of a patient's life than is necessary to cope adequately with his needs.

Each professional service has its limited aim defined by legislation or professional ethics, but problems of living cannot always be divided along these artificial lines. In some instances, the clinical medical treatment takes the patient back to his former good health. In others, financial assistance may be all that is necessary to meet a social need. Others again need counselling or case-work to help to restore disturbed relationships. A single one of these processes may be enough. If several people are working at the same time and on the same problem, without adequate communication with one another, and without having some common aim, the result may be damaging.

Fragmentation of problems and of work is sometimes apparent at the time that some aspect is referred to the community mental health service. There are occasions when, despite our claims to be an integrated service, some fragmentation continues after a case has been referred to the local authority, and two departments of the same service may be approached at the same time. The following case will illustrate a number of points.

An unmarried woman, 28 years old, living with her widowed mother, had recently left the psychiatric wards of a Central London teaching hospital. A letter from the psychiatric social worker of the hospital was sent to the principal mental health social worker of the Newham service, giving the history, which was briefly as follows.

The girl had attended an ordinary school, had been employed for 2 or 3 years, and then for some 10 years had remained at home with her mother. No one had complained until about 18 months ago. She then became irritable with her mother, and had begun to suffer from a feeling of strangeness and of depression. She had been referred by her family doctor to the local psychiatric out-patient department, and from there, a placement had been obtained for her at the teaching hospital. She responded to medical treatment and was placed in an occupational therapy unit, where she began to work adequately. When attempts were made to help her find outside employment, in anticipation of her discharge, she left hospital immediately against advice. The psychiatric social worker of the hospital had been in touch with the mother and had felt that an overclose and possessive attitude was a factor in the pathology. The letter stated that the psychiatrist in charge of the case would write simultaneously to the medical officer attached to the adult training centre of the Newham authority. A recommendation was to be made that the girl should attend that centre, and it was requested that visits should be paid by one of the Newham psychiatric social workers to the home, in order to "attempt to modify the attitude of the mother".

Later, a copy of the psychiatrist's letter was made available to the intake conference of the community mental health service, but placement of the young woman at the centre was apparently being dealt with as a separate process.

The psychiatrist's letter referred to the clinical diagnosis of "depression and depersonalization", and ended with the opinion that the prognosis was likely to be bad, as a good deal of social work which had been done with the mother had been unsuccessful.

It was evident that some co-ordination of the treatment of mother and daughter would be necessary. Co-ordination of the processes needs a key figure, and it was thought that this should be the family doctor. One of the psychiatric social workers, therefore, telephoned the family doctor, asking if he would like to discuss the problem of this family with those who were going to take the next steps to help them. He demurred a little, saying that he did not have much time, and he would need to see the patient first. Would the psychiatric social worker go and visit the young woman, and tell her to come to see him, and, after that, he would get in touch with us? He sensed some hesitation, and repeated his request for the psychiatric social worker to go to the patient, saying that he himself could not visit without being asked, and also that he had not much time for consultations with other services. The psychiatric social worker asked if it would help if she and the consultant psychiatrist visited him at his surgery, at the same time as the patient. The doctor's tone changed immediately. "Would he do that?" he asked. "In that case, I will go and visit the patient this afternoon, and I shall arrange for us to meet", and he suggested a time 2 days later.

The story is perhaps spoiled by the sequel, which was that when the doctor visited the home, the daughter and mother together told him that they wanted no medical help, no psychiatric help, nor any attendance at the training centre. The young woman would herself get a job when she wanted one.

The staff at the training centre still felt that if only the girl could have been separated from her mother in some way, and had attended the centre, all would have been well. Had she not worked adequately in the occupational therapy unit of the hospital? The mother was no concern of theirs, if only she would let the daughter free. She needed to be told that she was not acting in the daughter's best interests.

The family doctor was prepared to accept the position that he would offer and arrange any help that was possible, when this family felt they needed it. Incidentally, it is never true that doctors have no time for psychiatric patients or those who need to talk about some problem. It is just that they have no time for what seems to have no purpose or end-product, or for anything that seems unimportant.

There were a number of diagnoses applicable to this case. There was the *clinical* one of depression with depersonalization, but the patient was supposed to have recovered from this. The depersonalization syndrome could have been expressed *in terms of psychopathology*, according to particular schools. At this level of diagnosis, the correct treatment would have been to provide psychotherapy—if this process was available—within the resources of a hospital or local authority service and acceptable to the patient.

The situation could be thought of in *cultural terms*, recognizing that, scarcely a generation ago, it would not have been thought unusual for a single young woman to continue to live with her widowed mother without going out to work. This seems abnormal in the present age, and medical attendants and officers of the various social services are inclined to apply pressures to fit individuals into a pattern that is acceptable to the culture of this age. At the same time, while considering this dimension, it might be conjectured that the patient's original symptoms were associated with an attempt to break out from the outmoded culture within her home.

The next level of diagnosis is that of *family interaction*. Here, the treatment would aim at dealing with the family process and would involve joint interviews of the mother and daughter. The attempt to deal with clinical and occupational treatment of the daughter as a separate process from social casework with the mother had failed. One should have expected such failure. The assignment offered for the community mental health service was to visit the mother, in order to induce her to adopt a more socially acceptable attitude to her daughter and to the outside world. There is no reason to expect that any individual who is conscious of being right will accept the need to question the standards of a lifetime.

So far, this case has been unsuccessful, but lessons can be learned from it, and even in this particular case, the ground has been prepared for an integrated approach through the family doctor when the next crisis occurs. It is to be expected that the conflicts of dependence and independence/separation, and union (Kahn, 1965), will have their vicissitudes; and the time will arise when mother and daughter together will feel the need of help. That will be the time for therapy on a family basis.

Amongst the levels of diagnosis, we should not neglect the insights given us by great poets and dramatists. Several months after the discussions on this case, there arose, from the recesses of memory, recollections of Tennyson's *Lady of Shalott*. Here, a house-bound (or castle-bound) woman who could not face the busy world, except in the reflection of a mirror, made an attempt to release herself and to enter into the ordinary community.

> She has heard a whisper say,
> A curse is on her if she stay
>   To look down to Camelot.
> She knows not what the curse may be,
> And so she weaveth steadily,
> And little other care hath she,
>   The Lady of Shalott.

Seeing her knight in the distance, she ventured to break away.

> She left the web, she left the loom,
> She made three paces thro' the room,
> She saw the water-lily bloom,
> She saw the helmet and the plume,
>   She look'd down to Camelot.
> Out flew the web and floated wide;
> The mirror crack'd from side to side;
> 'The curse is come upon me,' cried
>   The Lady of Shalott.

The poem goes on to say how she floated downstream to her death.

What was the whisper? In whose voice was it expressed? Many times, in the individual therapy of patients, I have been confronted with self-recriminations of those who accuse themselves of badness at the slightest attempt to find any independence, to assert themselves, or express themselves with vigour. The recriminations are their own, but when pressed, they reveal that the voice in which they are expressed is that of the mother.

In a figurative way, the syndrome of depersonalization could be expressed as the shattering of a mould which had been applied to the personality. When the mould is broken (the mirror cracked from side to side) there is no alternative image which the individual can recognize as representing the self. The personality has acquired no shape of its own. Cure is sometimes sought in a way that either attempts to fit the individual back into the old mould, or alternatively, there are always other individuals ready to find a new shape in which to compress the patient. Such a patient seldom has the resources, or the opportunity, to achieve an identity that is satisfactory. The pull of family (sometimes even after the death of parents) is too strong. These are the cases where family therapy needs to be a conjoint affair. They are most successful when they are multiprofessional. Many visits have been paid to homes by a combined team of psychiatrist, psychiatric social worker and a therapist, or instructor from one of the training centres.

Extending the Range of Child Guidance

The child guidance clinic, at the beginning, provided the inspiration for the multidisciplinary nature of the community mental health service. It is now receiving, in return, the benefit of the experience of communication with other services. There had already been a background of integrated investigation and diagnosis. The child psychiatrist in the child guidance clinic carries a responsibility for clinical diagnosis, but he does not make his diagnosis alone, on the basis of his own observations and written reports from colleagues. The relevant diagnosis is arrived at in joint personal discussion of the three participants. When communication has to be made with schools, with children's departments, and probation departments, it is equally necessary to recognize that a relevant diagnosis is not one which is made in the child guidance clinic and conveyed in writing to the other agency. If it is going to acquire meaning for other people who are working with the problem, they also need to share in the *making* of the diagnosis. This means that wherever the problem is one in which a number of people have to share the work, they also have to share the making of decisions.

The child guidance clinic carries out a considerable amount of work in the traditional pattern, but wherever it is thought necessary, visits are paid to schools and other departments in order to discuss problems.

Such visits are becoming increasingly welcome. At first, as was mentioned previously, it seemed that other agencies were more anxious to get rid of a problem than to understand it. Schools, naturally, look for help with the problem of children whose behaviour is unsatisfactory. The hope is that the undesirable behaviour is the equivalent of illness. Sometimes this is so, but it is not invariably the case. Undesirable behaviour may be a way of expressing emotional disturbance. It may be a reaction to an unsatisfactory environment, or it may be the failure to *acquire* normal standards of behaviour. It has to be emphasized that a child guidance clinic has not got a stock of "treatment", which will convert bad behaviour into good behaviour.

Visits to the schools are undertaken in order to discuss problems of particular children, and sometimes it is possible to find explanations which leave the problem within the educational field. These visits, too, are usually multi-professional. The educational psychologist is the essential member; a psychiatrist and psychiatric social worker, or both, may accompany him.

Joint Interviews with Patients

Health visitors and medical officers often come for help with regard to families with whom they have been working for a long time. Sometimes, it is only to discuss the problem. At other times, it is because one or more members of the family are thought to be in need of some kind of further assessment or of psychiatric treatment.

Many of these cases are inappropriate to the psychiatric hospital in-patient or out-patient investigation, and many of them, although exhibiting some psychiatric symptoms, can well continue within the field of work of the health visitor or medical officer at the Maternal and Child Welfare Clinic. In such cases, it is considered to be better that the interview with the family by the community care psychiatrist and psychiatric social worker should take place *in the presence of the original worker*. More and more joint interviews of this kind are being undertaken. The original professional worker is not a silent observer, but a participant, and the problem is neither taken over nor competed for.

Planning for Hostels

There is one field of work in which Newham has made no progress at all, although it is a statutory obligation. This is the provision of hostel accommodation for mentally disturbed and mentally handicapped children and adults. None has been built so far, because we do not know what to build.

The first thoughts were that different hostels would be built for children and adults with different categories of disturbances or defect, but we do not know how to translate the needs from a clinical diagnosis to a shape of living space. A good many types of residential accommodation already exist in the hospital and social services of the country. There are different kinds of hospitals for those who need medical and nursing care. There are residential schools for children needing special education; remand homes and approved schools for delinquents; children's homes for those deprived of parental care—and these may be institutions, cottage homes, or there may be boarding-out arrangements.

There is a lack of knowledge of how the residential part of any provision is related to the total requirements of some particular category of person or problem.

We shall be driven to experimenting with a number of different kinds of accommodation, e.g. small flatlets in the ordinary housing provision for the area; bed-sitting rooms in units that may have common dining or recreational facilities; and possibly adaptations of old houses, if these can be found in an area where there are very few houses of the larger type. Supervised lodgings in ordinary homes might be obtained. What we hope to do is to introduce, as the criterion for types of accommodation, the concept of functional diagnosis rather than of clinical categories. We shall have to ask, "What is the type of residential need for some particular person?", rather than, "What kind of a hostel is necessary for a mentally defective person, or a schizophrenic patient?". The question of supervision, and of clinical and social case-work support, will be as essential as the type of accommodation, and many local authorities have already experienced residential staffing difficulties in some of the cases where hostel provision has been made. When we make our first experiments, it will be with considerable trepidation.

Conclusion

Developments of community mental health services have been found necessary for the following reasons.

1. Progress in clinical treatment of mental illness has been so great that many patients are able to be discharged from psychiatric hospitals after a fairly short stay. Many of these patients need continued treatment, or supportive services, while living in their own homes. Many other mentally ill patients are able to remain in their own homes and in the community throughout the duration of the illness. Domiciliary treatment is possible only when supportive services are available, and when the community is tolerant to the presence of the mentally ill within its midst.

2. Mental illness is recognized as having expression in forms other than the symptoms which fit into categories of disease. Disturbances of thoughts, feelings and behaviour, and of interpersonal relationships, have psychiatric implications, but the persons in whom the disturbances appear may continue to be the concern of a variety of professions, who have to work in co-ordination with one another.

3. Notwithstanding the therapeutic advances referred to, mental illness remains a heavy burden on medical and social services, and on the community as a whole. The prevalence of mental illness is so high that the total range of the services that are available is never likely to cover the total needs. There is, therefore, a demand for preventive services.

Prevention is largely a non-psychiatric process and is a product of the work of every professional and non-professional worker who has any responsibility for nurturing, educating, training, or curing human beings.

The theoretical basis is an extension from psychiatry, and community mental health services carry the medical principles of prevention into other services.

The community mental health service provides a working model for co-ordination of professional practice which is involved with the many different areas of living activities. The problems are multidimensional, and the service is multidisciplinary.

The service is professionalized on the medical model of the successive processes of:

1. Investigation.
2. Diagnosis.
3. Treatment.

1. THE INVESTIGATION

The multidimensional nature of the problems requires that each aspect of the investigation be carried out by a professional worker, who has had training and acquired skill in his particular field.

The child guidance clinic system of working with a team of psychiatrist, psychologist, and psychiatric social worker can provide a prototype for a community mental health service.

2. DIAGNOSIS

It is only for the purpose of medical treatment that diagnosis in terms of clinical categories is useful. Other dimensions of diagnosis are relevant when action has to be taken by non-medical personnel, and these may be expressed in terms of disorder of function, or of relationships, or in levels of maturity.

Thus, a diagnosis in terms of educational disabilities and capacities leads to decisions on special educational provision. An occupational diagnosis leads to rehabilitative procedures. A social diagnosis may include descriptions of the ability to use material resources, or may be expressed in interpersonal relationships and is the basis of social case-work.

None of these diagnoses is ever complete in itself, and a comprehensive diagnosis is necessary for integrated action, which is the treatment.

3. Treatment

This is the action which follows from the investigation and diagnosis. It has been customary to confine the word "treatment" to medical procedures, but phrases like "occupational therapy", "remedial teaching", and "special educational treatment" now give recognition to the possibility of a variety of structured therapeutic procedures, which follow the making of precise diagnoses.

A community mental health service needs to have a range of therapeutic activities which may be carried out either within its own boundaries, or in co-ordination with other professions.

Types of Treatment

Clinical psychiatric treatment has not been mentioned here, as it is the responsibility of the hospital services, but all community mental health services depend ultimately upon the existence of the hospital medical service, which deals with the clinical aspects of mental illness at in-patient or out-patient level, and on the family practitioner, who maintains responsibility for the patient at all times.

The community mental health service supplies the *rehabilitative, supportive and preventive services*. These latter services, applied either to a patient or his family, may have to be co-ordinated with clinical treatment.

Psychiatric theory and practice make a contribution to the non-clinical services such as *occupational therapy* and *case-work*, dealing with a patient and with the members of the family.

The wide range of services needs a co-ordinator who becomes a key figure. The key figure may be the family doctor, psychiatrist, psychiatric social worker, or a member of another profession, such as a health visitor or child care officer. The selection of the key figure may depend upon the way the problem is first presented, and frequently it is a diagnostic assessment made by the community mental health service which enables some other service to retain, or resume, the primary relationship with some individual or family. Some professional service has to accept a continuing responsibility during the time that various other services take up and relinquish their specialist roles.

Interprofessional Consultations

These consultations may be a part of investigation, diagnosis and treatment. When a problem is referred by one service to another, the procedure may take any of the following basic courses.

1. Complete transfer of the responsibility.

2. Examination and reporting back to the original agency.

3. Conjoint examinations and treatment.

The last-named procedure depends upon the development of common aims and a common language, and requires confidence in one another.

4. The Mental Health Consultation. (This process takes place in the absence of the client or patient. Other professions seek help with specific problems. In discussion of these problems, general principles are arrived at.)

Finally, it is necessary to emphasize that all the processes which are at present being undertaken by a community mental health service need conceptualization and formulation. Phrases like "giving support" or "making a relationship" are applied indiscriminately to organized professional work, and to the unorganized interpersonal processes that exist between lay members of the community. Professionalization involves a *disciplined* use of relationships, and the study of the nature of the interaction between therapist and patient. Professional work must be capable of being taught, in order that the work should not die with its orginators. Systems of community mental health are new. Comparisons might be made between the development of a service and the life history of an individual.

Referring to the integrative processes which take place in the life of a child between the ages of 9 and 12, Henry Maier states (1965):

> The *child* brings into several systems the standards he has acquired and practised in the past. He also incorporates his elders' comments, standards and expectations. Basically, he relates fragmentary practices, hear-say and knowledge into one related, practical system, although the theoretical implications of the system will not be comprehended until later. [My italics.]

If, in the above passage, we substitute the word "community mental health worker" for the word "child", it would be a fair representation of the present level of community mental health work. Much progress has yet to be made before even its adolescence is reached.

References

CAPLAN, G. (1962), *An Approach to Community Mental Health*, London, Tavistock.
CLARK, D. H. (1964), *Administrative Therapy*, London, Tavistock.
EARLY, D. F. (1960), *Lancet*, **i**, 435.
FREUDENBERG, R. K., HARDING, W. G. and KAHN J. H. (1965), *Mental Health Services in the United Kingdom*, Geneva, W.H.O.
KAHN, J. H. (1963), In Freeman, H. L. and Farndale, W. A. J. (eds.), *Trends in the Mental Health Services*, Oxford, Pergamon Press.
KAHN, J. H. (1965), *Human Growth and the Development of Personality*, Oxford, Pergamon Press.
KAHN, J. H. and NURSTEN, J. (1964), *Unwillingly to School*, Oxford, Pergamon Press.
MAIER, H. (1965), *Three Theories of Child Development*, New York, Harper & Row.
MARTIN, D. V. (1962), *Adventure in Psychiatry*, Oxford, Bruno Cassirer.
QUERIDO, A. (1963), *The Efficiency of Medical Care*, Leiden, H. E. Stenfert Kroese.
TIZARD, J. (1964), *Community Services for the Mentally Handicapped*, Oxford Medical Publications, London, Oxford Univ. Press.

33. Developing a Community Mental Health Service*

ANTHONY R. MAY and S. L. WRIGHT

IT IS fair to say that in Great Britain we have crossed the threshold of social psychiatry, and have now accepted a concept of care for the mentally ill within the social and cultural confines of the community. In the past decade we have advanced financial, humanitarian and clinical arguments to support this attitude. But in retrospect, we can trace its ideological and practical evolution through the transition from custodial care to the therapeutic community of the mental hospital; from exclusively institutional to increasingly extramural psychiatry; from negative restraint of mentally disturbed behaviour to positive treatment; and from the boredom and overprotection of the isolated institution to the therapeutic stimulus of a normal social environment. These trends have been recognized by implication of the Mental Health Act (1959), but it has fallen to the professional staff working in this field to develop the new patterns of care, within a framework which seeks to integrate prevention, treatment and rehabilitation.

The application of these principles has raised practical problems for clinical psychiatrists and for local authority staff, in striving to achieve a goal which may be summarized as co-operation, co-ordination and communication, and which will incidentally provide for continuity of care. The development of a comprehensive mental health service must be based on a multilateral approach to the clinical, social and economic needs of the patient and his relatives. This in turn requires a multidisciplinary team, with a unified direction of purpose (Caplan, 1964). Local conditions will inevitably modify the pattern (Mackeith, 1960), but in this paper we shall describe the organization of the mental health service in Croydon, which is a former county borough on the outskirts of London, with a population of 250,000. (It has now become a borough within the Greater London Council.) This description of a joint enterprise refers mainly to adults who are mentally ill.

The Aims

In planning a comprehensive service, it is necessary to clarify the broad aims, and these may be defined as follows:

*Based on papers read to the Mental Health Group of the Society of Medical Officer of Health (A.R.M.) and to the Health Congress of the Royal Society of Health (S.L.W.).

1. To provide for prevention, recognition (diagnosis), treatment and rehabilitation of different types and different stages of psychiatric disorder presenting in a community.
2. To provide a range of treatment possibilities, and to avoid isolation and segregation of patients in a psychiatric hospital wherever possible.
3. To promote community and family support and tolerance, which will facilitate extramural management of the patient.
4. To foster integration and co-operation between diverse professional and lay organizations with responsibilities for mental health and illness in a community.

If we accept these aims, it will be apparent that they cannot be achieved without producing initial resistance on the part of staff who are required to modify their traditional roles. It is especially important to ensure harmonious integration between those whose training has emphasized the clinical aspects of mental illness, and those who are most concerned with the impact of disturbed social behaviour in a community context. These different orientations are responsible for most of the difficulties which stand in the way of progress to a unified service, and are epitomized in the attitudes of psychiatric hospital and local authority staff.

Barriers between Mental Hospital and Community

Within the mental hospital, nurses and doctors tend to adopt a mainly clinical approach to the patient, often without due reference to social factors. Admission is viewed as a circumscribed clinical episode, and the patient as a sick person who has come to be "cured". This concept of "individual" medicine, in which the patient has a special and dependent relationship with hospital staff, is one which derives from the treatment of physical illness. But, as in the management of tuberculosis, it cannot be applied exclusively to the mentally ill, since the social background is often all-important. Furthermore, the trend to earlier discharge makes it all the more necessary for proper evaluation of the social adjustment of patients who are required to face once more the stresses of a competitive community. Assessments of recovery which are based on hospital standards of conformity may not be valid in terms of normal society, especially when the judges are themselves accustomed to the artificially low requirements of the sheltered institution (May et al., 1963).

Lack of consideration for the social stresses operating on a patient, or within his family, may result in relapse and re-admission. Where clinical recovery is equated with social stability, insufficient attention is paid to the burden on family and relatives, and responsibility for social adjustment is often handed over by clinicians to local authority staff without proper consultation.

On the other hand, general practitioners, social workers and health visitors often show unrealistic expectations of clinical possibilities in psychiatric treatment. It is understandable that family and relatives find it difficult to tolerate deviant behaviour which they cannot understand, especially when they are without any form of support. But often, the patient is blamed for unreasonable and antisocial attitudes which are precipitated by environmental stress. In these circumstances, both clinical and social factors may interact and a combined effort is necessary to prevent admission to hospital, and to guard against subsequent disillusion when the expected therapeutic miracle is not forthcoming (May, 1961).

Duties of Local Authorities in Mental Health

The duties of local health authorities before 1959 were concerned almost entirely with the removal of psychiatric patients into mental hospitals. Dealing with them in the community is new and perplexing. In the field of physical diseases, tuberculosis offers the closest parallel. A chronic disease for which treatment was largely palliative and institutional, it was widespread, and not only was the patient at risk, but he could also be a danger to other people. The diagnosis carried the stigma of incurability and the suspicion of hereditary taint. Long-term supportive measures were needed for the patient and his family. To deal with this situation, the tuberculosis service joined prevention with treatment, care and after-care. Tuberculosis dispensaries were set up, where the doctor in charge linked hospital treatment and community care. He had a team of ancillary workers to support the family doctor, and access to rehabilitation facilities.

With the advent of successful chemotherapy, the cure of tuberculosis became possible. As a result, the stigma has largely disappeared, and the need for supportive services is steadily diminishing. One hopes that in the not too distant future, the treatment of chronic psychiatric illnesses will show a similar drastic change. Meanwhile, its social effects must be coped with, as chronic tuberculosis was formerly, by co-ordinating hospital and community care.

Planning the Hospital–Community Service

The social geography must first be studied. It is important that the catchment area of the hospital and the territory of the local health authority should coincide. This is not always so difficult as may appear at first sight. County councils, and county borough councils, the present local health authorities, were responsible before 1948 for providing mental hospitals. It is not uncommon, therefore, to find that although the mental hospital is some miles from the centre of the town, the boundaries of its catchment area are those of a county borough, or a section of a county. When the social geography is so convenient, or has been suitably adjusted, the local authority can then seek the co-operation of the medical staff of the hospital concerned, as advisers to the medical officer of health on community mental health services. There must be an indication, by reimbursement of salary, that this is not merely a façade of co-operation.

Joint appointments are clumsy expedients, but they are necessary with the present tripartite division of the health service. It is the only way at present by which the patient is guaranteed a full and adaptable service, and one which can deal not only with smooth progress from illness to recovery, but also adjust to any setbacks.

Having achieved co-ordination of planning, the domiciliary psychiatric team must next be provided.

The Mental Health Centre and the Community Psychiatrist

In connection with tuberculosis, the tuberculosis dispensary, which later became the chest clinic, must be mentioned. It provided accommodation for all concerned with the community care of the tuberculous, facilities for certain types of treatment, and ready access to advice and practical help for patients' relatives. The application of this idea to the mental health service is immediately apparent. The day hospital (Farndale, 1961) is emerging as a necessary component of a community mental health service, and the psychiatrist in charge is the greatest user of the social-work team (May and Gregory, 1963). The sharing of the services of this consultant by the regional hospital board and local health authority, with agreed reimbursement of salary, allows him to exercise, as the community psychiatrist, the essential clinical supervision of the psychiatric social-work team. They are seconded to him, in the way that the staff of the chest clinic act for the chest physician. Their office accommodation should, ideally, be in the premises used by the day hospital, and in this building should also be the facilities for the social clubs and day centre activities which are the responsibility of the local authority. The basic mental health centre has three components—the day hospital, the day centre, and office accommodation for the social-work team.

Problems of divided responsibility arise, and there will need to be an agreement between the regional hospital board and the local health authority about initial provision of the premises and sharing of running costs. If the policy is agreed, this is only a question of arithmetical calculation.

Other components of the mental health service may be added to the mental health centre; for example, a child guidance clinic (*Lancet*, 1963). It may adjoin the psychiatric unit of a general hospital (Little, 1963), but this is not essential.

The Social-work Team

Since psychiatric diseases are characterized by failure in social adaptation, trained social workers seem to be the proper officers for advisory and supportive duties.

The problem of co-ordinating hospital and local health authority social work is complicated by the long-established custom of mental hospitals employing their own psychiatric social workers. Furthermore, it is necessary to bring together those self-trained by long experience and others who have academic qualifications.

There can be little argument that the leader of the social-work team should be an experienced senior psychiatric social worker. This appointment should presumably be made by the local health authority. The first duty of the senior psychiatric social worker, who may be designated the Senior Mental Welfare Officer, is to ensure that all staff are used as members of a joint hospital–community service.

No simple formula can be suggested to regulate the allocation of work. There is a statutory duty on local health authorities to appoint mental welfare officers, so that one is always available to deal with urgent admission of a patient to hospital. There is also the statutory responsibility for the visiting of patients under guardianship, and for this, the division of the area into separate officers' districts may be desirable, to ensure continuity of supervision. A combination of service on districts and attachment to hospital clinical teams seems a workable solution.

Training of Social Workers

Whatever theories are put forward, any success must depend upon the recruitment of social workers. This was covered very fully in the report of the working party on social workers (Ministry of Health, 1959). The report calculated for the mental health service, one psychiatric social worker per 150,000 and four general-trained social workers per 100,000 of the population. This figure of about five social workers per 100,000 of the population is quoted as the number likely to be employed by local authorities in the Ministry of Health's Plan-development of Community Care (1963a). This seems to be a modest establishment to meet the estimated minimum case-load of mentally disordered patients, of 5 per 1000 of the population.

Local authorities cannot directly augment university training courses. They can only second staff on salary for such training. The Younghusband courses for general social workers are being arranged at colleges for further education. County and county borough councils can therefore set up training courses for these general purposes social workers.

As with the university courses, the local authorities have powers to second these staff on salary, in order to undertake the necessary training. In all this there is nothing new, and future developments may include the pooling of costs on the basis already established for midwives and health visitors, to ensure that all authorities contribute.

General Practitioners

It is the family doctor who has the responsibility for domiciliary medical care. A recent publication on the work of the family doctor (Ministry of Health, 1963b) devotes a section to mental health services. Two of the comments emphasize that comprehensive community mental health services are not yet available. Despite the statement, "It should be recognised that work in this field is very time-consuming and arduous and makes considerable inroads in the doctor's working day", there is a request that "all services provided by clinics, hospitals, local authorities, employment officers and voluntary workers should be co-ordinated through him (the family doctor)". It is wrong to place upon the family doctor the burden of social work. Taking the example of the tuberculosis service, family doctors have not resented the supervision and after-care given by chest physicians. Subject to their being kept informed, general practitioners have been pleased to leave specialized treatment and social work to the chest clinic staff. The essential factor is the acceptance by a consultant physician of clinical responsibility for the actions of the individual members of the team. The family doctor, knowing that he may contact the consultant physician at a local centre, and that his right to information and help will immediately be recognized, welcomes the assistance thus given in coping with a chronic illness.

This report also mentions, in connection with psychiatric illness, that "re-admission today is often more difficult than the effort to obtain admission in the first place. Rigid catchment areas complicate this." Removal of the power to enforce admission formerly possessed by duly authorized officers has increased difficulties in regard to re-admissions. The solution is the integrated hospital–community service, and the catchment area is basic to this concept. It does not preclude the voluntary acceptance by a hospital of a particular patient.

Domiciliary Nursing Service

Domiciliary visiting by their nurses has been developed by some mental hospitals. Introduced primarily because of a shortage of psychiatric social workers, it has been continued as a form of district nursing for psychiatric patients. Its value is not disputed, but power to employ nurses for such a purpose seems limited to Section 26 of the National Health Service Act. It could be provided by the ordinary local authority district nursing service, with assistant supervisors linked with the nursing staff of the mental hospital.

Hostels

Most authorities are approaching the provision of hostels for the mentally ill with some caution. Merely to replace hospital beds with hostel places seems a doubtful advance. A need for certain groups is easier to understand. Thus the elderly mentally confused patient, too disturbing for an ordinary old people's home, may require a special hostel, within the general provision of hostels for elderly persons. Younger patients, able to go to work, may need a period in a hostel before returning home, or to ordinary lodgings. Experience of these short-stay units proves that it is easier to admit than to discharge. The report on community services (Ministry of Health, 1963a) shows that local authorities are planning hostels for the mentally ill to give some 30 places per 100,000 of the population, excluding provision for the elderly mentally infirm.

Group Homes

Some authorities are experimenting with groups of 5 or 6 patients, selected as congenial companions and who are self-supporting, to share a house provided and furnished by the local authority. This avoids the need for costly purpose-built structure, and clearly permits great flexibility.

Boarding-out

A local authority boarding-out officer, able to guarantee board and lodgings charges, intensive social support services, and immediate removal of a patient in the event of unforeseen difficulties, can place successfully a variety of cases. The obvious advantages of living as ordinary members of the public in congenial lodgings need no stressing. The cost per patient, including salary of the boarding-out officer, is substantially less than for a place in a hostel. To succeed, such a scheme needs the backing of a co-ordinated hospital–community service, of the type described. From experience, a full-time boarding-out officer should be able to place and retain up to 25 patients in suitable lodgings (Wright, 1966).

Evaluation

Clearly, the development of community services for the mentally ill is at a very early stage. If one accepts the view that there have been no fundamental discoveries in the treatment of psychiatric illnesses, one can only hope to show that the services prevent the ill-effects on patients of long-continued detention in mental hospitals, without placing an undue burden upon their relatives or upon the community. Research projects to this end, however careful, have necessarily been against the background of meagre social care and after-care. The need to evaluate the structure of the new services must not be overlooked, but the urgent task is to construct the services themselves (Wright, 1963).

The Principles of a Comprehensive Service

Bearing in mind the aims of a comprehensive service, and some of the problems inherent in traditional attitudes towards mental illness, we have evolved certain principles, which we have followed in devising the framework of our service.

1. We have tried to ensure a co-ordinated clinical and social approach to patients. In effect, this has meant providing for the contributions of doctor, nurse and social worker in the assessment of cases at all stages of illness, rehabilitation and resettlement.

2. We believe that staff should be able to rotate through different treatment centres, so that they can gain direct experience of the role and function of colleagues with whom they will be working. To this end, the joint appointment of hospital and local authority staff facilitates the interchange between clinical and community setting, and tends to avoid professional isolation in specialized categories.

3. A comprehensive service has to be flexible, if it is to meet the needs of patients with different types and at different stages of illness. Sometimes clinical emphasis will be predominant, and at other times social factors are paramount. Appropriate treatment facilities and staff should be readily available to meet these reciprocal needs, while continuity of care depends on easy transfer of both patients and staff within the service.

4. At our present stage of development, we believe that over-all clinical direction is necessary. In a service which seeks to co-ordinate clinical, social and economic measures, the needs of the patient and the community are perceived in many different ways by different agencies. Each of these assessments may be accurate, though some are more limited than others (Susser, 1965). The "community psychiatrist" (who may well require special training) is usually in the best position to co-ordinate the available facilities, and is an acceptable leader where professional allegiance may otherwise diverge. In Croydon, a consultant psychiatrist from the local mental hospital works on a sessional basis under the Medical Officer of Health, and is also Psychiatric Adviser to the local health authority.

5. The final principle we have adopted is to place the headquarters of our mental health service within the geographical location of the community it serves. The isolated mental hospital is outmoded as the principal administrative and treatment centre of psychiatric services, quite apart from the problem presented by deficiencies in communication. We believe that the

local community mental health centre is the logical base for the clinical and social staff whose responsibility lies in the demographic area, and it also provides a focus for consultation and advice for general practitioners and for others concerned with patients and their relatives.

The Method

In following these principles, the practical steps we have taken include the integration of clinical and social facilities, the integration of staff, and the organization of certain centralized services, which are available to a variety of referring agencies (May, Sheldon and Mackeith, 1962).

Treatment facilities which are common to most areas of the country today include the local mental hospital, out-patient diagnostic and after-care clinics, a day hospital,* and often a psychiatric unit in the local general hospital. Instead of considering these as relatively autonomous units, we have tried to integrate them into a network, which can meet the needs of the individual patient at different stages of his illness. In practice, this has meant that staff as well as patients have unrestricted use of any of these facilities, and are able to follow their patients as they move from one to another. We have sought to avoid any firm distinction between clinical supervision in the hospital and social supervision in the community. In fact, where a patient lives, and where he undergoes treatment or rehabilitation are factors suscep-tible to a variety of permutations and combinations.

The Mental Welfare Department of the local health authority has also been integrated into the network. An increasing number of referrals from sources other than the general practitioner enter the service through this channel, and although they usually present as social problems, the close and regular association with the community psychiatrist provides for clinical assessment wherever necessary. Other departments of the local authority, such as Housing, Education and Welfare, find this a useful arrangement, as do the local voluntary social organizations. Cases requiring psychiatric treatment can be quickly admitted to the appropriate centre, or else the various sup-portive agencies can be easily mobilized.

Integration of staff has been assisted by the joint hospital–local authority appointment of social workers, and by arranging for psychiatrists and mental hospital nurses to work in the community (May and Moore, 1963), while local authority social workers continue to be involved with their patients in the clinical treatment centres. Under these circumstances, both hospital and local authority staff should work together as a team, and in regular ward-rounds and conferences, they have gradually developed a mutual considera-tion for each other's point of view.

The centralized services include provision for industrial and domiciliary

* See Appendix to this paper.

rehabilitation. Industrial therapy workshops have been established for some years in the mental hospital, in the day hospital and in the adult training centre for the mentally subnormal. In the last year, industrial work has been extended to the occupation centre for the severely physically handicapped, and at the same time, the local authority has rented factory premises in Croydon, which have become the headquarters and top-grade workshop of our unified industrial therapy organization. Those trainees showing the most aptitude in peripheral workshops can now progress to the sheltered factory, where they work together irrespective of mental or physical handicap, and where more realistic work pressures can provide a more accurate assessment of their potential (May and Smith, 1965). At all stages of industrial rehabilitation, social and clinical supervision is continued, but the local Disablement Resettlement Officer of the Ministry of Labour is co-opted into the team, to advise on past work record and future prospects of patients.

Domiciliary resettlement in the community often represents the most difficult phase in rehabilitation of the mentally ill. When patients cannot or should not return home, because of unsatisfactory and unalterable family relationships, alternative accommodation must be found. This will include a hostel or private lodgings, and in Croydon we have centralized arrangements for this. A boarding-out officer employed by the Mental Welfare Department attends any conference involving a patient who will need such help. This officer contributes to the team discussion, wherever it takes place, and her judgement and advice are invaluable, since she can correlate the clinical and social status of the patient with suitable vacancies. She forms the link between the mental health service and the local Mental After-Care Association Hostel, and maintains contact with some forty landladies, who have taken our patients as lodgers.

A useful addition to our centralized services has been the provision of an emergency "walk-in" clinic, based on the mental health centre. This is primarily a clinical facility, which enables general practitioners to obtain a psychiatric opinion on patients without the delay occasioned by our appointments system. But many referrals come from other sources, including social workers, nurses and various social agencies. For this clinic to be effective, the psychiatrist who runs it must have experience of all the supportive, treatment and rehabilitative facilities which are available, and must be able to call on these resources without delay.

Future Developments

The service we have described has evolved in Croydon over the past 4 years. It represents an attempt to meet new trends in management of psychiatric illness, to adjust community and hospital resources to the advantages of acutely ill as well as chronic ambulant psychiatric patients, and to provide a flexible frame of reference for staff concerned with clinical and social maladjustment in members of an urban industrialized society. In so far as Croydon is a compact geographical area, where local authority boundaries coincide with the catchment area of the psychiatric services, the administrative problems are less complicated than those of diffuse rural communities.

Even so, we are aware of the limitations of our current organization. The potential links with geriatric and child guidance services, and with health visitors, district nurses and voluntary social agencies, have not been fully exploited. Our aims for the primary prevention of psychiatric illness are at present subordinated to our efforts in secondary and tertiary prevention, though they merit important consideration in future planning.

We feel that a unified service embracing a population of 250,000, however compact, presents too unwieldy an administrative unit for the efficient deployment of our staff and facilities, and the dilution of these resources over the whole area places a constant strain on communication and co-ordination at the local level. We have, therefore, begun to divide the catchment area into geographical sectors, each with a population of 70,000–80,000, which will be the responsibility of clinical and social work teams based on local mental health centres. These strategically placed centres (of which three are currently designated) comprise day hospital facilities, and diagnostic and after-care clinics, and provide the headquarters for the staff working in the area. Liaison with local general practitioners, social agencies and relatives is much closer, personal contacts are improved, and the team effort is properly focused on *out-patient* care and treatment. Each sector has its own allocation of acute short-stay beds in the mental hospital, and together with the mental health centre, they form the treatment facilities available to the team of consultant, registrars, nurses and social workers. Team members are able to follow their patients before, during and after admission to hospital, but the organization differs from that of the hospital "firm", in that the administrative headquarters is not confined to the clinical setting of the hospital.

The Ministry of Health has emphasized the contribution which the general practitioner can make in early diagnosis and after-care of psychiatric illness, and the Gillie Report (Ministry of Health, 1963b), as mentioned above, suggests that the family doctor should co-ordinate ancillary and social services as the leader of the community psychiatric team. We have recently completed an investigation into the attitude of our local general practitioners, and there seems little doubt that these official expectations are overoptimistic. The average general practitioner feels that co-ordination of staff and services, especially in regard to chronic ambulant psychiatric patients, is the responsibility of the psychiatrist to whom he refers his case. If the general practitioner is to be integrated into the mental health team, he needs more practical experience of its scope and function, and this can perhaps be achieved more easily when he is in closer personal contact through a local mental health centre.

In conclusion, we should emphasize that co-operation between local authority and hospital services depends as much on personalities as on administrative ingenuity and expediency.

> He that complies against his will
> Is of his own opinion still.

References

CAPLAN, G. (1964), *Principles of Preventive Psychiatry*, London, Tavistock.
FARNDALE, J. (1961), *The Day Hospital Movement in Great Britain*, Oxford, Pergamon.
(1963), *Lancet*, **i,** 1007.
LITTLE, J. C. (1963), *Lancet*, **ii,** 1159.
MACKEITH, S. A. (1960), *Public Health*, **74,** 175.
MAY, A. R. (1961), *Lancet*, **i,** 760.
MAY, A. R. and GREGORY, E. (1963), *Public Health*, **78,** 19.
MAY, A. R. and MOORE, S. (1963), *Lancet*, **i,** 213.
MAY, A. R., SHELDON, A. P. and MACKEITH, S. A. (1962), *Lancet*, **ii,** 1319.
MAY, A. R. and SMITH, J. A. (1965), *Occupational Therapy*.
MAY, A. R., GREGORY, E., JONES, D. M. H. and BRUGGEN, P. (1963), *Lancet*, **ii,** 241.
MINISTRY OF HEALTH (1959), *Report of the Working Party on Social Workers*, London, H.M.S.O.
MINISTRY OF HEALTH (1963a), *The Development of Community Care*, London, H.M.S.O.
MINISTRY OF HEALTH (1963b), *The Field of Work of the Family Doctor*, London, H.M.S.O.
SUSSER, M. W. (1965), *Medical Care*, **3,** 52.
WRIGHT, S. L. (1963), *Public Health*, **77,** 218.
WRIGHT, S. L. (1966), *Public Health*, **80,** 164.

APPENDIX

THE DAY HOSPITAL IN A COMPREHENSIVE PSYCHIATRIC SERVICE

A. P. SHELDON and A. R. MAY

A day hospital has existed in Croydon since December 1956, with the part-time attendance of a psychiatrist and the services of a nursing sister and two nurses. It catered mainly for the daytime supervision and education of chronic psychotic and geriatric cases, and in this respect, functioned mainly as a long-stay "ward" of the mental hospital (Warlingham Park). Over the period 1957–61, 163 patients were admitted, with an average of 30 new admissions each year and an average daily attendance of 20. Some details of these patients are given in Table A1, showing that a preponderance of patients came from the older age groups and that the duration of stay was long, with a small turn-over of cases.

TABLE A1.

Details of 163 Patients, 1957–61

Diagnoses					Previous admission to mental hospital			Age				Duration of stay			
Schizophrenia	Affective psychosis	Organic psychosis	Neurosis	Other, incl. personality disorder	None	One	Two or more	Under 20	20–39	40–59	60+	<1 month	1–2 months	2–4 months	4 or more months
39	49	31	12	32	39	67	57	3	39	55	66	41	34	20	68

Present Facilities

This experience, which is not uncommon in day hospital practice, confirmed the need for a revision in policy, if we were to develop a treatment unit which would play a more active and effective role in the total district service envisaged (May, Sheldon and Mackeith, 1962). An opportunity to re-organize the day hospital arose in 1961, when the local health authority provided new premises in the form of a large house and garden, situated on a main 'bus route near the centre of the town.

At the same time, increased staff became available. This now comprises a part-time consultant, a full-time registrar, a nursing sister and two nurses, a full-time psychiatric social worker, a full-time occupational therapist, and part-time assistance from a psychologist. This staff is provided by Warlingham Park Hospital, except for the psychiatric social workers, who are all appointed jointly by the Hospital Management Committee and the local health authority.

The day hospital offers treatment 5 days a week, on a full-time or part-time attendance basis. It is open from 9 a.m. to 5 p.m., and the same premises are used each evening for after-care clinics, group psychotherapy, and patients' social clubs.

Accommodation is on two floors, with additional facilities for industrial and occupational therapy and for art therapy. On the ground floor are the dining room, club room and kitchen; on the first floor are offices for doctors, nurses, secretary and psychiatric social worker and two group discussion rooms.

Besides routine contact with medical staff, patients are divided into groups, which meet once a week at fixed times with a designated member of the staff. Groups are based on considerations of age, diagnostic category and personal problems. Depth of discussion varies with the group composition, but these meetings provide at the least a means of assessment of progress. Drugs are prescribed through the hospital dispensary. Electroplexy is carried out at the nearby psychiatric unit of the local general hospital.

The patients' programme includes occupational or industrial therapy, for which they receive token payment; lectures and demonstrations organized by voluntary agencies and business firms; play readings; cookery classes; and expeditions to shops or local entertainments. A midday meal is provided free, and tea on a nominal payment. Ambulance transport is available to those patients too ill or feeble to come by public transport, but we encourage patients to come independently whenever feasible. Bathing facilities are available at the day hospital for cases in need of toilet supervision, and a chiropodist visits regularly. A washing machine has been installed for use by patients themselves.

Referral and Treatment

Patients are referred from any part of the district psychiatric service including out-patient clinics, mental hospital, psychiatric unit in the local general hospital, out-patient nursing service, Mental Welfare Department of the local health authority, or direct by a general practitioner. In order to control the admissions, we hold a weekly pre-admission clinic at which all potential admissions are interviewed, but in fact the number rejected is very small, since our usual policy is to take every case for at least a period of assessment. When a patient is accepted, he is told about the treatment programme and what is expected of him by way of attendance and participation in activities. At the same time, both the referring agency and the general practitioner are informed.

At a weekly staff conference, individual treatment plans are formulated and reviewed from time to time. Special emphasis is laid on social aspects and relatives are always seen by the psychiatric social worker. Financial, economic and employment problems are considered, and local authority agencies are consulted where necessary. Provisions for employment or attendance at the local industrial rehabilitation unit are made through the disablement resettlement officer, who attends this conference.

As the patient improves, his full-time attendance is progressively cut to a few days in the week. After discharge, he comes to an evening after-care clinic or social club, and contact is maintained with relatives and employers in special cases.

The Patients

We have collected clinical and social details, and followed the outcome of treatment in the 186 patients who were admitted to our new day hospital in one year since its opening in 1961.

TABLE A2.

Clinical Details of 186 Patients, 1961–62

Diagnoses					Duration of illness (since 1st referral to psychiatrist)			Previous admission to mental hospitals		
Schizophrenia	Affective psychosis	Organic psychosis	Neurosis	Other, incl. personality disorder	< 1 year	1–2 years	> 2 years	None	One	Two or more
55	56	21	24	30	74	12	100	30	63	93

TABLE A3.

Social Details of 186 Patients

Age				Sex		Civil status			Social[a] class			Domi-cile		Distance from day hospital	
Under 20	20–39	40–39	60+	Male	Female	Single	Married	Widowed/divorced	1–4	Skilled	Unskilled	Lives alone	Lives with relatives	Under 2 miles	Over 2 miles
11	59	65	51	56	130	62	88	36	30	106	50	59	127	100	86

[a] L. S. Economics classification of jobs.

Clinical details are given in Table A2. The diagnostic range shows a preponderance of psychotic patients and of patients with a long history of illness and of previous admissions to mental hospital. Less severely ill patients are in fact in the minority, and this underlines the unselective nature of our admission policy.

Table A3 shows that these patients came mostly from older age-groups, and that two-thirds lived with a relative, either spouse, child or parent.

Details of referral (Table A4) show that the majority came from psychiatric sources, and in fact, the distribution of these referrals was spread evenly over all grades of medical staff from consultant to registrar.

TABLE A4.

Details of Admission of 186 Patients

Source of referral			aReason for referral				Duration of stay				
Mental hospital	Psychiatric clinic	Other, incl. G.P. domiciliary visit	Acute	Support	Convalescence	Relapse	1 month	1–2 months	2–4 months	4–6 months	6–12 months
61	75	50	38	22	44	82	71	43	15	16	41

aAcute   =   short-term active treatment.
Support   =   long-term including relief for relatives.
Convalescence   =   after discharge from mental hospital.
Relapse   =   clinical or social deterioration otherwise requiring re-admission
to mental hospital.

Discussion

The function of a day hospital varies widely from place to place, depending mainly on the policy of the psychiatric services for the area, which determines the role it is to play. Sometimes its function is to act as a long-stay "ward" for chronic patients whose illness is stabilized, but who need supervision during the day, although relatives are willing and able to tolerate them at night and over the weekends. This was the case with our own day hospital before 1961, and the stagnation in such a unit is demonstrated in our figures for this period (Table A1). Another difficulty in organization arises where the day hospital is without a defined catchment area. Not only is such a treatment centre denied the full support and co-operation of other agencies, but also the problems of liaison and of after-care of discharged patients must influence the type of patient accepted, as well as the quality of social and clinical supervision which can be offered. The importance of this is emphasized by our experience of the after-care requirements in those patients we discharged in 1961–2, where continuous social work with relatives was every bit as important as clinical supervision of the patient.

TABLE A5.

Status at 1 Year after Admission to day Hospital

Discharged			Still attending day hospital		Admitted to mental hospital		Died
	Domicile						
	Lives with relatives	Lives alone	Full-time	Part-time	1st admission	Re-admission	
Psychiatric supervision (by doctor, nurse, or P.S.W.)	70	6	13	6	12	31	6
No psychiatric supervision	38	4					
Total	118		19		43		6

The majority of day hospitals in this country are linked to a district psychiatric service and are able to call on all the facilities of the service when needed. Because of this, the admission and discharge policy of the day hospital can be flexible, and we believe this setting is essential if the criteria of patient selection are not to be dictated by too rigid standards of diagnosis, age or behaviour. An active treatment policy is necessary if stagnation is to be avoided, but at the same time, the day hospital should not be filled with patients who, though acceptable to the staff, could in fact be treated in an out-patient clinic.

In our opinion, the maximum number of patients under treatment should not exceed 45, nor should the size of the unit or the staff detract from close and easy interaction between all members, both staff and patients, who form the day hospital group. Consistency of staff attitudes is very important in such a closely knit community, and this is more easily achieved if formal and informal communication is fostered, on a basis of equal contribution and participation at the non-executive level.

Those who work in day hospitals recognize that the therapeutic atmosphere derives not only from its easily accessible location in the community (both for patients *and* their relatives) but also from the special status of those who attend. Patients do not lose contact with realistic social situations as they do in hospital, and they can therefore make a more vivid and socially dynamic contribution to group discussions. At the same time, the division between patients and staff is far less pronounced than it is in hospital, and there is much greater opportunity to influence family relationships, at the very time when these are likely to be of special importance. In a sense, the patient is a member of two families at the same time, and if he benefits from his membership of the day hospital "family", it is not surprising that he finds difficulty in severing his connections with it. We have found it better, therefore, to reduce attendance by stages as a patient improves, and since our after-care services are based on the day hospital premises, continuity of care after discharge is ensured.

The results we have achieved with a difficult class of patient, many of poor prognosis and prone to relapse, and re-admission to institutional care, suggests that the day hospital in a comprehensive psychiatric service should not merely imitate mental hospital practice in a community setting. Instead, it should take advantage of its unique relationship with the patient and his family, and strive to anticipate social as well as clinical requirements, to a degree that is not possible with other forms of treatment.

Reference

MAY, A. R., SHELDON, A.P. and MACKEITH, S. A. (1962), *Lancet*, ii, 1319.

Industrial Therapy and Rehabilitation, Croydon

Source of Referral	Site of Industrial Therapy Workshops	Special Factories for Assessment and Intensive Retraining	OPEN INDUSTRY

General Practitioner
Psychiatric Out-patient Clinic
Local Authority Departments
  e.g. Mental Welfare
    Public Health Nurse, etc.
Social Agencies
Relatives
          etc.
	Warlingham Park Hospital, 300 Patients	LOCAL AUTHORITY
		Sheltered Factory
		70 Patients
		Majority Mental H'cap
		Indefinite Stay
			(approx. 10% from Factory)

	Croydon Day Hospital, 30 Patients		
General Practitioner Junior Subnormal Training Centre Education Department Mental Welfare Department Ministry of Labour etc.	Local Authority Adult Training Centre for Subnormals, 60 Patients		
		MINISTRY OF LABOUR Industrial Rehabilitation Unit Majority Phys. H'cap 2 months limit	MINISTRY OF LABOUR Government Training Centre (specialized)
General Practitioner General Hospital Health and Welfare Department Ministry of Labour etc.	Local Authority Occupational Centre for Physically Handicapped, 30 Patients		

Domiciliary Resettlement, Croydon

Warlingham Park Hospital
Living in hospital, but
working out in community
[hospital = hostel]

Group Homes
5–6 patients living in
houses rented from
the local authority

Voluntary Assoc. Hostel
10–15 beds
subsidized by
local health authority

Lodging in Private House
Landladies subsidized
and supervised by
local health authority

Psychiatric Out-patient
Clinic
Day hospital
Mental Welfare Department
Other Social Agencies,

etc.

(Relatives)

(Relatives)

(Relatives)

34. The Burden on the Household in an Extramural Psychiatric Service

J. Hoenig and Marian W. Hamilton

Introduction

There have been efforts, throughout history, to maintain the psychiatrically ill in the community outside hospital, for instance, the boarding out system in Scotland or the community at Gheel in Belgium. The success of Querido's work in Amsterdam (Querido, 1955) brought renewed stimulus to the idea of extramural care, and it aroused the interest of the Ministry of Health (Maclay, 1958) in this country. However, apart from sporadic efforts made by individual hospitals, such as Graylingwell (Carse et al., 1958), it fell to the Manchester Regional Hospital Board to experiment systematically with extramural types of care on a regional scale.

This regional effort has been going on now for some 15 years and Regional Hospital Board statistics show that 73·5% of all new patients (both in- and out-patients) incepted in the region as a whole are dealt with by the new General Hospital Psychiatric Units instead of the older mental hospitals. The remaining 26·4%, who are dealt with by the conventional mental hospital services still operating in the region, are drawn mostly from those parts of the region where general hospital psychiatric units are planned but not yet in existence.

From an administrative point of view it has been shown quite conclusively that this extramural type of psychiatric care does work (Smith, 1960). The units can look after patients not only at inception but for long periods afterwards (Hoenig and Hamilton, 1965). It has been suggested by Jones (1962) that extramural management is "unsuitable for the majority" and can only deal with selected patients, but this clearly is not so, as has been shown by a number of investigators (Leyberg, 1959; Silverman, 1961; Freeman, 1963; Hoenig and Hamilton, 1965, etc.).

Critics of the service have pointed out that if the psychiatrically ill do remain in the community and are not admitted to hospital for long periods, the burden of care is merely shifted onto others, particularly the patient's family. In this connection, Wing et al. (1964) indicated that patients could only stay in community care if, in many instances, the families were prepared to act as nurses. This is clearly a problem that needs to be examined, and as these new psychiatric units develop, more attention is being directed to this aspect. Investigation of family burden, however, is relatively new and scientific work upon it is in its infancy. Methods of assessment have still to be developed. In this paper we describe an investigation into family burden and our own attempt to evolve some reliable method of assessing it.

The Investigation

The investigation took place in relation to patients treated at two general hospital psychiatric units in the Manchester Hospital Region. The units operated within a catchment area of approximately 170,000 and 280,000 inhabitants respectively. The consultant psychiatrists in charge of the units did not share the same enthusiasm for this pioneer extramural service, and the two areas they served, though typical Lancashire communities, differed in that the one was a much more industrialized area (mainly textiles) than the other, and also had a more static population.

We took all patients incepted for the first time by these two units over a 12-month period (1 November 1958 to 31 October 1959 and 1 May 1959 to 30 April 1960 respectively). We included all such patients, irrespective of whether they were incepted as in-patients, out-patients, on domiciliary visits or other. From this clinic population a sample was drawn of 273 patients. In order to see difficulties at their maximum, the sample was stratified in such a way that it was loaded with patients who had the worst prognosis and presented the severest problems of management. The stratification is set out in Table 1.

TABLE 1.

	Clinic total	Sample	%
Patients over 60 years of age 　All diagnoses	178	89	50
Patients under 60 years of age 　Organic psychosyndromes	13	13	100
Epilepsy	10	10	100
Schizophrenia	58	58	100
All other diagnoses	700	103	14·7
TOTAL	959	273	47·4%

It will be seen that the organic psychosyndromes, the epilepsies and the schizophrenias in the under-60 age group were more numerously represented (each 100%) in the sample as were the over-60 age group (50%).

This stratified sample was then followed up 4 years after inception by a research psychiatric social worker. The interview with the patient, and with the relative where practicable, lasted 1½ hours and was semi-structured. The findings in each unit were separately analysed, but results proved so similar that it is possible to present them here as one.

Our concern here is the effect of the patient's illness on his family, although in the course of our main investigation a great number of other clinical and social factors also came under review. How the patient himself fared through the 4 years and what use was made of the medical and social services have been described elsewhere (Hoenig and Hamilton, 1965). It was found that over the period, patients were very little in hospital, though they remained chronically ill and the work adjustment was only fair. In view of this, the sample lent itself particularly well to an investigation of family burden.

Assessment of Family Burden

The main problem was how to assess the way in which patients affected their household and to what extent they did so. Grad and Sainsbury (1963) used the word "burden" to describe this effect and we have adopted the expression. It does, however, require some care in its usage, because the investigator and the investigated may have different conceptions on the matter. To meet this point, we have defined "burden" in the following way.

We selected certain specific effects on the life of the household, and also noted the occurrence of certain abnormal behaviour traits in the patient. We called these the "objective" burden. When both these aspects were put together, we used the expression "combined objective burden".

We then inquired whether the households themselves had felt that they had been carrying any burden in a subjective sense. This we called the "subjective burden". It will be shown that these two types of burden do by no means coincide.

Having made this distinction, we related the two types of burden, subjective and objective, to a number of clinical and social factors that seemed relevant.

Finally, we inquired of the relatives to what extent they had received any social agency care and whether they felt that more could have been done to help them over the four years, by either the medical or social services.

Findings

I. Objective Burden

(a) Type 1: *Effects on the household*

Table 2 shows the particular effects which were looked for in our inquiry. They were grouped together under four main headings of (1) financial effects on the household, (2) effects on the health of any household member,

TABLE 2.

Adverse Effects on the Household (%)

Type of objective burden caused by patient's illness	No	Yes		Not applicable or not known
FINANCIAL				
Financial status of the patient or the household has suffered	67·9		16·5	15·6
Any member of the household lost earnings	56·0		6·6	37·4
Any member of the household had to start going out to work	51·2		5·1	43·7
HEALTH				
Physical strain on any member of the household, due to nursing the patient	66·1	Some Marked	4·4 1·5	28·0
Poor health in any member of the household caused by patient's illness	66·4		6·9	26·7
CHILDREN				
Separation of children under 16 from their parents	12·4	From mother Father Both	7·3 5·1 0·4	74·8
Distress in children under 16	20·5	Distressed Neurotic	2·1 0·4	77·0
GENERAL				
Disruption of the life of any member of the household	27·3	Some Much	25·7 12·8	34·2

(3) effects on the children, and (4) effects on family routine (e.g. interference with social life, with children going to school, etc.).

It will be seen that the effects in the last category (4) were the most common. The figure here is as high as 38·5%. If, however, only severe effects are taken into account, the figure drops to 12·8%. Financial loss to the patient or household comes next with a figure of 16·5%. The remaining effects all show a relatively small percentage of the households involved. Other members of the family lost earnings in 6·6% of the cases, and in 5·1% they were forced to start work because of the patient's illness to make up loss of income. In 5·9% of the households the nursing burden was heavy enough to cause physical strain; in 1·5% this reached a severe degree, while in 6·9% health was actually affected.

The figures as they stand in Table 2 illustrate the various burdens as carried by our sample as a whole. As a large percentage of patients had no children in their household, it is perhaps more meaningful to calculate the cases where children were separated from their parents or suffered distress in relation only to the actual population at risk. In calculating the burden on this reduced total, we discounted separations that lasted only a week or less. In spite of that, we found that the risk of separation was high. In 40·7% of the families at risk, children suffered separation, and although actual distress was only recorded in 8·1%, this is by no means a negligible figure.

It will be appreciated that there was a certain amount of overlap in the various individual burdens and that several effects might coincide in one household. When all the households are counted in which *any* effect had been operative, it is found that 49·4% carried some burden, whereas 28·0% did not. (In 22·0% the questions were either not applicable or full information could not be obtained.)

Comparison between the individual findings is difficult and only allows for restricted comment. There seemed to be a large number of households where the routine of family life was disrupted in some way and the financial loss suffered was not inconsiderable. The most noteworthy effect, perhaps, is that on the children. The other effects seem relatively small, although, if it is borne in mind that several of these effects might coincide in any one household, the total burden might prove quite large.

Further analysis of the households that appeared to carry *objective* burden in this sense showed that neither age, sex, social class nor civil status played any significant part in causing such burden. It did seem to matter, however, what kind of household the patient stayed in: whether he lived with his parents, spouse, sibs or other kin, grown-up children or alone. This can be seen from Table 3 (col. A).

TABLE 3.

The "Total Burdens" by Type of Household (%)

Type of household	A Total objective burden caused by adverse effects on the household		B Total objective burden caused by abnormal behaviour	
	No burden	Burden	No burden	Burden
With parents	18·2	19·3	17·8	22·0
With spouse	45·2	62·2	58·0	50·0
With siblings or other relatives	10·2	6·6	8·5	9·0
With grown-up children	5·2	8·1	3·6	12·0
Alone or at no fixed abode	21·2	3·8	12·1	7·0
All patients	100·0	100·0	100·0	100·0

Table 3 (col. A) shows that the various types of household are not very differently distributed in the burden and no burden groups, with the exception of the conjugal homes, which seem to suffer the most. Whereas the no burden group contains only 45·2%, the burden group shows 62·2%. The difference, however, does not reach statistical significance.

TABLE 4.

The "Total Burdens" by Diagnoses (%)

	A		B	
	Total objective burden caused by adverse effects on the household		Total objective burden caused by abnormal behaviour	
	No burden	Burden	No burden	Burden
Organic psychosyndrome	12·3	14·8	9·4	20·9
Schizophrenia	20·3	25·2	17·0	32·7
Affective psychoses	28·3	21·5	26·9	21·8
Epilepsy	5·1	2·2	5·3	2·2
Personality disorder	22·6	28·1	30·4	16·8
Abnormal psychogenic reaction	10·1	5·9	10·5	3·9
Others	1·3	2·3	0·5	1·7

As can be seen from Table 4 (col. A), diagnosis also plays a part in that schizophrenia and personality disorder are slightly over-represented in the burden group, although the differences again are not statistically significant. The burden group shows schizophrenia in 25·2% of the cases as against 20·3% in the no burden group, and personality disorder in 28·0% as against 22·6% in the no burden group. Affective psychoses (21·5% versus 28·3%) and abnormal psychogenic reactions (5·9% versus 10·1%) are, on the other hand, under-represented in the burden group.

If the morbidity rate (duration of illness) is considered, we find that the longer the patient has been ill over the 4 years, the more likely he will be to create adverse effects for his household. This applies particularly to the patients who have been ill for more than 2 years. The findings are set out in Table 5 (col. A).

Whereas the patients with the shortest duration of illness (less than 6 months) form 34·4% of the no burden group, they are only 12·5% of the burden group ($p < 0.001$).

Those who have been ill for more than 2 years form only 40·5% of the no burden group compared with 61·7% of the burden group ($p < 0.001$). The distribution switches over with the patients who were ill for 1–2 years (6·3% in the no burden group and 14·3% in the burden group ($p < 0.001$)). All these differences are very highly significant.

We also measured the "total hospital time", that is, the amount of time the patient spent as an in-patient, either at the general hospital unit or in

TABLE 5.

The "Total Burdens" by Duration of Ill-health during the 4 Years (%)

Length of illness during the years	A Total objective burden caused by adverse effects on the household		B Total objective burden caused by abnormal behaviour	
	No burden	Burden	No burden	Burden
1–6 months	34·4	12·5	38·1	4·3
7–12 months	18·8	12·5	20·2	9·7
1–2 years	6·3	14·3	10·7	11·8
2 years and over	40·5	61·7	31·0	74·2
All patients	100·0	100·0	100·0	100·0

TABLE 6.

The "Total Burdens" by the Aggregate In-patient Time during the 4 Years (%)

Aggregate in-patient time during the 4 years	A Total objective burden caused by adverse effects on the household		B Total objective burden caused by abnormal behaviour	
	No burden	Burden	No burden	Burden
None	38·4	16·5	36·6	12·9
1–4 weeks	26·1	28·1	31·8	18·9
5–12 weeks	24·7	30·4	23·8	25·8
13–52 weeks	7·9	17·0	5·5	31·6
53 weeks and over	2·9	8·0	2·3	10·8
All patients	100·0	100·0	100·0	100·0

the mental hospital or in both. This is an aggregate figure, calculated over the 4 years, and does not necessarily mean one consecutive period of stay.

It will be seen from Table 6 (col. A) that those patients who never went into the unit or mental hospital as in-patients are under-represented in the burden group (16·5% as against 38·4% in the no burden group ($p < 0.01$)), while those who stayed 13 weeks to a year or more are over-represented in the burden group (25·0% as against 10·9% in the no burden group ($p < 0.02$)).

In conclusion, therefore, it seems that this type of burden depends slightly on diagnostic criteria and to a greater extent on the length of illness and hospital stay. Of the social factors, only the type of household seems to have some relationship, indicating that the conjugal household tends to suffer the most.

(b) Type 2: *Abnormal behaviour traits*

It was further recorded whether patients had at any time during the 4-year period shown abnormal behaviour traits to any marked extent while out of hospital. We assumed that any such behaviour, which the patient displayed more than occasionally, must needs constitute a form of burden.

TABLE 7.

Abnormal Behaviour

Types of abnormal behaviour	Number of patients per 100, showing abnormal behaviour				
	None	Occas-sional	Periodic	Constant	Not applicable or not known
Noisy or wandering at night	50·5	1·1	4·7	3·6	40·1
Dangerous to themselves or to others	45·0	4·7	7·7	4·7	37·9
Unacceptable sexual behaviour	58·3	—	0·7	0·7	40·3
Generally restless, noisy or talkative	52·7	21·2	7·3	0·7	18·1
Unresponsive	52·8	1·5	4·1	2·5	39·1
Apparently wilfully unco-operative	44·0	2·1	10·0	5·1	38·8
Used odd speech or expressed 'unusual' ideas	44·5	3·3	11·3	4·4	36·5
Hypochondriasis	54·0	0·7	0·7	4·4	40·2
Requiring physical nursing care	44·0	2·7	4·4	10·6	38·3
Demanding excessive companion-ship	49·8	2·1	3·3	5·5	39·3
Other unusual behaviour	35·1	3·3	14·6	10·9	35·1

Table 7 lists the various types of abnormal behaviour, which were recorded. The types were graded as to whether they were shown by the patient occasionally, periodically or constantly during the 4-year period. Most types of behaviour showed a fairly low incidence, amounting to about 10·0% of the patients, if the categories periodic and constant are taken together. The traits which occurred more frequently than this are, first, those grouped under the heading other unusual behaviour (25·5%). This consisted of a number of miscellaneous traits which seemed to fall broadly into the following categories: (1) hostile, irritable, morose behaviour, (2) behaviour traits calling for supervision and watchfulness (i.e. the forgetfulness of dementing patients, etc.),

(3) offensive personal habits, (4) extreme seclusiveness and withdrawal. The three other more frequently recorded traits were as follows: apparent wilful unco-operativeness, odd speech and unusual ideas (i.e. deluded patients) and those requiring nursing care. All these latter three traits had an incidence of approximately 15·0%. Unacceptable sexual behaviour, on the other hand, was recorded in only 1·4% of the households.

Table 7 does not, of course, show whether a patient displayed only one or several of the recorded traits. However, if *all* types of abnormal behaviour are taken together, discarding those shown only occasionally, we find that 37·0% of the patients displayed some abnormal trait to a sufficient extent to be recorded as periodic or constant (i.e. burdensome) while 27·8% did not. (In 35·2%, uniform data could not be obtained.)

Further analysis again shows that, as with the previous type of burden, age, sex, social class and civil status played no significant part in the total picture.

As can be seen from Table 3 (col. B), the various types of household are fairly evenly distributed between the burden and no burden groups. The only marked difference shown is in those patients who lived with their grown-up children; those who caused burden were 12·0% as against 3·6% of those who caused no burden. The absolute figures, however, are small and the differences are not significant.

With regard to the diagnostic groupings, as can be seen from Table 4 (col. B), both schizophrenia (32·7% of the burden group and 17·0% of the no burden group; $p < 0·01$) and the organic psychosyndromes (20·9% and 9·4% respectively; $p < 0·01$) shows a higher incidence than expected in the burden group, whereas the personality disorders show a lower incidence (16·8% versus 30·4% of the no burden group). The difference in the latter, however, is not significant. The other diagnostic groupings are fairly evenly represented.

The morbidity rate, as can be seen from Table 5 (col. B), shows there is a correlation between the incidence of abnormal behaviour and the duration of the illness. Whereas patients with the shortest illness (under 6 months) form 38·1% of the no burden group, they form only 4·3% of the burden group ($p < 0·001$). The longer the illness, the more the burden due to abnormal behaviour. Where the illness lasted more than 2 years, the figure in the burden group has swollen to 74·2% compared with 31·0% in the no burden group ($p < 0·001$). These differences are highly significant.

From Table 6 (col. B) it will be seen that the total hospital time spent as an in-patient is also related to the frequency of abnormal behaviour. The figures for those patients who showed little or no hospitalization (up to 4 weeks) were 31·8% of the burden group as against 68·4% of the no burden group. The figures for the longer-stay patients (13 weeks and over) had reversed (42·4% of the burden group and only 7·8% of the no burden group; $p < 0·001$). This relationship can probably be understood to mean that periodic or constant abnormal behaviour displayed by the patient tends to lead to prolonged hospitalization.

In conclusion, therefore, while objectively burdensome abnormal behaviour seems related to such clinical factors as diagnosis and morbidity rate and can itself affect the length of hospitalization, the social factors do not seem to play any significant part.

(c) *Comparison between the two types of objective burden*

The two types of total objective burden in respect of (1) the adverse effects on the household, and (2) the abnormal behaviour traits shown by the patient, lend themselves to comparison with each other. Although so different in nature, they seem rather similar in most other aspects with the exception of their actual incidence and their relationship to diagnosis and the total hospital time spent by the patient.

In the first place, the total amount of burden inflicted in respect of Type 1 (adverse effects on the household) affected $49 \cdot 4\%$ of the cases, whereas in respect of Type 2 (abnormal behaviour traits) the total burden was recorded only in $37 \cdot 0\%$ of the cases ($p < 0 \cdot 001$). The first type of objective burden therefore seems the more widespread.

Secondly, in respect of diagnosis (Table 4), the two types of burden differ as regards the burden connected with the personality disorders. These disorders are represented in Type 1 burden to a perhaps unexpectedly high degree, but in Type 2 burden they appear comparatively to a much less extent than is the case with the other diagnostic groups. As regards the organic psychosyndromes and schizophrenia, these appear to be associated more with Type 2 burden than with financial loss or other such adverse effects listed under Type 1 burden.

In the third respect (amount of hospitalization) the difference between the two types of burden is only one of degree. In both types the longer the aggregate in-patient time, the more burden is recorded, but in the case of Type 2 burden the gradient is even more marked than in Type 1. This seems again to suggest that the periodic or constant recurrence of abnormal behaviour traits is a more disturbing form of burden, bringing the patient into hospital more readily.

(d) *Combined objective burden*

The data thus accumulated were very varied, yet as the differences in most relevant aspects between the two types of burden were so slight, it seemed justifiable to put them together into a single total. We accordingly drew into one group all those households where *any* type of objective burden had appeared, irrespective of the individual categories. Thus emerged what we have called the "combined objective burden", which represents the sum total of the two types of burden which we had previously analysed, i.e. the total burden due to adverse effects on the household and the total burden due to the incidence of various abnormal behaviour traits (Tables 2 and 3).

We found that there were 152 cases ($55 \cdot 7 \%$) where some objective burden had been recorded, as against 121 cases ($44 \cdot 3 \%$) where no objective burden had appeared (including those cases where full information could not be obtained). Having thus established the overall incidence, it seemed important to find out what were the factors related to objective burden in this general sense.

Sex of the patient, it appeared, was not an important factor; age had a slight relationship, though not to a statistically significant degree. Patients over 60 years of age comprised $39 \cdot 0 \%$ of the burden group as against $25 \cdot 1 \%$ of the no burden group, suggesting that objective burden in general tends to arise rather more frequently if patients are in the older age group. Neither civil status nor social class played any significant part. The situation with the type of household was rather different.

TABLE 8.

The Combined Objective Burden by the Type of the Patient's Home ($\%$)

	With parents	With spouse	With siblings	With grown-up children	Living alone	No fixed abode	Total
No burden	28·1	38·8	7·4	4·1	8·2	13·4	100
Burden	18·4	59·2	5·3	8·6	4·6	3·9	100

Table 8 shows that those patients who lived with their parents formed only $18 \cdot 4 \%$ of the burden group as against $28 \cdot 1 \%$ of the no burden group ($p < 0 \cdot 05$). Those who lived with their spouses showed a reverse trend, namely they seemed to be over-represented in the burden group with $59 \cdot 2 \%$ as against $38 \cdot 8 \%$ in the no burden group ($p < 0 \cdot 01$). The same trend appears where patients lived with their grown-up children, but there the difference is not significant. Thus the parental home tends to suffer less than the average, whereas the conjugal home, in particular, tends to suffer more. The other types of household did not seem to affect the issue to the same extent. The fact that those who lived alone, with or without a fixed abode, are comparatively more prominent in the no burden group is mainly due to the absence of any household group, who could have carried any burden through the 4 years.

As regards clinical factors, the difference between the patients who created burden and those who did not is not so uniformly great as might have been expected. The diagnostic groups are fairly equally represented in both the burden and the no burden group, and the differences that exist are not significant.

TABLE 9.

The Combined Objective Burden by the Aggregate Length of Morbidity during the 4 Years (%)

Aggregate duration of illness	1–6 months	7–12 months	13–24 months	25 months and over	Total
No burden	45·9	23	8·1	23	100
Burden	10·8	11·6	12·4	65·2	100

The morbidity rate, however, seems rather more significant. Patients who were ill for more than 2 years comprise 65·2% of the burden group, as against 23·0% of the no burden group ($p<0·001$). There is a consistent decrease in the burden group, the shorter the illness lasted, until the group of patients ill for less than 6 months are only represented by 10·8% in the burden group but by 45·9% in the no burden group ($p<0·001$). The differences shown in Table 9 are very highly significant. Thus, the longer the patients are ill, the more likely they are to constitute some form of objective burden to their households. The quickly recoverable conditions, independent of diagnosis, cause least upset.

TABLE 10.

Combined Objective Burden by Aggregate Time spent in Hospital during the 4 Years (%)

	Nil	1–4 weeks	5–12 weeks	13–52 weeks	53 or more weeks	Total
No burden	42	28	22·3	5·2	2·5	100
Burden	16·4	26·3	30·9	18·6	7·8	100

The total hospital time spent by the patient also seems related to the amount of burden. It will be remembered that the total length of time spent as an in-patient was assessed throughout the whole 4 years, irrespective of whether the patient's stay was consecutive or intermittent, as indeed it was for the majority. As Table 10 shows, those who had been in-patients for more than 3 months comprised 26·4% of the burden group as against 7·7% of the no burden group. The figures in the 5–12-week group show the same type of difference, but less marked. However, those who had not entered hospital at all showed the largest difference, viz. $16\cdot4\%$ in the burden group and $42\cdot0\%$ in the no burden group ($p<0\cdot001$). It is not easy to interpret these figures. It is possible that hospitalization is a result of burden, meaning that if burden arose, hospitalization tended to be resorted to, and if it arose with any frequency, then the aggregate hospital stay would lengthen. On the other hand, if one thinks in terms of financial loss, separation of children, etc., it is possible that hospitalization could then have been the cause of the burden.

It is most likely, since we are dealing with such a complex entity, that these factors each play a part in a varying degree. Without being able to demonstrate the matter, we rather suspect that in this particular sample of patients the length of hospital stay is more an *indicator* of burden in the community rather than the *cause*.

In conclusion, as so little is yet known of the matter it is difficult to say whether the incidence we have found of the combined objective burden is unduly large or not. In absolute figures it seems considerable, affecting more than half the households. The fact that it is sensitive to such factors as type of household, duration of illness and possibly the aggregate hospital stay would suggest that, as such, it possesses some validity as a measure of the burden any chronic psychiatric patient's household may have to carry.

II. Subjective Burden

Having assessed the combined objective burden, we then made a special inquiry from the available informants as to whether they themselves thought their household had suffered some degree of burden over the 4 years as a result of the patient's illness. This inquiry, therefore, was directed at attitudes rather than at objective events. It was striking to find that the subjective attitudes of the informants by no means coincided always with what one would have expected from the objective assessment.

In 94 cases full information could not be obtained, mostly because there were no informants who could report over the 4-year period as a whole. The tables referring to subjective burden therefore refer only to the remaining 179 cases in our sample.

Table 11 shows that where no combined objective burden was recorded, the household did not complain of hardship, which is what would be expected, though of course, this category also included some cases where occasional burden had arisen. This slight burden was obviously accepted by the family and had not become a matter of complaint.

Where there had been more than occasional combined objective burden, informants had complained about severe hardship in $19\cdot6\%$ of the cases. Another $56\cdot7\%$ of them had complained of some subjective burden. Thus, in $76\cdot3\%$ of the cases where the patient had caused his household some objective burden, this had been experienced as subjective burden by his family. The

TABLE 11.

*Subjective Burden by the Incidence of the Combined
Objective Burden (%)*

Subjective burden	Combined objective burden	
	No burden	Burden
None	100·0	23·7
Some burden	—	56·7
Severe burden	—	19·6
All patients	100·0	100·0

most interesting group are those households where objective burden did arise, but this was not experienced as any hardship at all, nor was any complaint expressed (23·7%). This figure shows that nearly as many as a quarter of all the families who had a psychiatrically ill patient in their midst causing burden to the household accepted the situation uncomplainingly. It could be regarded, therefore, as a kind of measure of family tolerance towards the psychiatric patient.

It is reasonable to expect that the various individual objective burdens that have been listed would not meet with the same amount of tolerance. Abnormal behaviour traits, particularly characteristic of the psychiatric patient, may be tolerated differently from such troubles as financial loss, etc., which are not specific to psychiatric breakdown, but can be expected wherever there is any patient suffering from chronic illness.

In fact, the tolerance figures for the two types of objective burden do, indeed, differ. Where there was Type 1 burden, no subjective burden was reported in 17·4% of the cases; where the objective burden was due to Type 2 burden, the figure was only 12·7%. This seems to suggest that the effects on the household which the psychiatric patient creates, in common with other chronically ill patients, are more readily tolerated than the abnormal behaviour traits which characterize the psychiatric patient, although in the latter group a certain degree of tolerance does also exist. This is further borne out when one looks at the severe subjective burden alone, i.e. what one might call the "intolerance towards burden". There, we find in the case of Type 1 burden intolerance present in 21·5%, whereas the figure is 27·8% in the case of Type 2 burden.

As regards the sex of the patient, both sexes are equally distributed in the subjective burden and no subjective burden group. Age of the patient, however, does seem to play a certain part in that the more severe the subjective burden, the larger the incidence of the upper age group. Only 36·5% of the over-60's fall into the no burden group as compared with 50·5% of the under-60's ($p<0·05$). In the severe burden group, the figures are 21·6% for the over-60's and 10·0% for the younger group.

Civil status of the patient does not affect the issue to any statistically significant degree, although there is a significant trend if severe burden only is taken into account. The married patients comprise 76·0% of this latter group, whereas single patients (including the widowed, separated and divorced) comprise only 24% ($p<0·001$). This may well be related to the fact that the conjugal households carried a considerably larger amount of objective burden, particularly of Type 1.

TABLE 12.

Subjective Burden by the Type of Household (%)

Subjective burden	Type of household				
	With parents	With spouse	With siblings or other relatives	With grown-up children	Alone, or at no fixed abode
None	39·6	49·5	58·7	20·0	50·0
Some burden	52·6	33·7	35·3	60·0	37·0
Severe burden	7·8	16·8	6·0	20·0	13·0
All patients	100·0	100·0	100·0	100·0	100·0

Table 12 shows that the type of household in which the patient lived had some effect on the situation. Siblings and other kin complained least of subjective burden (41·3%). Fifty per cent of the spouses complained and 60·4% of the parents. The highest figure came where the patients lived with their grown-up children, namely 80·0% ($p<0·02$), but absolute figures are still small.

With those patients who lived alone, with or without any fixed abode, the question was not really applicable. It will be remembered that the parental home suffered least combined objective burden (Table 8). In spite of this, it appears to show almost the highest complaint ratio. This suggests that the parental home is more "intolerant" or reacts more severely than the other types of household.

The distribution of social class is interesting in that social classes I and II report a higher percentage of subjective burden, viz. 66·6% in class I and 62·0% in class II, whereas in classes III, IV and V, subjective burden is reported in 49·4%, 47·0% and 48·0% of all cases. There is a similar trend as regards severe subjective burden. The highest figure (24·0%) is in class II, then comes 16·8% in class III, 6·0% in class IV and 9·0% in class V. Although the trend is consistent, the differences are not statistically significant.

As regards the clinical factors, there are some differences in relation to diagnosis, though nowhere do they reach statistical significance. The greatest number of cases where subjective burden existed were among the epilepsies (75·0%). This percentage may be spurious, because the absolute figures are very small. Next come the organic psychosyndromes (70·0%), followed by the schizophrenias (60·4%). The affective psychoses (46·5%), the personality disorders (44·3%) and the abnormal psychogenic reactions (41·3%) are all very similar to each other. As regards *severe* subjective burden, this occurred most frequently among the organic psychosyndromes (37·0%), affective psychoses (17·5%) and schizophrenia (9·4%). It is interesting to note that the schizophrenias caused so little severe subjective burden, as compared with the organic psychosyndromes and the affective psychoses in particular. Since we know that the objective burden for the schizophrenias was fairly high (Table 4), there seems to be a particular tolerance towards them. These patients seem somewhat accepted in the home, constituting no more than a mild irritant (i.e. only *some* subjective burden) to other members and give rise to severe complaints in only a relatively small group.

It is also rather surprising that the personality disorders and abnormal psychogenic reactions, though lowest on the list, are still complained of as causing subjective burden. The other diagnostic groups are too small for analysis.

The morbidity rate has a clear relation to subjective burden, as is shown in Table 13.

TABLE 13.

Subjective Burden by Aggregate Morbidity during the 4 Years (%)

Subjective burden	Duration of illness during the 4 years (months)			
	1–6	7–12	13–24	25 and over
None	16·0	45·0	12·5	21·1
Some burden	33·0	35·0	81·5	50·5
Severe burden	—	20·0	6·0	28·4

The least subjective burden appears related to those patients who were ill for less than 6 months (33·0%) ($p < 0·001$) and those ill from 7–12 months (55·0%). The patients who were ill longer show a higher rate of subjective burden, namely 87·5% in those who were ill from 1–2 years. The differences are just significant ($p < 0·05$). Once, however, the 2-year period is over, there is a slight fall to 78·9%, suggesting that some adjustment may have been made by the households concerned.

As regards severe subjective burden, however, apart from the fact that there was none among the families of those who were ill for less than 6 months, the general trend is not maintained quite as clearly, as there was a considerable amount of severe complaint where the morbidity was from 7–12 months' duration (20·0% as against 6·0% in the 1–2-year group).

TABLE 14.

Subjective Burden by the Aggregate In-patient Time, during the 4 Years

Subjective burden	Aggregate in-patient time during the 4 years (weeks)				
	None	1–4	5–12	13–52	53 and over
None	62·0	55·0	41·5	21·8	10·0
Some burden	31·0	35·3	32·0	74·0	70·0
Severe burden	7·0	9·7	26·5	4·2	20·0
All patients	100·0	100·0	100·0	100·0	100·0

When the total hospital time is considered, we find that the proportion of cases where subjective burden is recorded rises consistently with the length of in-patient stay. Table 14 shows that those who had never been in hospital were complained of in 38·0% of the cases; those who were there only up to 4 weeks in 45·0%. Those who were in hospital for 5–12 weeks were complained of in 58·5%. After this, there is a steep rise to 78·2% for those who stayed up to 1 year and to 90·0% for those over 1 year ($p < 0·01$). As regards severe subjective burden, the gradient disappears somewhat; the highest percentage (26·5%) appearing in the 5–12-week group; the over 1-year groups coming out with 20·0%.

In conclusion, the discrepancy between the combined objective burden and the subjective burden is most striking. Subjective burden does not necessarily occur in those types of household that carry the most objective burden. The diagnostic categories affect subjective burden much more differentially than is the case with the combined objective burden. It is noteworthy that with regard to the length of illness and the total hospital time, there seems to be a levelling-off effect after the second year in each case, suggesting that some adjustment has taken place in the household and tolerance developed.

III. The Services and the Subjective Burden

Any investigation of subjective burden would be incomplete without relating it to other factors, in particular the help given to the household during the 4 years. It goes outside the scope of this paper to give a full account of the different services, though this has been done elsewhere (Hoenig and Hamilton, 1965). Here we shall only indicate one or two main findings.

TABLE 15.

*Subjective Burden by Care rendered to Patient or the Household
by any Social Agency (%)*

Subjective burden	Any social agency care given to the patient or the household	
	No	Yes
None	60·0	31·5
Some burden	30·0	51·1
Severe burden	10·0	17·4
All patients	100·0	100·0

Table 15 shows that there was a relationship between subjective burden and social agency care. The latter heading included the main statutory and voluntary services (approximately fifteen in number). When such care was recorded, it was found that in most cases subjective burden had indeed been present (68·5%); when no such care had been recorded, the figure was only 40·0%. This might indicate that the social agencies were sensitive to the presence of subjective burden, but though the differences in the figures seem large, they do not reach statistical significance. Only if those cases alone are taken into account, where subjective burden is severe, does the correlation with social agency care become highly significant ($p < 0·01$).

The one social agency which could be expected to be the most active was the Local Authority Mental Health Service and, indeed, one finds the same trend as above in operation, but somewhat more pronounced (Table 16). In those cases where the Mental Health Service intervened, 73·8% complained

TABLE 16.

*Subjective Burden by Mental Health Service Care given to the
Patient or the Household (%)*

Subjective burden	Care given to patient or the household by the Mental Health Service	
	No	Yes
None	56·0	26·2
Some burden	33·9	52·5
Severe burden	10·1	21·3
All patients	100·0	100·0

of subjective burden, whereas 44% did so where the Mental Health Service had not operated ($p < 0.01$).

Although there is a correlation between subjective burden and social agency care, there still remains a group of cases (40·0%) where subjective burden was reported but no social agency care had been given—not even from the Mental Health Service. Particularly striking is the group where no social agency care was given, not even from the Mental Health Service, although *severe* subjective burden appeared to have existed.

In view of the above discrepancies between the need and the care given, the views of the relatives were also sought as to whether they felt more could have been done to help. This question was intended to include not only social agency care, but medical care also.

TABLE 17.

Subjective Burden by Informants' Opinion whether more Help should have been given (%)

Subjective burden	Should more have been done?	
	No	Yes
None	53·8	—
Some	38·0	80·0
Severe	8·2	20·0
Total	100·0	100·0

These attitude polls are, of course, not very reliable and need to be interpreted with care. Table 17 shows that, as one might expect, all those informants who thought more could have been done had also complained of subjective burden, including 20% who had felt that the burden was severe. In no case without subjective burden was it suggested that more should have been done. It will be remembered that the combined objective burden was more frequent than the subjective burden (Table 11) and therefore the group who felt no more should have been done must have included some households where objective burden existed, and yet no subjective burden was reported, nor were they dissatisfied with what had been done. In fact, this was so in 6·0% of the cases. What is surprising is that the group who felt nothing more should have been done also included 46·2% where subjective burden was present, and in 8·2% this was even severe. This latter group includes patients where medical and social agency care had been given, as well as some where no social agency care had been given. The fact that severe subjective burden persisted in this way makes one wonder why the patients were, nevertheless, satisfied with what had been done. The figure of 8·2% can be taken as a kind of measure of the minimum level of expectancy, i.e. what help the community feel is available to them with their plight in looking after the psychiatric patient in their home.

Discussion and Conclusion

The group of patients studied all lived in areas which had relatively homogeneous mental health services, each centered on a single general hospital psychiatric unit. Because of the policy of these units, which was to keep the patients in the community, wherever possible, we had a group of unselected psychiatric patients who spent much more time with their families than would commonly be the case. This presented us with an excellent opportunity to investigate the effect of these patients' illness on their families. It also enabled us to experiment with finding a method that would measure this effect.

A comprehensive follow-up of this nature over a 4-year period has never been done, so far as we are aware, yet the usefulness of our own method can only be assessed fully when similar studies are forthcoming for comparison. Nevertheless, we feel that for a number of reasons, the method we have used does have a certain degree of validity:

(1) It was tried out in two areas which were sociologically and to a certain extent administratively different, yet the results of our investigations proved quite comparable. The individual types of burden and the overall burden carried by the patients' households seemed similar in extent.

(2) The various characteristics of the different burdens seem broadly similar in the two areas, particularly in the way they related to certain clinical and social factors.

(3) Such variations as occurred seemed quite meaningful, i.e. they were in line with many observations made in other studies using quite different methods.

The final proof can, of course, only lie with further studies. While the above reasons cannot be taken as final evidence of the validity of our method, we feel they are at least promising enough to make further investigations on similar lines worth while.

The final operative entity of all the different types of objective burden recorded in our study was the combined objective burden, as we have termed it. This was shown to be considerable, affecting more than one-half of the households.

It would be interesting to see how this compares with, say, a group of patients whose illnesses are managed in a different type of service, where more emphasis is laid on prolonged hospitalization. This would, indeed, be a most profitable application of this method, in helping to decide which type of psychiatric service is the preferable. It would also be interesting to find out how this objective burden might appear in the households of patients with chronic physical illnesses. Indeed, such an investigation may throw light indirectly on the previous question, but none has so far been done, so that one can only speculate. From the way in which the combined objective burden was arrived at, we found certain hints that some differences between psychiatric and non-psychiatric patients can be expected.

One part of the combined objective burden which we called Type 1 burden (adverse effects on the household) consisted of items which are not specific to the psychiatric patient and perhaps may be found in many types of non-psychiatric illness. The other part, Type 2 burden (abnormal behaviour traits), is more characteristic for psychiatric patients, though not entirely so, as it includes such items as "behaviour requiring nursing care", etc., which, if anything, is more characteristic for the physically ill.

This would suggest that Type 1 burden would be equally characteristic for psychiatric and non-psychiatric patients, whereas Type 2 burden would be more characteristic for psychiatric patients as such. Although there is a good deal of truth in this, it nevertheless would appear too superficial an assumption in the light of all our findings. It seems that both types of burden can be variously influenced by all kinds of factors—clinical ones such as diagnosis, morbidity rate, total hospital time, as well as social ones—and the variations found were quite marked in both types, even though we were dealing with psychiatric patients only. These did not appear to be at all a homogenous group, in relation to these types of burden.

It has been shown in relation to the personality disorders, for instance, that while they show a considerable amount of burden in the sense of Type 1 burden they showed considerably less in the way of Type 2 burden. However, with the organic psychosyndromes and the schizophrenias, the two types of burden occur with an equal frequency. Thus, when comparisons are made with non-psychiatric patients, it would be necessary to compare individual diagnostic groups rather than psychiatric patients as such.

In particular, those patients with personality disorders and abnormal psychogenic reactions, who are if anything psychiatric patients *par excellence*, are found to cause a very considerable amount of objective burden in absolute figures, apart from comparisons. This finding suggests that the name "*minor* psychiatric illnesses", which is often used to describe them, seems hardly justifiable.

It is interesting to find that Type 2 burden was more highly related to length of hospitalization than Type 1 burden. If it *can* be assumed that this type of objective burden is to a certain extent more characteristic of certain types of psychiatric patient, this would appear to throw some light on why chronic mental illnesses tend to be managed on in-patient lines to a greater extent than non-psychiatric illnesses.

The combined objective burden showed a clear relationship to the type of household in which the patient lived, namely that the parental home suffered least burden, whereas the conjugal home suffered most. At first glance, this finding seems at variance with what has been found by others in relation to the chances for successful rehabilitation of schizophrenic patients returning home from the mental hospital (Carstairs, 1959; Wing *et al.*, 1964; Cooper, 1961; Mandelbrote and Folkard, 1961, etc.). These investigators found that patients who returned to a parental home were more likely to be readmitted to hospital than patients who returned to the conjugal home. Indeed, the same was found to apply to schizophrenic patients in the present group (Hoenig and Hamilton, 1966). Some light, however, is thrown on this problem by our further findings in relation to what we have called subjective burden. Here we find clearly that the parental home, although it suffered least objective burden, nevertheless was the more complaining; more so than the conjugal home, though the latter in fact carried more objective burden. Thus it is shown that successful rehabilitation may well depend more on the subjective burden sensed by the family than on the objective burden.

This differentiation between objective burden and subjective burden proved quite illuminating in several other aspects also.

It is most important to realize that subjective burden is less widespread than objective burden and particularly so if only *severe* subjective burden is taken into account. As we have shown, Type 1 burden is more widespread than Type 2, but subjective burden is lower than either of these. The difference between objective burden and subjective burden, i.e., the number of cases where objective burden definitely exists but is not complained of, then becomes an index of tolerance in the community towards the chronically ill patient and the psychiatric patient in particular. It can be seen that the tolerance extended to Type 2 burden is smaller than that extended to Type 1 burden and to the extent to which Type 2 burden is characteristic of certain psychiatric illness, these illnesses are the less readily tolerated in the home.

Tolerance was found to be of a different magnitude in different types of homes and in relation to diagnostic categories. It also showed a varied relationship to the length of the illness; whereas objective burden increased consistently with the length of illness, subjective burden showed a levelling off, resulting therefore in greater tolerance towards the very chronic patient.

As regards the total hospital time spent by the patient as an in-patient, whereas the combined objective burden seemed to rise with the length of the aggregate time spent in hospital, the subjective burden again showed a levelling off effect. This means, perhaps, that where there is combined objective burden, prolonged hospitalization provides a relief which leads to a reduction of the subjective burden.

Considering the burden on the household, it seemed an obvious step for us to relate it to the help that had in fact been given, in particular by the social services. Indeed, we found a large number of households did receive social agency care, though there were many (40%) who, although they complained of some or severe subjective burden did not receive any. This is an aspect which demands further investigation, and our findings will be published in due course. Many relatives who felt distress and had not received social agency care did, indeed, feel that more should have been done. A great deal has been written about the help that should be extended to the families of psychiatric patients if they are to keep the patient in their midst rather than have him confined to hospital for long periods, and this finding points up the necessity for it.

What was surprising, perhaps, was the attitude of many relatives towards what further help could be expected. There were a considerable number—in fact nearly one tenth—who although they suffered severe subjective burden, felt that nothing more could have been done to bring them relief. This figure of 8 % we called the level of expectation, or rather the level of lack of expectation. It would be interesting to find out whether the frequency of this attitude varies in other communities and in particular, whether it varies with differences in the psychiatric services available in different localities or with the degree of sophistication in the public served.

We are hoping to apply this method of assessing burden on the household to psychiatric patients in other settings, and hope we will be in a more satisfactory position to judge the validity of the findings and the usefulness of the method when further studies on similar lines have emerged.

Summary

1. With different types of psychiatric services coming into use, where the patient is expected to live in the community with the minimum of hospitalization, it becomes increasingly necessary to investigate the effect of the patient on his household and the attitudes that prevail in the community towards the patient and his illness.

2. 273 patients and their households were investigated, who were served exclusively by a new type of general hospital psychiatric unit in the Manchester Hospital Region. The new type of psychiatric administration consisted mainly in avoiding long-term hospitalization and managing the patient while he remained in the community.

3. An attempt was made to evolve a method of assessing the burden supposed to devolve onto the community in such an extramural service.

4. To this end, a distinction was made between objective burden in terms of (1) adverse effects on the household, and (2) abnormal behaviour traits shown by the patient, on the one hand, and the subjective burden felt by the household, on the other. The two types of objective burden were spoken of collectively as the combined objective burden.

5. The distinction between the types of burden on the household proved

useful, as they occurred to different extents and showed different character-istics. These are described in detail.

6. Comparison between objective burden and subjective burden allows an assessment of the tolerance which exists in the community towards the psychiatric patient. Objective burden existed but no subjective complaints were made in 23·7% of families.

7. Examination of the relationship between subjective burden and social agency care received by the household illustrates the usefulness of the concept of community expectation regarding what help can be rendered by the medical and social services.

Acknowledgements

The research was carried out with the help of a grant by the Manchester Regional Hospital Board. The field inquiry was made by Miss Nancy B. Young, psychiatric social worker.

We wish to thank Dr. Peter Sainsbury and Dr. J. Grad, Dr. M. Susser and Dr. Zena Stein for their co-operation in compiling the interview schedule. We also want to thank Dr. E. T. Downham and Dr. R. S. Ferguson and their respective staff for the help they extended to us throughout.

References

CARSE, J., PANTON, N. E. and WATT, A. A. (1958), District mental health service: The Worthing experiment, *Lancet* i, 39–41.
CARSTAIRS, G. M. (1959), Social factors in the outcome of mental illness, *Proc. R. Soc. Med.* 52, 279–83.
COOPER, B. (1961), Social class and prognosis in schizophrenia, Parts I and II, *Brit. J. Prev. Soc. Med.* 15, 17–41.
FREEMAN, H. L. (1963), Community mental health services: some general and practical considerations, *Compr. Psychiat.* 4, 417–25.
GRAD, J. and SAINSBURY, P. (1963), Mental illness and the family, *Lancet*, i, 544–7.
HOENIG, J. and HAMILTON, M. W. (1965), Extramural care of psychiatric patients, *Lancet* i, 1322–5.
HOENIG, J. and HAMILTON, M. W. (1966), The schizophrenic patient in the community and his effect on the household, *Int. J. Soc. Psychiat.* 12, 165–76.
JONES, K. (1962), *Mental Hospital at Work*, Routledge & Kegan Paul, London.
LEYBERG, J. T. (1959), A district psychiatric service: the Bolton pattern, *Lancet* ii, 282–4.
MACLAY, W. S. (1958), Experiments in mental hospital organisation, *J. Canad. Med. Ass.* 78, 909–16.
MANDELBROTE, B. M. and FOLKARD, S. (1961), Some factors attached to the outcome and social adjustment in schizophrenics, *Acta Psychiat. Scan.* 37, 223–5.
QUERIDO, A. (1955), The Amsterdam psychiatric first aid scheme and some proposals for new legislation, *Proc. R. Soc. Med.* 48, 741–8.
SILVERMAN, M. (1961), A comprehensive department of psychological medicine; the problem of the in-patient case load: a 12 months' review, *Brit. Med. J.* ii, 698–701.
SMITH, S. (1960), Report to Manchester Regional Hospital, *Manchester Regional Hospital*.
WING, J. K., MONCK, E., BROWN, G. W. and CARSTAIRS, G. M. (1964), Morbidity in the community of schizophrenic patients discharged from London mental hospitals in 1959, *Brit. J. Psychiat.* 110, 10–21.

35. The Burnley Psychiatric Service

E. T. DOWNHAM

THE concept of psychiatric care in a general hospital is not new and is not peculiar to any one country. However, the progressive encouragement and development of general hospital departments offering comprehensive psychiatric services as a planned policy is unique to the Manchester Regional Board area in Great Britain. Such units are close to the population they serve and to the local authority community and after-care services with which they must co-operate. Their development has been neither uniform nor standardized, and ample scope was allowed for the different approaches and attitudes of the psychiatrists in charge. Various reports have been published, analysing briefly what this means for the services concerned (Leyberg, 1959; Freeman, 1960; Silverman, 1961).

In 1964 ten of the general hospital units in the region, containing 863 short-stay beds, admitted 5294 patients as compared with five mental hospitals containing 9038 beds (2051 for short-stay cases) which admitted 3945 patients. There has been a gradual run-down of the mental hospitals, from a 12,500 in-patient population in 1949 to 9000 in 1964. In 1964 41% of admissions in the Manchester Region were made to the major mental hospitals and 59% to the general hospital units.

For the past 9 years, Burnley General Hospital has almost completely contained the out-patient and in-patient psychiatric needs of a population of 171,000, in addition to accepting an average of 22% newly incepted patients

TABLE 1.

Totals of New Patients incepted to the Unit

November 1956–December 1957	801
January–December 1958	652
January–December 1959	688
January–December 1960	691
January–December 1961	709
January–December 1962	705
January–December 1963	648
January–December 1964	610
January–December 1965	604
Total:	6108

636

from outside the catchment area. Seventy active beds became available gradually for this purpose, representing 0·4 per 1000 of the population in the catchment area. No new cases have been refused inception as in-patients or out-patients to the unit during the period January 1957–January 1966, and only 31 have been transferred to a major or special mental hospital—a proportion of approximately 0·5%, 6108 cases, representing all types of psychiatric illness, have been treated by the department during this period.

The catchment area, covering approximately 100 square miles, consists of the County Borough of Burnley and the surrounding division of Lancashire County Council, situated in the north-east corner of Lancashire. The chief industries are light engineering, textile manufacture and processing, and coal-mining.

Development of the Department

Although the general principles underlying the needs of a general hospital psychiatric unit were known at the beginning of this period, their detailed evolution could not be governed and planned. Expediency and economy were frequent and important factors. The psychiatric wards at Burnley were locked and mainly custodial in their function until 1956. There was little active therapy or out-patient work. The darkly painted, dimly lit wards still employed seclusion and restraint. Knives, forks, razors and mirrors were not allowed, and the nurses were definitely custodial in their attitude.

By January 1957, with new medical and lay staff appointments, an open ward was in use and the department began to control its own records and organize its own appointment system. These steps, enabling complete administrative control and confidentiality to be present in the department from the start, are imperative for a psychiatric unit. A good medical secretary and a capable senior nursing sister of warm personality are equally important.

At this time, a basic medical staff structure of one part-time consultant, one registrar and one senior house officer was established. Further secretarial and clerical assistance was added, the nursing establishments were improved and staff training began. It was found that the medical, nursing and lay staff must work as a team and attention must be given to the co-ordination of all levels of staff function in order to ensure the essential flexibility which the treatment of the psychiatric patient demands. The protective aspects of care can be maintained without rigidity and traditional attention to protocol. The main problem in this respect has been the divided nature of the appointment and control of the various staff involved as a result of the administrative structure of general hospitals. This still requires attention.

In the first 6 months of these changes, a local branch of the National Association for Mental Health was formed, a therapeutic social club opened, two further mental welfare officers appointed by the local authority, a mental health exhibition took place in the hospital, and in May 1957 the seclusion register was finally closed. By April 1959 the last hospital patient was de-certified and no long-term compulsory admission has been required since. The wards were gradually modernized and redecorated, and in November 1960 a new out-patient and treatment unit was opened. A day-care service and small industrial workshop were also added.

The out-patient and treatment centre was designed for maximum use and flexibility. Attention was paid to comfort and informality, both in design and decor. Three consulting rooms, four treatment rooms and a large convertible general purpose room were provided, in addition to good waiting, reception and utility accommodation. An evening out-patient clinic proved a most needed service, enabling patients or their relatives to attend without losing time from work. During the evening clinic period, group therapy sessions can run concurrently. Another diagnostic and decision clinic has been held during a weekday and each is attended by three doctors, a senior nurse and a receptionist. Treatment sessions for psychotherapy, abreactive and analytical procedures, supportive measures and physical treatments are used by all medical staff throughout the week. It is important to appreciate that once a decision is made and a programme of treatment offered to the patient, it is essential to provide adequate staff, time and space for this treatment to proceed. Thus, it has been found that the ratio of treatment to diagnostic sessions is in the order of 6 to 1. Voluntary workers, often former patients, provide tea services at most sessions, adding an element of both reassurance and informality which patients appreciate. Table 2 illustrates the use of these services:

TABLE 2.

Psychiatric Out-patient Attendances

	New	Old	Total
1957	406	1652	2058
1958	389	2504	2893
1959	436	2685	3121
1960	491	2947	3438
1961	581	4136	4717
1962	587	4726	5313
1963	515	4765	5280
1964	543	4555	5098

The wards have remained completely open, without any security or re-straint rooms, since 1957. On both male and female wards, a pattern has emerged. For each sex, there is an acute admission ward area, a planned short-stay area and a psychogeriatric area. A mixed ward for both sexes became part of the short-stay area. The acute admission wards accept patients not previously seen by the department, those admitted on compulsory orders and those considered to be in need of protective measures or special nursing care. A trained nurse is in charge of each division, responsible to the departmental sisters. The short-stay planned admission wards were arranged as self-care units under nursing supervision as part of the rehabilitative plan. All patients are consistently encouraged to accept informal admission. These changes are reflected and illustrated in Table 3.

TABLE 3.

Psychiatric Admissions, 1950–64

	Female	Male	Total
1950	85	82	167
1951	67	73	140
1952	72	88	160
1953	58	70	128
1954	87	95	182
1955	86	81	167
1956	139	79	218
1957	228	136	364
1958	311	159	470
1959	390	257	647
1960	396	253	649
1961	429	233	662
1962	447	248	695
1963	434	298	732
1964	439	284	723

Development of Special Features

In 1959, because of the increasing demands for beds for elderly demented patients, a senile dementia day-care service was started. The object was to relieve the burden upon the family by offering supervision and care from 8.30 a.m. to 6 p.m. on 1–5 days a week, according to need. The selection of cases was usually made on a domiciliary visit and consideration was especially given to families with young children or work responsibilities. A maximum of eighteen patients is accepted daily and the composition of this group and their subsequent disposal is shown in Tables 4A and 4B.

So far, there is no evidence of any significant increase of chronically ill or elderly psychiatric patients needing to remain in hospital. The occupancy of the psychogeriatric wards has been reduced and there has been no unmanageable increase in demands on the day-care service. It must, however, be appreciated that other ancillary services were expanding at the same time. Local authority hostels for the elderly and mentally ill, rehabilitative workshops and social services have accepted an increasing responsibility. Adequate

TABLE 4A.

Day-care Patients. Diagnosis and Disposal, 1959–64

Diagnosis	No. of Cases	Workshop		Home		Hostel		Chronic sick		Died		Re-admitted		Currently attending	
		F.	M.	F.	M.	F.	M.	F.	M.	F.	M.	F.	M.	F.	M.
Affective disorders	56	4	1	20	6	4	1	3		8		3	1	4	1
Schizophrenia	9	1	0	3							1	3	1	1	
Pre-senile dementia	6			1		3	2	9	1	2	1		1	4	
Senile dementia	35			3	1	4		3	5	11	1	2		4	1
Arteriosclerotic dementia	35	1		4	4					7	2		2	1	1
Paranoid states	8		1	4		2		1		1			1	1	
Organic psycho-syndrome	6		1	1		1								1	
Psychogenic states	2		1			1									
		6	3	36	11	14	3	16	6	29	4	8	6	12	3
Total	157	9		47		17		22		33		14		15	

TABLE 4B.

Day-care Patients. Age and Diagnosis, 1959–64

Diagnosis	No. of Cases	Under 50		50–70		70–90	
		F.	M.	F.	M.	F.	M.
Affective disorders	56	13	—	24	6	9	4
Schizophrenia	9	7	1	1	—	—	—
Pre-senile dementia	6	—	—	4	2	—	—
Senile dementia	35	—	—	6	—	24	5
Arteriosclerotic dementia	35	1	—	8	6	12	8
Paranoid states	8	3	1	3	—	1	—
Organic psycho-syndrome	6	2	1	1	—	1	1
Huntington's chorea							
T.L. epilepsy, epilepsy post-leucotomy (2)							
Alcoholic dementia							
Psychogenic states	2	—	1	1	—	—	—
		26	4	48	14	47	18
Total	157	30		62		65	

geriatric services and beds in the general hospital have also made their contribution. These facilities are shown in the figures given in Table 5 in relation to disposal.

Rehabilitation

More purposeful rehabilitation and occupational therapy has been introduced both on the wards and in the occupational therapy department. Several contracts for work from outside firms were carried out, and in 1961 an industrial therapy workshop was built which also incorporated the developing day-care service. At night, it is used for meetings of the Psychiatric Social Club, the Ladies Sewing Group and the Alcoholics Anonymous. Patients attending the industrial therapy workshop are mainly those who have been discharged from the ward and are not fit to return to work. The working conditions and activities are made as realistic as possible; work is accepted on contract basis, at normal industrial rates and is very varied. Patients are expected to work for 25 hours a week, 10 a.m. to 12 noon and 2 p.m. to 4.30 p.m. During the lunch period discussions, musical appreciation sessions and group meetings are arranged. Out-patients receive bus fares, lunch and tea, and are able to earn up to £1 15s. per week, according to their output, in addition to their National Insurance or National Assistance benefit. Those requiring medication are supervised in this respect by the

TABLE 5. *Chronic Sick Patients*

	Male	Female
1. Number in residence 1956	28	37
2. Number in residence 1964	16	22
3. Remaining from (1) in 1964	9	11

Diagnosis and Disposal of Chronic Cases since 1957–63

	No.	Died	Remain	Home	Medical	Chronic sick	Mental hospital	Mental Def. Hospital	Hostel
MALE									
Schizophrenic	20	1	7	4	—	—	2	—	6
Subnormality	17	3	4	—	—	—	4	4	2
Dementias									
(a) Neurosyphilitic	2	—	1	—	—	—	—	—	1
(b) Epileptic	3	2	—	—	—	—	—	—	1
(c) Alcoholic	4	1	—	1	—	1	—	—	1
(d) Acute confusional	6	1	—	4	1	—	—	—	—
(e) Senile and arterio-sclerotic	12	3	4	—	—	4	—	—	1
Total	64	11	16	9	1	5	6	4	12
FEMALE									
Schizophrenic	4	—	1	—	—	—	2	—	1
Subnormality	8	—	7	—	—	—	1	—	1
Affective disorder	7	—	2	—	—	—	1	—	4
Prefrontal leucotomy	3	—	—	1	—	—	—	—	1
Dementia	25	11	9	1	—	1	—	—	3
Cerebral tumour	1	—	—	—	—	1	—	—	—
Paraphrenia	2	—	2	—	—	—	—	—	—
Total	50	11	21	2		2	4	—	10

workshop supervisor, who is also a trained nurse. One of the more senior medical staff takes responsibility for the patients in the workshop and day centre. Admission to the workshop is arranged for patients needing:

1. Encouragement and help in returning to their employment.
2. Rehabilitation and training towards seeking employment or towards regaining self-respect and a sense of belonging, if found to be unemployable.
3. Assessment in relation to potential working capacity.
4. Simple support and activity, if unemployable initially.
5. Assistance through work therapy with personality or psychogenic disorders.

During the first $3\frac{1}{2}$ years (October 1961 to May 1965), this workshop accepted 212 patients, 64 of whom returned to open industry. The diagnosis of these patients has been examined in relation to the patients' age, length of stay, earnings and disposal, and is shown in Tables 6A, 6B, 6C.

It has been suggested that general hospital psychiatric departments often have no definite catchment area, with its concurrent responsibilities, and are usually selective in their patient population. However, the catchment area of this service has already been described and defined. During the past 9 years, the number of patients who have not been treated by the Burnley Department of Psychiatry or have been subsequently transferred to other hospitals is negligible. Knowledge of this fact has been gleaned from the local authorities (through whom compulsory types of admission have to be arranged), statistical returns made to the regional hospital board, information from

TABLE 6A.

Workshop Patients, October 1961–May 1965

	No. of Cases		Under 20	20–40	40–60	Over 60
	M.	F.				
Paranoid states	—	3	—	—	1	2
Epilepsy	6	3	—	1	4	4
Subnormality	9	2	2	3	5	1
Personality disorders	17	5	2	8	11	1
Dementia	2	1	—	—	—	3
Abnormal psychogenic states	5	12	—	3	13	1
Schizophrenia	45	26	6	38	24	3
Affective disorders	25	34	—	12	32	15
Others	6	11	—	5	6	6
	115	97				
Total	212		10	70	96	36

TABLE 6B.

Workshop Patients, October 1961–May 1965

	No. of cases		Length of stay (months)					Earnings				
	M.	F.	3	3–6	6–12	12–24	24 and over	Very poor	Poor	Average	Good	Very good
Paranoid states	—	3	1	1	—	1	—	—	1	1	1	—
Epilepsy	6	3	4	—	3	—	2	—	5	4	—	—
Subnormality	9	2	4	—	5	—	2	1	6	3	1	—
Personality disorders	17	5	11	3	6	2	—	—	6	9	5	2
Dementia	2	1	1	1	—	1	—	—	3	—	—	—
Abnormal psychogenic states	5	12	7	2	4	4	1	1	7	4	4	1
Schizophrenia	45	26	34	12	7	11	7	4	30	23	10	4
Affective disorders	25	34	36	4	6	6	7	—	18	25	9	7
Others	6	11	8	7	2	—	—	—	9	6	2	—
Total	212		106	30	33	25	18	6	85	75	32	14

TABLE 6C.

Workshop Patients, October 1961–May 1965. Diagnosis and Disposal

	No. of cases		Discharged, no improvement	Home	Hostel and L.A.W.	Work in comm.	Admitted to wards	Currently attending	Died
	M.	F.							
Paranoid states	—	3	1	—	—	1	—	1	—
Epilepsy	6	3	—	2	2	2	—	3	—
Subnormality	9	2	3	1	1	3	—	3	—
Personality disorders	17	5	6	2	3	8	—	3	—
Dementia	2	1	1	—	—	—	—	—	2
Abnormal psychogenic states	5	12	3	2	—	6	—	6	—
Schizophrenia	45	26	—	6	4	32	11	18	1
Affective disorders	25	34	3	20	3	12	8	12	—
Others	6	11	1	7	3	—	—	5	1
Total		212	18	40	16	64	19	51	4

general practitioners and personal knowledge of the area. It is accepted that a small number of patients will always seek and obtain treatment outside the area. In order to try to meet some of the doubts that have been expressed over the type of patient the general hospital unit can accept, a diagnostic break-down of cases is presented here, with a table of the transfer to major mental hospitals (Tables 7A and 7B).

Local Authority Services

It is important to appreciate the contributions of the local authorities who have been evolving their own services during the same period. The establish-ment of mental welfare officers was increased and arrangements made for them to attend university courses so that they could receive professional training. In April 1960, the Burnley Health Department converted an open-air school into industrial workshops for handicapped subnormal and psy-chotic patients. Within 12 months, 62 patients (15 females and 21 males with subnormality and 8 females and 18 males with psychosis) were engaged in such activities as light engineering, carpentry, nylon fur mitten manufacture and a car-washing service. An average of 70 trainees are now accepted annually and 26 per annum have gone into open industry. These patients receive a maximum of 30s. a week in addition to National Insurance or National Assistance benefit, and are provided with meals. As a pilot scheme,

TABLE 7A.

Diagnostic Breakdown of Case Sheets raised, 1958–9

AFFECTIVE DISORDERS 232		ORGANIC REACTION DISORDERS 55	
Manic depressive psychosis	20	Arteriosclerotic dementia	17
Endogenous depression	34	Epilepsies	12
Involutional depression	76	Senile dementia	9
Puerperal depression	20	Associated with neoplasia	6
Senile depression (over 65)	23	Associated with toxic and infective	
Re-active depression	59	factors	8
		Others	3
ABNORMAL PSYCHOGENIC RE-ACTIONS 252		PERSONALITY DISORDERS 64	
Phobic anxiety states	90	Alcoholism	17
Neurotic depressive reactions	56	Sexual deviations	15
Psycho-somatic reactions	41	Psychopathy	32
Hysterical reactions	36		
Obsessional neuroses	11		
Behaviour disorder	18		
SCHIZOPHRENIA 21			
PARANOID STATES 29			
SUBNORMALITY 10			
NIL PSYCHIATRIC 12			

TABLE 7B.

Breakdown of Transfers to Major Mental Hospitals from August to September annually

	Male		Female		Totals
	Vol.	Cert.	Vol.	Cert.	
1951	4	27	1	27	59
1952	3	22	1	19	45
1953	5	19	5	17	46
1954	4	13	2	12	31
1955	2	12	2	20	36
1956	2	6	0	11	19
1957	0	3	0	4	7
1958	0	3	1	2	6
1959	0	0	2	0	2
1960	0	0	0	0	0
1961	0	0	1	0	1
1962	2	0	3	0	5
1963	3	0	1	0	4
1964	4	0	1	0	5
1965	1	0	0	0	1

in April 1962, a halfway house hostel with accommodation for 16 male or female patients was opened and in 2 years 24 patients have been discharged, through this, to the community.

General Hospital Psychiatric Care

There is no doubt of the benefit in terms of earlier diagnosis and treatment, quicker return to work and reduced economic hardship, to the patients and families, consequent upon the local development of a fully comprehensive psychiatric service. At times, doubts have been raised about the effectiveness of the intensive short-term admission and treatment policy described here. Recently, this question has been investigated by Manchester University Department of Psychiatry through a follow-up study (Hoenig, 1965). The preliminary results appear to indicate that this policy is effective and that it does not make undue demands on the community.

This question of reduced economic hardship is an important one, which has not been sufficiently stressed. Patients will accept earlier admission to the general hospital they know, near home, and less overall time is lost from work by both patients and relatives. Far too often, even today, psychiatric illness impairs economic and social standards in the home, thus further increasing the burden. There has been an undoubted improvement in the attitude of the community towards the mentally ill and an increasing use of the services available. Medical, social and geographical factors have been all in favour of this development. At the beginning of the period described here, the psychiatric service was minimal in this area and the nearest large mental hospital was 26 miles away. Yet the degree of use of the new service, the co-operative attitude of general practitioners, the high reliability rate of their case references (in terms of psychiatric need), and the acknowledgement of the unit as an integral part of the general hospital, suggest that the community was ready to accept this new concept. There have never been any pressures to keep these patients further away, nor any serious objection to the relatively special favours, in terms of upgrading of facilities and staff, granted to the psychiatric department. Other specialties, with equally pressing needs, recognized those of the psychiatric patient and the former neglect they suffered.

The advantages of a comprehensive psychiatric unit in a district general hospital, as opposed to the large special psychiatric hospital, may be considered as:

(1) *Medical.* Closer links with general practitioners and consultant colleagues, both in daily work and in social and academic settings, undoubtedly inspire confidence in the ability of psychiatry to offer something definite to the patient. Because the department is in the local community, earlier referral, diagnosis and treatment follow, and with this, a reduction of the frequency with which people require to be admitted, under forms of compulsion or in states of severely disturbed behaviour. As the service has developed, with improved community, professional and staff attitudes, incidents of impulsive, unpredictable and violent behaviour have been so reduced as to become a distinct rarity. The fact that the unit is accessible and open to the community, both lay and professional, allays fear, prejudice and doubt and encourages individual interest and confidence. The service available is less impersonal, involving known people, rather than paper references. The general hospital unit will therefore deal with about four local authorities, involving ten people, rather than many authorities, and many unknown persons, as in the case of larger hospitals. The doctor–patient relationship is enhanced and is more consistent; this relationship, which must be dependable and enduring, is of paramount importance. This is still one of the most potent therapeutic agents, notwithstanding modern chemotherapy and physical methods of treatment. Continuity of care is also more certainly ensured in the smaller unit, from a relatively small number of staff members.

By its example, the psychiatric unit may influence other departments in the hospital in the understanding of emotional factors in disease. Any steps which bring psychiatry to the general body of medical thought and actions must be regarded as valuable.

This proximity is a good influence, too, upon the psychiatric staff, both medical and nursing; they are less divorced from, and so more aware of, the general organic problems of medicine and surgery and more capable of managing them. Special medical needs are more easily met and handled in the general hospital milieu. Cases of neurosis, with presenting physical symptoms and psychosomatic disorders, are more easily seen; arrangements for the screening and treatment of attempted suicides are facilitated, and such developments as the senile dementia day-care service and rehabilitative workshop can be realistically organized in close proximity to the patients' homes. Similarly, arrangements for visiting, weekend leave and holiday admission are simple and economical. It is therefore possible to encourage the patient to make contact with, and live in, the more normal environment of his home and town than in the artificial one of an isolated hospital. Arguments are put forward that only the large special psychiatric hospital can provide for the special medical needs of the mentally ill. This can be countered by pointing out that the amenities provided are often unreal, over-supportive and superfluous. If the community accepts the concept of psychiatric illness as one requiring consideration and encouragement, without condescension, then automatically, access can be provided to the patient's usual environment, which is a more realistic measure.

Architecturally, there must be adequate living space and special consideration of the needs of psychiatric patients, but this does not require separate, special institutions. Experience in Burnley and in the Manchester region generally shows that the provision of $0 \cdot 5$ beds per 1000 population is ample. Emphasis should be upon function, flexibility, economics and the needs of patient and staff. Generous out-patient space is absolutely necessary for individual interviews and treatment sessions, as well as any group procedures. In the wards, there is a place for single rooms, but communicating units of three to six beds each, allow better supervision as well as improved social contacts, between patient and staff. Special facilities, such as quiet rooms, games rooms, day space and workshop areas are essential. In these smaller, compact units, staff teamwork is enhanced. Uniformity of aim and purpose can be engendered, in both staff and patients, by the lead given by the clinical director. Finally, it is essential that there are adequate geriatric beds and social services, the latter in the form of home helps, nightsitters, wardens, meals-on-wheels and hostel accommodation. Given such facilities, it has been our experience, in the past 9 years, that chronic in-patients do not accumulate.

(2) *Social.* The department is in the local community and becomes part of it, subject to the same criticism or praise as any other institution. Normal out-patient reference methods encourage the acceptance of advice, treatment and, if necessary, admission. Useful and successful therapy begets confidence, which is soon spread locally. Day-to-day contacts between hospital, general practitioner and local authority staff promote appreciation of each other's

contributions and problems. Special problems can be considered at a realistic case conference level, with all associated workers present, and the effect of decisions can be readily checked. The access of patients and their relatives to senior nursing and medical staff is purposely encouraged and seldom abused.

The therapeutic social club is less hospital-orientated than many, since most members are past or present out-patients, and some also from the wards. Their programmes bring in local organizations and these contacts have produced good catalyst reactions in support of psychiatric patients, whose behaviour and outlook have surprised many a visitor.

(3) *Geographical*. There would not seem to be any valid point or advantage in perpetuating the segregation and isolation of sick people, away from their community, because they are mentally ill. This is not a contagious disease.

Our experience over 9 years is that at least 98 % of all types of psychiatric illness can be treated in a comprehensive general hospital department of psychiatry. Because of the relative smallness and intimacy of such a department, very occasional disturbing cases may require transfer. As there is no facility for strict custodial care, certain cases referred by the courts are not acceptable. But in any case, the provision of prison and remand centre psychiatric hospital accommodation and staff must be the solution here. Rarely, the difficult epileptic or psychopath becomes too much of a problem, and the unco-operative alcoholic outwears his welcome.

There seems no doubt that with a policy of early admission and early discharge to the community, a higher recurrence rate will occur in a small group of people. Indications are that this group mainly comprises patients who, under the old conditions, would have been permanent or very long-stay admissions. Acceptance of their recurring problems, by good staff attitudes, helps their periods of remission in the community, while mutual trust leads to earlier re-admission and less deterioration. There has been no significant increase here in chronic patients requiring to be retained 2 years or more. In fact, this population and accommodation have been almost halved, with the help of the senile dementia day-care service, now in operation for 4 years.

Summary

The planned development of a comprehensive psychiatric service in a district general hospital is described, including its experiences over a period of 9 years and certain general findings and principles. The essential needs of the department and the special developments of a senile dementia day-care service and industrial workshop are outlined. The advantages of such a department in a general hospital, in terms of medical, social and geographical factors, and the range and types of cases which can be accepted, are described and discussed. There is considered to be good evidence that such units can meet the main needs of a population of about 200,000. This has been proven in Burnley during the past 9 years, with seventy active beds, a ratio of $0 \cdot 35$ per 1000 of the population. Adequate geriatric and social services, both in the hospital and the community, are essential, together with realistic co-operation and a sense of joint purpose.

Acknowledgements

I would like to acknowledge the support of the Manchester Regional Hospital Board and particularly of Dr. F. N. Marshall, Senior Administrative Medical Officer, Dr. Pigott, Chairman of the Board's Mental Health Committee, Dr. S. Smith, member of the regional board and Medical Superintendent, Lancaster Moor, for the sustained interest and enthusiasm they have shown in the development, regionally, of the general hospital psychiatric service. My special thanks are due to Dr. J. S. B. Mackay, Deputy Senior Administrative Medical Officer of the Board, the active architect and developer of this regional policy. I also wish to acknowledge the support and assistance locally of the Burnley Hospital Management Committee and their officers. Finally, I wish to thank my staff past and present for their loyal help and co-operation and particularly my most patient secretary, Mrs. C. Bladen, for all she has done.

References

LEYBERG, J. T. (1959), *Lancet*, **ii**, 282.
FREEMAN, H. L. (1960), *Lancet*, **i**, 218.
HOENIG, J. (1965), *Lancet*, **i**, 1322.
SILVERMAN, M. (1961), *Brit. Med. J.*, **ii**, 698.

36. The Psychiatric Rehabilitation Association

John Denham

THE aim of all rehabilitation is the adaptation of the patient to society. He is taught to give up the status of a sick person and restart his life without over-emphasis or any residual disability. To further this aim, the Psychiatric Rehabilitation Association was set up in the East End of London and at Long Grove Hospital in 1960.

Membership of the Association includes psychiatric patients in hospital and in the community, their relatives and friends, and any other interested persons in the community or in the mental health services. To make it effective, patients are enrolled early in their period of treatment. They are invited to introductory meetings, where free membership is offered, and exposition of the Association's purpose is found to be acceptable, even to the seriously thought-disordered.

Theoretical Considerations

The mentally ill belong to a minority group. As a result of their illness and disability, they are rejected by society and placed in institutions which are remote from their community, so that they become socially isolated. Psychiatric patients in hospital, like any other group of people who spend long in an institution, develop defects of personality, amongst which loss of initiative appears to be the most noxious. It is common knowledge that this process of institutional neurosis (Barton, 1959) may proceed at a rapid pace in patients with insecure personalities and backgrounds.

Treatment of the acute psychiatric patient is a professional process, but rehabilitation is a social one. Social rehabilitation aims to reverse the process of social isolation and institutionalization. The first task is the integration of patients into groups. These groups have a definite purpose—rehabilitation, and they are reminded of it incessantly. After a period of acclimatization, patients will be made aware, first of their immediate, and later of their more distant social environment. They will examine their status as psychiatric patients, and thus be able to identify with other members of the group. This is the first break in social isolation, and the beginning of group-work proper. The groups, originally led by professional group-workers, will demonstrate their own initiative and then assume their own leadership.

Rehabilitation would not be complete without preparation of the community to accept and welcome back the patients after their discharge from hospital. Group-work with relatives and friends is started at an early stage, experiences with their disturbed family members exchanged, anxieties about their return brought out, and the isolation of the families of psychiatric patients reduced. The in-patient and community groups are joined together for mutual understanding and assistance.

Some theoretical considerations about leadership may be appropriate here. The psychiatric hospital, like many other institutions of the welfare state, has a patriarchal structure. Leadership is vested in those who know best; it is sapiential. In practice, it will either take a course of power or one of influence. Psychiatric patients are only too ready to submit to the magic of the omniscient. The dependency needs of patients often set psychiatrists an impossible task. In rehabilitation, patriarchal attitudes must give way, and patients' initiative receive encouragement. Leadership will pass from the professional to the patients during group-work, and turn against the cherished regulations and tradition of the institution.

In patient-groups, a similar process applies in miniature. As leadership passes from the professional to the patients, it gets into the hands of the most vocal—mostly the paranoid or the psychopathic. Both are liable to provoke indignation in the groups, which may well be one of the most stimulating motives in group activity. The stage has then been set for pathological leadership, but it is not allowed to become pathological by the patients. The group of patients will follow such a leader while he remains within the bounds of reality, but withdraw their support on each occasion that his demands become frankly morbid.

Group-work

The method of social rehabilitation is group-work. This is distinct from group-psychotherapy, where emotional integration and insight is achieved through multiple transference. In group-work, longitudinal explorations are replaced by examination of the present-day existence of a minority group consisting of psychiatric patients. Such groups cohere through shared feelings of rejection and resentment against common prejudices. Through group-work, the patients change from regarding themselves as specially deprived and in need of extraordinary facilities and concessions, to a state where they refuse to be singled out through special treatment. Painfully, they recognize that psychiatric illness cannot be disguised as "nerves", but is a disorder of function, like any other disease of the human body. They then realize that mental disorder is not a sign of personal weakness, to be condemned, but an illness, with all its hazards of recovery and disablement. By comparing the handicaps caused by physical and psychological complaints, their sympathy and concern will extend to others and breach their isolation.

This represents a rough outline of the re-motivation to be achieved by group-work, which we found to be equally applicable to regressed schizophrenics and to verbally agile neurotics. Three stages of group-work may be described: the first is activation, whereby the patients' awareness of society and social functions is aroused; the second is the acclimatization of the individual to the group situation; and the third represents a return of initiative.

During activation, the patients are stimulated to examine their immediate environment and to compare it with social institutions at large. In a group of verbally active patients, this will represent no difficulty. When the members are severely withdrawn and/or psychotic, remnants of social awareness have to be sought in the group. Sessions may then more resemble a junior school class. Photographs and film strips of public places, persons and familiar objects may help to stimulate interest, but have to be accompanied by repeated reminders that the purpose is rehabilitation, even if it seems to arouse no response. Groups of withdrawn patients also join with other groups, which increases their activation, prepares them to adjust to the larger group, and in turn produces social consciousness in the more active patients. The latter are made aware of the plight of those more ill, more isolated, or more handicapped. In hospital they are encouraged to visit the infirm and elderly and, at home, the physically disabled. The mixing of physical and psychiatric rehabilitees may be essential for the success of industrial rehabilitation units.

Activation also leads to the well-known phenomenon of releasing hostility and directing it against the institution and its employees. This takes the form of numerous complaints about food, treatment or regulations, and allegations of cruelty, or demands for extra comforts and privileges. These moves have to be recognized as the beginnings of group formation, rather than suppressed as signs of imminent rebellion. In such a *milieu*, the psychopathic and paranoid patients will gain a short-lived ascendency, while just and unjust criticism will soften the rigidity of the institution.

With increasing identification, group-formation will progress, its purpose being to seek general understanding and solutions of the problem of mental health. At all times, discussions are in general terms, and individual explorations are discouraged by the group-worker. During this stage, the stigma of psychiatric illness will be the background against which adjustment has to be found. Patients' concern about being accepted in work and home situations is a recurring topic, and conformity to general standards of conduct and wage-earning are frequently expressed aims. Their aspiration to gain equality, and to prevent it from being impaired by the stigma, is their main anxiety. It is of great import for them to learn that efforts at concealing mental illness, when looking for work or accommodation, are as futile as confiding it too readily. Failure in such situations may only represent a secret wish to retain the protected status of a patient.

Socio-drama

Common situations of conflict are acted out in hospital in socio-drama, through spontaneous role-playing. The same distinction as between group-work and group-psychotherapy exists between psycho-drama and socio-drama; portrayal of individual trauma is replaced by situations of potential social conflict. Interviews with future employers, landladies, officials and doctors are portrayed in turn by several pairs of patients. Usually, they portray the interviewer as kindly and weak, although he is feared for his harshness and rigidity. This allows the other performer to conceal his fear of failure. The inappropriateness of the performance is received by the group with great good humour. Defects are pointed out, and corrected in subsequent attempts. Staff should remain passive throughout, to prevent comparison with patients which would enhance their feelings of inferiority. Jocular acceptance by the audience is reassuring to all, and identification with those taking part is of equal importance. The value of socio-drama lies in demonstrating that the interaction of two or more people determines the content of their communications.

Inquiries by patients about the causes, treatment and course of psychiatric illness will increase, and provide evidence that they are able to face the realities of their illness, in a social setting. The psychiatrist must be prepared to talk about these subjects in a factual manner, avoiding technical terms. Refusal to give information, or softening the harsh facts, undermines patients' search for confidence. An alternative mode of introducing discussion on mental health is through one of the many psychiatric films. Although a few may protest that some subjects should not be shown to patients, experience has indicated that they are well able to appreciate them and to discuss them intelligently. Such discussions are led by experienced staff members, who will be able to lead the group to understand the relevant factors of the film. In discussion of methods of treatment, most patients (including the psychotic) will look in preference to insight-giving therapy, voice popular misgivings about drugs acting on the central nervous systems, and query empirical forms of physical treatment. The discussions will be of a high level of intelligence and understanding, and may appear to be superior to those of professional groups. This could be explained by the high degree of concern with the subject and the strength of motivation of patient-groups. They also expect the information they receive to be of high quality, when outsiders like public leaders and officials are invited to address them.

As the patients' isolation diminishes, with increasing identification in the groups, their sense of personal inferiority and failure will decrease. They will be able to regard themselves as responsible individuals. This sense of responsibility is generally regarded as the most integral faculty of human existence and is endangered or lost during psychiatric illness. Society demands responsibility, and mistrusts all those who are liable to lose it. As the patients learn to regard themselves as responsible, both in groups and as individuals, initiative is regained. In rehabilitation, initiative expresses itself through positive social action. As such, it may be misinterpreted, both in the hospital and in the community, as unwarranted rebellion. In hospital, the groups will encounter the barriers of institutionalization, while in the community they will show up the deficiencies of local authority provisions and may initiate after-care themselves. It is the task of the psychiatrist to recognize initiative and its therapeutic importance, encourage it, and reassure his staff and associates that patients' initiative will increase rather than diminish their status.

It is important to mention group-leadership and its relationship to professional staff. Attitudes towards doctors and nurses are recognized, examined and utilized, both in individual and group psychotherapy. The same tenets apply in group-work, where dependency needs have to be changed into-initiative, and the paternalism of the institution give way to group activity. Professional leadership must encourage and influence personal initiative from the patients, not just passively allow them. Initially, therefore, group leadership will be professional, until group formation has succeeded, and leaders have emerged spontaneously. Peer-leaders can influence groups more effectively, and should therefore receive some training in the aims of rehabilitation. This has been done through activation of peer-leaders in special groups, which have the responsibility of planning the group programme. As they develop their initiative and confidence, they work alongside professional group-workers, and eventually participate in the preparation courses for voluntary workers.

Group-work also aims at social agencies, where a wealth of goodwill exists, together with fear of doing harm through a faulty approach to the psychiatric patient. The essence of group-work with members of the community is to show that interaction with psychiatric patients need not be the prerogative of the expert.

Activities in Hospital

The Psychiatric Rehabilitation Association was first set up in Long Grove Hospital, Epsom, Surrey, and the East End of London in 1960, to bridge the 25-mile gap between the community and the hospital that served the area. It provides within the hospital:

(i) *Groups for recent patients on individual wards*

These take place once a week on individual admission wards in Long Grove and St. Clement's hospitals. Nursing staff and all patients—however disturbed—are invited, and between twenty to thirty attend at each meeting.

Patients with minor psychiatric illnesses will concern themselves with common social problems, while those with major disorders tend to concentrate on mental illness, its cause, prognosis and stigma. With recently admitted patients, the stage of activation is short, their social isolation being less complete, though often an intrinsic feature of their personality. Groups devote most of their attention to current social problems, and benefit mainly on return to their home. Four obstacles—or crises—to resettlement can be distinguished on leaving hospital: the actual leaving of the shelter of the hospital and giving up of the status of a patient; the return to work, which tests their sense of responsibility and exposes them to the doubts of their fellow workers; and, finally, when adaptation seems to have been established for several months, but when they realize that many of the expectations will never be fulfilled. They may then break down and again seek the shelter of the hospital.

(ii) *Groups for chronic patients*

These are held weekly on the rehabilitation ward at Long Grove Hospital, with all patients and staff. Activation is the main concern of group-work with chronic patients. According to severity of illness and length of stay in hospital, such groups require simple educative measures. This has been initiated by group-workers, and will be continued by nursing staff for prolonged periods, to prevent reappearance of the well-known signs of chronicity.

(iii) *A large combined group for all*

For the weekly evening meetings, of up to 100 members from the recent and chronic patients group, an agenda is prepared in a group meeting of peer-leaders. The meeting is conducted on a formal basis, with chairman and secretary elected by the combined group from the group peer-leaders. A report of activities is given and minutes are read. A main speaker—usually a professional worker from inside the hospital or from outside social agencies— addresses the meeting and leads the discussion. In these group meetings, the basis of the whole rehabilitation effort is established. There, policies are discussed, new enterprises developed and "better" patients encouraged to help the "bad" ones. The fear of chronic mental illness is present in most of the recent admissions; they shun and dread the chronic wards. If they take this fear home with them, they may become phobic or "house-bound", or relapse under the most minor stress. When they have learned to help those less well then themselves, their ego will be strengthened and their social conscience aroused. Of particular interest was a scheme for younger patients to visit elderly ones, who had no visitors. This added to the comfort of the elderly and the self-confidence of the young, though it sometimes interfered with ward routine.

(iv) *A news letter*

This is published monthly, compiled in the Psychiatric Rehabilitation Association's office in the East End of London, and contains news of activities progress and projects, the programme and location of community centres, and a short article relevant to psychiatric rehabilitation. (A previous effort of a patient-produced magazine ceased publication because editor and assistants could only be recruited from short-stay patients. The necessary continuity was lacking, and occasional controversial material, in the absence of censorship, aroused opposition in the hospital.)

(v) *Visits of in-patients to groups in the community*

In spite of distance, three regular visits have been arranged by coach of groups of thirty patients from Long Grove Hospital to meetings in the community. The current patients participate in ex-patient and relatives' groups. There, they gain confidence, by meeting and listening to former patients, and also give reassurance to their friends and relatives that they are on the way to recovery and full responsibility. In addition, they take part in discussions, led by community-leaders and officers of the various welfare departments.

(vi) *Experience for nurses in group-work techniques*

Participation of nursing staff is on an informal basis, and is particularly useful for junior nurses who are not burdened by the care and responsibility of the senior staff. The nurse is given an opportunity to observe patients in the setting of a group, to listen to free expression and discussion by the patients. Often in a group-setting a new facet of the individual patient emerges and provides a new insight for the nurse. Thus in group-work sessions many patients exhibit a good deal of knowledge and understanding of the problems of psychiatric nursing in a rational manner. In group-work general topics of mental health and rehabilitation replace the more individual and therapeutic approach of the staff and ward meetings of "therapeutic community". In both cases participation of nurses was found to be beneficial to ward and patient management and to give an added incentive and interest to all grades of staff. If aptitude is shown, nurses participate as group-workers.

Activities in the community

In East London, the Psychiatric Rehabilitation Association entered the field of community care shortly before section 6 of the Mental Health Act of 1959 became operative. It has therefore concerned itself—generously supported by the London County Council—with pioneering after-care facilities, in addition to its prescribed purpose of preparing the ground for the reception of the returned patients into the community and their rehabilitation there. The Psychiatric Rehabilitation Association's functions and provisions in the community include:

(i) *Group-work with discharged patients, out-patients, patients' families and friends*

This is being done in four centres in East London. The site of each centre has been chosen mainly for convenience to patients and relatives living in the vicinity. Local authority and church halls are being used, free of charge. Patients who joined the Psychiatric Rehabilitation Association during their stay in hospital are invited to attend and to bring their families and friends with them. Their attendance is registered; regular attenders who fail to turn up are visited by one of the voluntary workers. These groups are also joined by selected out-patients from psychiatric clinics in the area. The main criteria for selection are the patients' isolation, loneliness and their personal need for social rehabilitation.

Group-work follows exactly the same lines as described above. Activation is carried out by a professional group-worker. These groups are also used for the training of voluntary workers to take over eventually some of the work carried out by the professional. A meeting lasts approximately 2 hours; the first half-hour is occupied with casual conversation and cups of tea. The formal programme lasts 1 hour, and an additional half-hour is usually required for short interviews with patients and relatives. This type of interview allows an informal approach and collection of valuable information about patients' progress.

Once a month each group receives a visit from patients still in hospital, and a combined programme is arranged. These meetings allow also for the meeting of in-patients with their friends and families. On average, each of these groups has an attendance of 30, although on evenings when in-patients visit, this number may increase to 80 or 100. Visitors from the various social agencies are frequent, and social-work students come as part of their training.

(ii) *Coach service for visitors to hospital*

As Long Grove Hospital is at a distance of 25 miles from East London, visiting is usually restricted to once a week through distance and cost of travelling. One of the earliest efforts was to establish a coach service, and a coach has since been hired on every Sunday. One of the patients, or relatives, acts as conductor, and visitors are picked up at three different points in the

area. This reduces the time and expense of the journey, and at the same time
allows for considerable interactions of patients' families and friends.

(iii) *Day centres*

The Psychiatric Rehabilitation Association was able to pioneer the first
Day Centre for chronic patients in the community, which was opened at
Hackney Downs Chapel in 1962. The need for such a centre was shown by
the investigation of Enid Mills (1962). Chronic patients often used to use
public libraries and parks to pass their time. Spontaneous groups may be
formed to support each other, where they would share their meagre incomes.

Day centres were opened not only with the aim of providing a haven for
the chronic patients and a relief for their families during the day, but also
with rehabilitation in mind. This depended on an active and co-operative
community attitude. The centres have to provide a climate which encourages
the patients to enjoy their work, leisure and loyalty to each other. The first
day centre operated on 5 days a week in a church hall. Patients were accepted
from out-patient clinics, doctors and social workers, whatever their psychiatric
condition. There was a need for occupation and minor industrial work was
introduced. In the absence of funds, this day centre initially relied entirely
on voluntary help. Voluntary workers would act as day-centre supervisors
to the limit of time they could afford to spend there. Ideally, staffing would
be two (full time) per session. It is important to have one full-time staff
member to supervise the staff work of the centre while the others visit and
establish the first contact with the patients before they join the group. At a
later stage art and craft classes were introduced with the help of the education
authorities. Combined creative activity led to more rapid integration of the
patient into groups. They were encouraged to take an active interest in the
management of the centre in the provision and execution of the work done,
and to help those patients who are less able to adjust to the activities. Patients
often would call and escort each other to the centre and follow up those who
ceased to attend. The earnings of the group were discussed and members
decided whether to share or save their earnings for a group holiday or some
other project.

In an area where the relapse rate is high, where many patients live in
inferior lodgings and often are regarded as unemployable, the day centres
have shown themselves valuable places for assessing five groups of patients.
Firstly, they are an important aid to patients recently discharged from
hospital who are symptom-free but have not found employment, especially
for those who are living alone. Secondly, there are those patients who have
been discharged but are not yet fit for work; they are kept in a mood of
activity and prevented from becoming unemployable. Thirdly, there are those
patients who have been chronically ill and who are recovering from acute

illness, where the day centre presents the first step towards an industrial rehabilitation unit of the Ministry of Labour. Fourthly, there are the chronically disabled patients who will require permanent sheltered conditions and who are a heavy burden on their families. These patients benefit greatly from the day centres, while a reduction of stress in the home increases the relatives' tolerance and makes them less anxious to return the patient to hospital. Finally, there exists a fifth group of patients who have been on the list of the Disablement Resettlement Officer at the Ministry of Labour for many months and years. These patients show no overt psychiatric disability, but are unable to hold down any ordinary employment for more than a short time. They have usually entered and failed various courses of rehabilitation. Not many patients in these five groups are suitable for existing rehabilitation centres, either because they are not stable or because they only require immediate and short-term attendance at the day centre.

It is essential that the day centres be placed in those areas where a high geographical incidence of mental illness exists. By far the largest group of chronic patients live in areas which are overcrowded, have low rateable value and specialize in sub-letting of furnished rooms.

(iv) *Sheltered employment in industry*

Unexpected progress amongst chronic patients living in the community necessitated the provision of employment of a more regular and competitive nature. With the help of the Rotarians, groups of patients found employment in local industry. Small groups attended whole or part time according to their personal ability. In the initial phase, a voluntary worker went to work with the group. The Psychiatric Rehabilitation Association was paid for the work of the whole group and the money distributed amongst the patients according to the time each had been able to work in the factory. Progress in this was rapid, and most of the patients were soon offered whole-time employment at the usual rates.

(v) *Residential centre*

This has been set up in collaboration with the Cheshire Foundation and accommodates 30 patients, recently discharged from hospital, in 3 Old Nichol Street, London, E. 2. The premises had previously been used by a religious body as a hostel and settlement. It required considerable renovation and decoration, most of which was carried out by patients from the day centres and by ex-patients during their free time. Groups of young people from the International Voluntary Service, Community Service Volunteers and Toc H assisted at various times in decorating and preparing the centre for use. Resident Staff consists of a warden (preferably with psychiatric nursing experience) and a deputy warden. In addition a full-time domestic help and a part-time cook are employed. Most of the patients are accepted directly from hospital on discharge and are expected to be employable and be able to contribute towards the cost of their maintenance. Usually, a request is made by the discharging doctor to the local authority to sponsor the patient at this hostel and to guarantee the maintenance cost, up to £6 per week on a sliding scale. During the first 9 months, 36 patients entered the residential centre; 7 had to be readmitted to hospital while the remainder were able to find full-time employment and, after a period of approximately 3 months, to return to their families or alternatively find suitable lodging with selected families. Most of the latter group keep in touch with the centre, frequently visit it and join in the activities of the resident group of patients. The residential centre also accommodates a Psychiatric Social Club every Saturday evening and a Sunday Lunch Club. It has been planned to provide there a resettlement unit which will be a combination of a sheltered work shop and day centre.

(vi) *A resettlement unit*

A resettlement unit is under active planning. Premises are available at the Residential Centre in Bethnal Green. Work will not be on a sub-contractual basis, since planning, design, production and marketing are envisaged as taking place within this unit. A paid supervisor and an assistant will deal with at least ten patients, who will attend for a full 8-hour day. A grant has been made for this project by the Queen Adelaide Fund, and it is expected that it will be recognized by the Ministry of Labour as a rehabilitation centre so that patients will qualify for the usual allowance.

(vii) *Art group*

The value of the art classes in the day centres in integrating patients into groups was such as to result in the setting-up of a separate art club in the Geoffrey Museum under professional guidance. This caters for 10–15 patients, some of them may never have had any experience in drawing, painting or sculpturing before.

(viii) *Music group*

Music also has been found useful in group-formation, and therefore two music groups were started. The aim is to make patients aware of the emotions aroused in the appreciation of music and to encourage them to compare their personal experiences. This leads to a freeing from emotional inhibitions and helps them to adjust in social settings.

(ix) *Sunday lunch clubs*

The weekend was found to be the most difficult period for patients living in the community. None of the usual facilities are available, and patients are exposed to tensions in the family whilst everybody is at home. For this purpose, a Sunday Lunch Club was started by the patients. Room and cooking facilities were provided free in a local church. They collected 2*s*. 6*d*. from each member. Two of the members do the shopping on Saturdays, while another two do the cooking on Sundays. Two such clubs exist and cater for up to fifteen patients each. They are run entirely by the patients and a meeting lasts 3–4 hours.

(x) *Group holidays*

Great difficulty has been experienced in obtaining recuperative holidays for chronic patients in the community. The members of the various groups decided to arrange for such holidays themselves. Members' subscriptions and help from interested groups in the community enabled thirty patients to have a holiday in a boarding house at a seaside resort. The patients' main emphasis was that they should have a holiday under the usual holiday circumstances, and not be placed in a special home. A whole boarding house was hired at the beginning of the holiday season and the group travelled there, together with a group-worker and voluntary helpers, who helped to make this venture a success. A further three holiday periods have since been arranged.

(xi) *Emergency fund*

This was provided to assist patients in their first week after discharge from hospital. It was found that the usual National Assistance allowance was not sufficient to enable patients to obtain lodgings and food for the first week, even if they were working. The stress of the first week often interfered with their occupational adjustment, and early return to hospital became likely. The patients' attendance at groups in hospital led them to call at the Psychiatric Rehabilitation Association's office in such periods of stress, and a special fund was set up to make loans up to £2. So far, none of the patients has failed to return the loan in due course.

(xii) *Group-work training centre*

With the help of the King Edward Fund, it was possible to set up a Group-work Training Centre in Hackney. The main emphasis has been to provide training for voluntary workers in the management and activation of groups, rather than teaching psychiatric case work. Voluntary workers, some of whom may have been psychiatric patients, come from all walks of life—school teachers, salesmen, manual workers and clerks. They eventually fulfil a useful function in a wide range of activities, from statistical work to tea-making. The training is in the basis and methods of group-work. It enlarges the outlook of the participants and creates greater confidence, providing them with valuable experience in group activities.

The course has been prepared and directed by Mr. J. Wilder, Secretary of the Psychiatric Rehabilitation Association, who has been accepted by the Inner London Education Authority as a Senior Lecturer in Sociology. Representatives from the University of Wales, Chiswick Polytechnic, and various public schools have attended these training sessions and group-work demonstrations, and have used them increasingly for secondment of under-graduate and postgraduate students, as part of their in-service training.

(xiii) *Liaison*

Liaison with Ministry of Labour, National Assistance Board, Ministry of National Insurance, local authority health and welfare departments, employers associations, personnel officers, trade unions, religious bodies and voluntary organizations has been of material assistance in the rehabilitation effort.

(xiv) *Social investigation and surveys, research*

In a practical sphere, the first aim was to assess the potential needs of discharged patients. Preliminary surveys showed that 30% of male patients discharged from Long Grove Hospital did not return to the address from which they had been admitted, highlighting the need for hostels and foster homes. Objective assessment was made of the social needs of 100 consecutive admissions to hospital. Half of the patients had no social problems; in a quarter, they were minor; in 20% they were appreciable; and in the remaining 5% they appeared severe and insoluble. In a hospital with an active treatment programme, the re-admission rate tends to be high. Follow-up inquiries were sent to 100 discharged patients, but only half replied. A third of those who replied expressed gratitude for what had been done in hospital and said they required no further help; a further third expressed various needs, while the remaining letters showed obvious mental disturbance. When those who failed to reply were visited, they were found to be reasonably well, but socially isolated, and despondent about the prospects of their future mental health; they had all been in hospital more than once. The males were mostly schizo-phrenics and a few psychopaths; the females were all unattached or foreign-born. A tendency to relapse showed high correlation with obvious loneliness. The collection of figures for admissions and discharges from the various districts within the area was found to be essential for the planning and siting of community facilities. Progress was estimated by an initial increase in re-admission rates with a subsequent decrease proportional to the provision of out-patient treatment without waiting lists, together with active home visiting. Most of these surveys were only rough indicators of social factors and needs; they were rapidly changing, and could hardly be subjected to statistical analysis in the absence of great resources for research.

(xv) *Visiting scheme*

The visiting of patients recently returned from hospital has aroused most controversy. The Psychiatric Rehabilitation Association invites every patient to attend group meetings, either alone or with interested relatives and friends. This invitation is taken to them by voluntary workers, who are instructed to make no inquiries of the patient or the family, but to be ready to listen to any information or demands. They report their visits briefly, and in suitable cases continue their calls and maintain contact. Often, they are able to persuade the isolated to join in group activities, or escort the phobic or the fearful in their initial journeys to shops and welfare offices. From the patients' angle, there have been no difficulties; they accept a lay visitor without suspicion, and rejection of visitors has been a rare exception. The visitors know where to turn if the patients require professional help, although they may be received with suspicion and anger by social workers who may feel that their function has been usurped by untrained "do-gooders". In this respect, it is essential to remind them that the community support given by the voluntary worker cannot be given by the professional, while the care and casework of the social worker is a far more specialized task, to be reserved for those who require it most, in view of extreme staff shortages.

Shaping of a Comprehensive Service

The development and progress of the Psychiatric Rehabilitation Association in East London provided an object lesson that rehabilitation could be undertaken in the community. At the same time, the Observation Ward at St. Clement's Hospital was converted into an Early Treatment Unit (Benady and Denham, 1963). Whereas previously two-thirds of the patients admitted to the Observation Ward were transferred for further treatment and care to the appropriate mental hospital, increasing numbers received treatment, and two-thirds were able to return directly to their own homes. This proportion has now been increased to 99%. Thus it has been found possible to treat 350 patients in 24 beds annually, requiring an average stay of 23 days. Easy and frequent visiting led to relatives' participation, while improvement of the patients and general tolerance increased proportionally. Resettlement of patients is facilitated by group-work and attendance at day centres during their stay in hospital. Medium- or long-stay beds are only needed for 1 % of the patients treated at St. Clement's Hospital. From 1 April 1965, St. Clement's has taken over one-fifth of the Long Grove Hospital catchment area. A link exists as regards geriatric patients who require long-stay accommodation not available locally.

It has been estimated that between 250–300 patients annually will require in-patient treatment from a catchment area of 100,000 population. The closeness of the hospital to the patient's home enables treatment to be given often on a day or domiciliary basis, and makes follow-up visits easy. St. Clement's Hospital, with 123 beds, now admits 1200 patients a year from the area served by Long Grove Hospital. This has shown that short-term treatment of all types of patients is possible without provision of medium- and long-stay accommodation, provided adequate rehabilitation facilities are available in the community, for both industrial and social needs.

Summary

The Psychiatric Rehabilitation Association is primarily a self-help organization. On a theoretical basis of integration of socially isolated patients into groups and into the community, it aims at the social rehabilitation of psychiatric patients and of their families. Towards this end, it furthers investigation into the social factors of mental illness, initiates experiments in after-care and rehabilitation, and arouses the community to take an active part in the resettlement of psychiatric patients. It has helped towards the shaping of a comprehensive psychiatric service, based on short-term treatment and rehabilitation in the community without medium- and long-stay beds.

References

BARTON, R. (1959), *Institutional Neurosis*, Bristol, John Wright.
BENADY, and DENHAM, J. (1963), *Brit. Med. J.* ii.
MILLS, E., *Living with Mental Illness*, London, Routledge & Kegan Paul.

37. The Local Authority Hostel as a Transitional Institution *

ROBERT APTE

SINCE the inception of the 1959 Mental Health Act, hostels have become one of the major responsibilities of the local authorities in providing "community care" for the mentally ill. The first local authority hostel was opened just at the time the Act was passed by Parliament. Since then, there has been a steady growth in the number of local authorities developing and providing these facilities. By the end of 1964, there were approximately forty in operation. The potential role and importance of the hostel in the future can be gauged by the fact that local authorities plan to open 251 hostels by 1974, providing places for 5243 residents with varying types of psychiatric disorders, not including the subnormal (Health and Welfare Plan, 1964). This would be equal to 6% of all psychiatric hospital beds by that time (Hospital Plan, 1962). This paper is based on data collected from twenty-four hostels which had already been in operation for at least 1 year by the end of 1963.

Although hostels are one of the basic segments of local authority responsibility in the mental health service, very little information has become available about them. In England and Wales there has been no detailed research on them, and little in the way of theoretical or conceptual thinking has been presented in the literature. This would not be so surprising, if it were not for the fact that hostels are not a new phenomenon in Great Britain. One large voluntary agency has been responsible for operating a series of hostels for the after-care of the mentally ill since 1879, and several others since the early 1950's. In spite of these eight decades of experience, little information and accumulated knowledge has become available for the use of the mental health planner. Up to 1965, on the completion of this research, not more than four or five authoritative articles had been published about the experiences of the hostels in England and Wales (Clark and Cooper, 1960; Harbert and Taylor, 1962; Adams and Gautrey, 1964; Burkitt and Walker, 1964; Morgan, 1964).

What are the purposes of hostels? Most local authority staff connected with their administration and operation describe hostels as "home-like"

*This research was carried out while the author was at the London School of Economics. It was supported partly by a fellowship from the United States Vocational Rehabilitation Administration and partly from the Nuffield Provincial Hospitals Trust.

environments, serving as a "bridge between hospital and community". They have been organized as transitional institutions for ex-patients of psychiatric hospitals, in order to assist them in their readjustment to community life. These may be individuals with no home to go to, or who need a further period of rehabilitation before being able to live independently. They may also be those whose homes hold little promise for their social betterment. In addition, hostels may serve as a temporary haven or asylum for emotionally disturbed individuals in the community, for whom it is thought that hospital care is not needed or desirable.

Brown, Carstairs and Topping (1958) have demonstrated that schizophrenics returning to the community do better in environments other than that of their immediate family. Hostels may have a potential for serving as long-term homes for this group of individuals, especially when the environment is constructed with this specifically in mind. One may assume that homes of this nature would be organized along different lines from those constructed as transitional institutions. They would be organized with the aim of establishing a satisfactory equilibrium among the residents, with the hope that they would be able to function with a minimum of supervision. To date, only a few local authorities have committed themselves to providing permanent homes of this nature, although it is becoming a trend.

The type of hostel that this paper will be mainly concerned with is the one that functions in the capacity of a half-way house. The majority of residents coming into these hostels have developed institutional syndromes of dependency, apathy and alienation. They are the patients who have been in hospital longest, and have often been rejected by the community. The challenge of the hostel is to help transform their social behaviour and attitudes into ones which are appropriate for living in the community, rather than in an institution.

Theoretically, the transitional process can be broken down into two separate but inter-related elements, *the grading of steps* (Schwartz and Schwartz, 1964) and the *grading of stress* (Cummings and Cummings, 1964). The first is that the social environment of the hostel be logically graded in a progressive manner towards the community. Restrictive controls over the patients, which are common to the hospital, need to give way to more permissive practices. This is similar to the concept used in medicine of progressive patient care. Here, the patient is allowed more responsibility for himself and is supervised to a lesser degree. Bowen (1961) describes this concept as the "salmon ladder". The second element, graded stress, is more individualized and requires that the staff purposely place progressively greater stress on the individual, by expecting him to take increasingly more responsibility, and to be faced with new and more demanding social situations. This applies both in the social environment and at work. Essential to the transitional process is qualified staff, who can individualize the resident's needs, and provide support and services for him while he is undergoing the new experiences. This can best be accomplished by the warden, psychiatrist, psychiatric social worker, and rehabilitation officer working together, to assist the resident to reach a pre-planned and realistic goal. Needless to say, this process takes professional effort, experience, and time.

Most of the hostels visited have some aspects of these elements, but none have all of them. These elements remain ideals, and a series of controlled experiments are necessary to determine the best way to apply the right combination of them in order to develop a *milieu* that will permit and encourage behavioural change in the individual. A host of important questions remain to be answered in this context on the effects of various sizes of hostels, their staffing patterns, staff qualifications, and the housing together of various diagnostic groups. As this research obtained information from a great variety of hostels, serving slightly different populations, the data cannot provide direct answers to these questions.

The twenty-four hostels included in this study represent 90% of the local authority hostels which had been in operation for 1 year by the end of 1963. Thirteen of them were situated in the north, five in the West Country and Wales, two on the south coast, and four in the Metropolitan area. All but two were sponsored by county boroughs. The average number of places was 16, but they varied in size from 5 to 30 places. Twenty-five per cent had 10 or less places, an equal number having 21 or more, and 50% having between 11 and 20 places. Eleven of the hostels were exclusively for females, eight were mixed and four were for males only. Fifteen of the authorities took over large old homes, converting them into hostels, and eight were in pre-existing buildings that had been used for either dormitories or hotels in the past. Only one hostel had been purpose-built. All but two were located within urban residential or industrial areas of the communities.

The Staff

The staff member most influential to the resident is the warden. The person holding this key position has the major responsibility for creating the "climate" of the hostel, and the greatest potential for bringing about change in the functioning of ex-patients. Faced with the need to unlearn institutional modes of behaviour, and to learn or re-learn effective social roles, the resident looks to the warden as the mature adult model, who sets the standards for behaviour. If the warden's position allows him enough time, and if he is aware of his potential role, he can be of great help to the resident, through providing him with encouragement and support, and making clear to him what the reality is, to which he needs to adjust.

Most of the wardens hired by the local authorities are in their fifties and sixties. Half of them are married, with their spouses also being employed in the hostel, usually in the capacity of deputy warden, cook, or supervisor of the domestic staff.

These positions were recruited principally from the fields of general or psychiatric nursing. Fifteen (62%) of the wardens had previous nursing experience in general or psychiatric hospitals, with an average of 18 years each. Of this number, 86% had some nursing qualification. Two additional wardens had experience working as assistants in non-medical institutions. The remaining seven had no specific experience or training related to the health or welfare field. With the majority of positions being filled by those with a nursing orientation (but without education in rehabilitation concepts), there is a threat that institutional ideologies, values, and modes of behaviour will become entrenched in the hostel *milieu*. Although some medical officers of health and mental welfare officers are becoming aware of this, little has been done so far to remedy the situation. There are no professional or semi-professional personnel available, schooled in rehabilitation philosophy and techniques, who are prepared to take on these positions.*

In addition to the warden and assistant warden, the other staff likely to be found in hostels are cooks, domestics, gardeners and maintenance men. As there are no established standards for the over-all staffing of hostels, the staffing ratios provided vary considerably in size. Two hostels have as few as one staff member for every 8 residents, while seven have one for every 3. The average ratio is one staff member to every 4·25 residents. Apparently, the reason for the difference in ratios is that local authorities have had no experience on which to base their staffing patterns. There is no model established of the "ideal hostel", so that each authority has evolved its own formula for staffing. It was interesting to find that the differing ratios are not related either to the social characteristics of the population served or the amount of individualized services given. They appear to be more related to the age and condition of the building, the size of the garden and the amount of building maintenance required.

Policies on Employment and Length of Stay

Twenty out of the twenty-four hostels had definite expectations that the residents be employed, as a condition of their stay. Experience has shown that many residents do not find work when they get to the hostel, and about half of them leave without having been in employment. Only one of the hostels has a training centre, and all of its residents are expected to attend there daily, until they leave.

An important issue is the policy on the maximum period of time a resident is permitted to live in the hostel. This has a direct bearing on the rehabilitation

---

*In 1964, the National Association for Mental Health held its first course for the training of hostel wardens.

process. When they opened, the majority of hostels had set limits on the length of stay allowed—usually 6 months. To their chagrin, they learned that this was unrealistic, as significant numbers of the residents did not leave. Most of the authorities have since modified their policies to the point where they have become very flexible. There is some evidence that the phenomenon of the dependent or long-term resident in many of the hostels is as much the effect of a lack of professional services to the individual, as it is of his illness.

Hostel Services

Only seven (29%) of the hostels provided social, educational, or recreational programmes as frequently as once a month or more. These activities included social club meetings, discussion groups, dancing and classes of various types. Very rarely did the residents leave the hostel with the warden to participate in social, cultural, or recreational activities. The warden's potential role of helping the residents return to the community culture has not been developed. Ten of the hostels had psychiatric social clubs in their communities, but less than 20% of the residents regularly attended them. Most of the wardens believed that it was up to the residents to find and provide their own activities, and local authority staff did very little to stimulate social or recreational activities within the hostels.

Community Services

Community psychiatric and social-work services are the responsibility of the Mental Health Department of the local health authority. Local authorities are in varying stages of building up these services, and due to a nation-wide shortage of professional staff, many of the hostels have operated with very little professional assistance. Fifty-eight per cent of the hostels had social workers available to provide services to the residents, but only one-third had regular service from a psychiatrist, either to deal directly with the residents or to provide the hostel staff with consultation on how to deal with the residents' problems more effectively.

The mental welfare officer is the one individual coming from outside that most frequently assists the warden with social and administrative problems. He often helps residents to find accommodation when they are ready to leave. The more difficult part of his task is advising on the management of behaviour problems within the hostels. Although there is usually a selection committee which may be made up of a medical officer of health and a consultant from the neighbouring psychiatric hospital, the mental welfare officer is the person most influential in determining who actually comes into the hostel and when they leave. Their attitudes, training and experience have a profound effect on the way the homes are organized and function. One-fourth of the mental welfare officers concerned with hostels in this study are qualified psychiatric social workers.

Classification of Hostels

To obtain a clearer description, the twenty-four hostels in this investigation were classified into two groups—those operating as long-stay hostels, and those operating as transitional hostels. The criterion used to distinguish the two types was whether or not the majority of the residents in the home during the period of the year left for the community, or continued to stay on. Those hostels where the majority left for the community within 1 year were considered to be transitional hostels, the remainder long-stay hostels. On this basis, sixteen of the hostels were transitional and eight long-stay.

It was found that the long-stay hostels were different in many ways from the transitional ones. In addition to 52% of their beds being blocked with long-stay residents, as compared with 25% in the transitional, they had older residents, more women, more individuals with the diagnoses of senility or organic psychoses, and fewer with schizophrenia. A significantly larger number of their residents returned to the mental hospital than did the transitional hostel residents—36% compared to 21%. The remainder of the paper will deal solely with the transitional hostel.

The Transitional Hostel

The sixteen transitional hostels have 262 places—164 for females and 98 for males. During the year 1962–3, 191 men and 276 women occupied these places, giving a turnover rate of 1·8 persons per place.

The average ages of the men and women residents were 38 and 43 years respectively. Only 22% of the men and 30% of the women had ever married. The residents came into the hostels from many different sources, the hospital being the principal one, providing 68% of the residents. Thirty-two per cent lived in the community before entering—a proportion that was higher than anticipated.

Forty-nine per cent of the group had schizophrenia, 20% depression or neuroses, 11% personality disorders, 11% subnormality, and the remaining 9% had diagnoses of alcoholism, senility or other psychiatric disorders with organic involvement.

The group as a whole can be characterized as one having a history of either long periods of hospital stay or of frequent admissions. Only 8% had never been in a mental hospital, and 55% had been in hospital two or more times. Of those who had been in hospital, 35% had stayed over 1 year during their last admission.

What was the outcome of the stay for the hostel residents during the period, 1962–3? Success cannot be judged by residents' movement into the community alone, nor can failure be judged by movement back into hospital. A resident moving from a hostel into digs might constitute more of a failure than an individual returning to the hospital, who has learned from the hostel that he is not ready to face the demands made in the community. With this caution in mind, data on outcome is presented in Table 1.

TABLE 1.

	Males	Females
Returned to community	64%	67%
Returned to hospital	15%	22%
Still in after 1 year	21%	11%
Total	100%	100%

Roughly the same percentage of males and females return to the community, but the percentage of males continuing on in the hostel after a year is twice that of the females. A higher percentage of women returned to the hospital than men. Of those residents returning to the community, 38% moved into lodgings by themselves, 27% moved on to other hostels or institutions, and only 35% were reunited with a member of their family or went to live with a friend. There is little doubt that for the majority of psychiatric patients, returning to the community from a hostel continues to mean either isolation or being placed in indifferent surroundings.

The inability of residents to form satisfying and meaningful relationships continues to be a major symptom of their illness, once they return to the community. As two-thirds of them become isolated from close social contacts, what has the hostel done to prepare them for this kind of solitary existence? Has it been a strong enough force to shape the way they will handle their feelings and social situations in the community? The answer to these questions can be illustrated in part by the way most hostels have handled the need for medication. It is the general practice to continue the residents on medication, during and following their period in the hostel. As it is known that a large percentage of them will be living on their own when they leave, it might be expected that the hostel staff progressively teach them to handle it themselves. This has not been the usual practice, however; 66% of the hostel staff continue to hand out the medication to them, usually three times a day, until the day they are ready to leave. This system, while it keeps the illness in check, teaches the residents little of what is going to be important to them in the future.

The re-establishment of the ex-mental patient in the role of a working person in the community is one of the principal aims of a programme of social rehabilitation. This is only somewhat more true for men than women because of the difference in their social roles. Because of the importance of employment as a criterion of rehabilitation, the experience of the residents with employment in the hostels becomes a crucial matter, in terms of the over-all success of the programme. Table 2 provides data on the residents' employment while living in the hostel.

TABLE 2.

	Percentage of time employed while living in hostel	
	Males %	Females %
Half-time or more	48·5	33·0
Less than half-time	6·5	25·0
Not employed	45·0	42·0
Total (191)	100% (276)	100% (365)

More than half of the total number of men and women were employed less than half-time, or not at all, while living in the hostels. Of those residents who had left for the community, 49% of them were either holding a job or had one to go to. The other 51% were re-settled in the community without employment.

The Transitional Milieu

Each of the sixteen local authority hostels, and the psychiatric hospitals from which most of the residents came, were studied to see how they differ, and how the transitional *milieu* has been organized. The specific wards on which the patients lived were compared with the hostels, on a number of identical items. A scale, composed of 65 items, was used to measure the number of restrictive institutional practices, and the degree to which the individual is encouraged or expected to take responsibility. The scale collects data on policies and practices, regarding several areas of daily activities which are characteristic of institutions. The types of restrictive practices on which data were collected include control over the residents' physical movement, personal belongings, care of body, dress, food, and social relations. Data were collected on the responsibility expectations in the areas of decision-making, seeking one's own medical and social services, organizing one's own schedules, and responsibility for handling one's own personal possessions. The maximum score an institution or hostel could achieve on the scale would be 65 points. This would be the most restrictive one—the type that would be likely to encourage dependency, or what is now called "institutional neurosis" (Barton, 1959).

In Table 3, the scores of the hostels and referring wards can be compared.

TABLE 3.

Hostel	Score	Ward	Score
A	9	A	57
B	14	B	47
C	16	C	34
D	18	D	46
E	18	E	56
F	22	F	55
G	24	G	39
H	26	H	50
I	27	I	41
J	28	J	27
K	29	K	41
L	29	L	49
M	30	M	47
N	32	N	48
O	33	O	55
P	37	P	59

Table 3 demonstrates that there is a great range among the hostels in the restrictiveness of their environments. Comparing the number of restrictive practices of the hostels with the hospital wards, it can be seen that some wards are less restrictive than hostels on these 65 items. Forty-three per cent of the hostels were more restrictive than the least restrictive ward. The data also suggest that there is no correlation between wards and hostels in the number of restrictive practices discontinued, with some hostels being almost as restrictive as, or even more, restrictive than, the ward from which the patient came. Conversely, there has been a failure on the part of a few local authorities to provide *continuity of care,* by designing hostels that are too *open* in relation to the referral wards. The social *milieux* of these hostels are too *laissez-faire,* in that insufficient social controls are maintained to help the residents organize their activities within acceptable limits. For example, one hostel had 48 items fewer of a restrictive nature (from 57 to 9 items) than were practised in the chronic ward from which the residents had come. Had it been more closely designed to offer a transitional experience for the resident coming from this ward, there would presumably be less of a gap in the number of restrictive practices.

It has been found from the results of the first 5 years' experience of local authority hostels, that the manner in which the social *milieu* of the home is constructed has a strong effect on how the home is used by the residents. It is clear that the phenomenon of the dependent patient and the blocked bed is closely associated with the degree of restrictiveness and low expectation of the environment. Freeman and Simmons (1963) have demonstrated a close association between familial expectations from the ex-mental patient and the degree to which they returned to hospital. It is believed that this relationship exists in the hostel, but in special reference to its silting up and blocking. Medical officers of health, the administrative staff of local authorities, and wardens need to pay greater attention to the manner in which their attitudes and values towards handicapped individuals eventually become expressed policies, procedures and practices. These may turn back upon them, like a dog biting his own tail, to defeat the original goal. An example of this—the way in which most hostels treat the residents' need for medication, was reported earlier.

Another major problem facing the hostel, which has a great effect on its ability to achieve an effective role, is the low rate of occupancy. There was little indication that local authorities had planned and built the hostels with specific knowledge of what the actual demand would be. From the appointment of the Royal Commission in 1954, until the time the first dozen hostels were opened, there was a dramatic change in the hospital population. Those long-term cases in the more progressive hospitals that were able to move into the community with the supports available had already done so. In the other hospitals, the patients remaining tended to become more chronic, and increasingly more difficult to rehabilitate. The hostels that were opening found fewer individuals being referred from the hospitals than anticipated, and many of these were not taken, as they were considered to be poor risks. As a consequence, the hostels have been inefficiently used. During the year 1962–3, 75% of the hostels were less than three-quarters full, and of these, 25% were less than half full.

Due to the large number of vacant places, the authorities began accepting residents from many sources other than the hospital, and in several cases the catchment areas began to be enlarged. Individuals with psychoneuroses, behaviour disorders, and mental subnormality were taken in from the community, and mixed freely with schizophrenics from the hospitals. While there is no proof of the mixing being either helpful or harmful *per se*, it creates a serious management problem for the warden. As the different diagnostic categories have different environmental needs, no one hostel can effectively cope with them all, and still have the optimum number of controls.

Another characteristic way in which the problem of the high number of vacancies has been dealt with in many instances, is that the residents have not been under any pressure from the local authorities to leave the hostel. The economics of the hostels has been such that it has been to the advantage of the authorities to keep the beds full. The operating cost of the hostel remains high, even though there are a large number of vacancies. All of the hostels are, to a varying extent, dependent upon payment from the residents to meet their budgets. Many of the hostels have kept patients on for longer than necessary, in a semidependent role, to help meet the organization's needs, rather than encouraging them to leave when they are ready. By doing this, the original aim of the hostel (of resettling the patient) is sacrificed, and their dependency role is fortified.

Fortunately, not all the authorities have been under pressure to keep their hostels full, and some have allowed vacancies, rather than accepting individuals who might distort the purpose of the home. The information presented so far about vacancies and the need for unique environments suggests that local authorities should come together, perhaps on a regional basis, and decide how they may each specialize in different kinds of hostels. Only the largest authorities would be likely to have the demand for and be able to afford a gradation of hostels.

Finally, the research has shown that the amount of supportive services from the local authority, and of psychiatric consultation which is given to the warden, plus the case-work services available to the resident, have a significant influence on both the kind of hostel environment that is eventually developed and the way the resident uses it. Those hostels with the highest amount of services of this kind are the ones that are the least restrictive, and they are also less likely to become blocked with long-stay residents. A detailed report of these findings will be provided in a future publication. While this finding is to be anticipated, it can be a useful *caveat* to those authorities now operating or planning services without providing sufficient professional staff and professional know-how.

References

ADAMS, A. C. and GAUTREY, B. (1964), *Medical Officer*, **111,** 109.

BARTON, RUSSELL (1959), *Institutional Neurosis*, Bristol, John Wright.

BOWEN, W. A. L. (1961), in *Hostels and the Mental Health Act*, London, National Association for Mental Health.

BROWN, G. W., CARSTAIRS, G. M. and TOPPING, G. (1958), *Lancet*, **ii,** 685.

BURKITT, E. A. and WALKER, J. V. (1964), *Medical Officer*, **112, 53.**

CLARK, D. H. and COOPER, L. W. (1960), *Lancet*, **i,** 588.

CUMMINGS, J. and CUMMINGS, E. (1964), *Ego and Milieu*, London, Tavistock.

FREEMAN, H. E. and SIMMONS, O. G. (1963), *The Mental Patient Comes Home*, London, John Wiley.

HARBERT, W. B. and TAYLOR, F. J. D. (1962), *Lancet*, **i,** 1064.

MINISTRY OF HEALTH (1962), *A Hospital Plan for England and Wales*, Cmnd. 1604, London, H.M.S.O.

MINISTRY OF HEALTH (1964), Health and Welfare, *The Development of Community Care*, London, H.M.S.O.

MORGAN, P. (1964), *Monthly Bulletin of the Ministry of Health and Laboratory Service*, **23,** 224.

SCHWARTZ, M. S. and SCHWARTZ, C. G. (1964), *Social Approaches to Mental Patient Care*, New York, Columbia University Press.

38. A Comprehensive Service for the Mentally Subnormal *

ALBERT KUSHLICK

IN THIS country, we are now participating in a dramatic extension and development of services for the mental subnormal. This is to be seen mainly in such local authority facilities as social-work services, training centres and hostels, special educational provision and diagnostic and out-patient clinics run both by regional hospital boards and local authorities. These developments make it an urgent necessity for all those involved to co-operate, and to ensure that their efforts result in the provision of a comprehensive service for the mentally subnormal and their families.

By a comprehensive service, I mean one that meets as effectively as possible all of the needs of the subnormal and their families for as long as they need it. In the case of idiots and imbeciles, this would appear to be from birth or early childhood and for the whole of their lives. In the case of the feeble-minded, it means at least from early childhood until the end of a prolonged adolescence.

The second major responsibility is that of evaluating the many different types of service which we are providing or may provide in the future. In other words, we must examine as objectively as possible what we are doing, and try to assess the advantages and disadvantages of different types of service, by measuring the extent to which they are meeting certain specific recognized needs of the clients and their families.

Terminology

In this paper, the term "subnormal" will be used to mean all grades of subnormality. The terms "idiot", "imbecile" and "severely subnormal" will be used to mean people scoring I.Q.s of under 50. The term "feebleminded" or "mildly subnormal" will be used interchangeably to mean people of I.Q. over 50 who are classified as subnormal.

The Prevalence and Prognosis of Severe Subnormality

In England and Wales, about 3·7 per 1000 of the people who survive to the age-group of 15–19 are likely to be severely subnormal. Kushlick (1961)

*Based on a paper presented to the Society of Medical Officers of Health, February 1965.

678

examined the records of all mental defectives known on 1 January 1961 to the Mental Health Department in Salford, a northern English industrial city of 153,000 people. Goodman and Tizard (1962) examined the records of all mental defectives known in 1961 to the Mental Health Department of Middlesex County, with a population of 2,231,100. They also collected details of children of I.Q. under 50 who were of school age, but who were not known to the Mental Health Department because they were still attending schools within the ordinary educational system, private schools and private homes. Kushlick (1964) examined the records of all mental defectives known on 1 July 1963 to the area served by the Wessex Regional Hospital Board. The three county boroughs, Southampton, Portsmouth, and Bournemouth, and the three counties, Hampshire, Dorset, and the Isle of Wight, had a total population of 1,740,000 people. The records were obtained from the mental health departments of the local health authorities, from psychiatric hospitals for the subnormal and the mentally ill, and from registered private homes serving the region. The prevalence of severe subnormality found in these surveys in comparable age-groups is shown in Table 1. The rates are very similar for both urban and rural areas.

TABLE 1.

Prevalence of I.Q. under 50 in Age-groups where All Subjects are likely to be Known

	Age-group	Total I.Q. under 50 rate per 1000	Mongol rate per 1000
England and Wales (Lewis, 1929) 1926–9: Urban Rural	7–14	3·71 5·61	0·34 N/K
Middlesex (Goodman and Tizard, 1962) 1960 1960	7–14 10–14	3·45 3·61	1·14 N/K
Salford (Kushlick, 1961) 1961	15–19	3·62	0·90
Wessex (Kushlick, 1964) 1964: County boroughs Counties	15–19 15–19	3·54 3·84	1·15 1·18
Onondaga 1955	5–17	3·6	N/K
Baltimore (Lemkau et al., 1943) 1936	10–14	3·3	N/K
Rural Sweden (Akesson, 1961) 1959	All ages	5·8	0·03

TABLE 2.

Prevalence of Subnormality by Age and Grade[a]

	Grade				All grades				
	Severely S/N		Mildly S/N						
	Salford 1961	England[b] 1926–9	Salford 1961	England[b] 1926–9	Salford 1961	England 1926–9 (From Penrose)	Baltimore 1936	Onondaga 1955	Rural Sweden 1955
0– 4	0·89	0·69	0·15	0·51	1·13	1·2	0·7	4·5	12·5
5– 9	1·62	3·09	0·36	11·41	1·98	15·5	11·8	39·4	18·4
10–14	2·55	4·35	0·29	21·25	2·84	25·6	43·6	77·6	37·2
15–19	3·62	2·84	8·63	7·96	12·27	10·8	30·2	—	14·2
20–29	3·44	2·07	4·16	6·33	7·66	8·4	7·2c	—	19·7
30–39	3·77	1·49	1·83	4·21	5·59	5·7	8·1c	—	22·7
40–49	2·47	1·22	2·56	4·18	5·04	5·4	8·3c	—	17·7
50–59	1·70	0·90	1·04	4·00	2·83	4·9	6·4c	—	17·6
60+	0·52	0·48	0·60	2·42	1·13	2·9	2·6c	—	8·4
							1·9c		
Totals	2·24	1·87	2·057	6·73	4·38	8·6	12·2	—	17·4

[a] See Appendix 1 for methods used in the surveys.

[b] Calculated from Lewis (1929), tables 17(A) and (C), and Penrose (1963), p. 23.

[c] Age groups are 20–24; 25–34; 35–44; 45–54; 55–64; 65+.

Prevalence rates of severe subnormality in the U.S.A. are similar to those found in this country, but differences in survey methods render comparisons with English survey results difficult.

The English studies suggest that distinct clinical entities are now contributing similar proportions to the condition of severe subnormality. Thus, Table 1 also shows that the prevalence of mongolism in the age-group of 15–19 is very similar in all the surveys. Most mongols are severely subnormal, although our findings in Wessex suggest that just over 10% of mongols have I.Q.s of over 50. From this, it can be seen that mongolism at present accounts for about one-quarter of all cases of severe subnormality in this age-group.

The means of identifying severely subnormal subjects is similar in all industrialized countries. In this country, most of them are excluded from school because they are deemed "unsuitable for education" in the ordinary school system by teachers, educational psychologists and school medical officers.

In this country, nearly all severely subnormal people who have survived to the age-group of 15–19 have been notified to mental health departments. Kushlick (1961) found that only a very small proportion of these subjects were notified for the first time after the age of 19. The reason for this appears to lie in the prognosis of people with severe subnormality. Only about 10% of these subjects are able to hold employment in open industry (Tizard, 1958). The remaining 90% appear at the present time to remain permanently dependent economically, and become known for this reason to the social agencies dealing with subnormality. This has been shown by follow-up studies and indirectly from other evidence.

Table 2 shows that the age distribution of severe subnormality remains fairly constant between adolescence and middle age, in contrast to the picture for mild subnormality, where the rates decline sharply after adolescence. It has also been shown that nearly all severely subnormal subjects who survive childhood are eventually admitted to hospitals for the subnormal. It is known that the waiting list for admission to these hospitals consists largely of the severely subnormal, and that once they are admitted to hospital they are seldom, if ever, discharged.

The Prevalence and Prognosis of Mild Subnormality

The I.Q. range 50–70 or 75 has been suggested as diagnostic of the grade of mild mental subnormality. This has not proved useful, either clinically or administratively. There are many people in this I.Q. range who are never dealt with as subnormal and who do not appear to have problems arising from their low intelligence, and there are people of I.Q. well over 70 who are being dealt with by the services for the subnormal. In this country there has never been, nor is there now, an upper psychometric limit to this degree of subnormality. On a test standardized to give a mean of 100 and standard deviation of 15, the proportion of the population scoring between 15 and 70 would be nearly 20 per 1000. In the Salford survey, the highest prevalence rate for mild subnormality was found among those aged 15–19; it was 8·7 per 1000, or just under a half of the rate expected on the criterion of I.Q. alone (see Table 2). Nor is the I.Q. level the sole determinant of who is to be classified as educationally subnormal (ESN) and given special education within the ordinary school system. The total number of children in special schools seldom exceeds half of the 2·0% to be expected, if all children of I.Q. 50–70 were to attend. Moreover, the Report of the Chief Medical Officer (Ministry of Education, 1962) shows that about 40% of children in the special schools scored over 70.

Unlike the severely subnormal, most of whom are excluded from the ordinary school system, the majority of the mildly subnormal first become so classified in this country when they are notified by the Education Authority to the Mental Health Department as in need of supervision on leaving school. Thus, 90% of the mildly subnormal people referred to Salford Mental Health Department between 1948 and 1960 were notified between the ages of 15 and 19 (Kushlick, 1961). This also explains why mental health department registers have very few mildly subnormal people aged under 15, and why there is a sharp rise in their numbers in the age-group 15–19 (Table 2).

There is much evidence that unlike severe subnormality, mild subnormality is a temporary incapacity, related largely to educational difficulties experienced at school. After leaving school, the majority of these people become socially and economically independent and are indistinguishable from the rest of the community. Moreover, unlike the severely subnormal, nearly all of whom appear eventually to be admitted to hospital unless they die whilst still young, only a minority of mildly subnormal subjects are ever admitted to hospital.

Inconstancy of the I.Q.

It has also been shown that people categorized as mildly subnormal or educationally subnormal continue to make I.Q. increments for some years after it is believed that I.Q. growth is complete (Clarke and Clarke, 1954; Stein and Susser, 1960). This observation is important because it questions the concept of the constancy of I.Q. as an assessment of innate "intelligence" among the mildly subnormal. Second, it complicates further any attempt to measure the prevalence of mild subnormality on the criterion of I.Q. Third, this phenomenon appears to be characteristic of mild subnormality in the absence of brain damage and may partially explain the good prognosis of these subjects after they leave school. Fourth, it suggests that the ability of the mildly subnormal to profit from education may indeed improve from the time they leave school, and emphasizes the need to provide them with adult education on leaving there.

While the data show that most of the severely subnormal subjects who do not die at an early age are eventually admitted to hospitals, this should not be taken to mean that this is the only or the best way to cater for their needs or those of their families. It is merely demonstrated that they appear, at present, to have a type of incapacity requiring a form of special provision for the whole of their lives, in contrast to the mildly subnormal, whose incapacities and needs are largely temporary. Second, the respective prognoses illustrated for the two grades are valid only for large numbers of cases, whereas the prognosis in an individual case requires the skilled consideration of many factors other than the I.Q. Third, while it is clear that those in the I.Q. category over 50 merge imperceptibly with the community at large, the medium-grade I.Q. range (20–49) contains within it a wide variation of capacity, which overlaps at the upper end with that of the category of I.Q. over 50.

The Causes of Mental Defect

The primary cause of the social and intellectual handicap of the severely and mildly subnormal also differ.

Thus, the primary cause among the severely subnormal appears to be observable pathology in the brain; on the other hand, such pathology is demonstrable in only a small proportion of the midly subnormal. There is evidence that social and cultural factors are very important in the aetiology of mild subnormality, occurring in the absence of obvious or presumptive brain pathology.

Crome (1960) examined the brains of 272 hospitalized imbeciles and idiots; definite abnormalities were found in 267. However, our knowledge of the causes of brain damage among these subjects is still very limited, and a definite cause is identifiable in only a minority of cases. Berg and Kirman (1959) examined the records of imbeciles and idiots who were consecutive admissions to the Fountain Hospital (Table 3). A definite causal factor was found in only 9·5% of cases, e.g. iso-immunization and prematurity kernicterus, tuberculous and influenzal meningitis, post-immunization encephalopathy, and recessive genetic conditions such as phenylketonuria, galactosaemia and cerebral lipoidoses. Probable factors were suggested in 4%, and possible factors in 56%. Twenty-three per cent of the subjects were mongols; these were included among the subjects with possible factors. In 31% no causal factor was identifiable. There are no comparable intensive studies of the clinical and neuropathological lesions among the mildly subnormal. Investigations of complete samples in defined populations face the problem of definition. The proportion of mildly subnormal subjects with brain damage

TABLE 3.

Aetiological Factors in 200 Consecutive Admissions

Group A: Due to known factor		19 (9·5%)
1. Environmental:		
Kernicterus due to rhesus incompatibility	6	
Kernicterus of prematurity	1	
Meningitis, tuberculous	4	
Meningitis, influenzal	1	
Pertussis immunization	1	
2. Genetic:		
Phenylketonuria	3	
Cerebral lipoidosis:		
Amaurotic family idiocy	1	
Unclassified	1	
Galactosaemia	1	
Group B: Probably due to factor indicated		8 (4%)
1. Environmental:		
Maternal rubella	1	
Therapeutic irradiation of mother	1	
Thiouracil treatment of mother	1	
Septicaemia, neonatal	1	
Septicaemia, with sinus thrombosis	1	
Gastro-enteritis with coma	1	
Encephalitis	1	
2. Genetic:		
Hypoglycaemia	1	
Group C: Other factors implicated		111 (55·5%)
1. Environmental:		
Birth trauma: probable	27	
Birth trauma: possible	9	
2. Genetic?		
Family history of mental retardation	18	
Family history of mental disorder, epilepsy,		
or other neurological abnormality	10	
3. Unknown:		
Mongolism	46	
Sturge–Weber syndrome	1	
Group D: No factors suggested		62 (31%)

varies with the sample source. About a quarter of these subjects selected in ESN surveys appear to have clinical signs of brain damage or sensory defects The remainder appear clinically normal.

Social Class and Mental Subnormality

It has long been known that in industrial societies, parents of severely subnormal children are evenly distributed among all the social strata in the society, while those of mildly subnormal subjects come predominantly from the lower social classes.

There is now evidence which suggests that mild subnormality in the absence of abnormal neurological signs, epilepsy, electroencephalographic abnormalities, biochemical abnormalities, chromosomal abnormalities or sensory defects is virtually confined to the lower social classes. Indeed, there is evidence that almost no children of higher social class parents have I.Q. scores of less than 80, unless they have one of the pathological processes mentioned above. This has been observed among ESN subjects, subjects referred to school psychological service and among 11-plus test results (Saenger, 1960; Stein and Susser, 1963).

The results of the Scottish Mental Survey of 1947 also confirm these findings. In this survey, there were no children who scored less than the equivalent of an I.Q. of 86 and whose fathers were in the professional class. Of children whose fathers were unskilled, the proportion rose dramatically to 26% (Scottish Council for Research in Education, 1953).

I have mentioned these social class differences mainly to stress the epidemiological differences between the two grades of subnormality. At the beginning of the century, this phenomenon was interpreted as being due to inherent genetic differences between I.Q. levels of the social classes. The prediction current at that time of "national degeneracy" or a fall in national intelligence due to the differential birth rate of the lower classes has not materialized. The Scottish Mental Survey showed that between 1932 and 1947, there had been no fall in the I.Q. of 11-year-old children. Moreover, there is now much evidence that this difference reflects on the one hand the differences in culture defined here as the way of life of the social classes, as well as the social and material disadvantages in the use of medical and educational services experienced by the lower social classes, which is now well documented. Nevertheless, many mental deficiency hospitals which were designed with a view to preventing the breeding of feebleminded patients by their segregation in colonies are ever-present reminders of the theory of "national degeneracy".

Selection of Subnormal Subjects who come to the Agencies

We have seen that virtually all people of I.Q. under 50 who survive long enough become known to educational and mental health authorities, require special services for all of their lives, and appear eventually to need residential care. However, only a minority of people in the I.Q. range 50–70 and some others of even higher I.Q. are classified and dealt with as mildly subnormal. Whereas among the severely subnormal, the main problems leading to their referral to the services are problems experienced by the family members, among the mildly subnormal, selection arises largely from behaviour disorders which create disturbances outside the family. It also appears that a large proportion of these behaviour disorders are caused by the child's rearing experiences in profoundly broken homes, and multiple placements in residential institutions or foster homes (Stein and Susser, 1960a).

These findings suggest that the social inadequacies of those subjects who fall into the hands of the social agencies, and who are classified as subnormal, may arise from a lack of social skills normally acquired by children within their own families (Parsons and Bales, 1955). Their problems may also arise from the possession of social skills learned in and appropriate to large authoritarian institutions, but which prove dysfunctional when the subjects have to adjust to the complexities of social relationships outside institutions (Goffman, 1957; Coser, 1962).

Is the Prevalence of Subnormality Increasing or Decreasing?

SEVERE SUBNORMALITY

Prevalence depends on trends in the incidence, on survival rates and on the prognosis of children with this condition. Differences between current prevalence rates and those found by Lewis in his classical survey of 1929 must be interpreted cautiously, because the expansion of services for the subnormal since then may have rendered the identification of such cases easier now than in 1926–9, and the standardization of the I.Q. tests used then and now may differ. Comparisons of current prevalence rates of severe subnormality from surveys in this country suggest that, in spite of increased survival rates of mongolism, the prevalence of severe subnormality has fallen since 1929. The apparent fall in prevalence may, however, be masking a real increase in the prevalence of severe subnormality as we now see it, i.e characterized by permanent severe incapacity. Thus, Goodman and Tizard (1962) (Table 2) showed that the prevalence of severe subnormality in the age-group 7–14 had decreased from Lewis's figure of 3·71 per 1000 in the urban areas to 3·45 per 1000 in Middlesex in 1961; in the same period, the prevalence of mongolism increased from 0·34 to 1·14 per 1000. They interpreted their findings cautiously, as reflecting an apparent decrease in the prevalence of non-mongol severe subnormality. Possible explanations for this apparent decrease are improved obstetric standards and reduction of infectious diseases. Similar apparent decreases have been found by Kushlick. The prevalence of severe subnormality in the age group 15–19 in Salford in 1961 was 3·64 per 1000, and in the Wessex county boroughs in 1963 it was 3·54 per 1000. Kushlick (1964) found the apparent decrease in the rural areas to be even higher. Lewis's 1926–9 rate in the rural areas was 5·61 per 1000 in the age-group 7–14, compared with the 1963 rate of 3·84 per 1000 in the Wessex counties in the age-group 15–19, in spite of the increased prevalence in 1963 of mongolism.

On the other hand, there is also evidence of an increase in prevalence. Table 2 shows that the total prevalence rates of severe subnormality and the age-specific rates for those aged 15 and over were higher in Salford in 1961 than those found in Lewis's survey. Kushlick (1961) showed that in Salford between 1948 and 1960, the total prevalence of idiots had increased by 83%, and that of imbeciles by 38%. Possible reasons for the increase are the observed increased survival rate of mongols and hydrocephalics, and the new problem created by the survival of very low birth-weight prematures and children with tuberculous meningitis, now the major cause of severe subnormality after mongolism.

The author favours this explanation of the paradox; that Lewis's sample in the age-group 7–14 might have included a large proportion of non-brain-damaged subjects with temporary incapacities, similar to the subjects with mild subnormality, whereas most of the children of I.Q. under 50 in the recent surveys are brain-damaged and permanently handicapped. Table 2 shows that the prevalence of severe subnormality in Salford remains fairly constant up to the age of 40, suggesting that these subjects continue to require supervision, in or out of hospital, until they die. However, the 1926–9 rates drop immediately after school-leaving age, like those for the subjects with mild subnormality. This suggests that some of the Lewis's severely subnormal subjects in the age-group 7–14 might, on leaving school, have adjusted sufficiently well to the demands of society, and that Lewis's rates in the subsequent quinquennium 15–19 are a truer reflection of the prevalence of severe subnormality characterized by permanent incapacity. It is of course possible, as Lewis himself suggests, that there were large numbers of severely subnormal people aged 15–19 unknown to the agencies he used as sources. Such agencies as the Labour Exchanges and the Public Assistance Committees might have been expected to know of the large numbers of unemployed imbeciles anticipated from the difference in rates between the age-groups 7–14 and 15–19 (the unemployment rate was very high at the time of this survey).

As the prevalence is likely to continue to increase until the survival rates have reached a maximum, the already overcrowded facilities for the severely subnormal will have to be enlarged.

Mild Subnormality

It is much more difficult to estimate the trends of mild subnormality, because of the problem of definition.

The results of the Scottish survey of the intelligence of 88,000 11-year-old children in 1932, and of 71,000 children in 1947, showed that the mean I.Q. had, if anything, increased from 34·5 to 36·7, due to the reduction in the proportion of low scorers (Scottish Council for Research in Education, 1949).

For other assessments of the trend of the problem of mild subnormality, we must rely on numbers of people receiving the services. This is an unsatisfactory method, as there has always been a shortage of these provisions, and increasing provision is more likely to reflect improvements in the quality of the services than real increases in the extent of the conditions. For example, provision for ESN children has increased.

The proportion of mildly subnormal people in hospitals for the subnormal has decreased since 1938, and there is evidence that the absolute number may also have declined since 1951. The fall in these numbers is probably due to a number of factors. The discharge rate of subnormal patients doubled in 1956 and has remained at this level ever since. The length of stay of those discharged has also decreased (1964: Registrar General's Supplement on Mental Health, 1960). Unless there is a high re-admission rate, the numbers of chronic, mildly subnormal patients should continue to fall.

Many of them were compulsorily hospitalized in the past because of the wide definitions of mental defect, and because of the large number of conditions which rendered mental defectives "subject to be dealt with" under the Mental Deficiency Acts. When such problems arise today, they are probably handled by social agencies not specifically concerned with mental defect.

The proportion of legally detained patients is now comparatively small. On 31 December 1963, in England and Wales, 5323 (8·2%) of the 65,000 subnormal people in psychiatric hospitals were legally detained and 1112 (1·7%) were detained in the special security hospitals, Rampton and Moss Side (Ministry of Health, 1964). There has been very little systematic study of this problem. It is likely that if the recent liberalizing of custodial régimes in the hospitals for the mentally ill is adopted by the hospitals for the subnormal, the difficulty of meeting the requirements of a minority of the subjects who require custodial care may be passed on to the state security institutions. Systematic epidemiological studies into the reasons for, and the effects of, custodial care of subnormal subjects are urgently needed.

At present in this country, people of limited capacity are, like everyone, benefiting from reasonably full employment. If, however, the introduction of automation is allowed to create problems of mass unemployment, as it has in the United States, it is clear that the mildly subnormal and other people in the social classes from which they come will be severely hit.

The Uses of Epidemiology in Assessing and Developing Services for the Subnormal

Before discussing the actual services, the following are some important qualifications in using the epidemiological data on severe subnormality.

1. The prevalence and prognosis of the condition is to some extent determined by the available services. Therefore, we will not know the true extent or prognosis of these people until first, the existing shortage of facilities has

been met; and second, until the methods of management have been evaluated, and affected people have been given the benefit of the best of those available. We may thus be seeing now not a "true" prognosis, but the results of the complications of the underlying organic process.

2. Some of these complications are avoidable, others may be. An obvious example is the retarding effect on emotional development, speech and verbal intelligence observed among children in large institutions (Lyle, 1959, 1960a, 1960b; Shotwell and Shipe, 1964). Moreover, the failure to provide adequate early counselling and relief to the parents of affected children may, by causing family tension, act against the child's development. Furthermore, we do not know the educational potential of these children in the hands of skilled qualified teachers, or even with the use of such aids as teaching machines. The present policy in England and Wales of excluding many of these children from the ordinary educational system, and the reluctance of many child guidance clinics to accept responsibility for their long-term care may well be to the disadvantage of the children.

3. The over-all prognosis for the severely subnormal is relatively poor, but even with the present facilities, their potential social and intellectual development in adulthood ranges widely from that of infantile behaviour to the ability to work in sheltered or open industry. This is particularly true of mongolism. Thus, Dunsdon, Carter and Huntley (1960) found that 6–7% of mongols scored I.Q.s of over 45 and that 1–2% scored 55 and over. Our own findings in Wessex suggest that just over 10% of mongols aged 15–19 had I.Q.s of over 50. (Miss Brooke of the Ministry of Health advised us to re-examine our data on this point after she had found this proportion in her hospital data.) There is also growing evidence that a proportion of phenyl-ketonurics (even untreated) may have normal or near-normal intelligence (Farquar, Richmond and Tait, 1963). Moreover, while it is possible to predict in early infancy with about 60% accuracy the non-mongol children who will have I.Q.s of under 50, the substantial remainder will do much better, and it is virtually impossible to predict the final development of individual children within the I.Q. range under 50 (Illingworth, 1961).

These facts emphasize the necessity for providing, at the earliest possible stage, the very best of facilities for children suspected of being subnormal.

The epidemiological approach lends itself to the development of a service which can both anticipate and deal with problems known to be present, a long time before they come to the notice of the existing services, and which are often worsened by delays (Morris, 1957). Numerous studies suggest that much of the therapeutic and social pessimism which surrounds the subject of subnormality is the result of ignorance on the one hand, and of lack of adequate facilities on the other.

There are systematic studies which have investigated the extent to which, and the reasons why, our sophisticated, diagnostic genetic counselling and social-work services are failing to meet the needs that exist (Holt, 1958; Tizard and Grad, 1961; Deisher *et al.*, 1962; Hudson, 1963) or failing to accept responsibility for long-term guidance (Rutter, 1964). Indeed, one of the most exciting fields for advance in modern medical care awaits the incorporation of the existing body of knowledge into the developing services for the chronically ill in general, and the mentally subnormal in particular.

Sociological studies of the changing structure and function of the "normal" family in industrial societies (Parsons and Bales, 1955; Young and Willmott, 1957) have revealed important mechanisms for the stress created by a chronically handicapped (deviant) member of the family (Susser and Watson, 1962). Moreover, other studies (Hollingshead and Redlich, 1958; Bernstein, 1960) have focused attention on unrecognized difficulties of communication which arise between professionals and their clients because of their different social class origins. These findings have led to systematic studies of the problems of families of the subnormal (Holt, 1958; Leeson, 1960; Tizard and Grad, 1961; Susser and Watson, 1962) and these are now well understood. Katz (1961) has described the evolution and function of the voluntary organization run by the parents of the mentally handicapped. It is now possible to deal with and relieve many of the family difficulties by the use of specialist services, whereas not long ago they were regarded as insoluble or remediable only by institutionalizing the subject. Similarly, outstanding advances have been made in the education and training of both the severely and the mildly subnormal (Ministry of Health, 1962; Tizard, 1964).

There are still major administrative problems involved in integrating the available professional skills into a single service, which would be able to provide continuous care to the subject and his family. However, the availability in sufficient numbers of the basic facilities required might go a long way to meeting some of these difficulties.

I will now discuss briefly:

1. The problems of the families;
2. The extent to which the services are meeting the needs;
3. A possible design for a comprehensive service for the subnormal, in which areas of 100,000 provide for all of the needs at least of their severely subnormal subjects. I will also suggest a way in which these services might be evaluated (Kushlick, 1965).

PROBLEMS OF PARENTS OF THE SEVERELY SUBNORMAL

The needs of the child are full diagnostic assessment, correction of remediable defects and a programme to help him realize his potential. During this period, he needs the care and socialization which is part of ordinary family life, or where this is not possible, of a substitute family.

One of the myths about subnormality which still has some currency is that the problems of the subnormal do not begin until the children reach school age. All of these children and their families need, from the stage at which the diagnosis is first suspected, the best available help from a team of paediatricians, cytogenicist, biochemist, educational psychologist, audiologist, ophthalmologist, psychiatrist and social worker. This care must be continuous, until neither the child nor the parents have further problems and, if necessary, in the case of the severely subnormal, for the whole of their lives.

The difficulties of the parents of a child with suspected subnormality begin from the earliest recognition that a problem exists. The first is that of facing the implications of the diagnosis. I will not labour the well-known point that this always comes as a profound shock to the parents. There is, however, evidence (Tizard and Grad, 1961) that the manner in which parents are at present told of the possible diagnosis, and the type of advice which they are given at the time, are often inadequate by any standards. It may produce in the parents a fear and resentment of orthodox services, with the result that the parents become isolated from these services and shop around for miracle cures, in a manner which reflects their misunderstanding of the child's problems. The evidence we have on the question, "When should the parents be told of a suspected diagnosis?" is that parents wish to be told early (Tizard and Grad, 1961; Leeson, 1960), but that doctors' opinions and practice on this question differ widely. There is also evidence that the parental depression which follows the diagnosis may often go unrecognized and untreated, although skilled psychiatric care may be needed.

Parents often suspect a genetic cause of the child's defect. More important still, they don't always raise the problem with their medical advisers, who do not always take the initiative in raising it themselves. There is evidence that many of these parents take unnecessary decisions to have no further children because of the fear of bearing another defective child (Tizard and Grad, 1961; Holt, 1958). There is also evidence that parents of phenylketonuric children are often unaware of its genetic causation and have further children, unaware of the high risks involved (Deisher et al., 1962). Studies have shown (Tizard and Grad, 1961; Leeson, 1960) that from the time the diagnosis is suspected, parents are anxious about future provision for the child, even to the point of thinking what will happen when they die.

These problems alone suggest the need for special diagnostic and supportive facilities, which will provide the child and family with continuous care. The need for a team of people with special skill in diagnosis, assessment of the child and management of the parental problem arises both from the diverse nature of the difficulties involved, and from the ever-present danger that conflicting advice may otherwise be given to families by professionals, when they are consulted individually (Tizard and Grad, 1961). Moreover, some members, at least, of the team should have a profound knowledge of the existing facilities, i.e. educational, training, residential care, as well as the services offered by other social agencies, upon which the family may draw in the future. This function might well be performed by the social workers in the team.

The second major group of family problems arise from the excessive demands made on the family by:

1. Prolonged stages of dependence on the family—particularly the mother;
2. The behaviour of the child.

For example, the mother will have to deal with a child who takes longer to walk, talk and become continent than the normal child. Thus, she may need, from a very early stage, extra domestic help from a mobile laundry to deal with incontinence and, when the child reaches 3 or 4 years old a day nursery or crêche. The facilities of a crêche allow her some time to make social contacts, perhaps to earn some money, and generally to preserve her physical and mental capacity to cope with the child's excessive demands. This purpose can also be served by a baby-sitting service.

I have laboured the points about the excessive demands on the family because they are (as shown by a number of well-conducted surveys) the main problem of severe subnormality, as seen by the families, and because they also cover some of the major problems faced by the teachers or training-centre staff when the children go to schools or centres. They are also the main reason for admission to hospital.

THE EXTENT TO WHICH WE ARE MEETING THE NEEDS

In this section the figures will be somewhat simplified. Let us take (Table 4) an arbitrary population of 100,000, with an annual birth rate of 16 per 1000 (the average in England and Wales for the past 16 years). The advantage of such a population is that one can easily work out the numbers of defectives in bigger or smaller populations, merely by multiplying or dividing these figures as is appropriate. Our results also suggest that it might be administratively convenient to run a service in an area of this size.

TABLE 4.

Calculation of the Number of Children of I.Q.
under 50 Who will be born in a Period of 16
Years in a Population of 100,000

Population	100,000
Birth rate per year	16 per 1000
Births per year	1600
Births in 16 years	25,600
Subjects of I.Q. under 50	$3 \cdot 7 \times 25 \cdot 6 = 100$

Our arbitrary population of 100,000 has therefore a minimum of 6 new cases of severe subnormality every year ($3 \cdot 7 \times 1 \cdot 6$). Table 5 also shows that over a 5-year period, there are about 30 cases. Because our rates are based on survivors to the age-group 10–19 years, we can assume that all of these cases survive to the age of 16. There would be a minimum of nearly

TABLE 5.

Expected Prevalence of Severe Subnormality among Children in a Population of 100,000 with a Birth-rate of 16 per 1000

Age	No. of children	Minimum no. of sev. sub.	Idiots	Mongols	PKU	TBM	Rh.	Rub.
0–4	8000	30	5	8 (+1)				
5–15	17,600	66	11	17 (+2)				
Total	25,600	96	16	25 +(3)	2	2	1	1

100 children aged up to 15 in our population; 30 aged up to 4 and 66 aged 5–15. About 1 in 6 of these children are probably idiots, i.e. they score I.Q.s of less than 20 (Kushlick, 1961).

It can thus be seen that:

1. The number of new cases of severe subnormality arising every year is comparatively small—about 6.
2. The proportion of such cases with clinical conditions diagnosable at birth or shortly after is comparatively small—just over a quarter. However, a substantial proportion of the remaining three-quarters will have clinical signs of a central nervous system disorder, such as epilepsy, cerebral palsy, defects of hearing and vision, or behaviour disorders, such as overactivity and milestone delay. These signs can be detected early and investigations and management begun. If, however, we are to detect at an early stage every case of severe subnormality, *all* children with epilepsy, cerebral palsy, defects of hearing and vision, and abnormal milestones will have to be identified, and investigated by a diagnostic clinic, dealing with all disorders of development. This means that the number of children and of families likely to make demands on such a service will be considerably more than 6 every year.

In our survey, we have found (Table 6) that of the 30 expected severely subnormal children in the age group 0–4 in our population of 100,000, 1 is at present in a training centre, 1 is already in an institution for the mentally subnormal, and 2 are living at home and receiving visits from the mental welfare officer. (One is on the waiting list to go into hospital.) This leaves 26 unknown to the Mental Health Department. We are at present looking for

TABLE 6.

Observed Prevalence of Severe Subnormality known to M.H.D.s Among Children in a Population of 100,000—Wessex Region (excluding Wiltshire) 1.7.63. Rates per 100,000

Age	H.C.	H.C. + T.C.	Inst.	Other	Total	Total expected	S/SN not known to M.H.D.
0–4	2	1	1	—	4	30	26
5–15	7	22	16	2	47	66	19
Total	9	23	17	2	51	96	45

H.C. = Home care, not receiving training.
H.C. + T.C. = Home care and attending training centre.
Inst. = Hospital care and hostels.
Other = Guardianship, approved schools, foster-homes.

these children, but we do not anticipate that many will have been tested yet. It is interesting to speculate on how much the families of these children know of the children's needs or of the services available to them.

Assuming that the 3- and 4-year-olds and their families might benefit from daily attending at a crèche, 12 places would be needed where, at present, only 1 is available.

Of the 66 expected severely subnormal children (Table 6) in the age-group 5–15, 22 are attending training centres, 16 are in institutions for the severely subnormal, 7 are living at home, receiving only visits from the mental welfare officers (2 are on the waiting list for admission to an institution for the subnormal). This leaves 19 unknown to the Mental Health Department because they are still attending ordinary or special schools. We are at present looking for these children in the schools, though many of them are likely to have been tested already. Until fairly recently, when diagnostic units and special classes have been made available for children under 7 years of age, the severely subnormal who entered ordinary schools therefore spent the first 2 years of schooling in ordinary classes of 20–40 pupils. Many still appear to do so; others attend local authority training centres as informal attenders, and some receive home teaching.

Table 7, which gives the prevalence of *all* grades of subnormal children known to the mental health departments in our population of 100,000, shows that there were also 13 mildly subnormal children known—6 in training centres, 3 in institutions, and 4 apparently at home and not attending training centres. This table also shows that a total of 13 children are at home, not attending training centres. It is likely that this figure overestimates the size of this problem, as some of these children may still be attending ordinary schools. The reason that those who have been excluded from school are not receiving training is that they are too severely retarded or too physically handicapped for the existing training centres. Special-care facilities will be needed for these children. Thus, assuming that all of these children have been excluded from school, 42 junior training-centre places will be required. In 1962 in England and Wales, 30% of local health authorities had more than 50 places per 100,000 population and in 1972, 53% plan to do so (Health and Welfare, 1963).

TABLE 7.

Observed Prevalence of All Grades of Subnormality known to M.H.D.s among Children in a Population of 100,000—Wessex Region (excluding Wiltshire) 1.7.63. Rates per 100,000

Age	H.C.	H.C. + T.C.	Inst.	Other	Total
0–4	3	1	2	—	6
5–15	10	28	18	2	58
Totals	13	29	20	2	64

H.C. = Home care, not receiving training.
H.C. + T.C. = Home care and attending training centre.
Inst. = Hospital care and hostels.
Other = Guardianship, approved schools, foster-homes.

THE NEED FOR RESIDENTIAL CARE

This arises when either the severely subnormal child makes excessive demands on its intact family, or when the family, handicapped by sickness, death or the birth of another child, is unable any longer to cope with his "reasonable" demands. These children then need a substitute family.

At present, when these situations arise, the child may be admitted for long-term care to institutions for the subnormal, often after being over a year on the waiting list. They are, for historical reasons, mainly situated outside the area where the family live. They are often a long way from the nearest town, and are usually large, particularly for the need they are supposed to be meeting of a substitute family. As these institutions are isolated from the rest of the community, they must provide, in addition to substitute families, their own medical and nursing care, psychological assessment (this is at present provided by only a minority), training and education services. A small proportion of the children in need of substitute families are fostered out to ordinary families.

Let us assume that our area of 100,000 people were to provide the residential facilities for these children within its boundaries. The results of the Wessex survey show:

1. How many places would be needed to house all of the children now in institutions for the subnormal and on the waiting list for admission to hospital;
2. The extent and character of the management problems of these children.

Looking back at Table 6, we see that of the 96 severely subnormal children expected in such a community, 17 are already in institutions and 3 on the waiting list for admission to hospital. Table 7, which includes children of all grades, shows that there are also 3 mildly subnormal children in hospital. Thus, our population could meet all of their needs by providing 25 such places. Let us assume further that they were housed in family units of 10 children each. We now know that each unit would consist on an average of 1 pre-school child, 3 aged 5–9, 5 aged 10–14 and 1 aged 15.

TABLE 8.

Social and Physical Incapacities and Behaviour Disorders (percentages) among all Wessex (excluding Wiltshire) Subnormal Children aged 15 and under in Residential Care on 1 July 1963 by Place of Care

Place of care	Incontinent only	Incontinent and bedfast	Incontinent and behaviour difficulties	Behaviour difficulties only	None of these	Total (per-centages)	N
Registered private homes	15	36	9	6	33	99	66
Hospitals	23	24	15	12	25	99	242
Whole region	22	26	13	11	28	100	321[a]

[a] Thirteen cases were in local authority hostels.

Table 8 shows the social and physical incapacities and behaviour disorders among the children in hospital. The children's incapacities were rated on a standardized schedule by the sisters and charge nurses in the hospitals, and by the people in charge of the registered private homes. Our family of 10 children would contain, on average, 3 incontinent bedfast children. Of the remaining 7 ambulant children, 3 would be continent and present no major behaviour problems, 2 would present the difficulty of incontinence only, and 2 would present at least two major behaviour problems, such as aggression, destructiveness, overactivity, self-mutilation or attention-seeking—one of these children would also be incontinent.

In the proposals to be submitted to the Wessex Regional Hospital Board about the setting-up of such experimental units, I am suggesting that the responsibility for the units might be that of the regional board, and we are now investigating the practical possibilities. They would thus be staffed by house parents and part-time assistants, who would function as substitute parents.

During the day, these children might attend local training centres and special-care units. They would receive their routine medical care from general practitioners and make use, as required, of the specialist services provided by the local authority and regional hospital board. If possible, their care would be the responsibility of the same team of people that I described earlier to deal with all of the children with developmental handicaps. This would ensure continuity of care between the family and the residential institution.

The accommodation required is an ordinary house fitted with minor modifications, e.g. a downstairs lavatory and bathroom. The part-time staff would be accommodated in houses in the neighbourhood. An ideal site for these units and staff accommodation would be a housing estate near the training centre. In rural areas, the units would be in the central rural town, or in the town which had the training centre.

We also know the extent to which the local training centre provision for children would have to be increased to meet the demands in the areas with a comprehensive service.

Table 7 shows that in our population of 100,000 30 children were attending junior training centres. In the area with the comprehensive service, a further 20 places will be required for those children now in institutions outside the area. A further 13 places might be needed for those subnormal children now living at home but not receiving any training. (The reason that many are not receiving any training is that they are too severely retarded or too severely handicapped for the existing day training centres. Once special-care unit facilities are available, their needs can be met.) Thus, training-centre places will, in the comprehensive service areas, have to be expanded by at least 33 (20 + 13) to 63 places.

This is a minimum estimate, because it is based on the number of cases known to mental health departments. We saw (Table 6) that 26 of the expected 30 severely subnormal children aged 0–4 were not yet known to the Mental Health Department. If crêche facilities are to be provided for the 3- and 4-year-olds, a further 12 places will be needed for them. I am not discussing in detail the problem of mild subnormality, but it is worth mentioning at this stage that crêche facilities or day nursery places are also needed for the slowly developing, mildly subnormal children of lower social-class origin from broken homes. It has been clearly shown that these children benefit considerably from a pre-school training programme (Kirk, 1958).

N.A.M.H.S.—Z*

EVALUATION

We would like to use the expansion of facilities in our region to try and evaluate different types of residential care. Thus, we intend to do this in two demographically comparable rural and urban areas, each of about 100,000 people. We anticipate from our results that the children in each area will constitute comparable experimental and control groups. In the experimental urban and rural areas, we intend to provide the comprehensive service I outlined earlier, together with residential units situated in the area where the children live. The control areas will have the same facilities, except that when children need residential care, they will go into the existing-type residential institutions, situated outside of the area.

We would like to compare in experimental and control areas:

1. The development of the children;
2. The problems of the families;
3. The administrative problems involved;
4. The costs.

Finally, our estimates are based on current prevalence rates and current rates of hospital use. We believe that the only way of verifying them is to test them experimentally. The type of service suggested is designed to be sufficiently flexible, so that fairly inexpensive adjustments can be made as we go along.

PREVALENCE OF ADULT SUBNORMALITY IN WESSEX

If we are to provide in experimental areas for the residential care of all the subnormal children currently in hospital, some estimate is required of the number of residential places required for severely subnormal adults in such an area, because places will be required for these people as they grow older.

We have found (see Table 9) that our area of 100,000 people could provide residential care for all of its adult severely subnormal subjects presently in hospital, if it were to make available 77 places (74 in hospital plus 3 on the waiting list) (Table 9); for example, in eight units of 10 beds or sixteen units of 5 beds.

The Wessex results suggest that there is at present a marked shortage of training-centre facilities for severely subnormal adults living at home. Thus, we found (Table 9) that there were 29 per 100,000 severely subnormal adults attending local authority training centres. (The rate for England and Wales in 1963 was 24 per 100,000—Ministry of Health, 1964.) In Wessex, 19 per 100,000 were for the severely subnormal. There were, in addition, 32 per 100,000 such subjects living at home and not receiving any training.

We have not yet analysed the physical and social capacities, and behaviour difficulties of the adults, but other follow-up studies suggest that people of

TABLE 9.

Prevalence of known Subnormality per 100,000 of the Total Population among Adults aged 16 and over by Grade and Place of Care on July 1963—Wessex Region (excluding Wiltshire)

I.Q.	Area	H.C.	H.C. + T.C.	Inst.	Other	Total	Waiting list	Population in thousands 1961 Census
Under 50	Counties	33	18	73	3	127	2	1172
	County boroughs	32	20	76	5	133	4	574
	Total	32	19	74	4	129	3	1746
Over 50	Counties	62	10	55	18	145	1	
	County boroughs	55	9	51	11	126	2	
	Total	60	9	53	16	138	1	
Not known	Counties	1	—	5	1	8	—	
	County boroughs	4	—	4	—	9	—	
	Total	2	—	5	1	8	—	
Totals	Counties	96	29	133	22	280	3	
	County boroughs	91	29	131	17	268	6	
	Total	94	29	132	20	275	4	

H.C. = Home care, not receiving training.
H.C. + T.C. = Home care and attending training centre.
Inst. = Hospital care and hostels.
Other = Guardianship, approved schools, residential employment, etc.

I.Q. under 50 fail to maintain employment on the open market (Ferguson and Kerr, 1955; Kushlick, 1961). Many of the 32 per 100,000 subjects would thus appear to need some form of sheltered employment.

The extent to which local training facilities will have to be expanded, if in the experimental area the 74 institutionalized subjects are to be housed within the local area, can thus be estimated.

As with the children, during the day the adults would attend occupation centres, industrial units, or sheltered workshops, or go out to work, depending on their incapacities. Their specialist needs would continue to be met by the team, and by all of the available educational and recreational services in the area.

CRITICISMS OF THE ADMINISTRATIVE PLAN

Some of the following criticisms have been raised.

1. The plan has been said to aim both at dispersing the traditional hospitals for the subnormal and at duplicating already-existing facilities. However, the main problem is not of replacing the existing services with something else, but of meeting unmet needs by providing new facilities. These are required to deal with the people who are now on the waiting lists, with the overcrowded conditions in the existing hospitals and, in Wessex, to provide in the region the number of beds now occupied by Wessex patients in hospitals outside the region. As these patients are discharged or die, their beds are filled with non-Wessex patients. Indeed, the fact that the two types of service will run alongside one another will make their evaluation possible.

2. It has been said that compared with the running costs of the traditional hospitals, the experimental units would be too expensive. The cost per bed of staffing and running the experimental units will, at the outset of the experiment, undoubtedly exceed that now obtaining in the traditional hospitals. This difference in costs may well narrow in the future. Thus, all authorities in the field of subnormality agree that if more adequate standards of care are to be provided, and if the existing overcrowding is to be ended in the traditional hospitals, radical improvements will be needed in their staffing ratios, as well as in their standards of accommodation and their facilities for education and rehabilitation. It is likely that the demand for improving conditions in the hospitals will receive increasing public support, as more public attention is focused on the services for the subnormal. Moreover, improvements of this sort are going on at present. These improvements will, in addition to raising the running costs, necessitate substantial additional capital expenditure. These are not only due to the provision of more accommodation for patients, but also, in isolated areas where other accommodation is not available, to the provision of houses for staff. In addition, new facilities such as schools, heating plant and catering facilities may become necessary when the existing services cease to cope with the demands of expanded accommodation. In comparing the costs of the two types of service, these items will have to be measured very carefully.

It has also been suggested that this is a way of passing financial responsibility from the Treasury to the rates. However, it is the responsibility of the doctor in preventive medicine, and particularly the epidemiologist, to:

    (a) Estimate the size of the problem;

    (b) Estimate the need; and

    (c) Look for a way of meeting these, and to convince people of its wisdom on the merits of the case.

The needs of the mildly subnormal adult are more difficult to estimate. We have seen that problems arise largely among those from broken homes, and that they occur mainly during adolescence. Stein and Susser (1960), and Tizard (1964) have estimated their need for hostel places during this phase of their development. There are, now, between 60 and 70 (Kushlick, 1965) mildly subnormal adult subjects per 100,000 of the population presently in hospitals for the subnormal. There is evidence, however, that when they are discharged or die, their places may not be taken up by other mildly subnormal people.

COMPULSION AND SERVICES FOR THE SUBNORMAL

The services for the mentally disordered have evolved from a stage where legal and bureaucratic authority was used to care for and control patients and their families, to the present time, when it is possible to use skilled professional authority and personal relationships to achieve these ends (Susser, 1961). The aspects of legal compulsion which remain, such as exclusion from school, removal of children from their families and detention of patients in hospital, need to be continuously evaluated, with the object of maximizing the place of skilled professional authority, accepted voluntarily by patients and their families because of their confidence in the service. The possibility that persons may be unnecessarily detained and deprived of their rights, as a result of being classified subnormal or severely subnormal, has led the Working Party of the British Psychological Society (1963) to recommend that among adults, the upper level of subnormality should be fixed at a W.A.I.S. I.Q. of 70 points, and that of severe subnormality, in which detention after the age of 25 years is easily affected, at 55 points. It is doubtful whether the implementation of this recommendation would do much to solve the problem. We have seen that the behaviour difficulties of the mildly subnormal (I.Q. 50–70) who are eventually admitted to hospitals for the subnormal, arise largely from their lack of socialization within a family during the first 10 years of their lives, rather than from their low I.Q. level. Their needs, like those of children with higher I.Q.s from similar backgrounds, would appear to require a combination of continuous specialized social work, and of psychological, psychiatric, educational and recreational services within a substitute family, until they have passed the critical stage of adolescence. In the absence of such a service, the individuals of I.Q. over 70 now dealt with as subnormal would, because of the minor acts of delinquency committed by the men and the promiscuity of the women, merely be diverted to social agencies like the prisons and local authority welfare departments. At present, none of these agencies is staffed or equipped to meet these subjects' needs. I believe that both scientific and humane interests in the field of subnormality will be best served by the continued study of the epidemiology of the condition, and by measuring how well the needs of the subjects and their families are being met.

Thus, from our knowledge of the epidemiology of mild subnormality, we can also see the limitations of the proposal in the early part of this century to lower the incidence of mild subnormality by a programme of compulsory sterilization. If every person in the I.Q. range 50–70 (about 2% of the whole population) were sterilized, the resulting decrease in the incidence of mild subnormality might be of the order of less than 10%. Thus, Penrose (1938) found that over 90% of the mildly subnormal in his hospital survey had parents of normal or dull average intelligence. The importance of family disruption as a cause of hospitalization of mildly subnormal subjects might even have led to an over-representation of his sample of subjects with mildly subnormal parents. No government other than that of the Nazis has ever suggested a hideous programme of this sort. However, some countries still practise compulsory sterilization of "certified", "ascertained" or hospitalized mildly subnormal people. Such a programme is unlikely to make any real impact on the incidence of the condition, because of the very small proportion of people in this I.Q. range who are ever "ascertained" or hospitalized. We have also seen (page 687) that there has not been any decline in the national intelligence, although social policy towards the mildly subnormal had been planned on the prediction of such a decline. Penrose (1963) has suggested that although environmentally induced increases in height and intelligence may be masking a genetic decrease, the risk of "national degeneration" is both speculative (because the evidence is to the contrary), and academic (because we cannot predict now the human qualities which will be needed by future generations). There is little doubt, however, that voluntary sterilization to limit family size may often relieve family problems, and this should, of course, be made available to people who choose it.

Finally, it has been shown by Belknap and Steinle (1963) that the quality of medical care in comparably staffed and equipped hospitals is very much higher in those hospitals where the influential political and economic figures in the locality participate actively in the hospital administration, and where the attitudes of these people favour the provision of a high standard of service to the community as a whole. This finding is probably of great importance to the services for the subnormal. In the present atmosphere of community tolerance of the subnormal and reasonably full employment, it is likely that radical improvements to the service might be possible, if there were to be a move in this direction by skilled and well-informed professionals in the field.

References

SCOTTISH COUNCIL FOR RESEARCH IN EDUCATION (1949), *The Trend of Scottish Intelligence*, London, London Univ. Press.

SCOTTISH COUNCIL FOR RESEARCH IN EDUCATION (1953), *Social Implications of the 1947 Scottish Mental Survey*, London Univ. Press.

A Special Census of Suspected Referred Mental Retardation (1955), Onondaga County N.Y., Technical Report of the Mental Health Research Unit.

The Health of the School Child, 1960 and 1961 (1962), Report of the Chief Medical Officer of the Ministry of Education, London, H.M.S.O.

The Training of Staff of Training Centres for the Mentally Subnormal (1962), Ministry of Health Central Health Services Council, Standing Mental Health Advisory Committee, London, H.M.S.O.

Report of the Working Party on Subnormality (1963), *Bull. of the Brit. Psychol. Soc.* **16**, 37–50.

Health & Welfare (1963): The Development of Community Care (Cmnd. 1973), London, H.M.S.O.

The Health & Welfare Services (1964), Report of the Ministry of Health for the year ended 31 Dec. 1963, London, H.M.S.O.

Supplement on Mental Health (1964), The Registrar General's Statistical Review of England and Wales for the year 1960, London, H.M.S.O.

AKESSON, H. O. (1961), *Epidemiology & Genetics of Mental Deficiency in a Southern Swedish Population*, Uppsala, University of Uppsala.

BERG, J. M. and KIRMAN, B. H. (1959), Some aetiological problems in mental deficiency, *Brit. Med. J.* **ii**, 848–52.

BELKNAP, I. and STEINLE, J. G. (1963), *The Community and its Hospitals; a Comparative Analysis*, New York, Syracuse University Press.

BERNSTEIN, B. (1960), Language and social class, *Brit. J. Sociol.* **11**, 271.

CLARKE, A. D. B. and CLARKE, A. M. (1954), Cognitive changes in the feebleminded, *Brit. J. Psychol.* **45**, 173–79.

COSER, ROSE L. (1962), *Life in the Ward*, East Lansing, Michigan, U.S.A., Michigan State University Press.

CROME, L. (1960), The brain and mental retardation, *Brit. Med. J.* **i**, 897–904.

DEISHER, R., BALKANY, A. F., PREWITT, C. D. and REDFIELD, W. J. (1962), Phenylketonuric families in Washington State, *Am. J. Dis. Ch.* **103**, 818–21.

DUNSDON, M. I., CARTER, C. O. and HUNTLEY, R. M. C. (1960), Upper end of range of intelligence in mongolism, *Lancet*, **i**, 565–8.

FARQUAR, J. W., RICHMOND, J. and TAIT, H. P. (1963), Phenylketonuria in pediatric practice: a review, *Clin. Pediat.* **2**, 504–16.

FERGUSON, T. and KERR, AGNES W. (1955), After-histories of girls educated in special schools for mentally-handicapped children, *Glasgow Medical Journal*, **36**, 50–6.

GOFFMAN, E. (1957), *The Characteristics of the Total Institution*, Walter Reed Symposium on Social Psychiatry, Washington, D.C.

GOODMAN, N. and TIZARD, J. (1962), Prevalence of imbecility and idiocy among children, *Brit. med. J.* **i**, 216–19.

HOLLINGSHEAD, A. B. and REDLICH, F. C. (1958), *Social Class and Mental Illness*, New York, Wylie.

HOLT, K. S. (1958), The influence of a retarded child upon family limitation, *J. ment. defic. res.* **2**, 28.

HUDSON, F. P. (1963), Phenylketonuria in the north of England, *Med. Off.* July 1963, 69–71.

ILLINGWORTH, R. S. (1961), The predictive value of developmental tests in the first year with special reference to the diagnosis of mental subnormality, *J. Child Psychol. Psychiat.* **2**, 210–15.

KATZ, A. H. (1961), *Parents of the Handicapped*, Springfield, Charles C. Thomas.

KIRK, S. A. (1958), *Early Education of the Mentally Retarded*, Urbana, University of Illinois Press.

KUSHLICK, A. (1961), Subnormality in Salford (pp. 18–48), in Susser, M. W. and Kushlick, A., *A Report on the Mental Health Services of the City of Salford for the Year 1961*, Salford Health Department.

KUSHLICK, A. (1964), *Prevalence of Recognized Mental Subnormality of I.Q. under 50 among Children in the South of England with Reference to the Demand for Places for Residential Care*. Paper to the International Copenhagen Conference on the Scientific Study of Mental Retardation, Copenhagen, August 1964.

KUSHLICK, A. (1965), Community care for the subnormal—a plan for evaluation, *Proc. Roy. Soc. Med.* **58**, 374–80.

LEESON, J. (1960), A study of six mentally handicapped children and their families, *Medic al Officer*, **104,** 311.

LEESON, J. (1962), *Demand for Care in Hospitals for the Mentally Subnormal*, Manchester Regional Hospital Board.

LEMKAU, P., TIETZE, C. and COOPER, M. (1942), Mental hygiene problems in an urban district: third paper, *Mental Hygiene*, **26,** 275–88.

LEMKAU, P., TIETZE, C. and COOPER, M. (1943), Mental hygiene problems in an urban district: fourth paper, *Mental Hygiene*, **27,** 279–95.

LEWIS, E. O. (1929), *The Report of the Mental Deficiency Committee Being a Joint Committee of the Board of Education & Board of Control: Part IV—Report on an Investigation into the Incidence of Mental Deficiency in Six Areas*, 1925–27, London, H.M.S.O.

LYLE, J. G. (1959), The effect of an institution environment upon the verbal development of imbecile children. (1) Verbal intelligence, *J. Ment. Defic. Res.* **3,** 122–8.

LYLE, J. G. (1960a), The effect of an institution environment upon the verbal development of imbecile children. (2) Speech and language, *J. Ment. Defic. Res.* **4,** 1–13.

LYLE, J. G. (1960b), The effect of an institution environment upon the verbal development of imbecile children. (3) The Brooklands residential family unit, *J. Ment. Defic. Res.* **4,** 14–23.

MORRIS, J. N. (1957), *Uses of Epidemiology*, Edinburgh and London, E. & S. Livingstone Ltd.

PARSONS, T. and BALES, R. F. (1955), *Family Socialization & Interaction Process*, Glencoe, Ill., Free Press.

PENROSE, L. S. (1938), (Colchester Survey) *A Clinical and Genetic Study of 1280 Cases of Mental Defect*, Sp. Rep. Scr. Medical Research Council, No. 229, London, H.M.S.O.

PENROSE, L. S. (1963), *The Biology of Mental Defect* (3rd edn.), London, Sidgwick & Jackson.

RUTTER, M. (1964), Intelligence and childhood psychiatric disorder, *Brit. J. Soc. Clin. Psychol.* **3,** 120–9.

SAENGER, G. S. (1960), *Factors Influencing the Institutionalization of Mentally Retarded Individuals in New York City.* A Report to the New York Interdepartmental Health Resources Board.

SHOTWELL, ANNA M. and SHIPE, DOROTHY (1964), Effect of out-of-home care on the intellectual and social development of mongoloid children, *Amer. J. Ment. Defic.* **68,** 693–9.

STEIN, ZENA and SUSSER, MERVYN (1960), Families of dull children.
Part II. Identifying family types and subcultures.
Part III. Social selection by family type.
Part IV. Increments in intelligence, *J. Ment. Sci.* **106,** 1296–1319.

STEIN, ZENA and SUSSER, MERVYN (1960a), The families of dull children: a classification for predicting careers, *Brit. J. Prev. Soc. Med.* **14,** 83–8.

STEIN, ZENA and SUSSER, MERVYN (1960b), Estimating hostel needs for backward citizens, *Lancet*, **ii,** 486–8.

STEIN, ZENA and SUSSER, MERVYN (1963), The social distribution of mental retardation, *Am. J. Ment. Defic.* **67,** 811–21.

SUSSER, M. W. (1961), in Susser, M. W. and Kushlick, A., *A Report on the Mental Health Services of the City of Salford for the year 1961*, Salford Health Dept.

SUSSER, M. W. and WATSON, W. (1962), *Sociology in Medicine*, London, Oxford University Press.

TIZARD, J. (1958), Longitudinal and Follow-up Studies, in *Mental Deficiency—The Changing Outlook*, London, Oxford University Press.

TIZARD, J. (1964), *Community Services for the Mentally Handicapped*, London, Oxford University Press.

TIZARD, J. and GRAD, J. C. (1961), *The Mentally Handicapped and Their Families*, London, Oxford University Press.

YOUNG, M. and WILLMOTT, P. (1957), *Family and Kinship in East London*, London.

Appendix 1

DETAILS OF METHODS USED IN SURVEYS QUOTED IN TABLE 2

Author	Area investigated	Date	Population sampled
1. Lewis (1929)	England and Wales	1926–9	6 rural and 6 urban areas of 100,000 people each.
2. Lemkau *et al.* (1943)	Baltimore	1936	Urban area of population 55,000.
3. Onondaga (1955)	Onondaga County	1955	Urban area of 116,000 children under 18 years.
4. Akesson (1961)	Rural Sweden	1959	10 rural parishes of total population 11,500.
5. Kushlick (1961)	Salford	1961	Urban area of 150,000.
6. Goodman and Tizard (1962)	Middlesex	1960	Urban area of 451,800 aged 0–14.
7. Kushlick (1964)	Wessex County Boroughs	1964	Urban area of 46,000 aged 15–19.
	Counties	1964	Urban and rural area of 90,000 aged 15–19.

How the subjects were identified

Children

1, 2, 3, and 4. All children both at school and known to social agencies.
5. Children known as mentally subnormal to Mental Health Department only.
6. As in 5, plus special schools, approved schools and private homes.
7. As in 5, plus hospitals, private homes and hostels.

Adults

1. All adults known to all social agencies—score I.Q. under 65.
2. All adults known to all social agencies diagnosed as mentally defective.
4. All adults in population scoring I.Q. under 70.
5. All adults known as mentally subnormal to M.H.D. only.

Criteria for grades

Only in 1 and 5 are grades recorded by age for all ages.

1. Children—I.Q. under 45–50; I.Q. 45–50 to 70.
Adults—I.Q. under 40–45; I.Q. 40–45 to 60–85.
5, 6, and 7. I.Q. under 50; I.Q. over 50.

39. The Northamptonshire Mental Health Education Project

An Experiment in Mental Health Education*

A. GATHERER

EVERY disease has its public image. Even the name of a disease conjures up in the mind a picture which will vary from individual to individual, with his experience and understanding of its cause and prognosis and with the folklore with which he has been surrounded. The public image of a disease can influence behaviour towards it. It can influence the demand for medical services, as is periodically seen in the panic for mass vaccination and public health action brought about by a small outbreak of smallpox. It can influence the prognosis as, for example, in the case of some types of cancer where fear of the disease can lead to delay in seeking medical advice. But the public image of psychiatric disorder brings with it a fear and prejudice which can influence the chances of recovery at almost every stage.

Nowadays, to treat an illness or to cure the symptoms of a disease is no longer sufficient. The aim is full rehabilitation. In psychiatric disorder this means that the symptoms are cured or alleviated, that the patient is back at home and that he has successfully picked up again the social links and relationships which were at first threatened by his illness and finally broken by his hospitalization. Rehabilitation can be partly brought about by doctors, nurses and social workers, but the rest depends upon the patient himself. He can only succeed if he is accepted and helped by understanding relatives, friends, workmates and, indeed, by everyone in the community. If relatives and friends are to be expected to play a part in the care and recovery of the psychiatric patient, they must understand their roles and must, therefore, understand something about mental health.

The importance of mental health education is underlined by the trend towards community care. Although initially due to the desire to avoid the effects of institutionalization in hospital, the rapid development of community care is being encouraged by the realization that it offers exciting possibilities of a new approach to the whole problem.

*Based on a preliminary report which appeared in the Annual Report for 1963 of the County Medical Officer of Health, Northamptonshire.

The care of the psychiatrically disordered in the community, however, will develop only as the result of public appreciation and education. The 1957 Royal Commission states:

> Community care of increasing numbers of mentally disordered will mean increased responsibilities for individuals, families and local authorities. . . . The general public will have to learn to tolerate in their midst persons with mild abnormalities of behaviour or appearance hitherto in hospital.

The importance of public attitudes was also emphasized by the Ministry of Health (1963) in its report on plans for the development of the health and welfare services of local authorities:

> The development of mental health services . . . should in turn increase the public's understanding of mental disorder and their sympathy with what the services are trying to do. Thus the expansion of the services and the growth of public appreciation of their objects must go hand in hand. In no other aspect of health and welfare is it so necessary to demonstrate the existence of the need in order to be able to meet it.

The need for mental health education of the public is so obvious that it is surprising so little has so far been done in this country. There are, of course, several difficulties which have to be considered in planning action in this field. The first is the lack of precise knowledge of the present attitudes. It is widely assumed that great strides have been made in improving public attitudes by the upgrading of the mental hospital, by the increased skills of psychiatry, and by the recent changes in legislation. There is an increased willingness to seek psychiatric help and a welcome frankness in discussion on mental health in press, radio and television. However, there are abundant indications that present-day attitudes still fall far short of the ideal. There is still the reluctance of out-patients to accept the need for psychiatric hospital treatment (Carstairs, 1963). To enter such a hospital still results in an invidious evaluation of the patient by his friends and relatives with his judgement, his ability to cope, his confidence and self-control all suspect (WHO, 1959). Such an evaluation is well recognized by the ex-patient (Mills, 1962), and, indeed, by astute members of the public, as was clearly shown during the mental health education campaign in Northamptonshire when one member of an audience asked why the village eccentric was accepted until he entered a psychiatric hospital and was then rejected. Public attitudes are revealed also by the resistance in many communities to training centres for mentally handicapped children and to the opening of community hostels for ex-patients.

Another difficulty involved in mental health education is that there is no single and simple message which can be publicized, nor is there a well-defined end result at which to aim. This contrasts markedly with campaigns aiming, for example, at increasing the number of people accepting vaccination and immunization, where the rate of acceptance can indicate the success or otherwise of the campaign.

There is also the problem of lightening the approach by using humour.

As one of the aims must be to expose the unfairness to the psychiatric patient of the joke approach to mental disorder, the methods used must be essentially serious. When dealing with a subject in which personal emotions amongst members of the audience may easily be involved, it is important that the overall impression should be one of honesty and sincere concern for the lot of the mentally disordered.

The creation of a demand for services which cannot be met is another hazard in mental health education. This is especially so at the present time, when there is a shortage of hospital and local authority staff and when the mental health services are in a state of flux.

The final difficulty is perhaps the most discouraging of all, and that is the great danger of arousing anxieties and feelings of guilt in the audience and, in fact, producing the opposite effect to that intended. The experience of the Cummings' so well described in their book (1957) has no doubt dissuaded many enthusiasts from embarking on a similar venture.

In advertising and in the audience research of the B.B.C. the danger of producing an "anti-effect" is well recognized (Belson, 1961). Every part of a campaign must therefore be carefully considered before it is launched, and procedures should be incorporated in the programme so that such an effect can be detected at the earliest possible moment.

The Northamptonshire Project

PREPARATIONS

The Project was a joint one between the County Health Department and the Northamptonshire British Red Cross Society. The detailed planning throughout was done by a Project Committee and the aim was to divide the work and responsibilities according to the particular attributes and availability of the members of each body. Membership of the Committee included a general practitioner as chairman, a consultant psychiatrist as adviser, two senior members of the B.R.C.S., a health education organizer, and the Deputy County Medical Officer as secretary.

It was considered important that the plans of the Project Committee could be interpreted and carried out at field level. To facilitate this, the county was divided into 56 localities and in each of these a local organizer was responsible for duties such as suggesting suitable groups for talks, publicity methods and generally promoting interest. Their activities were co-ordinated by area organizers, of whom there were 30. It was hoped that these would act as a link between the central organization and the field workers and that difficulties arising at the periphery would soon be picked up and referred to the Committee. Further co-ordination was obtained by the five district medical officers of health, each of whom formed a district committee with the help of senior administrative nursing officers and area organizers.

The aim was to overcome the difficulties imposed by geography in the planning of a complicated campaign in a predominantly rural county. The plan offered the opportunity of maintaining central control of the Project while at the same time encouraging local enthusiasm and participation.

The main worry of volunteers and, indeed, of Health Department staff, when asked to participate in the Project, was their strongly felt lack of expertise in the subject of mental health. It was therefore important to ensure that as full a programme of training as possible was arranged before anyone was involved in a job for which he or she felt inadequately prepared.

Training was especially required for interviewers and for speakers.

(i) *Interviewers*

The interviewers required an understanding of the principles of social survey work and a deeper knowledge of the rationale of the questions on the interview schedule. In order to give them the former, notes were drawn up outlining in some detail the rules which they had to obey concerning non-response, permissible prompting and general conduct of the interview. These notes were discussed, section by section, at one of the three training sessions which each interviewer was required to attend.

Each training session was repeated several times in different parts of the county so that the number of interviewers attending was seldom more than 8–10, and at all times the importance of the work which they were going to do was stressed. The schedule of questions was presented to them and each question in turn was discussed in order that they might understand the thinking which lay behind it.

(ii) *Speakers*

The original plan was to draw up in good time a panel of speakers who could be trained at leisure. However, the problems created by the hard winter of 1963 and by pressure of other work prevented this from being realized. It was also soon discovered that the training of lay people to act as speakers on a subject as difficult as mental health required very much more time and effort than could be spared. It was therefore decided that the speakers would be drawn mainly from the ranks of those already with some knowledge of this subject. In the event, most of the talks were given by the medical members of the Project Committee, other doctors and psychiatrists, psychiatric nurses, senior nurses in the Health Department, health visitors and B.R.C.S. volunteers. Occasionally the speakers went as teams, comprising a professionally trained person and a volunteer, and this proved an extremely successful arrangement because it gave the audience the benefit of an expert and, at the same time, the value of hearing from a lay person how the subject affected them as individuals. It was also beneficial in so far as the working link between the statutory and the voluntary speaker allowed each to see the particular value in the other.

The main problem was to standardize the approach and the message. This was achieved in three ways: in the first place by holding meetings between the speakers to discuss the relative emphasis to be placed on different aspects of the talk; secondly, by the use of an outline talk which was drawn up by the psychiatric adviser and the committee; and thirdly, by the use of agreed visual aids by the speakers.

The Aims of the Project

The original aims of the Project were formulated in October 1962 and comprised two main parts. The first one was to alter the attitude of the public to mental disorder in order to remove stigma, and the second was to attempt the prevention of mental illness by more intensive education of selected groups. It soon became apparent, however, that these aims were idealistic and over-ambitious and that the lack of knowledge of present attitudes in the community would hamper the first, while the second would require a very different approach and would better follow on at a later stage. It was therefore decided that the overall object of the Project would remain the altering of public attitudes, but that a clearer definition of specific aims would be required.

It was eventually agreed that these should be:

1. To make the public aware of mental disorder as a social problem;
2. To spread some knowledge of the aetiology (in general terms) of mental disorder;
3. To indicate the advances made in the treatment and care of the mentally disordered;
4. To explain what community care means, how lay people can themselves play a part and why it is, from the medical point of view, important that they should do so.

Once the aims had been clarified, the Project fell naturally into three parts. First a mental health education campaign with the aims as outlined above; secondly, an evaluation of the campaign; thirdly, the establishment of aids for community care.

The Methods of Approach Used in the Campaign

It was obvious that no single message could adequately cover the aims of the campaign and that the educational programme had to be carefully tailored to the understanding and interest of particular groups in the community. It was therefore decided to develop the approach to the public along three lines.

(a) *Voluntary societies*

The easiest channel of communication was to use existing voluntary society meetings and every society or group in the county known to hold regular meetings was offered a free speaker service. The talks given were varied according to the particular needs of the group with, for example, young wives' and mothers' clubs being told about the emotional development of children, and W.V.S. groups about the mental health aspects of loneliness in the elderly. Each talk had a basic outline—the problem; the modern approach; the Project and the part to be played by the public and, in particular, by the group being addressed.

(b) *Special groups*

In drawing up the programme, certain groups of people were selected whose opinions and attitudes were considered to be of particular importance in the care of the mentally disordered; to whom people turned in distress; or whose work enabled them to promote sound mental health. With these groups it was felt that special themes should be developed as a single talk would seldom be sufficient. Day or half-day conferences were arranged for these groups, with guest speakers to attract interest and group discussions to encourage the interchange of ideas. The groups covered in this way included the clergy, secondary school head teachers, industrialists, trade union officials, the police, and youth club leaders.

(c) *The general public*

The most difficult people to reach were the rest of the general public. Three methods of approach were tried:

(i) *Mass media*

The local press were approached at a very early stage. In February 1963 the County Medical Officer invited the editors and deputy editors of the two main local papers to an informal meeting where they heard a brief preliminary outline of the Project and met the members of the Project Committee. It was agreed that both papers would be invited to attend all open meetings and would have free access to the Committee, rather than obtaining all information through a press liaison officer. Press statements were therefore seldom used.

It was important to obtain the support of radio and television, and the news rooms of B.B.C. radio and television, and of A.T.V. (Midlands) were kept fully informed of all activities. It was realized that insufficient radio and television time would be granted to make a marked impact on the community as far as the content of the campaign was conerned, but, nevertheless, the frequent mention of the Project on television and radio aroused much interest locally.

(ii) *Exhibitions and open days*

A mental health exhibition was jointly organized with the staff of St. Crispin Hospital, and smaller exhibitions took place at various fêtes and flower shows. Open days were held at the four junior training centres in the county and also at the hospital.

(iii) *The ground level approach*

As it was realized that the approaches outlined above would reach only certain members of the community, an attempt was made to spread the information further to the ordinary man in the street by making full use of the local helpers. They were asked to talk about the aims of the campaign as much as possible in their districts, especially to those they considered to be local opinion leaders, in the hope that the latter would in turn influence others.

THE CAMPAIGN

The first public announcement of the Project followed the press meeting in February and was timed to precede by a few days the start of the first survey of public opinion. In order to prevent the initial publicity surrounding the news from influencing the results of the survey, the content was limited to a general statement. Nevertheless, there was an immediate and impressive local and national interest, with news reports on television and radio and in newspapers.

The inaugural meeting of the Project was held on 5 April 1963. The audience of over a hundred people included representatives from the Ministry of Health, the National Association for Mental Health, the Oxford Regional Hospital Board, all church denominations, and many local statutory and voluntary associations. The meeting was well reported in the local and national press.

The first month of the campaign had been deliberately kept free from too many engagements, so that final training and planning could be completed. Nevertheless, six organizations were addressed during that month and the pressure on speakers built up rapidly. The intention was that May and June would be active campaign months and that after a break in July/August, the peak months would be September/October, with the campaign finishing at the end of November. During these five busy months, 130 talks were given, the majority in the autumn.

On 9 May the B.B.C. television featured mental health and the Project in its Midlands' programme "Scan". Local reaction to the broadcast was excellent.

The first conference was held on 14 May 1963. It was arranged by the County W.V.S. and the theme was "The Mental Health of the Elderly". One of the main points emphasized was the importance of such activities as meals-on-wheels and visiting services and other work of W.V.S. volunteers in preventing many elderly people from sinking into social isolation.

On 6 June the second major conference was arranged by the Northampton-shire Churches Group Steering Committee, which was formed with the help of the Northamptonshire Rural Community Council to bring together representatives of churches of all denominations with members of the voluntary and statutory services. This conference began by considering the theme "Mental Disorder Today" and involved talks from a consultant psychiatrist, a general practitioner and a medical officer of health. The problems of the mentally ill in the community were outlined and the need for the public and voluntary societies to co-operate with the hospital, family doctor and the statutory community services was emphasized. The next part consisted of an address by Dr. Frank Lake, Medical Director, Clinical Theology Association, on the need for the clergy to extend their work for those with emotional difficulties. In the afternoon, the audience of clergy and social workers divided into groups for discussion.

For 4 weeks from the middle of June, the emphasis of the campaign was on the needs of the mentally handicapped. Open weeks were planned for each of the County Council training centres at Kettering, Northampton, Wellingborough and Corby, and as the pattern of the week was similar in each case, only one will be described in detail.

On 17 June the Open Week at the Kettering Junior and Adult Training Centres was inaugurated by a public presentation to the Adult Centre of a motorized cultivator by the Kettering Rotary Club. Organized parties visited the Centre by appointment on the Monday, Tuesday, Thursday and Friday while, on 19 June the centres were open to all parents, friends, and the general public. A film evening was held which was so successful that a repeat of the film/discussion had to be hastily organized because of the numbers present.

Towards the end of September, two evening conferences were held. The first of these was on 24 September and was organized in Northampton by the Knights of St. Columba. A large audience of voluntary workers of the Roman Catholic Church attended to hear the speakers outline the problem of mental ill health and the possible ways in which they could increase the help they were already giving.

The second evening conference was held 2 days later and was organized by the Northamptonshire Conference of the National Voluntary Youth Organizations for youth club leaders, the theme being based on the following extract from the Bessey Report on the Training of Youth Leaders: "The job of leadership is to help young people to grow up and to enjoy the process and to develop good personal relationships." The audience heard a specialist in child psychiatry talking about the development of relationships, and a wide-ranging discussion brought out many challenging aspects in which youth club leaders could play a major role.

The personal interest of the Chief Constable of Northamptonshire led to special meetings being arranged in each of the five police divisions. It was decided that the aim of these meetings should be to bring to the attention of the members of the police force the relevance to their work of some knowledge of mental health, and consisted of a general introductory talk by a doctor, a film on mental illness and a general discussion with the doctor assisted by a mental welfare officer. The American Embassy kindly lent a copy of the recently issued Chicago Police Training film entitled *The Cry for Help* which dealt with the handling of attempted suicide cases and this added to the interest of the evenings, although its content varied to a considerable and sometimes humorous extent from practice in this country. One outstanding conclusion was the great need for similar training films in Britain.

One of the highlights of the Project took place on 9 October with the luncheon at Knuston Hall Adult Residential College, at which the principal guest was H.R.H. the Duke of Gloucester. The occasion was a planning meeting arranged so that the senior representatives of the Health Department and the Northamptonshire Branch of the British Red Cross Society could hear a review of progress and consider future plans.

The campaign reached a climax during the week commencing 20 October, which was designated Mental Health Week. The first event was Mental Health Sunday, when a special service was held in the chapel of St. Crispin Hospital. A large congregation of representatives of statutory and voluntary bodies attended, with patients from the hospital. On the same Sunday, reference was made to the Project in other churches throughout the county and the Roman Catholic Bishop of Northampton arranged an octave of prayer.

On 21 October a large exhibition, organized by St. Crispin Hospital and the County Health Department, was opened in the Guildhall, Northampton, entitled "Hospital to Community—Focus on the Hurt Mind", and covered many aspects of diagnosis, treatment and rehabilitation of the mentally disordered. The exhibition was attended by just over 1000 people during the week.

For one day the exhibition was open to senior school children, and parties from two schools attended. The emphasis in the exhibition on machines and apparatus greatly interested them and many intelligent questions were asked.

On 22 October, a special one-day conference was arranged for the Project by St. Crispin Hospital Management Committee and was held in the hospital. The theme was "Industry and Mental Health" and the audience comprised industrialists, business managers and trade union officials. Much interest was engendered by this meeting amongst those engaged in industry, and a tour of the hospital, with the opportunity of meeting members of the staff, caused many of them to state that until then they had been quite unaware of the importance of sympathetic acceptance at work in the rehabilitation of the mentally disordered.

On 25 October St. Crispin Hospital held its annual Open Day and linked it with the Project.

In the evenings during Mental Health Week films were shown to invited audiences, and the subsequent discussions were led by senior nurses from the hospital, and mental welfare officers.

On another evening, the exhibition hall was given to the Northampton Branch of the National Society for Mentally Handicapped Children, who arranged a successful meeting, with the assistant secretary from the National Society's headquarters as guest speaker.

On the Wednesday evening the inaugural meeting of a Northamptonshire branch of the National Association for Mental Health was held. An enthusiastic audience representing many local societies and with people from all parts of the county, heard the Chairman of the Executive Committee of Cambridge-shire Mental Welfare Association talk about the achievements of her associa-tion. It was agreed that the Northamptonshire Association for Mental Health be formed, a significant result of the interest created by the Project and a logical step in ensuring the continuation of the process of mental health education.

A conference was held for secondary school head teachers and concentrated on attitudes, problems of mental ill health in school, and possibilities of promoting sound mental health. A panel discussion in the afternoon helped to show the enormity of the subject and its fascinating challenges to them.

The final conference was arranged by the Northamptonshire Federation of Women's Institutes. The organizers felt that a whole day on mental health matters was too much and so the morning only was spent on this subject. The afternoon, however, was on care of the elderly, and it soon became a discussion on the psychological effects of loneliness! The concept of com-munity care was well developed and the role of the Women's Institutes in the rural parts of the county was stressed.

In November a nation-wide radio broadcast entitled "My Brother's Keeper" was made, inspired by the Project. Concentrating on attitudes to mental illness, the broadcast set out to show that acceptance of the mentally disordered was seldom an easy or straightforward affair, especially from the point of view of relatives, and that community care was still not a universally accepted policy.

In describing the numerous meetings which took place during the months of active campaign, three specific points have not yet been covered. In the first place, the value of local enthusiasm in arranging a mass meeting was demonstrated by the success of a meeting in Daventry. Here, the district medical officer, with the help of a senior administrative nursing officer and local British Red Cross officers and cadets, arranged a film evening with the late Doctor the Honourable W. S. Maclay as principal speaker. The very large audience appreciated hearing about the modern mental health service from one of its principal architects.

The second point which should be mentioned is the tremendous help given to the campaign by certain societies with several branches in the county. The best example here is the St. John Ambulance Brigade, where the county headquarters drew the attention of their officers to the Project and thereby facilitated the arrangement of meetings all over the county. The main interests of the St. John Ambulance Brigade meetings was in the possibility of developing the idea of psychiatric first aid as a useful corollary to ordinary first aid.

Finally, the success of the village meetings must be mentioned. One of the obvious drawbacks to the method of approach used was that on several occasions, multiple meetings were arranged in certain villages, and the audiences inevitably overlapped considerably, with a fascinating permutation of officials. In some areas, the local organizer arranged a single meeting in the village with representatives from all societies and, where this happened, a particularly successful meeting resulted.

EVALUATION OF THE PROJECT

As previously mentioned, it had been decided that attempts would be made to evaluate the results of the Project. No single simple measurement could be made, as there were several different aspects of interest, for instance the impression, either favourable or unfavourable, which the campaign was creating in the community; the effectiveness of the campaign methods; and, most important of all, the effect of the campaign in achieving the aims of the Project.

(a) The impact

One of the constant dangers of propaganda is that it may produce effects which are very different from, and in fact the opposite of, those desired. Distortion and selective assimilation are well recognized hazards in communication, and any process of evaluation should attempt some measurement of these factors. This possibility of producing an anti-effect has already been mentioned as one of the difficulties in mental health education. It did not prove very easy to arrange a suitable method for detecting the development of such an effect at its earliest stage, but several steps were taken. In the first place, a careful check was made on the press coverage, in case editorial comments, letters and the general tone of articles, revealed any sign of antagonism, or lack of understanding. Secondly, the speakers were asked to note all questions from the audience and to send these to the Project Secretary; it was felt that this would give an indication of the most troublesome points on mental health in the minds of the audiences and, in addition, would reveal any marked failure to receive the information correctly. Also, the speakers were asked to state how, in their opinion, the meetings had gone and thus give a subjective assessment of audience reaction.

(b) *Effectiveness of methods*

It is virtually impossible to assess accurately the coverage achieved in a campaign of this nature because of the variety in the methods of approach over a relatively long time and large geographical area. Two steps were taken to try to give some estimate of the numbers reached by the campaign; first, details of the approximate numbers attending the meetings were kept and, secondly, a question was inserted in the follow-up survey to find out whether the persons interviewed had in fact heard of the campaign.

(c) *Evaluation of the effect of the campaign*

The major effort at evaluation concerned the measuring of short-term and long-term effects of the campaign. The aim here was to measure the existing knowledge in the community and, at the same time, the attitudes to at least some aspects of mental disorder. The scheme for evaluation included the following:

    base line measurements;
    practicable research design;
    a public opinion survey before and after the campaign;
    the analysis of the data collected.

(i) *Baseline measurements*

A survey of public opinion took place before the campaign started in order to establish a base line against which any variation in attitude or knowledge could be measured.

It was also important to establish that the mental health scene locally was in no way unique or unusual, as the type of mental health service available could easily influence community opinions either favourably or otherwise.

This point was discussed at length with the consultant staff at the local hospital and the conclusion was that the psychiatric services in the county, with a 1000-bed largely Victorian mental hospital with out-patient clinics in other parts of the county and, at that time, with no day hospital in operation, was in fact fairly typical of the mental health services in the region.

Another measurement undertaken to ensure that there were no obvious local factors to be considered, was a comparison of the county mental health statistics for 1962 with the national figures, including those which revealed the interpretation and use of the legislation under the Mental Health Act 1959, and the percentage of re-admissions and age-structure of new admissions. In each of these points the local figures did not differ to any significant extent from the national picture.

(ii) *The research design*

One of the questions which had to be answered early on was the usual one confronting anyone attempting a social survey, namely, how near to a fully scientific evaluation was it possible to get with the local limitations in staff, finance, time and specialist knowledge. Compromise between the ideal and the practicable was essential.

It was realized that the most worthwhile research design would mean an experimental and a control group, both of which would be surveyed before and after the campaign.

The difficulty was in getting a control group, for to be of value it would have to be essentially the same as the experimental group in every respect except that it had not been exposed to the campaign. Careful consideration was given to using two parts of the county, but this was found to be impossible because of the difficulties in getting two areas, one of which could be shielded from the campaign. The second possibility was to approach another county health department with a request that a control group from their area be surveyed, but this was again found to be impracticable.

Reluctantly, it was concluded that the research design could not include a control group, but would instead rely on a before-and-after survey in Northamptonshire.

The sampling method used was a random selection of one in 200 from the electoral roll, giving a sample size of 1000, the first number being obtained from a book of random numbers. The initial sample was made in February 1963 from the new electoral roll and the same roll was used for the second sample as the survey was to finish before the 1964 roll was issued. The geographical coverage of the sample was satisfactory and no part of the county was missed.

The collection of the data was by interview and, as previously mentioned, care was taken to train those taking part.

(iii) *The interview schedule*

The questions to which answers were required were divided into two groups: (1) those designed to measure knowledge, and (2) those aimed at eliciting attitudes.

(1) *Knowledge.* The information required was the interviewees' awareness of the size of the mental health problem; their ideas on aetiology; and their acquaintance with the modern approach to mental health services and with the implications of community care.

(2) *Attitudes.* In considering questions which would bring to light some indication of public attitudes to mental disorder, the basic assumption was made that most people were prejudiced in their feelings towards the mentally disordered in the same way as towards any minority group. Prejudice was defined as a hostile attitude towards a person who belongs to a group, simply because he belongs to that group (Allport, 1954). Three aspects of prejudice were distinguished (Sellitz and Barnitz, 1955):

the holding of stereotyped beliefs about the mentally disordered;
feelings against the group;
ideas about social provision for the group.

Suitable questions were then drawn up.

The personal data collected was the minimum considered necessary for sub-analysis and for sample comparisons. Age and level of education are invariably strong factors in community attitudes to mental ill health (WHO, 1959), and had, therefore, to be measured. The final question of acquaintance with someone who suffered from mental disorder was carefully considered before being used because of the danger of intrusion into private affairs. However, it seemed so necessary to have this information, however incomplete, that it was eventually included. Once the questionnaire was in draft form, detailed criticism was invited from several sources. It was then pretested twice, once with a group of 72 B.R.C.S. volunteers, and later with 30 clerical and administrative staff. The interviewers completed a trial interview and their forms were scrutinized; they were also given the opportunity of commenting on any apparently difficult or confusing question.

(iv) *The analysis of the data*

The completed schedules were coded by a small team of clerical staff and volunteers for subsequent analysis by electronic computer. It is intended that the results will be given in two main groups:

(1) the details of the first survey as an indication of state of present knowledge and attitudes in the county;

(2) the two surveys compared to measure any differences.

The detail results will be given in a full report on the Project.

Preliminary Impressions

A reliable estimate of the results of the Project will have to await the detailed statistics relating to the surveys and other measurements, but it is possible at this stage to give some initial idea of what has been achieved. The end results can suitably be considered under the following headings:

1. The establishment of aids to community care.
2. The effect of the Project on the mental health services.
3. The effect on those taking part.
4. The effect on the community.

Aids to Community Care

There is little doubt that the timing of the Project coincided with a considerable interest in mental health amongst the voluntary societies. Time and again it was found that the approaches made were met more than half-way, and the offers of help and goodwill were impressive. Several ways were suggested in which voluntary societies could help the achievement of the aims of the Project, for example, by considering carefully their collective and individual attitudes to the mentally disordered, by financial support of mental health research, and by increasing their own knowledge of the subject. Several societies approached the hospital with a view to arranging visits to patients, while other societies became more interested in the welfare of the mentally handicapped children at the training centres. In one part of the county the interest is likely to lead to the formation of the first social-therapeutic club in the area due to the initiative of the local branch of the British Red Cross Society. Amongst certain industrialists there has been an increased interest in mental health factors in industry and in the possible support which can be given to industrial therapy, and there is at present active interest in the formation of an industrial therapy organization in Northampton. The Rotary Clubs have formed an Industrial Advisory Board linked to the Henley Industrial Unit for mentally handicapped adults with the object of assisting and advising the Unit on job placement, suitable contract work and industrial methods. The interest created by the Project helped to launch a local Association for Mental Health with the dual purpose of encouraging the further development of mental health services in the area and continuing the process of mental health education.

THE EFFECT OF THE PROJECT ON THE MENTAL HEALTH SERVICES

The staff of the psychiatric hospital probably saw more immediate results of the Project than most, and some of them volunteered the impression that their work was being appreciated much more by the public than had previously been the case. The meetings for planning and discussion throughout the year led to a very close partnership between the hospital and the Health Department. At the same time the British Red Cross volunteers and, to some extent other societies, came to develop a deeper understanding of the problems of the psychiatric hospital.

As far as the community mental health services were concerned, it became clear that there was great need for a definition of the roles of the various types of staff. The part which the health visitors should play in the future development of the mental health services was raised in internal discussion, and the limits of their knowledge and training were also discussed. Perhaps the most impressive feature was their great potential as educators in mental health and as those who could be primarily concerned with the prevention of mental illness. The mental welfare officers took part in the Project as far as possible and their value in mental health education lay especially in the many human stories which they could recount to illustrate the important effects of present-day attitudes.

THE PROJECT WORKERS

The most obvious effect on those closely involved in the Project was undoubtedly profound exhaustion! The overtime which was required and the constancy of effort certainly created a strain on the whole Health Department and on the Red Cross Society. To a large extent this followed from the very success of the Project which evoked a demand for talks and meetings which stretched resources to the limit. By the end of the year it was apparent that the pressure could not have been maintained much longer without breakdown in the smooth running of the Department.

EFFECT ON THE COMMUNITY

The full effect of the campaign on the community can be adequately judged only after the detailed results of the surveys are known. They are, however, one or two definite results which can be mentioned now. For example, the interest created by the Project was marked, and it was encouraging to find that by the end of the year many people felt that they wanted more detailed information about various aspects of mental health. Another result was an approach to the Project Secretary by the area organizer for the Workers' Educational Association for a class on mental health and this, in fact, started in January 1964. It was so successful that demands for similar courses were received from several other parts of the county.

Some idea of the effect of the campaign on audiences was obtained from the questions which they asked at the meetings. In many cases these showed a surprisingly deep understanding of the problems of the mentally ill. At other times the audience was cautious about, for instance, the trend towards community care and, on several occasions, questioners raised the issue of too early discharge from hospital.

Conclusions

The experiment was well worthwhile even if the detail results and eventual evaluation do not reveal obvious gains. The difficulties in mental health education and the pitfalls to be avoided may discourage large scale attempts to alter public attitudes, but the rapid development of community care demands the co-operation of the public, and campaigns such as this offer a valuable opportunity to link the statutory and voluntary agencies in establishing community participation in health and welfare services.

Another lesson gained from this work was the importance of careful planning and sufficient time. It is undoubtedly true that, had the difficulties in the campaign been allowed to cause a postponement, it would in all probability have led to a cancellation of the Project. It was fortunate that the British Red Cross Society were determined that the Project should be held during their centenary year.

On the organizational side, the great benefit from close co-operation between local authority, hospital and voluntary society was impressive. It was plain that no one body alone could have undertaken an experiment of this magnitude.

Looking back over the Project as a whole, the most vivid impression which remains is that of the willing co-operation and complete dedication of those involved. It was as though the plight of the mentally disordered was accepted as a challenge to everyone in the community, with lay people playing a significant role, side by side with the professional. The genuine concern for the problems of mental ill-health and the eagerness to help tackle them revealed by the Project augurs well for the further development of community care.

Acknowledgements

I should like to acknowledge the considerable help I received at all stages from Dr. J. J. A. Reid, County Medical Officer, Northamptonshire.

References

ALLPORT, G. (1954), *The Nature of Prejudice*, Doubleday.

BELSON, W. A. (1961), *Communication and Persuasion through Broadcasting*, Reprint Series No. 133, Research Techniques Division, London School of Economics.

CARSTAIRS, G. M. (1963), in *The Distant Goal*, London, National Association for Mental Health.

CUMMING, E. and CUMMING, J. (1957), *Closed Ranks*, Cambridge, Harvard University Press.

MILLS, E. (1962), *Living with Mental Illness*, London, Routledge & Kegan Paul.

MINISTRY OF HEALTH (1963), *The Development of Community Care*, London, H.M.S.O.

Royal Commission on the Law Relating to Mental Illness and Mental Deficiency (1957), London, H.M.S.O.

SELLITZ, C. and BARNITZ, E. (1955), The evaluation of intergroup relations programmes, *International Social Science Bulletin*, **7**, (3).

WORLD HEALTH ORGANIZATION (1959), Technical Report Series No. 177, Geneva.

40. The Plymouth Nuffield Clinic*

K. F. WEEKS

with the assistance of

N. MATHESON, I. LANDY, J. HUNTER, S. CHAMNEY,
M. ANDERSON and J. HOLWELL

IN PLYMOUTH, for a number of years before 1961, the medical staff from the psychiatric hospital—Moorhaven—had devoted a considerable portion of their total medical time to the out-patient department, child guidance clinic and to examing patients in other hospitals and in their homes at domiciliary consultations. From 1959 time had also been spent with groups of general practitioners, school medical officers and health visitors, and probation officers.

It was in 1961 that we found the following suggestions made in a joint report issued by the Royal Medico-psychological Association and the Society of Medical Officers of Health:

> 1. Patients not resident in hospital should come under the care of an integrated service working from a special centre—a mental health centre—this could be the centre for diagnostic and therapeutic services—it should be the point at which all concerned with the work can meet, where conferences may be held, guidance and training given.
> 2. The psychiatrist and his staff from the hospital service should give all possible help and advice to the family doctor and to the local authority's staff and should carry out the psychiatric clinical work.
> 3. The social workers of various categories should pool their efforts as far as possible in each area, working closely with and for both Medical Officers of Health and hospital and making contact with the related organizations.

We must remember these related organizations include the voluntary services, who surely have a part to play in the mental health field and will be mentioned later.

Preparation

Discussions on the project of a mental health centre for Plymouth began in 1957; the senior medical staff of Moorhaven Hospital prepared a scheme which was discussed with the local authorities concerned and the South West Metropolitan Regional Hospital Board. Building began in 1962 after the Trustees of the Nuffield Provincial Hospitals Trust had approved the

*Based on papers presented to the Royal College of Nursing Conference held in London on 7 December 1965.

scheme and had most generously made a grant of £40,000 to build and equip the centre. The architects were asked to design a building providing accommodation for social workers from the hospital and local authority, a day hospital for different categories of psychiatric patients, therapeutic social clubs, rooms for individual psychotherapy, and a conference room. In another part of the building, with an entrance of its own, was to be a well-designed Children's Section. It was hoped that the centre—known officially now as the Plymouth Nuffield Clinic—would become the focal point of all the community mental health services and a meeting place where various groups of people might come for discussion. An imaginative move on the part of the Plymouth City Council was their decision to develop a part of the same site, which is within a few hundred yards of the main sections of the Plymouth General Hospital, as a new school health and dental clinic and a new maternity and child welfare clinic. The building of the Nuffield Clinic was completed in January 1963 and services have been provided since that time. The population served by the Plymouth Clinical Area Service is approximately 320,000 (220,000 in the City of Plymouth and 100,000 in West Devon) (Weeks, 1965).

A Joint Management Committee for the Clinic, composed of hospital and local authority representatives, was appointed and held its inaugural meeting in July 1962, and in October of that year one of us (K. F. W.) was appointed as Medical Director. The Joint Committee meets quarterly and is composed of two representatives from Moorhaven Hospital Management Committee, one from The Regional Hospital Board and three from the local authority (two from the Health Committee and one from the Education Committee). During 1964 they considered the following topics—to mention just a few:

> Ways and means of finding suitable industrial contract work for the day hospital patients.
>
> Recommending the appointment of a third psychiatric social worker and a second educational psychologist for the children's section.
>
> Approving in October a recommendation of providing special classes and a small hostel for severely maladjusted children—both have now been approved in principle by the local authority Education Committee.

Case Load

In 1965 the number of new patients seen in the Out-patient Department at the General Hospital had fallen slightly to 788, compared with 856 in 1964. If the patients need to be seen more than once, an appointment is made for them to attend one of the follow-up sessions held at the Nuffield Clinic. During the year the number of out-patient electroplexy treatments remained virtually unchanged compared with the ten previous years despite the wider

use of anti-depressant drugs. 205 patients were seen in their homes at domiciliary consultations, 150 in wards of the General Hospital and there were
146 Mental Health Act examinations. Throughout the year, the Children's
Section of the Nuffield Clinic had its resources fully extended and referrals of
new cases reached the high level of 380.

During the year there were 980 psychotherapeutic interviews at the
sessions for individual psychotherapy and 1623 interviews at the follow-up
sessions, all these being held at the Nuffield Clinic and amounting to nine
sessions per week. Our nursing after-care service began in 1957 and the figures
for 1964 were as follows:

Number of patients seen   165
Number of visits to the patient's homes   2870

At present there are five nurses who work in the community on a part-time
basis—they are all staff nurses. They visit patients regularly, always starting
with weekly visiting; the length of time between each visit is extended as the
patients' need allows.

Nursing after-care is only one of the many forms of after-care available.
A survey in 1964 showed that there were fourteen different forms of after-care
being recommended by the hospital psychiatrists—all the psychiatrists working at Moorhaven Hospital have weekly sessions at the Nuffield Clinic in the
Adult Department or the Children's Section or both. There are patients who
are independent enough not to need after-care, but this assumption can be
dangerous unless the decision is reached after very careful discussion.

Turning our attention to the patient who is referred to the psychiatric
service for the first time, this is a crucial point for the patient and family and
a testing time for the psychiatric team. A large number of patients do not
need to go to an in-patient unit. It has been shown that the Out-patient
Department in Plymouth in 1961 was carrying a major clinical load which
was of very diverse diagnostic composition. It is appropriate that the right
sort of management for these patients—in terms of time, space and ancillary
facilities—is selected so that they can receive the care they deserve. The
following details are for 1961 (Kessel et al., 1965):

80% of all new cases were first seen in the Out-patient Department;
14% were domiciliary consultations;
 5% were in general hospital wards.

Out of the total number of patients, 18% were referred by the psychiatric
service itself. They were mostly discharged in-patients for whom follow-up
was considered advisable, and a few were referred by psychiatric social
workers and the nursing after-care service. Of the remainder, by far the largest
number (78%) were referred by general practitioners, 15% were referred by
non-psychiatric hospital doctors, 2% by the local authorities, 1% by the

courts or probation service, 1% by the Ministry of Social Security and 1% were self-referrals. Regarding diagnoses, just under half the patients were neurotic and slightly fewer were psychotic. Personality disorders were noted in a small but appreciable number of men but not for women. Organic mental illness accounted for about 6%, schizophrenia for about 10% and subnormality 1%. The treatment recommended at the time of the examinations were noted. Half the treatments were physical, employing in four-fifths of these instances drugs designed to alter the mental state. Electroplexy was recommended for 8% of patients. A third of the treatments involved psychotherapy. Only a half of the domiciliary consultation patients required to be admitted as in-patients. Of all the new patients seen in 1961, 43% were admitted during that year, either directly or following their out-patient consultations. A follow-up study for 1964 has been completed by the Medical Research Council Unit and it is hoped that a further paper will be published this year. The broad aim of the 3-year research project was to study the extent of the psychiatric services in the area as they were prior to the operation of the Nuffield Clinic and to study changes in the patient contacts with the service following the opening of the Clinic.

Co-operation

Of those patients who do need to go to hospital, a higher proportion are seen first before admission by family doctor and psychiatrist. Before re-admission, the members of the team—psychiatric social worker, mental welfare officer or nurse—may be involved with the patient and the family. The family doctor is the one agent who can, if necessary, mobilize the whole psychiatric service.

For the group of patients who do not require hospital treatment, it is vital that the family doctor–psychiatrist team is working efficiently. Both have, or should have, the opportunity of calling upon other skilled staff when required. The family doctor is linked, or should be, to the health visitor, district nurse, midwife and, of course, the mental welfare officer. It would be an advantage if more of the staff of the community nursing services had been trained as psychiatric nurses. It is to be hoped that psychiatric nurses working outside the mental hospital—in the after-care service, day hospital, mental health centre, psychiatric unit in General Hospital—and those nurses working in the mental hospital, should be seen as one psychiatric nursing service to the area served.

Contact with other skilled staff and with colleagues working in other units has to be actively sought after. Both family doctor and psychiatrist can call upon the services of other specialist colleagues and other services such as family planning clinics, and the social workers and nurses involved should be able to seek the help of other social agencies.

If admission to hospital is required it should be planned—the proportion of patients going into hospital with inadequate preparation needs to be drastically reduced. Once the patient is in hospital, the advantages of regular case conferences cannot be over-emphasized. The "community" should be asked to prepare the ground for the patient's planned return to his or her home and work.

The extramural services must be of positive value to the patient and there must be no detrimental effect on other members of the family, upon the family as a whole or the community. The services outside the hospital must be extended as the number of psychiatric patients spending more of their time outside hospital is rising. In the 1930's, two-thirds of schizophrenic patients admitted to mental hospitals could expect to stay there for at least 2 years; in 1963 the proportion was only 10%.

In Plymouth, at the present time, we are concerned with seeking an increase in the establishments of skilled personnel for the service, the provision of a variety of hostel accommodation, the provision of a sheltered workshop and more meetings of those concerned in the mental health field. For children, we are pursuing the establishment of special classes, a small hostel, day hospital facilities and an in-patient adolescent unit, to be shared with Cornwall. These topics will be discussed by the Plymouth Nuffield Clinic Joint Management Committee at their meetings during 1966.

Services for the Subnormal

One of us (N. M.) has an appointment with the local authority with duties to administer—under the Medical Officer of Health—the local government side of the service and to undertake clinical work with the subnormal. Local health authorities have a duty to afford care and treatment for the mentally subnormal. The main effect of this in Plymouth has been the provision of junior and adult training centres. The Junior Centre is no new institution, but the numbers attending have increased from 24 in 1948 to about treble that number. It is housed in an adapted large suburban house. The Adult Centre is about 2 years-old, it occupies purpose-built premises and accommodates about half of the total number of trainees that should be provided for. The authority awaits the chance to extend it on a site already allocated but not yet available. The experience gained from the 2 years working will guide us in planning the extensions. The planning and building of the Adult Training Centre was taking place at the same time as the Nuffield Clinic. Local health authorities may also provide residential accommodation for the mentally disordered. Plymouth has made a start with a hostel for subnormal women who have no home or whose relatives are not able to care for them.

It is not yet clear what impact these extended services may have on the call for hospital beds. Several subnormal patients have been discharged to the community to take advantage of the provisions there. There has been no significant reduction in the numbers awaiting admission to hospital. There may well come about a change of distribution of patient types in the hospital population, with greater proportions of disturbed delinquent adults and low-grade children. With regard to these heavy nursing cases, destructive and grossly disturbed children remain perforce in the community for lack of hospital beds. In common with other authorities, we are trying to help families by providing special care units, and this aspect of the service needs to be improved. If regional hospital boards cannot provide residential accommodation, or if parents do not ask for that, then day hospital facilities should be provided (we have the precedent in the case of the mentally ill). These children do need nursing and medical care, and they should not be the responsibility of those in charge of training centres. Local authorities may be able to co-operate with hospital boards by providing premises and services linked to their training centres.

Some features of the Mental Health Service in Plymouth provide examples of dove-tailing. On the subnormal side, if a consultant's opinion is required, ready help is forthcoming from the staff of the Royal Western Counties Hospital, Starcross. A smooth working relationship is aided by one of us (N. M.) being a member of the Management Committee of that hospital. All the city school children are examined who are submitted for assessment in respect of backwardness at school. Recommendations are made about special educational treatment or perhaps they are found to be unsuitable for education at school. When a child leaves school for the Junior Training Centre, or is recommended for after-care as he reaches school-leaving age, the papers are received by the local health authority and one of us (N. M.) is already conversant with the case and is able to discuss it with the training centre teacher and/or mental welfare officer. In this work, many families are found who are in need of psychiatric help and, with the Children's Section of the Nuffield Clinic on the site, discussion with the above staff can readily take place. There is clearly an advantage in having the child psychiatry services closely linked with other mental health services. There is also a link between the Nuffield Clinic and a special department of the General Hospital, where there is a quarterly clinic for the very young deaf, attended by an E.N.T. surgeon, paediatrician, a school medical officer with special experience in the diagnoses and educational treatment of children with hearing defects, the head teacher from the local school for the deaf, and by one of us (N. M.) with an interest in the psychiatric aspect of the problem.

The local health authority encourages the work of voluntary bodies. The Mental Health Department convened the meeting that led to the formation of the Plymouth Society for Mentally Handicapped Children. This Society has the use of the authority's premises for their meetings. They, in turn, have given generously to the centres and hostel. The improvement in relatives' morale since the formation of the Society has shown the event to have been more value to the cause than any statutory enactment. The Adult Training Centre staff, as a voluntary service, run a social club for their trainees.

The social work service provided by the mental welfare officers on behalf of the subnormals is supervised by those experienced in that field, and in their work with the mentally ill there is direct contact with the psychiatrists. With regard to after-care for persons leaving hospital, we have held that a proper service could best be provided by a social worker who knew the patient and his family before admission and during the in-patient period. That worker would have direct contact with the doctors who had treated the patient and his work would be directed by the psychiatrist. In the early years of the service, this work was left to the hospital. In time, however, more and more mentally ill patients have been referred to the mental welfare officers for after-care, and they have been encouraged to identify themselves more and more with the whole treatment process. As the load became more than the hospital staff could cope with alone, the mental welfare officers have come to share after-care work with the psychiatric social workers and nurses.

In the field of the subnormal, there were in Plymouth, at the end of 1964, 450 subnormal and severely subnormal patients living in the community under the care of the mental welfare officers, and a further 395 were in psychiatric hospitals. With five mental welfare officers serving the city, each officer has some responsibility towards about 170 patients, varying from continuous support in the community to providing the occasional home report for the hospital. This is in addition to his duties as a statutory officer and his work with the mentally ill. This case load can only be reduced by increasing the number of staff.

The hostel for subnormal women patients and the Junior Training Centre are at present coping adequately with the demand made on them, but the Adult Training Centre is overcrowded and the waiting list is growing. This is because the trainees, many of whom are excellent workers, are failing to find and hold jobs. Two major factors may be important. Firstly, Plymouth is an area of relatively high unemployment and the mentally retarded trainees are in competition with normal school-leavers and others. Secondly, there is the apparent intolerance of industrial workers. The mentally retarded, placed in ordinary employment, although capable of doing the work required of them, seem to become the butt of jokes and teasing by other workers, with the result that they become unsettled and leave, or are dismissed for retaliating. The long-term solution seems to be more education and persuasion of industry, generally, in an effort to get it to accept the mentally handicapped as it already does the physically handicapped. A short-term solution might be the provision of sheltered workshops into which proficient trainees could move. A project of this kind is being considered in Plymouth.

The size of the list of patients awaiting beds in hospitals for the subnormal shows no sign of decreasing and, besides causing strain on the family, is disheartening for the social worker who has to try and persuade relatives to carry on under an almost intolerable burden. It would appear that hospitals for the subnormal, in the south-west at least, are the cinderellas of the hospital service.

Mental Welfare Officers

In the field of the mentally ill, the opening of the Nuffield Clinic has undoubtedly improved the service to the community. From the mental welfare officer's viewpoint it has brought most of the city's community mental health services under one roof. In the clinic, the five mental welfare officers have two offices and an interview room. The offices are next to the conference room on one side and on the other, next to the doctors' interview rooms, used for individual psychotherapy and follow-up sessions. Their interview room is next to others, used by the hospital social workers. The mental welfare officers now have almost daily contact with psychiatrists, psychiatric social workers, nursing staff of the day hospital and with the staff of the Children's Section.

Three of the mental welfare officers are at present attending an extramural social work course at Exeter University on one half-day a week. Some would like to attend a 2-year full-time course for a certificate in social work, but with the present complement of officers this would not be possible without a serious deterioration in the service now provided.

During 1964 some 302 mentally ill patients were referred to mental welfare officers with a view to admission to hospital and 272 were admitted—about 90%. This proportion is high compared with other areas because only the more severely disturbed patients are referred to mental welfare officers. The remaining 10% were dealt with by providing community care, out-patient treatment, admission to day hospital or referred to some other social agency. The admission rate via the mental welfare officer shows a surprising uniformity. Over the past 5 years, the number of admissions via mental welfare officers were: 1960, 258; 1961, 283; 1962, 265; 1963, 269; 1964, 272.

With the opening of the Nuffield Clinic it had been hoped to see a fall off in these figures, but this has not happened. We do know, however, that the proportion of patients admitted under Section 29 of the Mental Health Act is reducing as follows: 1961, 13·8%; 1962, 16·8%; 1963, 12·9%; 1964, 12·3%; 1965, 10·9%.

Although most after-care for the mentally ill is provided by the hospital psychiatric social workers, the mental welfare officers try to keep in touch with as many of their admissions as possible whilst in hospital and afterwards, unless some other social worker is already involved. However, pressure of other work, and the distance of the hospital from the city—14 miles—places a limit on this work.

The requirement of the Mental Health Act that a patient admitted compulsorily to hospital shall first be examined by a doctor having special experience in mental disorder has led to the medical staff of the psychiatric hospital seeing much more of patients in the community and of the social pressures involved. This, we are sure, has been to the benefit of all concerned. The number of Mental Health Act examinations carried out by the hospital medical staff in 1965 was 146 compared with 89 in 1963. This community experience has been extended to nursing staff and there are two schemes of this nature—the nursing after-care service and a scheme whereby psychiatric student nurses spend a short time working with a mental welfare officer.

Day Hospital

The day hospital accommodation in the Nuffield Clinic is designed for a maximum of sixty patients; it comprises two large and one smaller room, with toilets and bathroom and a small nurse's office with a built-in cupboard for occupational therapy materials. Bathing, shaving and hairdressing facilities are provided. Patients attending are provided with a midday meal for 1s., which is supplied by the School Meal Service and in holidays by the W.V.S. The cost of the meal is subsidized to the extent of 1s. 8d. Mid-morning and afternoon tea is provided free of charge. The day hospital caters for all types of psychiatric disorders, including geriatric cases but not subnormals. At 31 December 1965 there were 110 patients on the register with an average daily attendance of 55 patients. The day hospital is open from 8.30 a.m. until 5.30 p.m. on week-days. One-sixth of the total number of patients (that is one-third of the daily attendance) require transport either by ambulance or voluntary car service.

The patients are referred from Moorhaven Hospital by the hospital doctor, psychiatric out-patient clinics in the General Hospital, follow-up clinics held in the Nuffield Clinic (there are five sessions per week), following a domiciliary consultation and by psychiatric social workers, mental welfare officers and by the nursing after-care officers. Since the day hospital opened in February 1963, there have been 606 patients referred. In 1965 there were 200 admissions and 198 discharges. After admission to the day hospital, the patient remains under the care of the doctor and social worker who referred them. Appointments with the doctor and/or social worker are easily arranged, as the day hospital is an integral part of the comprehensive clinic.

The charge nurse is responsible for the overall administration of the day hospital; a deputy sister has a special responsibility for female patients. A male staff nurse has a particular interest in woodwork and, in addition to his duties in the day hospital, spends one day each week on nursing after-care duties and has at present a case load of 35 patients. There is a part-time female staff nurse who, in addition to nursing duties in the day hospital, spends 2 half days weekly visiting patients who have been discharged from the day hospital and has a case load of fifteen patients. There is a full-time female assistant nurse and always two student nurses from Moorhaven Hospital at the day hospital. There is one full-time occupational therapist. Patients are dispersed by the work they do rather than being grouped by age or diagnosis. The same case sheet is used for notes by the doctor, nurse and occupational therapist. The day hospital accommodation is also used for case demonstrations to student nurses from the General Hospital and for a weekly social club for out-patients every Wednesday evening. In December 1965 a club for disturbed adolescents was started and meets every Tuesday evening.

There is a short meeting of nursing staff, occupational therapist and patients each morning, before the patients divide into groups. Twice a week there is a longer community meeting with patients, doctors, nurses, social workers and occupational therapist, followed by a staff meeting to discuss patient management and to enable information and relevant change to be communicated. Only lack of medical time prevents there being a daily community meeting. The social activities are organized by a patient's social club committee which meets once weekly.

Once a week there is a meeting of doctor, psychiatric social worker and senior nursing staff to discuss admissions and discharges. It is at this meeting the policy for the day hospital is formulated, and it provides a suitable forum for ideas to be explored. Here the psychiatric social workers first discussed holding a weekly group meeting for widows attending the day hospital and a monthly social to be held in the evening for day hospital patients, their relatives, nurses and social workers.

Continuity of Care

The hospital social workers and the mental welfare officers from the City of Plymouth and Devon County Council attempt at all times to maintain the principle of continuity of care. Therefore, as far as possible, the social worker who may first encounter a family undertakes all the initial inquiry that is necessary, as well as the subsequent casework with the member of the family for whom it is appropriate. With those cases referred to the psychiatric service by the Children's Department of the local authority or the probation service, the psychiatric social worker's role may be one of delegating her task to the colleague who already knows the family. The child care staff and the probation staff may be able to carry on family case work of a similar kind to that of the psychiatric social worker, who can be there to support and advise in specific situation. The Nuffield Clinic has become the focus for the social workers to develop much sharing of knowledge and techniques regarding casework and student training.

On the preventive side, with the agreement of the Devon County Health Department, monthly meetings are held with the local medical officers of health, health visitors and social workers from the mental health services. Further, a psychiatric social worker is attached to each maternity and child welfare clinic in West Devon, in a consultative capacity, to discuss problems which may arise concerning families who may never need or reach a child guidance clinic or adult psychiatric out-patient department. Here, the health visitor often has the first close, supportive function with young mothers and pre-school children.

When nursing staff carry out after-care with patients, the selection of suitability is reached by discussion, based on the patients' needs. Each nurse can discuss problems of care with a psychiatric social worker and all information is channelled into informal meetings held in the Nuffield Clinic. Here, the respective roles can be examined in order to determine when it is appropriate to encourage the nurse to make use of other practical helping services, while the psychiatric social worker may be very firmly supervising the taking of medication or even bathing the baby. Such a system depends on a willingness to recognize statutory obligations, abilities in specific fields, an acceptance of the need to care for people outside the requirements of our own settings and not least, a good recording system with flexible and tolerant secretarial staff.

In Plymouth, there is a Guild of Social Service, which until recently embraced the more orthodox practical helping services. Now, with the advent of new social work staff, there are preliminary steps towards co-ordinating its efforts more effectively with the statutory services to help more families and to use the varying levels of skills more economically. To this purpose, voluntary visitors have been recruited who identify themselves with either the probation service, child care service or mental health service, to offer help and guidance under informal supervision. Their general training in the knowledge and function of the welfare state is under the organization of the Guild of Social Service, who recently appointed a training officer for this purpose.

Child Guidance Clinic

When the Nuffield Clinic project was conceived, the City's Child Guidance Clinic was housed in unsatisfactory premises. The psychiatrists were certain that the clinic for children should be included in the mental health centre and, after some time, this decision was accepted by the committee concerned and the staff of the Child Guidance Clinic saw the move as being stimulating and challenging. When the clinic moved to the Nuffield Clinic, it became known as the Children's Section; child guidance methods have continued to be used (Kahn, 1965). Some people had wondered how parents would feel about bringing children to a community mental health centre which included a day hospital for adult psychiatric patients, but in nearly 3 years only two mothers have expressed any anxiety on that account. The Child Guidance Clinic staff (psychiatric social workers, educational psychologist, secretarial staff) soon became aware, after the move, of being an integral part of a wider service. There has been a closer link with the Mental Health Department and the hospital social workers, who are to be found just along the corridor. The staff can more easily discuss the families in whom there is a mutual interest, and there can be joint interviews, so that a decision can be reached as to who should continue to work with the family. Of course, the Children's Section staff also work with other statutory and voluntary agencies. Occasionally, one of the adolescents who is attending, or a parent of a child known to the clinic, is admitted to the day hospital, and on these occasions the staff can continue to work with the nursing staff, continuity of care being preserved. The day hospital patients made a very useful fort for the play waiting room of the Children's Section, and an electric train set given by one of the children attending has been maintained by one of the nurses and a mental welfare officer.

One of the three psychiatric social workers in the Children's Section supervises a student from an Exeter University postgraduate course in social work and, for the first time, there is accommodation for a pre-nursing cadet from Moorhaven Hospital. These cadets have proved very useful indeed, and their duties include reception and looking after children while their parents are being interviewed. The children may be patients, siblings or friends. The cadet is encouraged to learn about play and what it means to the child.

The entrance to the Children's Section of the Nuffield Clinic is through glass doors to a large play waiting room. This is so attractive that we sometimes find children wandering in while their mothers are attending one of the other clinics on the site. The accommodation in the Children's Section consists of four rooms for psychiatric social workers, two for doctors, two for educational psychologists, and two well-equipped play rooms (one with sand and water) and an office for secretarial staff.

Health visitor teaching groups were started some years ago by the former Director of the Child Guidance Clinic. These now include the Senior Medical Officer for Maternity and Child Welfare, his colleagues from that department and the School Health Department and other workers interested in the family. These meetings are now also used for teaching health visitor students who are attending a full-time course of training at the Plymouth College of Technology. The staff of the Children's Section are also taking an active part in the courses of lectures required.

Records

Prior to the opening of the Nuffield Clinic, the Local Authority Mental Health Service kept case records of its subnormal patients, both in the community and in hospitals, together with minor details of mentally ill patients referred to mental welfare officers. Out-patient records for mentally ill patients were kept at the General Hospital.

When the Nuffield Clinic was nearing completion, after consultation with record officers from the Kings Fund Hospital Administration Staff College, it was decided that all psychiatric notes should be kept at the Clinic and be available to whatever agency needed access to them upon receiving a proper request.

All the existing local authority notes were perused and those thought to be "current" were given miscellaneous numbers. The general hospital psychiatric notes were amalgamated with any existing notes. The Child Guidance Clinic notes and those mentioned above were absorbed into the system, and one index card was made out for every case record. These index cards form the master index. When more than one member of a family is known to the Clinic, the index cards are cross-referenced. When a patient is seen at the Nuffield Clinic in any connection—at individual psychotherapy sessions, follow-up sessions, by mental welfare officers, psychiatric social workers, attending the day hospital, or being seen in the Children's Section, a Nuffield Clinic folder is made out. This contains all the relevant psychiatric notes and reports, previously contained in the miscellaneous file. Relevant notes include out-patient notes, mental welfare officers' notes, follow-up reports and discharge letters. General hospital notes are clearly marked that the psychiatric notes are available at the Nuffield Clinic, and will be sent to other medical staff on request—the psychiatrist in charge of the case is always asked first.

When a patient is admitted to the psychiatric hospital, the daily list of admissions is telephoned through to the Nuffield Clinic and any notes held at the Clinic are sent to the Hospital. These notes are returned to the Clinic, together with a discharge letter, when the patient leaves hospital. A copy of every discharge letter is sent to the Clinic regardless of the address on discharge. The details of these letters are entered in the master index. In a similar manner, when the general hospital prepare their psychiatric out-patient clinics for new referrals, they request the Clinic for any previous notes.

Finance

Lastly, a few words about finance, including the actual figures for the year 1964/5. Estimates for the Clinic are prepared in three categories: wholly local authority, wholly hospital, and joint. The first part covers the salaries of the staff in the Mental Health Department and Children's Section. The wholly hospital section provides for the salaries of the nursing staff, occupational therapist and the cost of occupational therapy materials. The joint expenditure covers the salaries of the secretarial staff, stationery, fuel, etc. These items are paid for from local authority revenue and a 50% adjustment is made between local authority and hospital finance staffs at the end of the financial year. To give a realistic "running" expenditure, the estimated cost of medical staff and psychiatric social worker's sessions at the Clinic is added to the above:

	£
Joint	9,649
Local authority	13,686
Hospital	6,628
Medical staff and P.S.W.s	17,628
TOTAL	£40,963

Conclusion

However it is organized, a psychiatric service has to show that it can provide effective care and treatment for individual patients and effective support for the family. The community must be satisfied that they have been cared for in a dignified and humane way and have had the opportunity to benefit from the best treatment techniques available for their particular illness.

In this chapter we have described some aspects of the developing psychiatric services in Plymouth including some details of a community mental health centre. The functions of such a centre remain the same as defined by a World Health Organization Technical Report 223 (WHO, 1961)—"the prevention and early detection of psychiatric disorder and social maladjustment and the organization of after-care and social rehabilitation. Such units could also serve as training centres for allied personnel and as public information centres".

References

KAHN, J. A. (1965), *Child Guidance and Child Psychiatry as an Integral Part of Community Services*, London, N.A.M.H.

KESSEL, N., HASSALL, C., BLAIR, R., GILROY, J. M., PILKINGTON, F. and WEEKS, K. F. (1965), *Brit. J. Psychiat.* **111**, 10.

WEEKS, K. F. (1965), in Freeman, H. L. (Ed.), *Psychiatric Hospital Care*, London, Baillière, Tindall & Cassell.

WHO (1961), Technical Report No. 223, *Programme Development in the Mental Health Field*, Geneva.

41. Day Hospital or Mental Health Centre?*

W. A. JAMES FARNDALE

THE idea of a day hospital once seemed revolutionary and slightly suspect. Could the psychiatrically ill be sent home in the evenings? They could, and are. The fact that a significant number of psychiatric patients can be treated by day has now become widely accepted. Epps and Hanes (1964) in the United States reported that it had been estimated that 50–75% of patients admitted to state hospitals could have been cared for in a day hospital. In Britain, Bennett (1964) considers that day treatment is making a numerically significant contribution to the treatment of psychiatric patients.

First Day Hospital

The Marlborough Day Hospital, London, which opened in 1946, was the forerunner of a complex growth of day units falling into three main categories: first, psychiatric day hospitals, where many of the patients attending would otherwise have been in-patients; second, geriatric day hospitals for physically infirm old people, many of whom may previously have been in-patients and who continue to attend for medical or social reasons; third, medical rehabilitation day centres which patients may attend prior to discharge after medical in-patient treatment. There are also, of course, general hospital out-patient departments with day wards. This paper deals with the development of psychiatric day hospitals and day centres in Britain, and is based for the most part on the author's previous research, published in 1961 and recently brought up to date.

Advantages to Patients

Day patients are not just out-patients; they are more than out-patients and have a status closer to in-patients. They are able to benefit to the full from the hospital treatment and facilities while continuing to live at home and travelling daily to the hospital unit. Most psychiatric day patients attend 5 days a week from about 9.00 a.m. to 5.00 p.m. They are provided with lunch and tea, as well as full hospital treatment free of charge under the National Health Service. The average length of attendance may vary from 6 weeks to

*Presented at the Health Congress of the Royal Society of Health, April 1965.

3 months, and, in fact, corresponds closely to the length of stay of similar in-patients. Medically, the treatment of certain mentally ill patients by day has certainly been successful. Patients in day hospitals run less risk of becoming institutionalized, and rehabilitation is easier. There are many social advantages: less stigma is involved, and the patient retains contact with family and friends, and remains, to a certain extent, in the community. Day treatment is thus an important part of community care.

From an administrative and economic point of view there are also advantages. Capital outlay is small in relation to in-patient units; beds are not needed and less space is required. Day hospital running costs will certainly depend on the quality of the facilities provided—costs will be high if treatment is of a very high standard. Where facilities correspond to average in-patient mental hospital facilities, day hospitals appear to cost less.

Day hospitals have the advantage of attracting good staff because they like the atmosphere and the regular hours of the units.

Selection of Patients

Few people would agree that day hospitals should entirely replace mental hospitals and psychiatric in-patient units. There is still a need for in-patient facilities. Some patients, for their own good, and sometimes for the good of society, are better treated for a period as an in-patient, and many psychiatrists prefer to treat acute cases, at least initially, in this way.

Careful selection of day patients and an equally careful planning of facilities will ensure that the right patients are treated in the right surroundings. Day hospital treatment is also a means of lifting undue stress from relatives, where a patient is not acutely ill and might otherwise remain at home all day. Some doctors have suggested that day hospitals should provide a handful of beds for overnight or weekend assessment of a patient's condition, or for people from some distance away who come for diagnosis; this is an excellent suggestion.

Selection of the right patients is the key to the value of day hospitals. Some doctors see day hospitals as a threat to the mental hospital, with its urgent need for modernization; others fear they may become long-term refuges for the chronically sick or those with inadequate personalities. The day hospital is neither superior nor inferior to the mental hospital. Psychiatric patients should be treated in the unit which best satisfies their needs, and both types of hospital should form part of a comprehensive treatment service.

It is important that day hospitals should be established in suitable catchment areas, so that the intake to mental hospitals can be reduced. Elder (1964) reports that the establishment of 2-day hospitals in Belfast has not materially affected the intake to the Purdysburn Mental Hospital. Conditions treated in the Belfast day hospitals are mainly psychoneuroses, early schizophrenia and endogenous depression. Only $4 \cdot 5\%$ of the 1963 patients had to be admitted subsequently to psychiatric wards. It is doubtful whether day hospitals will ever effect an exact corresponding reduction in mental hospital beds. Day hospitals are, in fact, creating a new clientele and may well be increasing the demand for psychiatric treatment. If they do, from an economic point of view this will tend to cancel out part of the potential saving implied in their lower capital outlay. But economic aspects, although they are important, should be subservient to the main object of treating a patient by the best possible clinical means.

An interesting fact that emerges from a study of the admissions and attendances of psychiatric patients between 1961 and 1963 (shown in Tables 1 and 2) is that while the actual numbers of new patients attending both day hospitals and out-patient clinics has increased, numbers of new day patients have more than doubled during this 3-year period—from nearly 6000 to nearly 12,000—while out-patients have simply increased by 20,000.

It is also significant that in 1961 attendances of day hospital patients measured only just over a quarter of out-patient attendances, whereas in 1963 the proportion had risen to almost half.

This upward trend in day patient attendances takes an added significance when seen against the background of in-patient admissions during the same period. Those rose by roughly 20,000 a year, but the percentage of the increase in relation to the total remained much smaller than the day patient percentage increase.

TABLE 1.

New Psychiatric Patients (Mentally Ill) 1961 to 1963

	In-patients	Out-patients	Day patients
1961	162,816a	145,000	5,700
1962	146,458	159,000	8,840
1963	160,405	166,000	11,588

a Figure denotes 14-month period.

TABLE 2.

Attendances at Out-patient Clinics and Day Hospitals

	Out-patients	Day patients
1961	1,028,000	322,848
1962	1,189,000	484,262
1963	1,227,000	681,527

The Demand for Transport

Views expressed as a result of the author's day hospital research (1961) were that psychiatric day hospitals and day centres are not relying unduly on ambulances for the transport of day patients who are not elderly, but geriatric day hospitals require transport for the majority of their patients.

The cost of providing ambulances for day patients is often marginal, and in many cases, where the demand has been small, there has been no need to augment the local ambulance service. There are indications, however, that the demand is increasing, although most local authority ambulance services are already hard-pressed and cannot undertake additional commitments.

In the case of psychiatric day hospitals and day centres, the ambulance authorities can provide the small amount of transport without much additional cost; therefore the cost of such transport does not necessarily nullify the savings that may be made by treating patients by the day instead of as in-patients.

In the case of geriatric day hospitals, the cost of transport is considerable and does cancel out to some extent the savings that might be shown on paper by treating a patient by day. However, patients at geriatric day hospitals or day centres do not usually attend every day, with the result that the cost of transport per patient or per member is small. Fundamentally, medical and social factors are more important than financial reasons when determining whether to treat patients by day.

Where regular transport is required, it is often more economical and more convenient for the centre to have its own vehicles, supplemented by hired or voluntary transport, or to be allocated a vehicle by the ambulance authority.

Vehicles carrying 9–12 passengers seem to be the most useful. Larger vehicles may be suitable in thickly populated areas but each journey would take longer. No journey should take more than one hour each way. For geriatric patients, the vehicle should be fitted with power-lift tailboard or ramp, which might save an attendant. Vehicles should preferably have some bucket-type seats facing forward, as well as clear glass, ample head-room, hand-rails, and safety straps.

Although day hospitals can operate successfully in a rural area, or can serve by expenditure on transport facilities, they are best sited in an urban area, near good public transport facilities.

The ambulance services have expanded rapidly, but still appear to be over-worked and subject to increasing demands. The problem of their organization, rationalization and expansion may have to be considered on a national basis. Hospitals are regionalized, but in England and Wales ambulances are localized, and there is some consequent overlapping of services. A Ministry of Health circular states: "In practice, it is found that whether the day hospital is a separate building or simply part of the day accommodation of the main hospital, it seldom functions efficiently unless it is situated within a radius of about five to ten miles of the homes of the patients who attend it, unless it is possible to provide a five-day hostel for those whose homes are further away."

The Hospital Premises

There are three main categories of psychiatric day units: (a) psychiatric day hospitals and day units; (b) day hospitals for the mentally subnormal; and (c) psychiatric after-care day centres.

Psychiatric day hospitals conform administratively to one of five types:

(i) small, detached psychiatric units linked to a parent mental, general or teaching hospital, with day hospital facilities, in-patient beds and an out-patient department. Examples are Uffculme; Birmingham; Whiteley Wood Clinic, Sheffield; and Ingrebourne Centre, Hornchurch, Essex.

(ii) day wards or day departments, separately accommodated within the grounds of the parent hospital. Examples are Bethlem Royal Hospital; the Maudsley Hospital, London; Mapperley Hospital, Nottingham; Cheadle Royal Hospital; and the Southern General Hospital, Glasgow.

(iii) day hospital facilities provided in in-patient wards and departments of the hospital. There are such facilities at De La Pole Hospital, Hull, Yorkshire.

(iv) an independent day hospital, not linked to a parent hospital, with an out-patient department but no in-patient beds. The Marlborough Day Hospital, London, is the only example in this country.

(v) detached day hospitals linked to a parent mental or general hospital, with no in-patient beds. Examples are at Bristol and Liverpool; Paddington Day Hospital, London; Stepping Stones House, Bromley, Kent; and Worthing Day Hospital.

The most firmly established trend is towards the creation of psychiatric units linked to general or teaching hospitals. The Manchester Regional Hospital Board was one of the first to develop these units, and has had a long experience of their successful operation. General hospitals wishing to develop a full psychiatric service might first establish psychiatric out-patient clinics and then develop a day ward and in-patient unit. Day patients could be taken into the existing occupational therapy department, although separate premises will ultimately be needed. Some psychiatric units attached to general hospitals are often initially similar in size and clinical facilities to the small detached units described in (i) above and have similar advantages.

This idea has recently been developed further by the South East Metropolitan Regional Hospital Board, Scotland, in conjunction with the Victoria Hospital, Kirkcaldy. A psychiatric day hospital linked to the Victoria Hospital will be the first stage in the construction of a "Day Hospital Complex" which will eventually have space for 50 psychiatric day patients, a geriatric day hospital and a day hospital for children.

The detached psychiatric units in (i) above, linked to a parent hospital and with full in-patient and out-patient facilities, usually have only about 30 beds, and a similar number of day places. These also provide continuity of treatment and care, and offer wide scope for the patient's changing medical and social needs, since his status can vary between in-patient, day patient, out-patient and club patient. Crockett, of the Ingrebourne Centre, has found that mixed in-patient and day-patient therapy is at least as good, statistically, as traditional methods, and the system has the advantage of catering for three times the number of patients who could have been treated otherwise. He feels strongly that new psychiatric units that are built should be primarily day patient centres with beds, rather than in-patient units with day patient facilities, and there is much to be said for this change of emphasis.

Day hospital facilities in in-patient wards have therapeutic and economic advantages. Day patients bring a breath of fresh air and outside life to the ward, and they require little additional expenditure, although they may cause an overcrowded ward, especially at meal-times. Many hospitals could initially offer such limited day hospital facilities for both psychiatric and geriatric patients without straining their resources. De La Pole Hospital at Hull is a good example of this type of development. The hospital, a psychiatric one, has 1000 beds, with facilities for 250 day patients, and serves a population of 300,000. It is significant that attendance of day patients has gone up from 2386 in 1955 to 46,204 in 1963, about 40% of whom are psychogeriatric patients.

Detached day hospitals, both independent and those linked to a parent hospital, undoubtedly represent a great advance on traditional mental hospitals. They have developed a very good atmosphere, there is a good ratio of medical and nursing staff to patients, the approach is informal and the appearance non-clinical. Patients are encouraged to take responsibility for some of the organization and running of the unit.

Marlborough Day Hospital, which is completely independent, (iv) above, and therefore does not fall into the category of the "catchment" day hospitals, aims to provide "a full psychiatric clinical and community services necessary for an area" (Bierer, 1963). This includes every possible service for the psychiatrically ill, including clubs and self-governed hostels and workshops. Bierer sees it as a genuine "community" hospital, organizing all the services in the mental and social fields at present split up between various authorities. There are as yet no self-governed hostels at the Marlborough, nor have Bierer and his staff been able to achieve the unification of overlapping services, but they have developed a successful combination of day, night, weekend and full-time services in one unit, described as the "Turno" hospital.

Independent day hospitals, which are not linked to a parent unit, are likely to be more expensive. For this reason, and because many psychiatrists prefer to be associated with an in-patient unit, day hospitals linked to a parent hospital are more likely to develop in the future, especially in residential areas which are some way from the "parent" hospital. This has already happened in Liverpool, where two psychiatric day hospitals have been opened since 1961 in East Liverpool, and Birkenhead, in addition to the South Liverpool Day Hospital. Egan, of the South Liverpool Day Hospital, feels that a day hospital is most successful when it is under the control of one consultant psychiatrist, who acts as director, rather than a number of consultant psychiatrists.

Local health authorities and local general practitioners can use detached hospitals of this type ((v) above) as "mental health centres", since the unit can work closely with other community mental health services. It is possible that the success of some of these hospitals may cause them to be expanded by the provision of a few in-patient beds, which will create a more flexible system.

Designing the Day Hospital

The optimum size of a detached day hospital, from an economic point of view, is over 40 patients for a catchment area with a population of 100,000. Many doctors prefer 30, although this entails a high weekly cost per patient. The Ministry of Health (1964) suggested a ratio of 50 to 100,000, "although the adequacy of this ratio is dependent upon the development of the services provided by the local authority". The author believes that, even where these services are good, more than 50 day places per 100,000 will eventually be required. There is no reason why the 50 places should not be divided among more than one day hospital, and, in fact, hospitals and local health authorities which work closely together are already discovering a need to provide both psychiatric day hospitals and psychogeriatric day centres for elderly patients. In Nottingham, where there is a very well-integrated mental health service, there is a day occupational centre for the elderly who have shown signs of mental instability, geriatric day units at Mapperley and St. Francis Hospitals, and day places for all age groups at Mapperley Hospital. As a result, Nottingham has a high ratio of day places to the population of 400,000.

One advantage of a day hospital is that it does not have to be purpose-built. As pointed out in a report made by a patients' committee at a Belfast day hospital, a large old house can be suitably adapted, and, in fact, adds to the informal family atmosphere, while the grounds can be used for gardening and recreation as well as for building extensions or occupational therapy huts. One converted sports pavilion with outlying huts has created a "club" atmosphere most successfully.

Accommodation required for a day hospital includes an out-patient facility;

a treatment facility including E.C.T. equipment, rest rooms and rooms for psychotherapy; a large room for occupational therapy, perhaps split into bays for the various occupations, and rooms for industrial and craft work for men; recreational facilities for games, sports, dancing and social activities; administrative offices and interview rooms for the consultant, registrar, psychiatric social worker, psychologist, sister, clerk, and visiting staff; smaller sitting rooms and quiet rooms, doubling as group treatment and discussion rooms; dining rooms for both patients and staff, a kitchen with facilities for evening use by social clubs, and finally cloakrooms. Some small overnight accommodation would enable the day hospital to be used as a night hospital and to accommodate a few patients in hostel-type facilities.

It is always useful to have a day hospital near a park, playing field or sports facilities. There should be a good parking area for cars and for the unit's own transport. It is essential that it should be within easy access of public transport as most patients, except the elderly, travel by public transport.

The Establishment of Mental Health Centres

In a few parts of the country, mental health centres have been established by local health authorities, and sometimes detached day hospitals or day centres operate as mental health centres. Mental health centres were proposed in 1959 in a joint memorandum of the Society of Medical Officers of Health and the Royal Medico-psychological Association. In this type of centre, the hospital, local health authority and general practitioner services are brought together to provide diagnostic and therapeutic services, occupational therapy, sheltered workshops and social clubs for patients who are not resident in hospital.

The centres are largely run by local health authorities, but occasionally they are established by the regional hospital board, as was the case in Southampton, or run jointly by the local authority and the regional hospital board's psychiatric hospital, as is the case at the Plymouth Nuffield Clinic (the Plymouth Community Mental Health Centre) (Peirson and Pilkington, 1961). The day hospital forms the nucleus of this Centre, and there is also provision for geriatric patients and for patients with psychoses and severe or chronic neuroses. It also has a child guidance clinic, a research department, and facilities for educating the lay public on mental health. Weeks, in the 1963 Report on the Plymouth Nuffield Clinic, draws attention to the advantages of having a day hospital as part of the Mental Health Centre.

With all this developing experience, it should be considered which type of day hospital or day centre should be provided for the mentally ill. Can the wide variety of day hospitals be reduced, and should the emphasis be on developing community mental health centres run by local health authorities, or day centres within the grounds of a hospital, planned by a regional board and administered by the hospital management committee, in close liaison with local health authorities and family doctors?

Many doctors and administrators favour the development of detached day hospitals or attached day wards planned by hospital authorities, and the development at the same time of local authority mental health centres and day centres which have a close liaison with a hospital psychiatrist.

Specialized Day Hospitals and After-care Centres

In addition to the large number of day-training centres for the mentally subnormal, day centres for the mentally ill in the form of workshops or occupational centres provided by local authorities are to be increased from 27 (578 places) in 1964 to 78 with 2987 places in 1974. Social centres or clubs for the mentally ill are to be increased from 105 in 1964 to 220 in 1974. Within the next 10 years, the number of day centres for the elderly (including the elderly, mentally infirm) is to be increased from 217 to 386.

There is no doubt that day centres for the mentally ill could also provide a transitional stage between hospital and home. Given a sufficient number, many psychiatric and geriatric hospitals could discharge patients at an earlier date. Some could also develop into mental health centres, with day hospitals attached. The 30-place day centre at Willesden is a good example of this "half-way house".

At Croydon, Nottingham, Salford, Oldham and York, there is good integration between hospital and local authorities, including joint appointments of medical and social work staff. At Croydon (May et al., 1962) the local authority mental welfare department and the hospital are responsible for running all the psychiatric services in the mental health centre, including the day hospital, evening after-care, psychotherapy groups and social clubs.

The Hospital Plan, of course, provides for each district general hospital to have psychiatric in-patient and out-patient units and a day hospital. However, psychiatric units of this type will not be sufficient to meet the total demand for treatment, nor will they be near enough to the residential population. Psychiatric units in general hospitals and mental hospitals will need to be augmented by satellite day hospitals, day centres and mental health centres, some of which could be provided with beds to enable them to act occasionally as night hospitals.

Where the general hospital is centrally situated in relation to the population, it would be an advantage for the day hospital to be in the grounds, so that there is continuity of treatment and care by medical and nursing staff. Mental health centres and detached day hospitals might well lack the resources of the day hospital attached to a large, modern parent hospital. But it is essential first to appoint a dedicated consultant and let him evolve his own clinical facilities; there may well be regional differences, but a better mental health service will be provided.

Many doctors favour the development of specialized day hospitals and day centres. Connell (in press) supports the Ministry of Health circular in recommending psychiatric day units for adolescents, and suggests they be attached, depending on the age of the adolescent, to hospital out-patient child psychiatry departments or to an adult psychiatry department. He also points out the need for day hospitals for children. Others feel that specialized units are required for neurotic and borderline psychotic patients, adult patients with acute psychoses, chronically disabled patients, psychogeriatric patients, adolescent patients, and children. They feel that a number of small, specialized units are preferable to a multi-purpose day hospital, although some consider there is no need to separate the groups of patients, with the exception of children, adolescent and geriatric cases.

Under the National Health Service, the hospital service concentrates on treatment of patients and the local health authority on prevention and after-care. This is an artificial distinction, and the time may not be far distant when it has to be removed. Each district or region might be given one combined hospital, health and welfare authority to plan a comprehensive health and welfare service, which would include day hospitals and day centres. More use could be made of voluntary organizations and grants made to them for the provision of local centres.

The climate of public opinion now seems right for fresh Health Service legislation. What form it will take may depend on pressure from interested parties. For example, important proposals have been put forward for area health service boards in the report by the British Medical Association Committee under the chairmanship of Sir Arthur Porritt. Also Mr. Arthur Blenkinsop, M.P., Dr. J. F. Galloway and Professor Fraser Brockington have made some interim suggestions in a recent symposium on the National Health Service (Farndale, 1964), and a proposal for a National Health Authority has emanated from the National Association of Local Government Officers.

Single authorities could well make better and more comprehensive plans for hospital, health and welfare services, and, if required, a larger authority could be given powers of raising money and imposing taxes so that financial decisions could be taken without reference to central government (Farndale, 1965).

There is, fundamentally, a need for hospitals themselves, through their regional boards and teaching hospitals, to take more responsibility for the development of the mental health services, including day services and community mental health centres. As an alternative, or in addition to integration, hospitals should widen their horizon and extend their services to provide and staff some of the community services (Freeman and Farndale, 1963).

The term "hospital" is no longer big enough or wide enough to include the extra-mural services and day centres which are being developed with assistance from hospital staff.

Conclusion

There is at the moment a great variety in types of day hospitals in Britain. The day hospital should preferably be in or near the general hospital, centrally situated and with good transport facilities. In addition, mental hospitals and psychiatric units in general hospitals, as well as treating some day patients, may need a series of satellite day hospitals and day centres, often staffed by the hospitals, but sometimes provided and maintained by local authorities and used by their staff as mental health centres. There is a need for the development of day hospitals attached to psychiatric units of general hospitals, and so giving continuity of care. There is also a need for specialized day hospitals treating patients in different age groups and with differing degrees of illness.

Some new psychiatric units could be day units with a few beds, rather than in-patient units taking some day patients.

More day centres for the mentally ill should be provided by local health authorities, and some of these could become mental health centres, providing long-term care and after-care and rehabilitating chronic patients. Day centres and mental health centres are as important to the community as day hospitals, although they still form a relatively small part of the mental health services.

At the same time, too great a burden should not be placed on a patient's family; there must be careful selection of patients for in-patient or day treatment.

There may well be a need for a new look at the administrative structure of the Health Service, particularly in relation to the mental health services.

All are agreed now on the value and place of the day hospital, and the day centre in a comprehensive mental health service. Day hospitals are playing their part in keeping patients out of hospitals and hostels, and they may help to reduce the number of psychiatric beds in the long run. They are also helping to meet the increasing demands being made on the country's psychiatric services, and their lower capital outlay may well provide an answer to some of the economic problems of the hospital service.

Acknowledgements

The author wishes to extend his appreciation to Dr. A. T. Elder, Deputy Chief Medical Officer, Ministry of Health and Social Services, Northern Ireland, for suggestions and helpful advice, and to the hospital authorities and local authorities, which provided much useful information.

References

BENNETT, D. H. (1964), in Epps and Hanes (*infra*).

BIERER, J. (1963), in *Handbook of Community Psychiatry and Community Mental Health* (ed. Bellak, L.), New York, Grune and Stratton.

CONNELL, P. H., in *Trends in the Services for Youth*, Ed. Leicester, H. L. and Farndale, W. A. J., Oxford, Pergamon Press (in the press).

ELDER, T. (1964), *A Comprehensive Mental Health Service*, Roy. Soc. Hlth. Congress Papers, 55.

EPPS, P. L. and HANES, L. D. (1964), *Day Care of the Psychiatric Patient*, Springfield, Illinois, Chas. C. Thomas.

FARNDALE, W. A. J. (1961), *The Day Hospital Movement in Great Britain*, Pergamon.

FARNDALE, W. A. J. (1964), *Trends in the National Health Service*, Pergamon.

FARNDALE, W. A. J. (1965), *Trends in Social Welfare*, Pergamon.

FREEMAN, H. L. and FARNDALE, W. A. J. (1963), *Trends in the Mental Health Services*, Pergamon.

MAY, A. R., SHELDON, A. P. and MACKEITH, S. A. (1962), *Lancet*, **ii**, 1319.

MINISTRY OF HEALTH (1964), *Improving the Effectiveness of Hospitals for the Mentally Ill*, Memorandum H.M. 64, 4.

MINISTRY OF HEALTH (1964), *Revision to 1973–4 Plans for the Local Health and Welfare Services*.

PEIRSON, T. and PILKINGTON, F. E. (1961), *Med. Off.* **105**, 215.

PAVITT, L. (1963), *Health of the Nation*, London, the Fabian Society.

POWELL (1964), The Future of the Health Service, *Daily Telegraph*, 2 Oct. 1964.

42. Towards a Community Mental Health Service, 1954-65 *

HUGH FREEMAN and GEORGE MOUNTNEY

THE development of psychiatry in this country during the last 20 years has been steadily in the direction of creating comprehensive services, to serve defined communities. To a large extent, this has been a pragmatic process, in which many medical and social trends have found a common path. The most important of these is the existence of the National Health Service, which is comprehensive both in supplying all forms of treatment and care and in serving the whole population. Other factors include the introduction of physical methods of treatment and of psychotropic drugs, which have spread psychiatric treatment out from the psychiatric hospital to involve general hospitals, family doctors and public health services. There has also been progress towards the dissolution of the traditional rigidly hierarchical mental hospital, and of the barriers which divided it from the community it served. Community or District Psychiatry (May and Wright, 1967) aims to offer a continuous spectrum of services, from full-time care in an institution on the one hand to occasional support on the other. It is fundamental that there should be an easy and co-ordinated movement between these facilities, as the clinical and social needs of a patient change. This involves a determined on-slaught on administrative obstacles, and on artificial barriers to communication, which individual services tend to put up in self-defence, or out of habit. Some of the general principles in this field have been previously discussed by one of us (Freeman, 1963). Bennett (1965) has pointed out that hospital admission and discharge should not be determined by a transient social crisis or by the results of a short episode of treatment; they should occur at an optimal time, in relation to a continuous plan of patient management.

It is no accident that the community mental health service has been most fully developed up to now in medium-sized county boroughs. In the first place, these have a sufficiently large population to support a complete range of facilities (except for the most specialized). They are also compact enough to have all these services within fairly easy reach of the whole community. Rural areas have neither of these advantages, while the largest cities tend to include concentrations of intractable social problems and large immigrant

*An earlier version of this paper appeared in the Monthly Bulletin of the Ministry of Health, February 1965.

groups. The medium-sized urban areas—particularly in the north of England—are generally communities that have remained fairly stable over the past century, and which seem to have benefited from a high degree of social integration and tolerance of stress, though with quickening social and cultural mobility, this is a wasting asset. Finally, there is the importance of communication. With a medium-sized population, it is possible for all professional workers involved to remain in continuous face-to-face communication, without the need for a highly formalized system (which often tends to defeat its own ends). To apply the principles of district psychiatry to rural areas and to great cities is a major task for the future.

Experience in Salford

The city of Salford has benefited from progressive policy in both the hospital and local authority fields. It has a long tradition of initiating new measures in public health, and in mental health matters, the Medical Officer of Health has delegated much of the responsibility for the development and running of the service to key professional workers.

On the hospital side, Salford has been fortunate in that the Manchester Regional Hospital Board has pioneered the development of local psychiatric units in general hospitals, almost from the beginning of the National Health Service. Long before the Mental Health Act, and even before many of the current forms of treatment were in use, several areas of the Manchester region had already achieved the form of service which is the object of current planning elsewhere (Leyberg, 1959; Freeman, 1960; Silverman, 1961; Smith, 1962). These local units have been evolved out of the former mental observation wards of general hospitals (i.e. those which had been formerly public assistance institutions). Unfortunately for Salford, its observation ward at Hope Hospital was destroyed by bombs in 1940, so that this development could not occur, and the lack of hospital accommodation within the city has been a serious handicap subsequently.

Up to 1956, Salford was served—together with a number of other areas—by a mental hospital of some 3000 beds, located several miles away. Compulsory admission was the most common method of entry, not so much because of the severity of illness, but more from the understandable reluctance of patients to enter a hospital with a fearsome local reputation. A bed could only be obtained there by the Duly Authorized Officer, and this invariably required haggling with the Medical Superintendent, his secretary, or a medical officer (who quite often had little command of English). On admission, the patient would have all his clothes and personal belongings removed, and these would be returned to the relatives. Before leaving the hospital, the Duly Authorized Officer would be given a certificate, noting only the state of the patient's body on admission. The local authority Mental Health Department had no further contact with the patient until the receipt of a note from the hospital, giving the patient's name and age and the section of the Lunacy Act under which he had been discharged.

The city's former voluntary hospital (Salford Royal) contains one of the oldest established psychiatric out-patient clinics in the north of England. With the National Health Service, its work was extended to the other general hospital (Hope), where a few beds were provided for psychiatric patients in medical wards. However, none of the professional staff working in the general hospitals had any direct contact with the mental hospital. They made use of the local authority Mental Health Department by referring chronic, disturbed or suicidal patients, either for supervision at home by the Duly Authorized Officer or for admission to mental hospital. The Duly Authorized Officer was also called to see patients in the general hospital, if they had not responded to treatment within a reasonable time. He had to decide whether to make efforts to obtain a mental hospital bed, or otherwise take responsibility for the patient's discharge. Therefore, the Duly Authorized Officer had to accept a large measure of responsibility for decision making, which would in general be regarded as a medical prerogative. A great deal of his time was spent in duties associated with admission of patients to hospital. Few professional social workers were attracted to the statutory aspects of the work, and this resulted in senior positions being mostly held by officers without a social-work orientation.

In this situation, there were three separate agencies serving the needs of psychiatric patients. A general practitioner had to decide which was the most appropriate one to deal with any particular patient, and once this initial approach had been made, it was difficult to change the method of care. This was because each agency operated to a large extent in a watertight compartment, while communications between them were difficult and formally structured. As might be expected in such a situation, feelings of hostility and defensiveness readily arose between one agency and the others; there was a tendency to be preoccupied with barriers to entry for patients and with means of transferring responsibility. Artificial problems of communication wasted a good deal of time for the hard-pressed professional staffs of all three services.

DEVELOPMENT OF A SERVICE

The first step towards the development of a comprehensive community service was in 1954, when a joint-user arrangement was agreed between the Department of Social and Preventive Medicine at Manchester University and the Salford Health Department. Some time later, the University Lecturer (now Reader) was also appointed Medical Officer for Mental Health to the Salford Health Department. His interests lay in research, epidemiology and social psychiatry, and these led him to attempt a rational analysis of what was wrong in the local situation. Weekly case discussions helped to raise the morale of those professional workers who were conscious of the need for change, while hastening the departure of those who wished to maintain the *status quo*. These discussions have since been the main medium of in-service training for mental welfare officers, and were associated with the beginning of a large-scale research programme, which since 1959, has included a complete case-register of all city residents who come into any form of psychiatric care. In 1954 also, a day centre for female patients was opened on weekday afternoons, in one room of a child welfare clinic.

In 1956, there was a change of catchment areas and Salford patients have since been the responsibility of Springfield Hospital, a psychiatric hospital of some 700 beds, immediately adjacent to a general hospital in Manchester. At this time, nearly 90% of admissions of Salford residents were made through the local authority Mental Health Department. There were a number of other changes during the next few years—the day centre was opened for the whole of each weekday; the work of the duly authorized officers was based on general practices, rather than on areas; a social club began to function on 2 nights weekly, attended mainly by subnormal and former psychotic patients; hostels were opened, one each for subnormal and mentally ill patients, and a small number of psychiatric patients began to be accepted at the Senior Training Centre.

By 1959, 25% of referrals to the Mental Health Department were being dealt with by social case-work only. In this year, for the first time, there were more voluntary than compulsory admissions to the psychiatric hospital. When the Mental Health Act came into operation in 1960, the routine notification of mental hospital discharges ceased, and a sample check showed that over a 3-month period, only 4 out of 52 consecutive discharges were notified to the Mental Health Department. However, within the next 3 months, 20 of the 48 un-notified cases were re-referred to the department from other sources. It became clear that fundamental changes were needed in the organization of services for the area.

These became possible in 1961, as a result of two new appointments. Firstly, an additional consultant psychiatrist was attached to the two general hospitals in the city and to Springfield Hospital. He was subsequently appointed Consultant to the local authority Health Department. For the first time, a single psychiatrist had access to all the facilities for psychiatric treatment in the area. Secondly, a mental welfare officer who had been seconded to a psychiatric social worker course was appointed Social Work Supervisor, on his return from the course, and subsequently Chief Mental Welfare Officer. Without a professional social worker at the helm, it would have been almost impossible to attract suitable staff for community work, especially in a rather uncongenial industrial area such as Salford. An earlier attempt to attach untrained local authority workers to hospital clinics ended in failure, largely as a result of conflict with professional social workers employed by the hospitals (Susser, 1962).

Following these developments, there were a number of necessary changes within the hospitals. At Hope Hospital, an in-patient unit of 23 beds was created, sharing a ward with the geriatric service, and doubly-trained nursing staff were appointed to it. At Springfield Hospital, it was agreed that all patients admitted from the Salford area were to be automatically assigned to the care of the new consultant, unless their admission had been arranged by one of his colleagues. In practice, after a short time, the great majority of cases were first assessed outside—in an out-patient clinic or at their home— or the case had been discussed with the general practitioner or mental welfare officer concerned. In this way, once the patient had been referred to any psychiatric agency, there could be continuous responsibility by the same professional team, with free communications between the different services involved. At one stroke, the wasteful bargaining process between referring and admitting agencies was largely abolished, and waiting lists for acute cases were eliminated, except sometimes for senile patients. Apart from emergencies, all referrals were now discussed between general practitioner, mental welfare officer and consultant psychiatrist, as to the appropriate form of management. Through more effective use of the total resources, there was less pressure on

TABLE 1.a

	1956	1957	1958	1959	1960	1961	1962	1963	1964
1. Total notification to the Salford Mental Health Service	605	608	556	503	587	555	589	593	657
2. Total new patients referred to the Salford Mental Health Service	323	312	289	233	238	255	260	298	301
3. Total number of patients referred to Salford Mental Health Service	506	504	478	430	498	470	467	508	532
4. Compulsory admissions to hospital from Salford Mental Health Service as shown as a percentage of total notifications	—	32	31	24	30	26	13	21·5	20
5. Percentage of all patients referred to the Salford Mental Health Service who were admitted to hospital	60	46	50	52	48	45	35	41	40

a Figures in this table are taken from the Annual Reports of the Medical Officer of Health, City of Salford.

the hospital beds, where the length of stay was also reduced. Emergency and night calls were reduced, presumably because patients were being seen at an earlier stage of their illness.

The effects of these changes were seen in the statistics for 1962, when the percentage of compulsory admissions fell to half (Table 1.4) and the percentage of all referrals who were admitted by 10% (Table 1.5). Of patients referred to the Mental Health Department for the first time, 30% were admitted to hospital and of these, only one-fifth were admitted compulsorily. Seventy per cent of patients admitted to Springfield Hospital were discharged within 2 months, compared with 50% during the previous 3 years. Though too many conclusions should not be drawn from figures of this sort (which could be explained in several ways), they appeared to represent the effects of a developing partnership between psychiatric hospital, general hospital and local authority Mental Health Department. Mental welfare officers were welcomed in the hospitals, where they visited patients freely and met medical, nursing and social-work staff on an easy and informal basis. This has proved more economical and more effective than attempts to set up a formal conference structure, and artificial breaks in the continuity of social work have been largely eliminated. In particular, cases of attempted suicide admitted to the general hospitals are routinely visited after discharge by local authority social workers.

CURRENT DEVELOPMENTS

The changes just described consisted of using the existing staff and facilities more effectively, and removing artificial barriers. Whilst this accomplished a good deal, it made everyone concerned more keenly aware of the need for still more radical developments. At Springfield Hospital, following the Ministry of Health Circular on Psychiatric Hospitals, it became agreed policy that an independent unit should be set up within the hospital to serve the Salford area. (It is estimated at present that it will be some 15 years before the services can move to a comprehensive in-patient unit at Hope Hospital.) This is similar to the "Dutchess County" arrangement, well known in the U.S.A. (Snow, 1965).

As a first step, a clinical firm was set up, with one registrar assigned full-time to the consultant, and a full-time secretary for the unit office. A 20-bed female admission ward was opened, and is now also taking a group of day patients from Salford; it is hoped that the whole of a similar ward for male admissions will become available during the next few months. Very little use is now having to be made of the hospital's closed admission wards. A new psychiatric social worker, jointly appointed by the hospital and local authority, has commenced duties in the unit, and a similar appointment has been agreed between the local authority and the general hospitals. Plans are being prepared to create a self-contained unit in one wing of Springfield Hospital, and it is fervently hoped that lack of money and administrative delays will not put off this development for long. It is also intended that general practitioners (who are already playing an essential role in the work of the general hospital service) will have the opportunity to take clinical assistant sessions in this unit. Although public attitudes have improved considerably, there is still much local prejudice against Springfield Hospital, and it is hoped that the developing unit will gain a new image which can overcome this.

On the local authority side, a working group for male day-patients was begun in 1963, and has helped to rehabilitate many men for normal work. The day centre for females has expanded to take an additional group of younger patients and also a geriatric group (which includes one or two men). Mental welfare officers now visit many cases referred to the general hospital out-patient clinics, before their first attendance. A social history is provided, and the patient may be introduced to any appropriate local authority services. Mental welfare officers also attend the weekly group discussion for patients and staff in the Salford unit at Springfield.

One facility which has been sought for a long time is a large house to be used for bed-sitting rooms—one of which would be occupied by a supervising social worker—to which patients could progress from the hostels. This much-needed scheme is now in preparation, after many delays. Finally, the child guidance clinic, which had been under the aegis of the Education Department, has come administratively within the Health Department. It is hoped that this will strengthen the development of a unified social-work service and make possible further developments in preventive psychiatry, which should also involve health visitors and the other staff of maternity and child welfare clinics. Selected health visitors are already attending the Mental Health Department weekly case discussions, and one mental welfare officer is helping in the social work of the child guidance clinic.

STATISTICAL ASPECTS

In 1961, Salford had a population of 155,000. Analysis of the first 6 years of the case-register (Susser, 1964) showed that during this period, the rate at which Salford residents aged over 15 with any type of psychiatric disorder reached all psychiatric agencies for the first time ever (i.e. inceptions) averaged 3·2 per 1000 per year (Table 2). The average number of all episodes of psychiatric illness (inceptions and recurrences) for which aid was sought averaged 7·5 per 1000 per year. In this period, the statistics indicate a trend towards an increase in the work of the local psychiatric services as a whole. Whereas the number of inceptions of illness which reached psychiatric agencies increased by 6%, the number of episodes increased by 19%. However, these increases occurred outside the mental hospital sphere. The number of patients admitted to mental hospitals fluctuated and showed no uniform trend during the period under review. There was a fall in inceptions admitted during the second half of the period (1961–4), and virtually no change in the number of episodes admitted. To some extent, long periods of mental hospital admissions were replaced by repeated episodes, but the care of these was partly transferred to general hospitals, local authority services, general practitioners and patients' families. In 1961–4, there was a rise in inceptions admitted to

TABLE 2.

Distribution between Psychiatric Agencies of Inceptions and Episodes of Mental Sickness in Salford (1959–61) and (1962–4)

	1959–61	1962–4	% Difference
INCEPTIONS			
Mental hospital	300	259	− 14
General hospital			
Admissions	25	64	+156
Out-patients	551	549	− 1
Total	576	613	+ 6
Total admissions	325	323	− 1
Mental health service only	259	331	+ 28
Total	1135	1203	+ 6
EPISODES			
Mental hospital	883	905	+ 2
General Hospital			
Admissions	35	124	+254
Out-patients	774	927	+ 20
Total	809	1051	+ 30
Total admissions	908	1029	+ 13
Mental health service only	705	890	+ 26
Total	2397	2846	+ 19

Salford general hospital beds, compensating for the fall in admissions to mental hospitals, so that there was only a 1% fall in the *total* of inceptions admitted. There was also a considerable increase in the number of inceptions and episodes dealt with by the local authority service (often with the participation of general practitioners), without use of the hospital service. These rose steadily year by year and suggested that a new class of work was being undertaken by local authority officers and facilities, apart from the redistribution of responsibility referred to above (Susser, 1964).

Future Tasks

Though the hospitals participating in this service are working with impro-
vised accommodation, they may fairly be said to offer adequate facilities for
the acute and short-stay psychiatric patient. A number of alterations are at
present under way, which will help to improve the quality of psychiatric care
in the hospitals. Staffing is still inadequate—particularly at the junior level—
and it is inevitable that treatment of neurosis should generally have a "first-
aid" or supportive quality. In an unsophisticated industrial community, we
are inevitably conscious of the need to maintain realistic levels of functioning,
rather than attempting to mould personalities. The problems of complex and
long-standing character disorders throw great strains on a service of this sort,
and help must be sought for them from more specialized units elsewhere.
Nor is it our intention to concentrate future resources on the treatment of this
group, though we would wish to have more psychotherapy available, for the
minority of selected patients who can benefit from it.

However, the greater reservoir of unmet needs is found among patients with
chronic handicaps of psychosis or senility. (Similar problems occur with the
subnormal, but the present paper does not attempt to deal with this aspect of
the comprehensive community service.) At present, we can do little for these
except to treat episodes of acute disturbance, restore nutrition and general
health, and provide long-term supervision and encouragement. Those of
working age who have a reasonable degree of motivation may be helped by
the hospital industrial therapy programme or by one of the local authority
day centres. Many patients have been encouraged back to work after long
periods of idleness, often starting their employment from the hospital. But
all of these are unemployed, and many are virtually housebound.

Plans have been prepared for a special centre, where such patients might
receive a highly supervised programme of social and industrial rehabilitation.
But at present, there seems to be no possibility of finance to put these into
practice. Whilst such a programme would be very expensive, no one has
attempted to measure the immense cost to the community of these patients'
years of idleness. There are also, of course, many similar patients within the
psychiatric hospital, who are very unlikely to be resettled in the community
under present conditions. Sheltered work and accommodation is needed for
them on a much greater scale, and must offer a progressive series of steps, at
each of which the patient can gain a greater degree of independence (Early,
1965).

The problems of the elderly are correspondingly vast, and much more
progress has to be made here towards co-ordinating the services that exist.
This must be both within the local authority (between its different departments),
and within the hospital service (between psychiatry, geriatrics and other
specialities involved). With senile cases, much effort is still being spent on

passing the buck, and probably the most fruitful development would be to give more practical help to families who are trying to care for an elderly relative at home. Active consideration is now being given to setting-up an assessment unit within one of the general hospitals, where elderly patients could be examined jointly by psychiatrists and geriatricians, and agreement reached on their management.

Conclusion

This story indicates how the framework has been laid down for a comprehensive community mental health service, within the tripartite structure of the National Health Service. We believe that where there is the will to co-operate, administrative barriers can be overcome and that they are often blamed for too many of the problems that occur. What we lack now is adequate trained staff, and buildings to fill in this outline and to provide a service of higher quality for the individual patient. In an industrial area, problems of work and social conditions are constantly to the fore, and we need facilities for a much more imaginative programme of rehabilitation. If, in future, we have more than a shoestring to operate on, some of these goals may be reached.

Acknowledgements

We would like to thank Dr. J. S. B. Mackay and Miss M. Prager for their helpful comments.

References

BENNETT, D. H. (1965), Address to Conference for Mental Health Services Staff, London, National Association for Mental Health.
EARLY, D. F. (1965), In *Psychiatric Hospital Care* (ed. Freeman, H. L.), London, Baillière, Tindall & Cassell.
FREEMAN, H. L. (1960), *Lancet*, **i**, 218.
FREEMAN, H. L. (1963), *Comprehensive Psychiatry*, **4**, 417.
LEYBERG, J. T. (1959), *Lancet*, **i**, 282.
MAY, A. R. and WRIGHT, S. L. (1967), This volume, p. 592.
SILVERMAN, M. (1961), *Brit. med. J.* **ii**, 698.
SMITH, S. (1962), *Lancet*, **i**, 1158.
SNOW, H. B. (1965), *Psychiat. Quarterly*, **39**, 607.
SUSSER, M. (1962), In *Sociological Review Monograph No. 5* (ed. Halmos, P.), Keele, University of Keele.
SUSSER, M. (1964), In *Annual Report of the Medical Officer of Health for the City of Salford*.

Index

S
S